D1612172

NINETEENTH-CENTURY ORIGINS OF NEUROSCIENTIFIC CONCEPTS

NINETEENTH-CENTURY ORIGINS OF NEUROSCIENTIFIC CONCEPTS

Edwin Clarke
and
L. S. Jacyna

UNIVERSITY OF CALIFORNIA PRESS
Berkeley Los Angeles London

University of California Press
Berkeley and Los Angeles, California

University of California Press, Ltd.
London, England

Library of Congress Cataloging-in-Publication Data

Clarke, Edwin.
Nineteenth-century origins of neuroscientific concepts.

Bibliography: p.
Includes index.
1. Neurophysiology—History—19th century.
I. Jacyna, L. S. II. Title. [DNLM: 1. Neuroanatomy—history. 2. Neurophysiology—history. 3. Neurosciences—history. WL 11.1 C597n]
QP353.C57 1987 612'.8'09034 86–7069
ISBN 0–520–05694–9 (alk. paper)

Printed in the United States of America

1 2 3 4 5 6 7 8 9

Contents

Preface

This book is an attempt to trace the origins in the first half of the nineteenth century of certain anatomical and physiological concepts that have proved fundamental in the human neurosciences. In the period we have selected, the latter consisted almost exclusively of neuroanatomy and neurophysiology. We have sought to explore the connections between these changes in ideas of structure and function of the nervous system and the wider science and philosophy of the period; and in so doing we have uncovered areas of interaction that warrant further explanation. In fact, each chapter, which encompasses a major neuroscientific topic, could readily be expanded into a separate monograph by taking cognizance of the many influences, both scientific and nonscientific, that helped to create, mold, and establish the neuroscientific ideas we accept today and of the reasons why others did not survive.

Although this book has been written in close collaboration, L. S. J. is chiefly responsible for chapters 2 and 3, whereas E. C. is author of chapters 4 (except for 4.5.2), 5, 6 (except for 6.5), and 7. We have benefited throughout from each other's criticism and guidance.

We wish to thank the Wellcome Trustees for their generosity in providing us with research funds during the preparation of this book. We are also grateful to Eric J. Freeman, deputy director of the Wellcome Institute for the History of Medicine and director of its remarkable library, and to Stephen Emberton, who made available to us their invaluable resources during the preparation of this work. L. S. J. wishes to record his debt to Lawrence Pedersen, who guided him through the labyrinths of early nineteenth-century French philosophy.

Edwin Clarke
L. S. Jacyna

Preface

This book is an attempt to trace the origins, in the first half of the nineteenth century, of certain anatomical and physiological concepts that have proved fundamental to the nervous system. [illegible] we have selected the latter [illegible] and neurophysiology. We have sought to explore the connections between these matters in ideas of structure and function of the nervous system and the wider science and philosophy of the period, and in so doing we have uncovered areas of investigation that warrant further explanation. In fact each chapter [illegible] encompasses a major neuroscientific topic [illegible] could readily be expanded into a separate monograph [illegible] taking into account of the many influences, both scientific and nonscientific, that helped to create, mold, and establish the neuroscientific concepts we accept today, and of the reasons why others did not survive.

Although this book has been a joint and close collaboration, E. S. Clarke is responsible for chapters 3 and [illegible], whereas L. S. Jacyna is author of chapters [illegible]. We have benefited throughout from each other's knowledge and criticism.

We wish to thank the Wellcome Trustees for their generosity in providing us with research funds during the preparation of this book. We are also grateful to [illegible] Bynum, deputy director of the Wellcome Institute for the History of Medicine and director of its research [illegible], and to Stephen Emmerson [illegible] invaluable assistance during the preparation of this work [illegible] early nineteenth-century [illegible].

Edwin Clarke
L. S. Jacyna

1

Introduction

The first half of the nineteenth century saw a revolution in the understanding of the structure and function of the nervous system and during it anatomical and physiological ideas that had long been widely accepted were overthrown. In this book we shall be particularly concerned with those ideas formulated by Galen (A.D. 129–199) in classical antiquity and by Albrecht von Haller (1708–1777) in the eighteenth century. These outmoded ideas were replaced by new concepts of the nervous system, which have survived in modified form to the present day, and it is of great interest to note how many basic neuroscientific concepts were established during this brief half-century. We can, in fact, claim that by 1850 the foundations of modern neuroscience had been laid. There is, however, one exception to this generalization. The notion of brain localization, although adumbrated early in the century, did not achieve full expression and approval until the 1870s. We shall consider the reasons for this delay in chapter 6.

During the early nineteenth century, advancement in the neurosciences depended, as in all fields of science, upon conceptual and technological innovations. In the following pages we are primarily concerned with the genesis of revolutionary ideas, although we also take cognizance of others of less lasting importance. Above all, we have tried to show that the pattern of neuroscientific thought cannot be understood in isolation: it must be set against the background of wider trends in the sciences and in the philosophy of the time.

In particular, we argue that changes in ideas of the function and structure of the nervous system during this period were stimulated by the romantic philosophy of nature that exerted a major influence upon biological thought in the first half of the nineteenth century. The late eighteenth century saw the beginnings of a trend to search for synthesis, unity, and general laws in the life sciences rather than to concentrate solely upon narrowly conceived empirical studies and the accumulation of data for its own sake.[1] Above all there was a growing conviction among scientists of this period that the human organism could not be understood in isolation, but that its relations to the rest of the organic world and even with inorganic nature must be discovered if knowledge was to advance.

This wide-ranging and ambitious program for the life sciences found proponents in Britain and France. But it achieved its fullest expression in the German-speaking states. There the goal of a comprehensive science of life which would itself be part of a general philosophy of nature and man was pursued with the most energy.

The strongest version of this course of study was the school of *romantische Naturphilosophie* inspired by the writings of Friedrich Wilhelm Joseph von Schelling (1775–1854).[2] The school of *Naturphilosophie* has generally received a harsh judgment from historians.[3] If *Naturphilosophie* is allowed any influence upon the medical sciences, it is a purely negative one. We believe that this opinion must be revised in the light of our discussion of concepts and strategies drawn from *Naturphilosophie* in the work of such major figures as Jan Evangelista Purkyně (1787–1869) and Gustav Gabriel Valentin (1810–1883) (see chap. 3.2–4).

Many of the individuals whom we will discuss were, however, only fleetingly—if at all—committed to the full-blown doctrines of *Naturphilosophie;* they can nevertheless justly be described as exponents of romantic biology. Various strands of thought and research traditions within Germany can be discerned at this period. The *Naturphilosophen* themselves were a far from homogeneous group. Further, Dietrich von Engelhardt has pointed out that Georg Wilhelm Friedrich Hegel (1770–1831) insisted upon a distinction between his "speculative" philosophy of nature and the products of such romantics as Heinrich Steffens (1773–1845) and Lorenz Oken (1779–1851).[4] Timothy Lenoir, meanwhile, has argued that the influence of *romantische Naturphilosophie* pales into insignificance in comparison with the impact upon German biology of the research tradition that emerged in Göttingen at the end of the eighteenth century, a research tradition that drew inspiration from the philosophy of Immanuel Kant (1724–1804) rather than from Schelling.[5]

If one looks beyond Germany, different national styles in science must also be acknowledged. As E. S. Russell points out, there were significant differences between the work of the *Naturphilosophen* and that of the French school of transcendental or philosophical anatomy led by Étienne Geoffroy Saint Hilaire (1772–1844),[6] who declared that this type of anatomical study comprised the most profound principles of the science. These principles were to be discerned by reasoning a priori, and because they were themselves part of a reasoning process, they transcended sense experience. Thus, he believed that enlightenment could be achieved by means of acute intellectual intuition, which therefore transcended physical appearances and permitted spiritual and nonmaterial causes to be just as acceptable as material ones. In Britain both the German and the French version of transcendentalism were widely disseminated and combined in an eclectic manner.[7]

It is necessary to recognize this diversity if the nuances of the life sciences of this period are to be understood. However, an emphasis upon the divergent paths that the quest for a unified science of life took must not obscure the extent of concensus even among apparently disparate individuals over the goals and methods proper to biology. Lenoir, for example, noted that most of his vital materialists "always did have and continued to have much in common with *romantische Naturphilosophie.* Indeed both traditions had the same goal of constructing a dynamical morphology, and 'organic physics' as it was termed." Where they diverged, he adds, was in their opinion of how much pure speculation could contribute to this endeavor.[8]

Relatedly, Russell notes that certain key concepts were common to both the French and the German transcendentalists: "the fundamental concept that there exists a unique plan of structure, the idea of the scale of beings, the notion of the parallelism between the development of the individual and the evolution of the race."[9] Such concepts played a central role in the writings of the *Naturphilosophen;* but they were also important to a much larger body of workers who were striving to achieve a comprehensive scientific understanding of vital processes and structures. Moreover, whereas *Naturphilosophie* enjoyed a relatively brief vogue followed by a rapid decline,[10] the more general movement of a romantic biology pursuing this end with these means persisted until the mid-nineteenth century and beyond.

It is easy to ridicule the more egregious speculations of the *Naturphilosophen.* It is also likely that the wide dissemination of the tenets of romantic biology led many other scientists into false analogies and faulty reasoning. For example, the tendency among experimenters of this period to ignore species differences and to assume that phenomena observed in one animal must exist for all may well have been a product of an uncritical acceptance of the "unity of organization" principle. We will argue, however, that the endeavors of scientists working within the framework of and employing the concepts of romantic biology were of great importance in the transformation of neuroscientific thought with which we are concerned. Other factors were, of course, at work; but we have stressed the role of romantic biology because we consider this to be one of the most original results of our study.

Although our emphasis is on the conceptual side of the science of the period, the practical methods employed to verify or disprove hypotheses must also figure in our discussion. These methods will be discussed as we proceed; but this opening chapter will consider in general terms the various sources and techniques resorted to in attempts to explore the form and function of the nervous system in humans and animals. Such investigations formed a major, indeed a predominant, part of the physiology and anatomy of the period; and it is necessary first of all to account for this predilection.

1.1. THE PRIMACY OF THE NERVOUS SYSTEM

In 1835, Antoine Jacques Louis Jourdan (1788–1848) remarked that the nervous system occupied the premier place in the researches conducted by physiologists in the first few decades of the nineteenth century,[11] but a keen interest in the phenomena displayed by this system was by no means peculiar to the nineteenth century. Thus, the reasons for this preoccupation supplied by Thomas Willis (1621–1675) in 1664 also apply in our period.. He wrote that

> the anatomy of the nerves [that is, the nervous system] provides more pleasant and profitable speculations than the theory concerning any other part of the animal body: for by means of it, are revealed the true and genuine reasons for very many of the actions and passions that take place in our body, which otherwise seem most difficult to explain: and from this fountain, no less than the hidden causes of diseases and symptoms, which are commonly ascribed to the incantations of witches, may be discovered and satisfactorily explained.[12]

One of the reasons why the nervous system exerted a fascination upon late eighteenth- and early nineteenth-century investigators, as it did upon those of other epochs, was its intimate association with the phenomena of mind. As we shall see below, the precise "seat" of the soul in the nervous system, and the nature of the relation between this organ and the mind, remained highly contentious. Nevertheless, it was generally recognized that the nervous system did represent an interface between the material and psychic realms and was, therefore, an object of unique interest.[13] In chapter 6, we shall learn how Franz Joseph Gall (1758–1828),[14] at the turn of the nineteenth century, insisted that the mind was situated in the brain, to us a very obvious conclusion, but by no means universally accepted in the early nineteenth century.[15] His advocacy of this neuroscientific principle, his application of it to a cult of psychological testing called organology and later known as phrenology (see chap. 6.3), his widespread teaching, and his skillfully executed and publicized dissections of the brain, together with the labors of his colleague, Johann Caspar Spurzheim (1776–1832), all helped to focus the attention of the layman as well as the scientist on the nervous system and, in particular, on the brain. Gall's eminent contemporary, François Magendie (1783–1855), who was one of the greatest physiologists of his age, also agreed that it was necessary to regard strictly the phenomena of the human intellect as "the result of brain action and not in any measure to distinguish them from other phenomena which depend upon organic actions."[16]

J. E. Lesch has examined the various reasons why Magendie's main research interests concerned the nervous system, and we can take him to be representative of others, who, on account of similar motives, elected neurophysiology as their chosen field of scientific study.[17] In his case, there was, first of all, the profound influence of the celebrated French comparative anatomist, Georges Cuvier (1769–1832), whose classical investigations led him to insist upon the primary functional importance of the nervous system.[18] The provocative theories of Gall and Spurzheim on the properties of the brain referred to above also drew attention to it, just as the researches of Charles Bell (1774–1842) highlighted the specific properties of the spinal cord roots, as we shall see below.[19] In addition, the contributions of clinicopathological correlation to the elucidation of neurophysiological problems, or "pathological physiology" as Magendie named it, seemed to him most rewarding. We shall discuss this topic in more detail shortly. Finally, the experiments on drugs that affected the nervous system carried out early in his career made a deep impression on Magendie,[20] as they did on others.

Another reason for the primacy of the nervous system in physiological research was that many considered it to be, in fact, the most "noble," or in the words of Gottfried Reinhold Treviranus (1776–1837) in 1821, "the first" of the organ systems of the body; and for this reason especially demanding of attention.[21] To say that the nervous system was the "first" of the bodily systems could imply various claims. Treviranus probably referred to hierarchical ideas of nature, popular especially among those influenced by the *Naturphilosophie* of the early nineteenth century, which saw animate nature advancing through progressively more elaborate and elevated stages toward a preconceived goal. This pinnacle of perfection was the human body, but there was also hierarchy within the human frame. On these assumptions, the nervous system represented the apogee of organic evolution; the point to which nature was striving, and to which all other systems of the body were subsidiary and preparatory.

The popularity of the nervous system in the physiological investigation of the body's systems may have been due in part to the paucity of experimental techniques available in the early nineteenth century. Those that existed were suited to neurological research, as we shall see, but not to the more intimate study of respiratory, gastrointestinal, endocrinological, and renal functions, where elucidation depended, as we now know, on more sophisticated chemistry than was then at the disposal of the physiologist, and was not to be available until later in the century.

Other possible stimuli encouraging interest in the nervous system, were the several disputes over priority of discovery that erupted in the first half of the nineteenth century and will be discussed in subsequent chapters of this book.[22] The best-known controversy was between Bell and Magendie concerning the functions of the spinal cord roots[23] (chap. 4.3), and the others included Luigi Rolando (1773–1831)[24] versus Marie Jean Pierre Flourens (1794–1867)[25] on cerebral and cerebellar functions (chap. 6.4,6) and Marshall Hall (1790–1857)[26] versus several opponents, who accused him of plagiarism in his research on reflex physiology (chap. 4.4). There was also an ongoing debate throughout our selected period between those like Hall, for example, who advocated a materialistic interpretation of neuroscientific phenomena and those who preferred to invoke vitalistic principles.[27] The problem of the location of the mind also generated a great deal of contention, and because it spread into nonscientific disciplines such as philosophy and theology, the nervous system received much more publicity than the other systems of the body. As in any field of human endeavor, disagreement bred action either in defense of an opinion or in an attempt to refute it. Thus, the various polemics involving the nervous system evoked concern with, and investigation of, its form and function.

An ascription of preeminence to the nervous system might also imply that it exercised a dominant role in the functioning of the body in general, as Willis had inferred in 1664. In addition to the intellectual and somatic functions, the nervous system was also held to be involved in such operations as nutrition and secretion,[28] and we shall observe in chapter 7 how physiologists came to maintain that the vegetative (autonomic) nervous system brought about these and other autonomic functions by means of nervous control. Moreover, it followed that because all bodily properties thus derived from the nervous system, then dysfunction must likewise arise from the same source.

The conviction that all, or almost all, diseases had their ultimate seat in the nervous system was another potent factor in drawing the minds of nineteeth-century investigators in that direction. Early in the eighteenth century, Friedrich Hoffmann (1660–1742)[29] adopted and modified by further conjecture an ancient Greek idea that the brain produced a special substance, which circulated in the nerves,[30] and, together with the circulating blood, controlled the body's vital activities. It was also the source of all diseases. There were other components of Hoffmann's system, but his neurogenic concept of disease etiology gained great prominence toward the end of the century, despite competition from similar theories, as Rath has shown.[31] The most striking and original application of Hoffmann's speculation was by the Scottish physician, William Cullen (1710–1790).[32] The theory of disease causation that he formulated appeared first in 1772 and it survived, at least in Germany, until the middle of the nineteenth century. Like other eighteenth-century physicians, he was attempting, unsuccessfully as it turned out, to provide clinical medicine with scientific foundations and to simplify the genesis of disease by incriminating only one universal etiological agent. The latter was a nervous "power" or "property,"[33] and like Hoffmann's substance, it was responsible for all pathological as well as physiological phenomena in the body.[34] It emanated from the brain and traveled through the nerves to maintain the tissues' tone.[35] Thus, Cullen was able to account for all disease states and also to suggest appropriate medication for them. It followed that if the nervous system was omnipotent in the economy of the body, it was worthy of close attention: "The nervous system, as an organ of sense and motion, is connected with so many functions of the animal oeconomy, that the study of it must be of the utmost importance, and a fundamental part of the study of the whole oeconomy."[36]

Cullen, unlike most of his predecessors, succeeded in popularizing his hypothesis, which eventually became known as the theory of "neuropathology." For obvious reasons, historians now prefer to call it "neural pathology."[37] In the early nineteenth century, its acceptance was greatest in the German-speaking nations, mainly because it invoked a generalized life force or "vital principle" and therefore appealed to adherents of *Naturphilosophie,* a cardinal tenet of which was the existence of a universal vital power. It continued to receive attention there until it was demolished in 1858 by Rudolf Virchow (1821–1902) with his theory of cellular pathology, which forms the foundation of present day morbid anatomy.[38] Outstanding medical scientists had subscribed to neural pathology, and these included the renowned Friedrich Gustav Jakob Henle (1809–1885).[39]

Meanwhile, in France, from the beginning of the century, a very different approach to disease etiology was emerging.[40] This was the notion of clinicopathological correlation based on morbid anatomy that would become the basis of modern medicine. It would eventually destroy not only neural pathology[41] but all other eighteenth-century concepts of disease causation except homeopathy. There were, however, some in France who preferred Cullen's doctrine and among them was Jean Georges Chrétien Frédéric Martin Lobstein (1777–1835) of Strasbourg who, in 1821, addressed medical students on the preeminence of the nervous system.[42] He will be encountered later because he contributed importantly to the study of the autonomic nervous system (chap. 7.6). He pointed out the paramount role of nervous system function in the healthy state. "Thus," he declared, "in all vital actions and in the case of those that demonstrate the principle on which life depends, nervous action is constantly recognized as the primary factor."[43] The nerves were of fundamental importance, because they carried morbid impressions to the brain and solar plexus (see chap. 7.7.3), and also controlled the blood vessels, which as in Hoffmann's scheme shared with the nervous system the responsibility for both the healthy and diseased body. Thus, "[I]n the vast field of pathology we constantly find the nervous system in the forefront,"[44] and it was "the premier source of all pathological affections."[45] Following Cullen, Lobstein used this knowledge in attempts to contrive specific treatments aimed at neural structures and exhorted his audience to familiarize themselves with the nervous system. Echoing Cullen's words of 1785, he insisted:

> It remains incontestable that a most perfect analysis of the nervous system and a most precise determination of the role that it plays in the state of health as well as in disease is an object most worthy of the physician's attention.[46]

If they did so they would walk "on the road that leads to the perfection of which medicine is capable."[47] There can be little doubt that this kind of persuasion from respected medical men, at a time when various rival theories of a vital principle and doctrines of disease etiology were still competing for cognizance, must have drawn considerable attention to the nervous system, and may have inspired some individuals to investigate its properties, either morphological or physiological.

A British commentator noted in 1824 that "[N]o subject has excited deeper and more universal interest among the present physiologists of France, than the Properties and Functions of the Nervous System,"[48] and he adduced a peculiar reason for this. Whereas in Britain, he explained, it was understood among the scientific community that when a man discovered and pursued a new and profitable line of research others did not disturb his progress nor encroach upon his preserves, this was not the case in France where ethics were different and a new and fertile field of discovery could be invaded by the pioneer's scientific brethren. This development, the writer thought, must benefit science by allowing more rapid advancement in the area, because of the labors of several rather than one investigator, and also by providing the benefits derived from the possibility of comparing and contrasting their individual results. Such an outcome had, he pointed out, taken place in France in the case of neuroscientific research, as was evidenced by no less than six important publications describing and assessing new and novel studies on the nervous system that had all appeared in 1822, and which he proceeded to review.[49] This special interest extended beyond the period we are dealing with, because the American physiologist, John Coll Dalton (1825–1889) in 1875 explained that concerning the nervous system "[T]his department of medicine is now so extensive, both in its physiology and its pathology, that few subjects can be said to have received greater attention."[50] And seven years later this "special activity of growth"[51] was still continuing.

1.2. METHODS OF RESEARCH

We possess several contemporary accounts of the avenues open to students of the nervous system. For example, Amariah Brigham (1798–1849) in 1840 listed seven methods for determining the functions of the brain: "(1) chemical analysis; (2) dissection of the brain; (3) experiments on living animals; (4) comparative anatomy; (5) the foetal condition and growth of the brain; (6) pathological observations; and (7) external examination of the cranium."[52] The last of these is a reference to Gall and Spurzheim's organology or phrenology, a cult based on an unproven hypothesis that psychological and moral propensities could be assessed by palpating the skull (see chap. 6.3). Although it is mainly of interest to historians of the phrenological movement, and will be considered in detail later, it can for our present purpose be ignored. Chemical analysis likewise has no role to play in our present discussions, but for different reasons. It had revealed, in a crude way, the basic constituents of brain tissue, but as Brigham confessed, "nothing has been learned by analysing the brain that has added to our knowledge of its functions."[53] In general, it is true to say that chemistry contributed little to the neurosciences during this period for the same reason that it could not contribute to an understanding of such functions as respiration, nutrition, and secretion; chemistry was still in a relatively primitive state and quite unable to answer the questions asked of it.[54] Its application to the problems of nerve function in the late eighteenth and early nineteenth century will be discussed in chapter 5.2.3, but it provided little or no elucidation at that time. Similarly, chemical substances were widely used to stimulate nervous tissue along with mechanical and electrical irritation, but their mode of action was quite unknown. We should, however, note that a topic related to chemistry, experimental pharmacology as we now term it, had an indirect influence on neurophysiological research. It was applied to the elucidation of nervous system function, and the most outstanding proponent of the method during our period was Magendie. His classic experiments on living animals revealed that certain drugs, for example, those of the *strychnos* family, acted on the nervous system,[55] and this finding, as we noted above, profoundly influenced Magendie in his contention that this system was central to the animal economy. However, the contribution to neurophysiology per se was small, as was also true in the case of Flourens's investigations in 1847 of the excitability of the spinal cord and other nervous centers during ether anesthesia.[56]

The five remaining methods listed by Brigham constitute the chief means by which scientists in the first half of the nineteenth century sought to expand their understanding of the nervous system. We should add microscopy to this list which, from the 1830s onward, provided an important additional resource. Some investigators pursued their research almost exclusively by only one of these techniques; others used two or more of them. We shall attempt to illustrate the potentials and limitations inherent in each of these approaches to the nervous system by discussing the work of certain exemplars whose labors figure prominently in the following chapters.

1.2.1. Gross Anatomy

The pure, gross anatomical approach is exemplified by Charles Bell. He used this approach in his attempts to bring order to the chaotic state of contemporary knowledge of the nervous system. His statement of 1821 illustrates vividly the situation he and others faced:

> The endless confusion of the subject induces the physician, instead of taking the nervous system as the secure ground of his practice, to dismiss it from his course of study, as a subject presenting too great irregularity for legitimate investigation or reliance.[57]

Relying almost entirely on anatomical investigations, Bell set about formulating his *Idea of a New Anatomy*[58] hoping to establish "grand divisions" of the nervous system anatomically defined and functionally distinct. He failed to achieve his objective, and a similar fate befell a second enterprise aimed at creating a new arrangement of the nervous system, with special reference to the nerves of the face. Nevertheless, his studies revealed originality, talent, and ingenuity, and they contained much that was of permanent value to the neurosciences.

The main reason for Bell's failures lay in his belief that deductions must, in the first place, be made from a meticulous study of anatomical structure, relegating other methods to a subordinate status. He was first and foremost an anatomist carrying on the Hunterian tradition; but unlike John Hunter (1728–1793), he had no faith in experimentation as a source of knowledge. Whether this was due primarily to his aversion to experiments on living animals (which he shared with Gall and many other scientists of the period) is not known. Unlike devout experimental physiologists such as Magendie and Flourens, Bell judged vivisection procedures to be of secondary value, only employing them after his anatomical conclusions had been formulated—and then only to confirm them or to impress his opinions on others. The few experiments he carried out were intended only to verify the fundamental principles upon which his systems of the brain and nerves were established. Moreover, he believed that the anatomical method could also solve problems of function, but it is ironic that the results of the few physiological experiments he conducted, and upon which he placed the least reliance, have turned out to be partially correct, whereas his proposed classifications of the nervous system have long since disappeared.

There was another reason for Bell's lack of success in these endeavors. Although a talented artist, and therefore able to portray his anatomical discoveries superbly, paradoxically he exhibited a curious obscurity of expression in his scientific writings. Numerous opaque passages can be cited and his research protocols lacked the precise and terse style characteristic of Flourens and Magendie so that doubts and uncertainties must have arisen in the minds of his readers. At a time when a scientific language was evolving and photography unknown, a simple yet accurate literary style was essential, not only for the sake of comprehension, but also to allow others to repeat an author's dissections or experiments and thus to compare results.

Another early nineteenth-century medical scientist who used anatomy in a way that we regard as very strange was Gall. His method was the reverse of Bell's because he began by erecting physiological hypotheses collected from clinical and pathological observations, analogy, and speculation, but few vivisections, and then verifying them to his satisfaction by dissecting the brain and spinal cord. We shall study more closely this unusual approach to brain function in chapters 2 and 6. We can note here, however, that he claimed in 1825 that "the anatomy of the brain serves only as confirmation of physiological discoveries."[59] This was three years before his death, indicating that his life's experience and that of others had not altered a belief he had accepted in the 1790s. Gall must not be dismissed for this inverted research method, because he not only helped to establish the notion of punctate brain localization (see chap. 6.3.4), but he also made a number of important anatomical discoveries (chap. 2.1), and he did not hesitate to attribute the credit for them to his research method:

> I owe almost all my anatomical discoveries to my physiological and pathological conceptions; and it is only from these, that I have been able to convince myself of the perfect agreement of moral and intellectual phenomena, with the material circumstances [that is, morphology] of [that is, underlying] their manifestations.[60]

Historians have emphasized Gall's contributions to the anatomy of the nervous system,[61] and among them Neuburger has claimed that "[T]he work of anatomists especially of Gall is the pedestal on which the physiology of Flourens stands."[62] Gall's contemporaries were equally laudatory as, for example, Herbert Mayo (1796–1852) in 1827: "The most serviceable impulse that has been given to the study of the anatomy of the brain of later years we may attribute to the theoretical account given by Drs. Gall and Spurzheim."[63] In chapter 3.5.2 we shall discuss further this "physiological anatomy," as particularly applied to the microscopical study of nervous tissue and the relationships established between the latter and physiological concepts. Thus, scientists were attempting to elucidate function by means of microscopical structure, and, as we shall point out, this method of physiological investigation, although not as yet adequately researched by historians, was of great importance for the development of neurohistology.

But as well as Bell, Gall, and others who applied their gross anatomical research in what we consider an unusual manner, there were many neuroanatomists in the early nineteenth century who pursued a more orthodox anatomical pathway. These included Pierre Augustin Béclard (1785–1825), Marie François Xavier Bichat (1771–1802), Karl Friedrich Burdach (1776–1847), Achille Louis Foville (1799–1878), Johann Christian Reil (1759–1813), Antonio Scarpa (1752–1832), Samuel Thomas Soemmerring (1755–1830), and Benedikt Stilling (1810–1879). Their influence was felt throughout our selected period, and they will be referred to repeatedly below. Many of them contributed to new ways of examining the brain and spinal cord, but Reil's improved method of fixing neural material and Gall's technique of examining the central nervous system functionally, that is, by tracing the white matter fibers from below upwards rather than by random slicing (see chap. 2.1), were particularly rewarding. Samuel Solly (1805–1871) in 1836 judged that the older procedures superseded by Gall and Reil were "totally inadequte to impart any real information in regard to the structure of the organ [brain]," and that "this circumstance has contributed essentially to retard the diffusion of sound knowledge in regard to the anatomy and physiology of the most important system of the body."[64]

1.2.2. Physiological Experiments

Following Brigham's list we can now consider two outstanding proponents of experiments on living animals. We have already referred to Magendie and Flourens who were the second and third in a dynasty of French experimental neurophysiologists that began with Julien Jean César Legallois (1770–1814) and that led by way of them to François Achille Longet (1811–1871), Claude Bernard (1813–1878), and Charles Edouard Brown-Séquard (1817–1894). The first of these eminent men, Legallois, was concerned mainly with spinal cord function, but he also took a broader view of the application of the experimental approach to the nervous system. Thus, concerning the problem of the sympathetic trunk, he stated that "all the questions, I say, insoluble until now by means of anatomy are completely resolved by the experimental approach."[65] Unfortunately, the interpretations derived from his experimental results did not equal in quality the skills he demonstrated as a vivisector nor was his optimism reflected in his overall achievement. Nevertheless, he inspired others, and many of his contemporaries agreed that the perfection of physiology was close to hand.

However, Magendie, who was the real pioneer of the experimental movement, did not share these expectations, and in an article dated 1809, he pointed out that physiology as a subject could only advance if the eighteenth-century type of research, whereby the vital forces and powers responsible for physiological phenomena were vainly sought, was abandoned.[66] In its place there must be a relentless search for explanations. As Albury has shown, Magendie shared with Cuvier a new way of looking at life, which brought about "the elevation of functions to a status of priority over anatomical structure."[67] This revolutionary approach, the reverse of that adopted by Bell and Gall, is the one we accept today.

We have indicated already the effect of contemporary philosophy on biological and medical thought, and Magendie is another example of this influence. As a young man he was connected with the ideologues, a group of intellectuals who were intent on creating a science of ideas that aimed at replacing existing metaphysical systems.[68] Temkin has traced this aspect of Magendie's background;[69] and we shall make further reference to the impact made by it and other schools of philosophy in early nineteenth-century France (see chap. 6.5). Suffice to mention here that Magendie's physiological method, in keeping with the ideologues' doctrine, was to accumulate by experiment as many new and true facts as possible, and, eschewing vague opinions and speculation, he believed that if facts were acquired in large numbers they would eventually lead to an integrated theory concerning the physiological phenomenon under scrutiny. In the chapters below we shall encounter some of his neurophysiological discoveries and observe how he typified the experimental investigator par excellence. His approach, therefore, could not have been more different from that of his contemporary and contestant, Charles Bell, as illustrated by the problem of spinal root functions.[70] Magendie denounced all forms of anatomical deduction and his general attitude is well exemplified by the following statement from his book on the functions and diseases of the nervous system:

> But concerning the nerve, what do you understand of its uses by examining its tissue? . . . There is nothing to indicate that it has one use rather than another . . . You prick it and the animal manifests pain. There, you are starting on the track of its functions; but in this case note that it is no longer a question of the scalpel or of meticulous dissections; you are in the field of experimental physiology.[71]

In effect, Magendie was finally destroying the anatomically based concepts of structure-function relationships in favor of the notion of a function as the product of several organs. The physiological systems of earlier centuries based on speculation and analogy applied to structure were to be replaced by empirically developed physiological ideas derived from systematic vivisections and accurate observations. This process was to find full expression in the many classical studies of Claude Bernard and was embodied in his equally classical book on experimental medicine.[72]

Magendie had much in common with Pierre Flourens, who was ten years his junior. Both were remarkably dexterous, perceptive, and articulate experimental physiologists, whose activities, although ranging over the whole subject, were particularly directed at the nervous system. In each, their experimental prowess owed something to the French surgical tradition that had begun in the eighteenth century, and in the case of the nervous system had shown that brain lesions could enlighten physiology, as we shall see below. Another factor responsible for their way of reasoning and their technique was the new anatomical approach to disease, founded in Paris during the early 1800s and forming the foundations for our method of clinicopathological correlation. They were also both deeply influenced by the philosophical thought of their time, and, as will be seen (chap. 6.5), in the case of Flourens, this accounts for a change of attitude to brain activity that is otherwise inexplicable. His main contribution to neurophysiology was threefold: he located the *noeud vital,* the respiratory center (chap. 6.4.1); he reached erroneous conclusions on cerebral function with immensely deleterious effects (chap. 6.4); and he identified correctly the cerebellar function of coordination (chap. 6.6). He claimed correctly that most of his success was due to a close attention to experimental method. We can also appreciate in the following passage his epigrammatic style referred to above:

> In experimental research everything depends upon the method; for it is the method that produces the results. A new method leads to new results; a rigorous method to precise results; a vague method has always led only to confused results.[73]

He repeatedly emphasized this basic principle, and he was one of the few physiologists during our period who wrote on "[T]he experimental method employed in my researches on the brain."[74] But, like Magendie, he was concerned to amass experimental data, declaring that "[T]he art of discerning simple facts is the whole art of experimentation."[75] To collect these facts, Flourens insisted that first the part of the brain under investigation should be adequately exposed; and that the ambiguous, contradictory results of his predecessors such as Haller and his school and Rolando were due to the relative crudeness of their techniques. Second, the part being studied must be ablated precisely, and it was Flourens who established this as a neurophysiological procedure of the greatest value. Third, complications must be recognized and avoided. "In physiology," he commented, "when a mistake is made, it is nearly always because all of the possible complications have not been recognized."[76] Their variety and significance will be discussed shortly. But as Young has pointed out, the quality of Flourens's surgical procedures was not equaled by his unsophisticated and limited postoperative observations on changes in behavior and by his controlled testing nor were his sweeping conclusions always warranted by the evidence he accumulated.[77] Nevertheless, we can agree with Neuburger's accurate general assessment of Flourens's contributions to neurophysiology:

> Flourens's work eclipsed that of his predecessors and contemporaries to the extent it did because of the fundamental reform in experimental physiology of the central nervous system that he brought about. He created a new method, he formulated problems in a new way, and he endeavored to substantiate his clearly defined ideas with plain facts.[78]

At the same time, we must not, however, despite Magendie's strictures, denigrate the important work of anatomists for we have already noted that according to Neuburger Flourens's physiology was based on it.

Flourens was not alone in paying little attention to the examination of changes in mental functions following experimental interference with animals' brains; appropriate methods of testing them were not to be introduced until almost the end of the nineteenth century.[79] Early in the century the Cartesian notion of animals being mindless automata still had an effect upon experimentalists and must have discouraged some from adopting these means of inquiry. In 1836 it seemed to Solly a hopeless task to investigate phenomena such as volition, instinct, and understanding, for he admitted that "it is obvious from what has now been said that a very scanty amount of information has been obtained, or seems likely to be obtained, by means of mutilations practised on the lower animals."[80] There were, in fact, no systematic attempts at psychological testing during our period.

Finally, concerning the types of physiologists, we should mention the emergence at the end of the 1840s of the full-time, pure physiologist, who, unlike the majority of his predecessors in this field, had no clinical practice and devoted all his time to research on the nervous system and to the teaching and training of students and assistants. We shall encounter them in chapter 5 and find that they established the discipline of biophysics. However, their main influence was after 1850.

In the chapters that follow, we shall refer on a number of occasions to the possible reasons for the frequent appearance of contradictory results among those practicing vivisection of the animal nervous system during the first half of the nineteenth century. We can discuss them briefly now with profit, but although by viewing them retrospectively and judging them by present day standards, it is not our intention to censure experimenters who were usually working under primitive conditions, with inadequate and crude apparatus, and with no substantial reservoir of experience to bolster their pioneer endeavors. First, there were factors attributable to the investigator himself, such as defective experimental methodology, an imperfection about which Flourens was so vocal. This would include a lack of dexterity, resourcefulness, and presence of mind (attributes just as important at the experimental as at the operating table); a faulty knowledge of anatomy; and inadequate powers of observation to detect the immediate and late effects on the animal of the procedure carried out. Other personal factors would comprise the inability of the investigator to plan experiments meticulously and to reason logically and without prejudice; whether he approached his selected problem objectively or with preconceived opinions and massaged his data consciously or unconsciously in order to achieve the outcome he preferred; and his willingness to extrapolate beyond his results and to indulge in analogy or speculation in order to supplement faulty or inadequate findings. The scientist's lack of skill at presenting his discoveries to his colleagues and students was another hazard, and we have already mentioned it. Finally, there was the problem of interpreting his results, and one of the commonest errors was to base an opinion on only a few experimental or clinical observations. Although statistics were in use in public health, clinical medicine, population studies, longevity, and so forth, as Francis Bisset Hawkins (1796–1894) attested to in 1829, they were rarely, if ever, applied to experimental physiology.[81]

Then there were the defects, hazards, and complications of the experimental procedure itself, both during the performance of it and after its completion. As we have noted, Flourens, in particular, warned against the various known complications, but there were some that he did not recognize, or did not fully appreciate their significance. The commonest error was to injure parts of the brain or spinal cord other than the one at which the experiment was directed. This was an inevitable outcome of the pre-Flourentian technique whereby areas of brain were attacked blindly, often without opening the cranial cavity. It was to avoid these common and potentially very confusing secondary effects that Flourens adapted the wide-exposure method so that ablation or irritation could be conducted accurately. Concerning the latter, there were three ways of stimulating nervous tissue: by mechanical, chemical, or electrical excitation. During our period, the last of these was the least reliable; because of technological inadequacies (see chap. 5), the stimulus was either weaker or much stronger than the physiological kind, with inevitable erroneous results in each case. Its unreliability in the early 1820s is demonstrated by Flourens's statement in 1824 that he had employed it, but regarded it, like chemical irritants, as a special agent and would report on its use later.[82] As far as we can discover, he never did. However, with advances in the physics and technology of electrophysiology (see chap. 5), electrical excitation became a powerful experimental tool that eventually produced spectacular results. J. C. Dalton could report in 1882 that "[I]t is hardly possible to overestimate the change thus introduced into the study of the nervous system, and the facilities which it supplied for further investigation."[83]

Other known complications to be avoided were damage to blood vessels during the operation which could produce severe bleeding and hypotension or postoperative manifestations of brain compression by an intracranial hematoma. Obviously these sequelae would seriously affect any attempt to examine the results of the procedure that had been performed. In 1824, Magendie gave a dramatic demonstration of the results of intracranial bleeding and of its relief when visiting William Hyde Wollaston (1766–1828) in London.[84] The effects of surgical shock during extensive and painful operations conducted on conscious animals were also known, but the etiology was not appreciated, and it was probably thought to be due to excessive hemorrhage, with which it was often associated.

The occurrence of shock and a hypotensive state must have been almost universal, and yet the experimenter expected to be able to examine the animal immediately for the effects of the mutilation or stimulation of the central nervous system. Such acute experiments must have accounted in part for the highly variable results reported by physiologists, and yet few seemed to be aware of the hazard. One of those who discussed this problem was Gall, and his astuteness in this regard was noteworthy. He was contesting Flourens's opinion that injury of the cerebellum produced incoordinated movements, and pointed out that no accurate assessment of the animals' movements could be expected, because they were, in fact, dying from the general effects of the surgical procedure.[85] Flourens claimed, however, that he did not carry out his postoperative tests until the general effects of the operation had worn off.[86] It is difficult, nevertheless, to believe that the acute pain from the trauma inflicted would readily subside. Besides, some of his experimental protocols belie this intention.

Another consequence of open procedures on the central nervous system was fully recognized, but its origins were not known. This was the fatal meningitis or wound infection that afflicted the animal that survived the experimental table. Like the immediate postoperative sequelae, this must also have been very common before the introduction of antiseptic and aseptic measures later in the century, and its effect on the various functions being examined postoperatively would have been considerable. Two British neurophysiologists in 1887, twenty years after the revolutionary application by Joseph Lister (1827–1912) of the germ theory of disease to the operating room, could warn that "all experiments upon the brain in which these [aseptic] precautions are neglected are not only liable to be lacking in definiteness and precision, but may even be expected to yield illusory results."[87] Fatal postoperative infection together with the immediate effects of surgical trauma, shock, and uncontrolled hemorrhage combined to make chronic, as opposed to acute, experiments rare events. Flourens was aware of most of these complications and tried to keep his animals alive as long as possible, but he was able to achieve success in only a few instances.[88] In fact, concerning the cerebellum it was not possible to carry out chronic experiments on its function until much later in the nineteenth century, when the postoperative complications could be avoided or overcome and the animal's survival greatly extended so that much more accurate and trustworthy observations could be made.[89]

Perhaps one of greatest sources of confusion among these early nineteenth century experimentalists was their disregard for the differences in the form and function of the nervous system in the various species of animals (chap. 1.2.3). From this stemmed many of the conflicting results and opinions that we encounter in the literature of the time. Equally disconcerting to us is the ease with which they could make totally unwarranted extrapolations from lower animals to humans, an error that began with Aristotle (384–322 B.C.) and can still occur today. Young has drawn attention to the fact that Flourens was guilty of this, even though he possessed a deep knowledge of comparative anatomy.[90] Thus, Flourens formulated sweeping generalizations concerning human brain function, based on animal material only (see chap. 6.4). In this regard Gall's comments on Flourens's studies are again enlightening:

> Besides, these cruel experiments, when they are carried out on animals of a low enough order, are hardly ever conclusive for [application to] man. In hens, pigeons, rabbits, guinea-pigs, and even in newly born animals of a higher order, all of the animal [somatic] life is not by any means under the domination of the brain.[91]

Few seem to have taken heed of this sage advice and warning. The age of the experimental animal, as Gall mentioned, was another hazard not widely appreciated in the early nineteenth century. Admittedly, Flourens preferred younger specimens, but his choice was made on practical grounds and based mainly on the fact that their cranial bones were soft so that access to the brain was easier.[92] On the whole, however, the significance of age was not appreciated, and it was taken for granted that the immature brain reacted like the mature brain, which is not so.

These, then, were the complications and hazards facing the experimental neurophysiologist early in the nineteenth century, and such was the number and variety of variables involved that it is small wonder that their field of research was bedeviled by dissenting and inconsistent opinions leading to discord and bitter polemics. But despite the potential risks awaiting them, they were able to pursue their studies with a considerable degree of success, as will be related in subsequent chapters of this book. Toward the end of our chosen period William Benjamin Carpenter (1813–1885), an influential British physiologist, underlined the practical problem of the experimenter:

> Every one who has been engaged in physiological experiments, is aware of the amount of difference caused by very minute variations in their circumstances; in no department of enquiry is this more the case, than in regard to the Nervous System.[93]

1.2.3. Comparative Anatomy

In a memoir of 1828 presented to the Académie des Sciences in Paris, A. L. Foville recognized that the methods students of the nervous system employed depended in part upon wider tendencies within the life sciences: different techniques had been used, "according to the different manner in which the subject has been considered; and also according to the progress of biology, or the science of life."[94] Resorting to the lower animals in order to settle questions of human anatomy and physiology was a well-established practice, which can be said to have begun with Aristotle and Galen, and Thomas Willis's contributions to knowledge of the nervous system in the seventeenth century by using animals were considerable.[95] The late eighteenth and early nineteenth centuries saw a growing emphasis upon comparative studies as the royal road to enhanced knowledge in all departments of biology, due in part to the studies and teaching of John Hunter and Georges Cuvier. Thus William Lawrence (1783–1867) in 1818 held that "a continuation of this method will place physiology on the solid basis of experience, and build up science on ground hitherto occupied by fancy and conjecture."[96] This was especially true in the neurosciences. Solly declared in 1836:

> There can be no question but that the only philosophical method of simplifying and giving a character of general interest to the anatomy of the human brain, is by commencing with the structure and functions of a nervous system in the lowest and simplest forms of animal existence, and from this rising by degrees to the highest, carefully observing each addition of parts, and the relationship borne by these to an addition of function.[97]

In the same year another commentator announced that "it [comparative anatomy] must henceforth be considered as the grand basis of physiology."[98]

This stress upon comparative studies owed much to the movement in the early nineteenth century to ascertain the general laws of life and organization. The romantic philosophy of nature to which we have referred above maintained that underlying the complexity of the living world there was simplicity. The most elaborate forms of organization were developments of simple types; the "highest" and "lowest" organisms were therefore constructed upon a uniform plan. The task of the biologist was to identify the simple type of a given structure and to trace its progressive elaboration in the *scala naturae,* culminating in its fullest expression in humans. Jacob Henle, in a retrospective review written in 1846, described this as the "genetic method" (*genetische Behandlung*) by means of which "an entirely new field of research was opened up."[99] Henle stressed the intellectual pleasure to be derived from seeing "the same idea embodied in a thousand forms, the most complicated structure developing from the simplest origins"; and he held that this approach had yielded novel insights into the functions of bodily parts, as well as fresh insights into the essential forms of compound organs.[100]

In the case of the nervous system, this "genetic" approach is well exemplified by the efforts of Gall to understand the structure of the brain by reference to simpler nervous structures in the human body and by comparison with the lower animals (see quote, n. 91, above). We will consider the momentous consequences of Gall's work for concepts of the cerebrospinal axis in chap. 2.1. We must note here that in this book we always use the word "genetic" in the sense outlined above rather than in the sense more familiar to modern biologists.

1.2.4. Developmental Anatomy

Brigham's fifth method was "[T]he foetal condition and growth of the brain." Comparative studies of the structure of adult organisms were, in the first half of the nineteenth century, accompanied by an intense interest in embryology. Connecting the two fields of investigation was the theory that the growth of the human embryo in some way paralleled the pattern of development evident in the animal series.[101] On this assumption, embryology and comparative anatomy were studies which must proceed hand in hand: embryology supplied a complementary means of seeking the typical structures that united the most complex with the simplest organisms.

The outstanding application of these methods to the nervous system is found in the writings of Friedrich Tiedemann (1781–1861) and his English follower John Anderson (fl. 1837), both of whom figure in chapter 2.2. In his 1816 study of the fetal brain, Tiedemann pointed out that the embryology of the human brain had been neglected previously; and he claimed that a study of it should "give an explanation regarding the fashioning and formation of the brain that, in its perfect state, is so complicated."[102] Moreover, "it allows many explanations for the structure of the brain that seem to me to be not unimportant."[103] Tiedemann also took a keen interest in comparative anatomy, maintaining:

> In my opinion the only two paths that can lead to a knowledge of the structure of the brain, but that are still infrequently used, are those of comparative anatomy and the anatomy of the fetus; for [the investigation of] this labyrinth they are like the thread of Ariadne.[104]

Although this comparative and developmental strategy received novel emphasis in the nineteenth century, it had possessed advocates in earlier periods. Nicolaus Steno [Stensen] (1638–1686) in 1665 recommended the use of both comparative anatomy and embryology in the study of the brain, arguing that "it is necessary to dissect and examine as many heads as there are different species of animals and different conditions in each species. In the Fetus of animals one sees how the brain is formed."[105] But apart from Willis, few heeded this advice.

1.2.5. Pathology Elucidating Physiology

Henle, who as we observed was sympathetic toward the theory of neural pathology, held that the physiologist possessed a further resource: the natural experiments that arose from the effects of disease. In particular, what little was known of the functions of the different parts of the brain derived, he claimed, chiefly from pathological observations. In view of the many difficulties attached to the pathological method which will be discussed shortly, we would wish to qualify Henle's claim. Nevertheless there is no doubt that in our period pathology did enlighten physiology.

By 1800 the process was well established; in particular there was Thomas Willis's selection in 1664 of the corpus striatum as a motor center on the grounds that degeneration of it was often present in patients who had suffered a contralateral palsy.[106] Also, certain French surgeons in the eighteenth century found that lesions of the brain, usually traumatic, could teach them something of its normal functioning; their conclusions often "contained more truth than the superficial shadowboxing of the pseudophilosophers and medical philosophers," as Neuburger put it.[107] He also believed that "[A]t all times the advances made in surgery in comparison with those made in anatomy had a fertilizing influence on experimental physiology."[108] In the early nineteenth century, the influence of the French school of morbid anatomy and clinicopathological correlation also increased the likelihood of clinicians and others being able to accumulate information on normal functions by observing the abnormal in humans, both in the hospital ward and in the morgue.

As we shall learn shortly, certain individuals in addition to Henle believed that this technique of elucidating physiology by means of pathology was "well calculated to extend our knowledge of the nervous system."[109] Unfortunately their enthusiasm could not always be justified, and the majority of investigators, on the basis of similar observations, denied the claims that a knowledge of abnormal functions and structures could throw light on the normal, and that it provided one of the main lines of inquiry into the physiology and anatomy of the nervous system. In their denials they cited mainly diseases of the brain, in which the pathological processes were rarely so precisely located or their influence so well defined that they affected only one of the brain's functions. A punctate lesion producing the early symptoms and signs of cerebral dysfunction usually spread, so that at autopsy its original site could not be defined; a similar sequence of events long delayed the diagnosis of appendicitis during life. It follows that it was impossible to correlate the presenting clinical picture with the primary lesion, and thus with the properties of the part of the brain where the latter resided. Moreover, in general, many diseases in their unhindered progress manifested secondary effects and complications. The outstanding French clinicopathologist of the nervous system, Claude François Lallemand (1790–1854), explained the impasse thus: "It is easy enough in *theory* to consider diseases in their simple state, to isolate them in our study, but in practice nothing is more difficult than to meet with a disease exempt from complications."[110]

In retrospect, however, we can recognize that the most serious deterrent was the relatively primitive state of the clinical and pathological investigation of the patient. In the case of the former, only the grosser manifestations of dysfunction of the nervous system could be detected, because the systematic assessment of the neurological and mental features of disease by special tests, as well as ancillary diagnostic methods, was not introduced until much later in the nineteenth and in the twentieth centuries. Morbid anatomical techniques, both macroscopical and microscopical, were similarly limited, and it was freely admitted that part of the ignorance regarding the connection between diseased structure and disordered function was due to the superficial nature of the postmortem examinations then being carried out. The clinician in the first half of the nineteenth century was therefore faced with a chaotic array of symptoms, signs, and pathological findings, and, on the whole, little advance was made in dividing them up into precise disease entities, let alone deriving physiological knowledge from them.[111]

Arising from this ignorance of the clinical and morbid anatomical features of neurological disorders was a most perplexing problem that was responsible throughout the century for confusion and contradiction among those attempting to delineate disease pictures, and also those who hoped to gain physiological insight from natural experiments in humans. In the case of diseases of the brain or spinal cord they encountered a bewildering paradox, rarely seen in other organs of the body. Thus, a patient could demonstrate very obvious evidence of a lesion, but at autopsy either no abnormality or only a trifling one could be detected by naked-eye or very limited microscopic examination. The reverse also occurred so that a patient shown to have harbored a florid pathological process of the brain or the congenital absence of part of it, might during life have revealed little clinical evidence of such gross morbid change. The opinion of Adolph Wilhelm Otto (1786–1845) in his textbook of 1809 must have expressed the feelings of many. He confessed that "[N]owhere else but in the brain do we encounter greater difficulty in making the results of an autopsy agree with the preceding [clinical] features of disease."[112] As for physiological inferences, neurologists today are amazed to discover individuals who lack, for example, most of their cerebrum and yet present tolerable intelligence, whereas some of our personal acquaintances possess a complete cerebrum, but have no pretensions to intelligence.[113] We can, therefore, appreciate the bewilderment of earlier scientists, who were attempting to prove that the cerebral hemispheres were the seat of the intellectual processes, induced by such cases. Another excellent example of the turmoil engendered by attempts to solve anatomical and physiological problems by studying the effects of disease in humans is the long, drawn-out controversy over contralateral innervation.[114] It began with the Hippocratic Writers (c. 460–370 B.C.), but was not resolved until anatomists in the nineteenth century could trace the whole motor pathway and verify the presence of a decussation of the tract that some clinicians had assumed to exist.

These various experiences must have dismayed investigators and discouraged the search for physiological enlightenment from human disease. As one observer asserted, rather than records of cases throwing light on the attempts of physiologists to ascribe motor and sensory functions to particular parts of the brain, "On the contrary, they are decidedly hostile to every hypothesis hitherto advanced."[115] Other early nineteenth-century investigators echoed this unpropitious situation with similar despondent comments. Solly, on the basis of extensive experience, complained "that there are few investigations more unsatisfactory and disappointing in their results than those which have diseases of the nervous centres for their subject, in reference to a connexion betwixt disordered function and diseased structure."[116] He did, however, correctly caution his readers against dismissing in despair an apparently unrewarding and even fallacious method of studying the physiology of the nervous system. "Nevertheless," he advised, "we should not entirely reject such aid, but merely remember how imperfect it is at present, and not therefore expect too much from it."[117] For the time being, pathology in the field of clinical neurology was "a most uncertain guide in physiological investigations of the kind we are so anxious to further."[118] Future developments would justify Solly's wise counsel.

Johannes Müller (1801–1858), the most outstanding, versatile, and respected medical scientist of the first half of the nineteenth century, held much the same view, which he expressed in his widely influential textbook of physiology that began its serial publication in 1833.[119] "After all," he declared, "the results of pathological anatomy invariably can have only a limited application to the physiology of the brain."[120] He assembled a few examples of confusing neurological syndromes to support this conclusion, each of which we can now explain satisfactorily.[121] Müller's arguments at that time were cogent and his prudence, like that of Solly, was praiseworthy, especially when we find that much later in the nineteenth century similar problems led to contradictory and disconcerting results due to a lack of the discretion he had advocated.

But despite pessimistic judgments and unrewarding experiences, clinicopathological correlation did occasionally lead to important neurophysiological deductions during the early decades of the nineteenth century. An outstanding example of this has been discussed by Lesch, in the case of Magendie.[122] We observed above that the latter had used the term "pathological physiology" to designate the method of investigation by means of which clinical medicine and morbid anatomy could enlighten physiology; it must, however, be distinguished from its modern counterpart, which implies the study of functional aspects of disease processes. By means of this procedure Magendie was able to demonstrate that the functions of the spinal cord roots and the nature of the cerebrospinal fluid and its circulation could be better understood. Thus, the judicious correlation of experimental findings with observations made on patients both at the bedside and at autopsy was in his opinion a fruitful technique. As we have stated above, Magendie was concerned primarily with the nervous system, as was another prominent French physician, Philippe Pinel (1745–1826), who also practiced and praised this research method.[123] As Lesch points out, Pinel seemed to be even more enthusiastic than his younger contemporary concerning the potential value of pathological physiology in the investigation of the nervous system:

> The application of pathological physiology to the elucidation of brain functions alone can give positive results; only it can complete an understanding of them; and it can correct a number of errors. These researches therefore deserve all our solicitude and attention.[124]

In retrospect it seems likely that Magendie's successful exploitation of pathological physiology was mainly due to his selection of the problems to which he applied it: spinal root properties and the circulation of the cerebrospinal fluid. Had he chosen instead to elucidate brain functions, his advocacy of pathological physiology might have been less ardent.

However, the best known and most significant example of pathological physiology was a proposal made by Jean Baptiste Bouillaud (1796–1881), in 1825, who nevertheless shared the skepticism of his contemporaries regarding the value of brain disease to physiology:

> Thus, although we cannot deny that cerebral pathology may be a precious means of elucidating the mysterious functions of the brain, we cannot but at the same time allow that this method of research is surrounded with great difficulties.[125]

Nevertheless, he was able to establish a firm association between a motor disturbance of speech and a frontal lobe lesion, which was to play a prominent role in the creation of the basic neuroscientific principle of punctate brain localization (see chap. 6.7). Bouillaud inferred another physiological principle from the process of correlating clinical with morbid anatomical findings when he concluded that "the precise part of the brain the injury of which produces derangement of the intellect is the cortical substance of that organ."[126] A contemporary, Jean Baptiste Maximilien Parchappe de Vinay (1800–1866), confirmed and extended this, using the same technique and arguing that the mental deterioration of patients suffering from a variety of neurosyphilis, general paralysis of the insane, was due to the decay of the cortex over the frontal lobes that he had discovered at autopsy. He concluded that this was the seat of mental as well as speech function (see chap. 6.7). His success was a triumph for both the morbid anatomical theory of disease and the possibility of pathology elucidating neurophysiology. Baron Dominique Jean Larrey (1776–1842), Napoleon's most prominent battle surgeon, also practiced pathological physiology and in 1829 could, he believed, detect specific dysfunctions following localized cerebral injury in humans.[127] He was, however, like Bouillaud, attempting to verify Gall's theory of punctate cortical localization of psychological functions, which, as we shall learn below, was demolished by Flourens's more accurate, but equally erroneous, animal experiments (chap. 6.4). Whereas Larrey's interpretations were proved wrong, Bouillaud's were later shown to be correct (chap. 6.7).

Finally, we shall refer briefly to one of the most perplexing lesions of the brain: the congenital anomaly of anencephaly. In earlier centuries it had placed traditional beliefs of nervous system function in jeopardy, for if the brain produced motion, how could these monsters move as they did? In the nineteenth century it also threatened the veracity of certain fundamental neuroscientific concepts, so that physiologists felt equally threatened. For example, Lallemand, an outstanding neuroscientist, declared on the basis of the few cases then reported that:

> These observations suffice to prove that the brain is not *the unique source of nervous power,* as Haller believed, nor *the unique center of the nervous system of animal [somatic] life,* as Bichat thought. They will prove once more that movements independent of the will are not under the influence of the cerebellum, if such [a refutation] is needed today.[128]

Anencephalics could, therefore, refute three prominent neuroscientific concepts, the first being that of Haller who claimed the brain was the motor center. Concerning Bichat's doctrine of two strictly separate nervous systems, the cerebrospinal and vegetative (see chap. 7.4), anencephalics were seen to confirm it by showing that the vegetative nervous system could exist and function independently of the brain. However, Lallemand here asserted that the theory designating the brain as the sole source of motor power within the cerebrospinal system was disproved by anencephalics. The third was Willis's theory that the cerebellum initiated all involuntary, vital (i.e., autonomic), movements. The second and third were subsequently shown to be incorrect and this pathological evidence contributed to their demise, but the first helped to establish present day views. The brainless monsters usually had a small amount of brain stem, and Lallemand could therefore argue that because they could move, it followed that this structure was able to instigate muscular movement. The realization, therefore, that the brain stem can play such an independent and vital role was in part due to the application of pathological findings to a physiological problem.

These were some of the ways in which observation of the abnormal facilitated the understanding of the normal during the first half of the nineteenth century. As the century progressed and as clinical neurology, neuropathology, and neurophysiology advanced, more benefits from the technique were forthcoming. In particular, surgeons were eventually able to study diseases of the nervous system at an early stage of their evolution and, consequently, the functions of the parts affected. The excellent advice given by Solly in 1836 when he counseled cautious application rather than disillusioned rejection of the method was thereby shown to be fully vindicated.

1.2.6. Microscopical Anatomy

As we have noted, Brigham, when preparing his list of methods for studying the nervous system in 1840, did not include microscopy. At that time it had only been in existence as a legitimate scientific technique for about seven years. Although some important advances had been made (see chap. 3) throughout the period we are surveying, the value of the microscope to medical science remained a controversial topic, mainly because of technological inadequacies. All discoveries before midcentury were made with relatively crude microscopes and there were no effective staining or other histological techniques. We shall survey below the studies carried out on the nerve cell concept (chap. 3), on the fine structure of the spinal cord as it concerned the physiology of the spinal reflex (chap. 4.6), and on the complexities of the fiber and cell arrangements in the vegetative (autonomic) nervous system (chap. 7.7.5). We shall also discuss (chap. 3.5.2) the influence of physiological thinking on the significance and role of microscopical structures, and the general interaction between physiological and anatomical reasoning which characterized mid-nineteenth-century neurohistology.

1.2.7. Conclusion

We have now reviewed the principal means available to students of the nervous system in the first half of the nineteenth century. But technology, however sophisticated, is only one element of scientific creativity; indeed, great results have been attained by the use of relatively crude techniques and deficient instruments. The human element in science is paramount: the investigator must frame meaningful questions, devise programs of research, and draw fruitful conclusions if there is to be any significant contribution to knowledge. The greater part of our effort in this work has, therefore, been directed at elucidating the intellectual background to the seminal achievements in the neurosciences accomplished during our selected period. We hope, above all, to have shown that the history of medicine and science cannot be divorced from an understanding of the general preoccupations and assumptions of an epoch.

2

The Cerebrospinal Axis

2.1. THE COMPARATIVE PERSPECTIVE

The modern concept of the nervous system is of a unity in multiplicity. The cerebrospinal axis is made up of a number of homologous units, each of which is capable of a measure of autonomous action, but which are integrated by various mechanisms into a functional whole. This view of the organization and relations of the spinal cord and brain first became established in the early decades of the nineteenth century; it replaced a contrary system of great antiquity.

This earlier system was usually designated the "Galenic" model of the anatomical and functional relations of brain and spinal cord. Richard Dugard Grainger (1801–1865) summarized its chief tenets in 1829. "Anatomists, from the time of Galen downwards," he declared, "have very generally regarded the brain as the sole origin and centre of this [nervous] system, and in accordance with this idea, the spinal cord and the nerves were described as prolongations of the cerebral organ, and even the great sympathetic [nerve] was viewed in the same light."[1] J. C. Spurzheim concurred that "the brain has very generally been regarded as the sole and common origin of every part of the nervous system. . . . In their [the old anatomists'] eyes, the spinal cord was a prolongation of the cerebral mass, and the great sympathetic, and the nerves of the abdomen and thorax, were continuations of the encephalon and spinal cord."[2]

This doctrine of the anatomical primacy of the brain was mirrored in prevailing views of the way the nervous system worked. In Charles Bell's words, "From the age of Galen . . . down to the present time, the hypothesis has been maintained with little variation, that the brain presides over the body through the spinal marrow and nerves."[3] Legallois had in 1812 emphasized the way this physiological doctrine followed from the Galenic notion of the anatomy of the spinal cord: as long as the cord was regarded merely as "a large nerve derived from the brain," then the brain naturally appeared as the source of all nervous power and as "the unique seat of the principle of life."[4] According to such reasoning, Carpenter observed in 1846, that the brain "was accounted, not merely the centre of all motion and sensation, but also of all vitality; the different processes of nutrition, secretion, etc., being maintained . . . by a constant supply of 'animal spirits,' propagated from the brain along the nerves, to each individual part."[5]

The Galenic model of the nervous system continued to attract considerable support, especially in Britain, as late as the 1830s and, in isolated cases, even later.[6] However, from the turn of the nineteenth century it had been subjected to criticism and revision on various grounds. By 1846 Carpenter was able to speak of the Galenic system as a superseded theory: he noted the process of "gradual limitation which has taken place in the physiological idea of the functions of [the brain]; from the period when it was considered as the centre of the whole life of the body . . . to the time of our present writing, in which the real extent of its agency is so much better understood."[7] This shift in notions of the function of the nervous system relied to a great extent upon different ideas of its organization. Carpenter listed the principal sources of change.

The first step was the withdrawal of the organic or vegetative (autonomic) functions from the control or support of the brain.[8] This concept of the complete autonomy of the vegetative from the cerebrospinal nervous system with its own nervous power was first sponsored by Bichat in 1800, and we shall discuss his doctrine in chapter 7.4 below. Vegetative bodily operations were now regarded as regulated by the ganglia of the vegetative nervous system alone. In the words of Maurice Krishaber (fl. 1846), following Bichat, "the [autonomic] ganglion was elevated to the rank of a nervous center."[9] Carpenter went on to mention changes in ideas of the properties of the spinal cord which had also detracted from the sole dominance of the encephalon. In particular, the experimental studies of Robert Whytt (1714–1766), Legallois, Marshall Hall, and others had demonstrated the "independent endowments" of the cord; that is, its ability to execute reflex movements even when separated from the brain (see chap. 4.2–4).[10]

There was, however, a further source of change. Ideas of the structure of the cerebrospinal axis underwent a revolution betwen 1800 and 1840. Quite literally, an inversion of previous modes of conceiving the axis took place: instead of proceeding from above downwards and seeing the spinal cord as a process of the brain, anatomists began to go from below upwards and to describe the brain as the culmination of the spinal cord. The new view was clearly expounded in volume one of the textbook by Robert Bentley Todd (1809–1860) and William Bowman (1816–1892) of 1845:

> The brain and spinal cord, in the vertebrate classes, form a central axis with which all other parts of the nervous system are connected. The former is evidently an aggregate of gangliform swellings, each possessing the characters of a nervous centre, but so connected with the others, that their functions are in no small degree mutually dependent. The latter has throughout its entire length all the characters of one uniform nervous centre, of cylindrical shape; but experiment has shewn that, if divided into segments in animals tenacious of vitality, each portion may exert an independent influence on that segment of the body whose nerves are connected with it. From this fact we may properly regard the cord also in the light of a ganglion compounded of smaller ones, which have been, as it were, fused together.[11]

This quotation indicated something of the mechanism of the change in question. The concept of the "ganglion," considered at that time on the basis of macroscopical evidence only to be an accumulation of gray matter, that had previously been confined to the spinal cord roots and the vegetative nervous system, was now extended to the cerebrospinal axis. A "genetic" approach was adopted whereby from this simple element more complex organs were evolved ("genetic" is used here and hereafter in the sense defined in chap. 1.2.3). The spinal cord ceased to be a mere cable of nerves flowing from the head. Moreover, the brain itself was now seen as a conglomeration of ganglia, as a more complicated version of the structures found below. This fragmentation of the organization of the axis had a physiological corollary: each "ganglion" was a partially independent center of nervous activity. The encephalon was a congeries of such centers, analogous to those of the spinal cord, each with its peculiar function.[12] There were, in effect, many "small brains" in the cerebrospinal nervous system, and we shall learn in chapter 7.5 that the same idea was held with regard to the ganglia of the vegetative system.

By 1845, when Todd and Bowman wrote, this way of seeing the nervous system seemed natural and to require no special justification. However, thc transfer of the ganglion from the vegetative to the cerebrospinal nervous system was not an obvious move to many earlier anatomists. Bichat himself had recognized no analogy between the two departments of the nervous system, but had remained wedded to the Galenic notion of the brain and spinal cord. Some of his followers strenuously resisted what they regarded as false analogies between different parts of the human nervous system and between the cerebrospinal axis and nervous structures in other animals. Thus, Béclard held that the macroscopical texture of the vegetative ganglia and of the brain was quite distinct. Nor could analogies be drawn with lower animals in order to establish the proposition that the human "brain and spinal cord are assemblages of ganglia."[13]

What overrode such preconceptions and biases and, more than anything else, overturned the Galenic model, was the rise to prominence of a comparative approach to questions of human structure and function.[14] As Charles Bell wrote in 1830, "if men look upon the same object in one unvarying aspect, they will receive a similar impression, and describe what they see in nearly the same words." For example, until recently, the practice of anatomists seeking to establish the paths of the nerves had been "to trace the nerve from the brain, and taking the instance of the human body, that is, the highest and most complicated form as the foundation of the system, instead of tracing nerves through the changes they exhibit in different animals."[15] During the late eighteenth and early nineteenth century several workers sought to supplement the traditional resources of medical science by undertaking extensive studies of the structure and function of the lower animals (see chap. 1.2.3). John Hunter in Britain and Félix Vicq d'Azyr (1748–1794) and Georges Cuvier in France were among the most prominent of this group. These men approached comparative studies not merely to improve the science of zoology, but also to cast light upon the nature of the human body. William Lawrence summarized their assumptions when in 1818 he claimed that the "varieties of organisation" evident in the animal kingdom "supply, in the investigation of each function, the most important aids of analogy, comparison, contrast, and various combination; and the nature of the [physiological] process receives, at each step, fresh elucidation." It was on "such researches and studies, on a foundation no less extensive than the whole empire of living nature, [that] the science of medicine must be established; if, indeed, it be destined to occupy the rank of a science."[16]

Michael Gross has shown how the new emphasis upon comparative studies did more than cast fresh light upon perennial problems of anatomy and physiology: it led to a reformulation of the basic questions with which these sciences were concerned. Specifically, the comparative approach led to efforts to achieve a general physiology and anatomy; to attain concepts of structure and function applicable to all or, at least, to most animals.[17] Investigations of the nervous system occupied a leading place among those engaged in this endeavor; many scientists insisted that it was only by reference to the larger world of life that this branch of medical knowledge could advance (see chap. 1.2.3). An anonymous reviewer expressed this conviction in 1837:

> In our researches into the structure of the nervous system, we may derive particular assistance from the information with which comparative anatomy supplies us; since by tracing the gradual appearance and development of its different portions, as we ascend in the animal scale, we can arrive at much more correct and definite notions of the arrangement and connection in that most complicated of all organs, the human brain, than can be acquired by the examination of it alone.[18]

In 1824 Friedrich Tiedemann went as far as to assert that "knowledge of the structure of the nervous system has principally been gained through comparative anatomy and made progress for which twenty years ago one could have scarcely dared to hope."[19] Among these achievements, it was widely agreed, the revision of old notions of the relation of brain to spinal cord was preeminent. When the French physiologist Frédéric Joseph Bérard (1789–1828) declared in 1823 that the "vulgar ideas of the general organization of the nervous system are incompatible with the notions of comparative anatomy," he had particularly in mind the theory that the brain was the source of all other structures in the system and of all its power.[20] Above all, Bérard held, it was Gall who, by taking a broad comparative outlook, had corrected earlier misconceptions. Gall had established that

> the brain, the spinal cord and the nerves do not proceed from a common origin in the course of their formation; but these different portions of the nervous system arise from a particular collection of gray matter, which constitutes their nutritional matrix; that each nerve, along with its ganglion, forms a partial and independent system, which has its origin in itself or in its gray matter, and that all these [isolated] systems form an unity, through simple means of communication.[21]

Gall was, indeed, a central actor in the revolution in concepts of the cerebrospinal axis that took place in the early nineteenth century. He, more than any other individual, popularized the notion that the axis should be conceived "genetically"—from below upward—rather than in the opposite direction.[22] This change in perspective was embodied in the method of dissection and exposition which Gall and his collaborator Spurzheim adopted in their many public demonstrations of the organization of the brain.

The generally adopted method at the beginning of the nineteenth century of dissecting the brain was recognized by later anatomists to be seriously defective, as we have already noted in chapter 1.2.1. In the words of one commentator, this method was "founded on the most erroneous and irrational principles."[23] The procedure was to begin "with the upper surface of the organ, cutting across the hemispheres, so as to expose the cavities and the objects which they contain, and then proceeding by successive sections to the base or lower part of the brain."[24] John Elliotson (1791–1868) lamented that, even in 1815, "while students are not instructed to dissect limbs and trunks by slices, as we cut brawn, they should be taught no other mode of examining the brain, and thus be left in ignorance of its true structure." Elliotson also remarked that it had been the activities of Gall and Spurzheim that had begun the reform of this state of affairs: he held that "some of the most candid anatomical lecturers of London have confessed that they knew nothing of the anatomy of the brain till they saw it dissected by his [Gall's] pupil Dr. Spurzheim."[25] Among the others who attributed to these demonstrations a far higher order of understanding of cerebral structure than they had previously possessed were Samuel Solly, J. C. Reil, Christian Heinrich Ernst Bischoff (1781–1861), and Johann Wolfgang von Goethe (1749–1832).[26]

In 1809 Gall and Spurzheim described the method that generated such enthusiasm and interest:

> In public demonstrations of the brain, we are accustomed to begin by the exposition of several general laws of the nervous system; we proceed next to the spinal cord, to the medulla oblongata, and lastly to the cerebellum and cerebrum, always faithful to the principle of following all of the parts in connection and in the order which nature seems to us to have established herself.[27]

This quotation makes clear that underlying this method of dissection was a definite theory of the structure of the nervous system. As Bischoff and Christoph Wilhelm Hufeland (1762–1836) put it, Gall believed he was "guided by nature" in proceeding from the spinal cord to the brain.[28] At the basis of his and Spurzheim's concept of the nervous system was an "anatomical etiology,"[29] which gave "genetic" priority to the lower elements of the cerebrospinal axis and which saw the brain as an elaboration of these.

Spurzheim himself said that "in our anatomical inquiries, the origin of the nervous system is the first consideration." He reviewed the Galenic notion that there was a "common origin of the nervous system"—namely the brain considered as "the origin of the spinal marrow and of the nerves." But he discarded this theory as incompatible with the facts of comparative anatomy.[30] It was necessary to seek another origin—or, rather, a class of origins—for the nerves, which would be equally applicable to humans and to the lower animals. The task of "anatomical etiology" would be to show how this common origin of the nervous system developed through the animal series, so as to bridge the apparently vast gap between human beings and molluscs. This task Gall and Spurzheim attempted in the first volume of their *Anatomie et physiologie du système nerveux* (see chap. 6.3.7).

Before the publication of this work in 1810 they submitted a memoir outlining their principal anatomical ideas to the Académie des Sciences in Paris. A Commission, headed by Cuvier, was appointed to report on these theories, and in 1809 Gall and Spurzheim in turn published a reply to the comments of the Commissioners (see chap. 6.3.7). Before considering in detail the system of Gall and Spurzheim, these documents deserve careful attention. They reveal that neither a commitment to nor a knowledge of comparative anatomy was in itself sufficient to produce the notions of the structure and function of the nervous system that Gall and Spurzheim propounded. Indeed even the questions they asked were not obvious to some contemporaries who were at least as learned in comparative anatomy as they. It was only when comparative studies were directed and informed by certain assumptions about the nature of the living world that they led to the new view of the cerebrospinal axis that Gall and Spurzheim achieved.

The Commissioners found much to commend in Gall and Spurzheim's anatomy of the nervous system; but they took issue with two crucial aspects of the system. The first of these was Gall's and Spurzheim's claim that the human spinal cord was composed of a sequence of discrete "ganglia." The Commissioners were initially unable to see any trace of the "swellings," which according to Gall and Spurzheim signified the existence of such ganglia, except at the points where the nerves to the upper and lower limbs issued from the cord, the cervical and lumbar enlargements.

After Gall and Spurzheim had produced their own preparation of the cord of a calf, the Commissioners grudgingly admitted the appearance of "a sort of swelling lying between each pair of nerves."[31] The Commissioners appointed one of their number to conduct his own research to settle the point; his conclusion was that there were no visible swellings even among quadrupeds closely allied to the calf.[32] At most, therefore, Gall and Spurzheim had identified an idiosyncratic feature of this particular mammal; they had not demonstrated a structure common to all vertebrates.

The Commissioners also took exception to an analogy Gall and Spurzheim had drawn between the animal and vegetable realms. They had suggested that nerves passing through the gray matter of ganglia were augmented in their volume, an observation first made by Johann Friedrich Meckel (1714–1774) the Elder in the eighteenth century (see chap. 7 n. 99). In this respect the ganglia were, Gall and Spurzheim held, like the nodes of trees from which new branches grew,[33] employing an analogy proposed by Thomas Willis in 1664 (see chap. 7 n. 56). The Commissioners were unimpressed with what Gall and Spurzheim had presented as a striking resemblance: it was impossible "to find anything other than an accidental resemblance" between the two classes of phenomena.[34]

These two areas of disagreement reflect major theoretical divergences between Gall and Spurzheim and the Commissioners. More precisely, the Commissioners lacked certain preconceptions that structured Gall's and Spurzheim's observations and reasoning. The Commissioners were handicapped, Gall and Spurzheim maintained, not by faulty methods or deficient materials, but by the inadequacy of their ideas. Their comments proved "how difficult it is to see well, as long as one is not guided by general laws."[35] What, above all, the Commissioners lacked was an adequate concept of the unity of the animate world, and of the fact that nature "never deviates from her primary type."[36] Because of this deficiency they asked meaningless questions while ignoring the essential principles that could alone guide research on to profitable lines. This was particularly evident in the Commissioners' remarks on the allegedly ganglionic structure of the spinal cord.

The historian Jules Soury (1842–1915) remarked that neither Cuvier nor any of the other Commissioners fully realized the central position of the concept of the ganglion in Gall's and Spurzheim's scheme.[37] Above all, the Commission missed the full significance that the notion of the ganglionic composition of the vertebrate spinal cord played within this system. The notion that the spinal marrow consisted of discrete segments was an indispensable axiom for Gall and Spurzheim: the logic of their system demanded it, and this imperative outweighed the difficulties of supplying conclusive visual evidence of the phenomenon. Unlike the Commissioners, G. G. T. Keuffel (fl. 1811), in an 1811 discussion of the anatomy of the spinal cord, fully recognized this fact. Keuffel too failed to observe the swellings to which Gall and Spurzheim referred; but he added that "if we follow theory alone, we must very readily admit that Gall's view greatly appeals to us, and that we can very well think of the spinal cord as composed of many nervous ganglia." In short, all difficulties of observing these ganglia must be set aside because the "necessity of this existence" was demonstrated by certain "general laws" to which at least some anatomists subscribed.[38]

The exchanges between Gall and Spurzheim and the Commissioners of the Académie des Sciences reveal the existence of two incommensurable paradigms. This division manifested itself not only in the field of neuroscience: it was also apparent in more general disagreements over the theoretical foundations of the life sciences. For example, in the well-known debate between Cuvier and Geoffroy St. Hilaire, the argument did not center upon facts; rather, "as [Geoffroy] himself admitted, his explanations were based on a completely different mode of seeing those facts. 'It is a question of philosophy that divides us.'"[39]

How much anatomists were prepared to see in the human body was determined by the theoretical framework within which they operated and this can be illustrated by the case of one scientist who passed from one model to another. Antoine Louis Dugès (1797–1838) confessed that it was from Cuvier that he had first derived a taste for comparative studies. In keeping with his preceptor's biases he was initially skeptical about the ideas of such "transcendental" or philosophical anatomists as Geoffroy and Étienne Reynaud Augustin Serres (1786–1868),[40] who declared, as we have noted earlier, that the type of anatomy they purveyed comprised the most profound principles of this science. His first paper on the nervous system showed the effects of this skepticism. Dugès subscribed unequivocally to the Galenic notion of the spinal cord as "a large nervous trunk" proceeding from the brain. Dugès was acquainted with Gall's opposing view of the cord, but held that "it is impossible to discern the series of ganglia of which it is supposed to be composed."[41]

After he came to Paris, however, and became better informed of the ideas of Geoffroy and Serres, Dugès's basic scientific outlook changed radically: he became (much to Cuvier's disgust) a convert to the principles of transcendental anatomy.[42] This change was especially evident in his views of the cerebrospinal axis. In stark contrast to his earlier statements Dugès declared that

> We therefore continue to see, along with Gall and many others, nothing in the spinal marrow except a series of ganglia which have coalesced and are manifested by the roots of each pair of nerves; *even though, at all ages, our senses are unable to discern this elementary composition.*[43]

It was therefore only workers within a certain paradigm that was variously described as the "transcendental" or "philosophical" approach to the science, who pioneered the revolution in ideas of the cerebrospinal axis. Those scientists who did not share these premises failed, even when viewing identical materials, to see the structures and relations others so confidently described. The following section seeks to delineate the main features of the model that had so profound an influence upon neuroscience.

2.2. THE INFLUENCE OF ROMANTIC BIOLOGY

Erna Lesky, the authority on Gall, has written that the "intellectual climate provided by the natural philosophy and anthropology of [Johann Gottfried] Herder [1744–1803]" provides "the real key to Gall's world, and with it we can reach, from within, a true understanding of his ideas and their genetic context."[44] (See chap. 6.3.5.1) Herder's thought must in turn be considered as an aspect of the movement in early nineteenth-century culture known as "romanticism." To invoke romanticism as an explanatory concept is also to summon a host of difficulties: the term is notoriously vague and resistant to definition. Nevertheless, it is possible to point to certain trends in the life sciences around 1800 that derived from a view of man and nature to which the term "romantic" is applicable. Such notions were especially prevalent in Germany, but were also current in France and Britain (see chap. 1).[45]

The fundamental axiom of the romantic philosophy of nature was its stress upon the unity of nature and, in particular, of the living world. Commitment to the idea of unity supplied scientists within this tradition with a regulative principle that guided research on to certain lines while excluding other possibilities. Thus Goethe, one of the most important precursors of romantic biology, premised his scientific investigations upon a belief in the unity of nature; conversely, "he was prepared from an early stage to rule out of order any scientific hypothesis, theory or principle which seemed to him to be incompatible with this traditional scheme."[46]

Treviranus made the axiom of unity the basis of the new science of "Biologie" that he attempted to launch in 1802;[47] it was this stress upon the analogies and interconnections between vital phenomena that distinguished the "biologist" from the mere "natural historian." The new science of life would seek to organize the manifold aspects of animal and plant life into "a whole, wherein the spirit perceives unity and harmony."[48] Treviranus was quite explicit about the a priori character of the principle he had enunciated: he declared that "the spirit strives towards unity in multiplicity, and obtains this through supposition, when experience cannot supply it."[49] Various French and British scientists were also prepared to make this supposition and to arrange their empirical observations in accordance with it.[50]

An especially important feature of the romantic stress upon the unity of nature was its implications for man's place in the cosmos. Human beings were seen as included in the great organic whole: in Goethe's words, "man is animal, an animal with a difference, singled out for higher things, but formed by nature 'nach einem Hauptplasma der Organisation' along with the other animals."[51] In this regard, therefore, romanticism had a decidedly naturalistic tendency; it eroded the strict distinction found in Christian thought between human and other living beings and instead sought ways of affirming their basic affinity. For instance, Goethe himself conducted comparative research into the cranial structures of humans and animals in an attempt to obviate one supposed difference between them. His delight at discovering the human intermaxillary bone derived from thus "bringing man and animals together, tracing them to be one."[52]

Despite their naturalism, however, the romantics were not content to say that man was merely natural; he must be allowed a special, elevated position in the creation. This demand created a dilemma:

> First there is the endeavour to find a place for man in the animal kingdom, to break his isolation, to bridge the gap between him and *other* animals. . . . Second, there is the endeavour to assure man, as an animal and despite his "identity" with his fellow creatures, a privileged position at the top of a newly conceived hierarchy of nature.[53]

This dilemma was resolved by an emphasis upon development as central to the organization of the living world.

The romantic conception of nature was not of a static hierarchy. It was, according to G. G. Valentin, pervaded with "the idea of becoming, of the restlessness in nature, the idea of endless, ever modifying and even thus, life-constituting processes."[54] Because they regarded the living world in these dynamic terms romantic biologists envisaged organisms not as "finished, terminated, static," but "in the phases of their development or in their metamorphoses."[55]

The omnipresent movement of the world was, moreover, progressive. All natural things showed a "yearning" to advance to a higher state of existence. This *conatus* could be understood teleologically: lower beings were "a preparation for a superior existence. To be a plant means to be ready for the life of an animal."[56] Similarly, lower animals were, so to speak, necessary preliminaries to more advanced varieties of life. With each step forward, "the powers and impulses of each branch of creation grow more manifold"; finally, Herder claimed, "they all unite in the figure of man, so far as this can contain them. At man the series stops."[57] In this way the romantic dilemma was overcome. Despite his intimate relation to other animals man remained supreme because he was the most developed; he was the end to which the rest of creation strove.

This conception of a dynamic hierarchy had several important implications. One of these was stated by the French physiologist Julien Joseph Virey (1775–1846) in 1835: man *qua* "the most perfect animal of all, exhibits the sum total of inferior structures, vertebrate and invertebrate."[58] Or, to use the words of Ignaz Döllinger (1770–1841), man, "the pinnacle" of the organic series, "combines in himself all lower levels of organization."[59] Conversely, the lower animals were partial representations of the human body; the entire animal series could, therefore, be conceived as a succession of "transitional forms," all tending toward their complete representation in human beings. Indeed, plants, too, could be included within this general dynamic conception: there was "a single force which develops plants and animals, and one law according to which this force acts." Consequently, certain modes of formation found in plants were repeated in animals and could even be discerned in humans.[60]

The same law that structured the animal and vegetable kingdoms was, moreover, at work in the development of each individual. For this reason a parallelism was apparent between the biological series and the embryogeny of the higher animals:

> just as each individual begins with the simplest form and throughout his metamorphoses develops and evolves itself, so also has the whole animal organism [that is, kingdom] begun its unfolding with the simplest animal form or with the animals of the lowest classes.[61]

Both series then progressed in step, each gradually attaining greater perfection. Because of this correlation an animal would pass through the permanent stages of beings lower in the series before attaining its proper form. Man, the pinnacle of creation, necessarily passed through all inferior stages.[62]

Embryology, in close conjunction with comparative anatomy therefore held a preeminent position among romantic biologists, as we have already learned: it supplied the chief method of discerning the way in which the human organism was generated through a succession of intermediate states. With the embryo, Döllinger declared, "we are at the source of life, and no one flatters himself to possess a knowledge of the human organism, until this origin has become clear to him."[63]

Perhaps the most distinguished of the scientists who undertook embryological studies within this interpretative framework was Tiedemann. In his *Éloge* of Tiedemann published in 1862, Flourens contrasted the philosophy of the German embryologist with that of his own master, Cuvier; and this appreciation will stand as a summary of the romantic approach to the phenomena of life described above. Cuvier, Flourens held, began from a philosophy of:

> particular facts and from individual and exclusive entities. M. Tiedemann began, on the contrary, from the philosophy of general ideas and from reified (*réalisées*) abstractions. He imagined a *general organism,* which he postulated as a real being: particular beings were no more, hence, than simple

> stages, simple *arrests of development* of this [general] organism. Apart from their [degree of] complication, all beings are similar; the different classes are nothing but different ages of a single [being]; man passes through all the inferior forms before arriving at maturity; he begins by being a polyp; next he is a worm; then a mollusc; then a cold-blooded vertebrate; then a warm-blooded vertebrate; an inferior animal is merely the embryo of a higher one.[64]

For our present purposes Tiedemann is an interesting figure for a further reason. He, like many others of a similar theoretical persuasion, saw a particularly fruitful and important application of the principles of romantic biology to lie in their relevance to the nervous system.

In romantic biology, the unity of the living world was evinced not only in the overall forms of animals, but also in the constructions of their particular organs. There were, Treviranus maintained in 1802, a certain number of "ground plans" in nature, by the "various combinations of which all other forms" were built. Because of this unity of type, Treviranus added, the "highest" and the "lowest" of nature's creations were bound together.[65]

By the 1830s such views had achieved a wide currency. John Fletcher (1792–1836) provided a particularly full statement of their implications: the "organs of the higher and those of the lower tribes, if not of plants, certainly of animals," were, he claimed essentially the same:

> the nucleus or structural elements of each organ in the former, not only existing, but being in fact in all their essential characters identical with those of the corresponding organ in the latter.[66]

In short, nature did not progress by introducing wholly new structures into her creatures; rather, it was "by means of the complication of [pre-existing] elements . . . that nature attains . . . this progressive ascent."[67] A result of this "genetic" continuity was that organic forms retained basic similarities, even in apparently disparate animals. The "elements" of composition were, as one commentator put it, "everywhere identical, disposed according to invariable rules."[68]

This doctrine had implications for human beings. From Herder onwards, writers in the romantic tradition regarded the human frame as constructed from elements which, although more fully developed in man, were also to be found in the lower animals.[69] In Fletcher's words:

> as the more elevated tribes of animals embrace generally, in a greater or less degree, every improvement successively made on the moulds of the several organs of the tribes below them, the splendid human organism itself consists merely of the same organs, regarded fundamentally, as exist in the polype, the differences consisting chiefly in their different degrees of elaboration.[70]

Momentous methodological principles were derived from these assumptions. "In virtue of this great law of the animal creation," declared Richard Grainger in 1842, "we are enabled by a judicious selection of those classes of animals which exhibit the simplest structure, to seize the essential typical form of organs, which, in man, although fashioned on the same model are obscured by their amazing intricacy."[71] The complex was to be understood by means of the elementary. Thus, Tiedemann held that an essential step in acquiring physiological knowledge was the "observation of vital appearances in the various tissues, organs, systems, . . . firstly in the simpler animals, and then, by way of the more complex [proceeding] to the most perfect."[72] This route, William Carpenter insisted, was the only one to an understanding of the "laws of life": the various perplexities that had plagued physiology for centuries could only be resolved when biological phenomena were "reduced to their simplest form," and then traced through the degrees of complication which culminated in humans.[73]

To illustrate this "genetic" approach to human structures Grainger took the example of the vertebral column and skull. In humans, the cranium appeared as distinct from the spinal column. In simpler animals, however, its true nature was evident: the skull was seen to be a modified extension of the vertebral chain.[74] Grainger here referred to one of the most famous achievements of transcendental anatomy—the vertebral theory of the skull which Goethe, Lorenz Oken, Carl Gustav Carus (1789–1869), and later Richard Owen (1804–1892) developed.[75] This theory supposed a community between the human skull and that of the lower vertebrates. But, in addition, it posited a unity within the body. Homologous elements were, it was claimed, deployed throughout the organism, "not only symmetrically and on each side in bilaterally-organized animals, but also longitudinally, one extremity reproducing the other."[76]

The law of serial repetition was taken to ludicrous lengths by some of the *Naturphilosophen,* notably, Oken. But more sober authors maintained that despite the "fantastic treatment of this subject by certain writers," the doctrine was of the highest value to osteology. It could, moreover, be applied to other organ systems such as the muscles.[77] However, as Treviranus affirmed unequivocally, for anatomists and physiologists of the first half of the nineteenth century, "the first among the organic systems of the animal, in respect of its origin and of its importance, is the nervous system."[78] Given the preoccupation of early nineteenth-century physiology with the nervous system, it was inevitable, therefore, that the proponents of romantic biology should seek to apply their principles to elucidate the structure and functions of this preeminent system.

Indeed, there was a widespread agreement that the nervous system provided a paradigmatic case for the vindication of romantic principles. It was here, more than anywhere else, that the unity of living beings was apparent: as Fletcher affirmed, "of all the organs of the body, none affords stronger evidence in favour of the doctrine of the unity of organic structure."[79] The nervous system displayed, moreover, to a high degree the progressive development that was supposed to pervade nature. Johann Friedrich Blumenbach (1752–1840) wrote in 1805 that "in no other class of functions in the animal economy is there so plausible a gradation from the simplest to the most complex evident, as in the [nervous system]."[80] This evolution of the nervous system, Müller asserted, was an aspect of "the true physiological concept" which dominated romantic biology: that is, of the "development, which constantly manifests itself . . . in all of nature."[81]

In consequence of these facts, the nervous systems of the various animals could be seen as so many partial approximations to that of humans. Further, according to the doctrine of parallelism, this series must be paralleled in human embryogeny.[82] Throughout its various metamorphoses, however, the unity of type of the system persisted. As E. R. A. Serres said of the brain, "the basic organ always remains the same."[83]

Among the individuals adhering to these principles were Gall and Spurzheim. It was by reference to such supposed "general laws" that they met and criticized the objections which the Commissioners had raised to their views. They affirmed their conviction in the "uniformity and invariability of the laws of nature," and, specifically, in that of the unity of type.[84] Their whole system was an attempt to vindicate these laws in respect of the nervous system. In particular, their "anatomical etiology"—their concern with the origins of nervous structures—derived from the "genetic" approach to anatomy outlined above.

To understand the complex, William Bennett (fl. 1826), the translator of Tiedemann's *Anatomie und Bildungsgeschichte des Gehirns im Foetus des Menschen* (1816), held in 1826 that it was necessary to comprehend its simpler anticipations: "to arrive at a knowledge of a compound organ, the most rational method of pursuit would be to examine its earliest state of development, and proceed in our inquiries from the simple to the compound."[85] Gall and Spurzheim also declared themselves "to be faithful to the maxim, that in all research one should proceed from the elementary to the complex"; and they proposed to treat the nervous system in this way.[86] Thus, although they were particularly concerned with the brain, in order to attain a proper conception of "the laws of this, the most noble of all the parts of the nervous system we treat, to begin with, simpler and less elevated systems."[87]

Indeed, if the implications of the "genetic" approach to anatomy were followed fully, the scientist should begin by identifying the simplest forms of the nervous system. To consider, in the words of John Anderson "the earliest stage of development of the nervous system—what shape, and of what texture, should we expect to find the most lowly organized animal forms."[88]

Romantic theoretical assumptions, therefore, presented the student of the nervous system with a central problem: to identify the "type"—the basal element—of nervous organization. It also demanded that he show how, in the zoological and the embryological series, this type became progressively elaborated. Ultimately, he had to show how the human nervous system could be considered as a compound and highly developed version of these typical structures.[89]

Analogies between the brain and nerves of human beings and other vertebrates were not unknown in earlier periods.[90] However, what was demanded now was something far more ambitious: a "genetic" account that would comprehend the nervous systems of all animals, vertebrate and invertebrate. To many anatomists, especially those in the Cuvierian tradition, such a transcendence of the obvious differences in structure between major classes—let alone between subkingdoms—was simply impossible.[91] Treviranus acknowledged the difficulties of assimilating vertebrate and invertebrate nervous structures; but he insisted that the a priori assumption of the unity of nature must override these problems. The disparities between vertebrates and invertebrates notwithstanding, "the brain of the lower animals is nevertheless, by the demand of reason, to be derived from the same primitive type (*Urform*), according to which the brain of mammals, birds, amphibians, and fish is built.[92]

Gall and Spurzheim were in 1810 satisfied that they possessed the means to mediate between the most distant forms of nervous organization. In the lower invertebrates the emergence of a heart and intestinal canal was accompanied by the appearance of accumulations of a "gelatinous substance" which gave origin to nerve fibers. These visceral nervous structures of simple animals were not based on microscopical examination, but they were, Gall and Spurzheim declared, "the type of systems of the same organs in animals of superior organization."[93] Moreover, as Gall's and Spurzheim's subsequent statements showed, these ganglia, together with their derivative fibers, were the type of all nervous structures in higher animals.[94]

Such a view was not peculiar to Gall and Spurzheim, although they did much to give it wide currency. J. C. Reil in 1808 had also sought the elemental manifestation of nervous structure in the lowest animals, and concluded that "at the lowest stage, in molluscs, the gray matter collects itself into round ganglia, which are distributed (*ausgefaet*?) asymmetrically, and the marrow shoots out from them in radiating and straight bundles."[95] In the same year, Tiedemann held that in the articulata, in molluscs, and in certain annelids, the only form of nervous system consisted of "ganglia from which the animals' nerves emerge." He added that in lower invertebrates, such as polyps and echinoderms, even this elementary nervous structure disappeared.[96] Tiedemann later decided that starfish were not, after all, bereft of a nervous apparatus: a ring of ganglia connected by fibers was visible around the mouth of these creatures.[97] Subsequent writers took this *Schlundring* as the most primitive manifestation of the nervous system and set out to show how other, more complicated forms could be seen as derived from it.[98] All these observations, like those of Gall, were macroscopical only.

This strategy was already evident in the 1816 work by Johann Lucas Schönlein (1793–1864) on the brain,[99] and was greatly elaborated in later years. Thus, John Anderson declared that the ganglionic ring found in certain radiata "is that form which, according to the laws of philosophical anatomy, we shall hereafter recognize as the essential base of even the most varied forms of the nervous system."[100] The primary ring could be developed in a number of ways. The ganglia could be diffusely distributed, as in molluscs, or arranged serially, as in articulata. In both cases there was a tendency for ganglia to become unequal in size and disparate in function. Thus in the higher molluscs a dorsal, supra-esophageal ganglion assumed a predominance over the other nervous centers; a similar process occurred in some insects where the most cephalad of the members of the ganglionic chain became larger than the rest. This structure, Anderson maintained, represented "the first appearance of a medullary mass corresponding to a brain."[101]

The concept of the ganglion, conceived as the basic form of central nervous organization, served therefore to unite the diverse forms found in the invertebrate classes. The next step was to demonstrate how this "typical" structure could account for the brain and spinal cord of vertebrates and so fully corroborate the principle of the unity of animate nature. This transition was affected by an account of the development of the brain and spinal cord that showed how these, too, were "ganglionic" organs.

It was argued that the development of the nervous system needed to be placed in its wide biological context. In particular, the analogies between this process and the growth of vegetables had to be recognized. Gall's and Spurzheim's use of such comparisons, as mentioned above, provoked incredulity in the members of the Commission appointed to consider their theories. However, Gall and Spurzheim were not merely resorting to a quixotic metaphor when they compared the growth of the nervous system to that of a plant; they were invoking one of the central axioms of romantic biology—the principle of the basic unity of plant and animal life. Thus, C. A. Philites (fl. 1809) wrote in 1809 that the heart was "initially developed in a *plant-like* way. The new organ springs forth from the germ of the higher animal, in the same way as the organs of plants multiply through sprouts and buds."[102] Gall proposed, in a similar fashion, to show the intimate relations between the growth of the nervous system and that of vegetables. This move was justified on the assumption that "nature follows the same type in the organization of the vegetable kingdom as in the animal kingdom."[103]

Specifically, in both cases growth proceeded from below upward and was achieved by means of the superimposition of new systems on top of existing ones. In the case of plants, new branches sprang from ring-shaped swellings; in the nervous system, accumulations of gray matter, or ganglia, performed the same function.[104]

Such reasoning vitiated the complete separation of the vegetative nervous system and the cerebrospinal axis, upon which Bichat and his school had insisted (see chap. 7.4). The latter no less than the former was composed of a number of ganglionic centers; the two systems were distinguished only by the different arrangement of these elements. While in the vegetative nervous system (which was seen increasingly as the embryologically most primitive part of the vertebrate nervous system), the ganglia were dispersed; in the cerebrospinal axis they were concentrated to a degree where their separate identity became difficult to discern. In this regard, the human nervous system epitomized the progression also found in the zoological series. In the lowest animals the nervous system was diffuse, but in the higher animals, it became gradually more concentrated.[105] Indeed, Tiedemann remarked, the lower animals could be viewed as so many stages in the advance toward the form of nervous system found in human beings.[106]

Upon such reasoning it ceased to be a question whether there were analogies between the human nervous system and that of invertebrates; all that remained to be decided was which structures in humans corresponded to what form of nervous organization found in these lower animals. The determination of these homologies occasioned much controversy, but an overall consensus did finally emerge. Basic to the theory that prevailed was the idea that the spinal cord of vertebrates and the ganglionic chain of articulata and annelids were homologous structures.

2.3. RENEGOTIATING THE "GANGLION"

Johann Heinrich Ferdinand von Autenrieth (1772–1835) in 1807 declared that "the spinal marrow appears in the lower animals still merely as a series of ganglia, with fibrous diverging nerves, and nerves going along its length uniting themselves into a continuum." The division of the spinal nerves of vertebrates into distinct pairs should, he argued, be seen as "the traces of an earlier division"; that is, as vestiges of the distinct ganglionic masses found in the lower animals.[107] Gall developed this theory, maintaining, in effect, an identity between the spinal cord and the ventral chain of insects and worms. Much of his insistence upon the ganglionic composition of the spinal marrow derived from a determination to demonstrate its affinity with the invertebrate form of organization. Just as the abdominal cord of the caterpillar presented a row of discrete ganglia, so "the swellings of the spinal marrow may . . . be regarded as so many ganglions"; in both cases, a pair of nerves issuing from each ganglionic mass.[108]

Not all anatomists found Gall's argument convincing. Louis Antoine Desmoulins (1794–1828), for example, held in 1825 that Gall based himself upon "a badly observed analogy in order to assimilate to the spinal marrow the double ganglionated chain of insects and annelids."[109] A decade later Joseph Swan (1791–1874) also questioned the doctrine of the unity of type as applied to the nervous system.[110] At least one reviewer approved of these reservations. He noted the ubiquity of the ganglionic form of organization in the invertebrate classes, and acknowledged that the ventral cord of articulates "may be regarded as the representation of the spinal chord in the vertebrated classes." But he added that this analogy was by no means as complete as some had implied: "between the structure and position of the parts now mentioned and the brain and spinal chord of Man, and the whole Mammalia, the resemblance is faint and the analogy incomplete."[111]

The very tone of these remarks, however, indicates that they represented the view of a dissenting minority, who were arguing against an established orthodoxy. Thus, another reviewer of Swan expressed amazement at the archaic character of his opinions on the comparative anatomy of the nervous system. In particular, the reviewer was "astonished" that Swan should be unaware that "the complete identity of the nervous chords of articulata, and the brain and ganglia of mollusca, with the cerebrospinal system of man and the higher animals, has been so fully made out by such authors as [Johann Friedrich] Meckel [the Younger (1781–1833)], Cuvier, Blumenbach, Gall, Spurzheim, Serres, [Karl Asmund] Rudolphi [(1771–1832)], and Ernst Heinrich Weber [(1795–1878)], and still more recently by Johannes Müller, Treviranus, and others."[112] Such authors as Treviranus were not oblivious to the problems in assimilating the ganglionic chain to the spinal cord: in particular, there was the fact that, whereas the former ran below the digestive tract, the other passed above the gut. But, given their commitment to the principle of organic unity, they exerted all their ingenuity to circumvent these cruxes, rather than abandoning the attempt to bridge the gap between the nervous system in the two animal subkingdoms.[113]

A succession of authors who were receptive to romantic conceptions of the living world proclaimed the identity of the spinal cord and the nervous systems of invertebrates in the period after Gall's and Spurzheim's publications. After describing the nervous organization of invertebrates, Burdach announced that "this ganglionated cord" unmistakably expressed the "*antetype (Vorbild)*" of the spinal cord.[114] Similarly, Fletcher wrote in 1835 that "the prototype of the Spinal Cord of Man may be considered to be the lines of nervous knots, connected by a double or single cord running down the body of most avertebrated animals."[115] Anderson insisted that the nervous system of insects led "us by strict analogies to the Vertebrata."[116] Solly considered in 1836 that "the structure of the nervous cord of the lobster is particularly interesting to us as affording a very perfect type of the spinal cord in man."[117] In 1847 he asserted that "the spinal cord is a series of ganglionic centres, structurally homologous and functionally analogous to the jointed ganglionic cord of the articulata."[118] By the 1840s, this doctrine had become sufficiently established to appear in medical textbooks without apology or defense.[119]

Once the principle of identity was accepted the way was open to further analogies between the spinal cord and the ganglionated chain. Thus, John Goodsir (1814–1867) in 1856 wrote that when the homologies between the two were understood, "we may legitimately employ the annulose animal in the morphological investigation of the vertebrate skeleton."[120] As we have seen, concepts of the morphology of the vertebrate nervous system were also affected by such comparisons. The Galenic notion of the spinal cord as a mere prolongation of the brain was set aside in favor of the view that it comprised a series of distinct, although coalesced, ganglia. Moreover, ideas of the functional properties of the cord were also altered by the invertebrate analogy.

Gall's own view of the functions of the cerebrospinal axis are elusive. He was much more interested in its "genetic" relations and in showing how brain structure corroborated his views on the nature of mind. As Henri Marie Ducrotay de Blainville (1777–1850) justly remarked, "the physiology of the brain, as Gall conceived it, is nothing more than what is called psychology."[121] Spurzheim, in contrast, did hold a more dynamic conception of the nervous system than his colleague Gall and tried to bring together anatomical and functional considerations. One of his principal conclusions was that it was highly improbable that "the spinal cord and its nerves are mere conductors of sensation, and of volition in reference to motion. I rather conceive that they aid in maintaining the powers of those parts to which they are distributed." In short, Spurzheim did not "believe that the only office of the spinal cord, with its nerve roots, is to establish a communication between external impressions and the brain and the instruments of motion." In addition to this commissural function, the spinal cord possessed an intrinsic power.[122]

Other commentators also concluded that (from the point of view of the new anatomy of the cerebrospinal axis that was becoming current) the Galenic notion of the actions of the spinal cord had become untenable. A new conception was needed; one which recognized that "the spinal cord is not a mere conductor of sensation and voluntary motion, but that it also aids in maintaining the vital energies of those parts to which its nerves are distributed."[123] This fact was seen as a necessary inference from the analogies that had been established between the cord and structures in the lower animals. In many invertebrates there was no "brain"—no dominant ganglion; sensory and motor functions were performed by the ganglionic chain alone. Because the spinal cord was the homologue of this chain, it too must possess comparable "peculiar and highly important properties."[124]

Moreover, in invertebrates, the anatomical separateness of the nervous centers coincided with a greater or lesser degree of functional autonomy and specialization. In higher animals, the tendency toward fusion and concentration obscured the structural distinctness of the ganglia; nonetheless, William Carpenter insisted, the vertebrate spinal cord still retained some of the physiological characteristics of the nervous system of insects and worms. Were not, he asked, "the segments of the spinal cord as independent of each other, in regard to their power of ministering to the reflex actions of the nerves proceeding from them, as are the distinct ganglia of the ventral cord of the articulata?"[125]

In effect, a metameric organization and functioning was ascribed to the spinal cord on the grounds of its zoological homologies. A similar conclusion could be derived by reference to the "law" of serial repetition. As noted above, in the early nineteenth century, the skeleton was often conceived as composed of a sequence of like elements that had undergone a variety of modifications. Autenrieth suggested in 1807 that the brain and spinal cord might be governed by the same principles as those that governed their bony containers. Just as the spinal column was divided into distinct vertebrae, so were the spinal marrow and its nerves correspondingly segmented. Even the muscles and the blood vessels of the back conformed to the same pattern. As a result there were "no long arteries, no long nerves, but short arteries and nerves, which appear on the back."[126] Fifty years later Louis Pierre Gratiolet (1815–1865) enunciated an identical theory:

> The relation which exists between the nervous centers [of the cerebrospinal axis] and the vertebral column is remarkable. The vertebrae . . . are to the skeleton as a whole what the segments are to the body of articulate animals. . . . Thus there are segments in the skeleton, there are muscular segments. The peripheral nerves in turn conform to this segmentation, and observation shows that similarly there are segments in the central nervous system.[127]

This mode of organization, Gratiolet continued, had physiological consequences. Each "segment of the spinal marrow can be considered as a particular center of action." However, the functional fragmentation this engendered was counteracted by connections that extended the effect of the irritation of one segment to the rest of the cerebrospinal axis. There was in consequence "at the same time, in the nervous axis, multiplicity and unity." Gratiolet, therefore, agreed with Gall that facing "each vertebra is a particular nervous segment. But the segments interconnect and, in the vertebrates, their individuality seems to be absorbed into the unity of the system."[128]

Gratiolet was especially anxious to show how the views of the spinal cord thus obtained from the principles of comparative and transcendental anatomy harmonized with and corroborated results gained from another source: vivisection. In particular, he claimed, Gall's theory of the segmentation of the cord was confirmed and, in its turn, gave an anatomical explanation for the experimental results of Legallois and Hall (see chap. 4.3 and 4.4, respectively).[129] In 1838, Dugès had already brought together the theory of the segmented structure of the spinal cord, as revealed by analogies with the invertebrates and the corresponding organization of the spinal column, with the work of these experimentalists. Both forms of investigation had, Dugès claimed, proved equally fatal to the Galenic and Hallerian notion of the brain as the sole source of power in the cerebrospinal axis. It was true that in the higher animals the brain did dominate and coordinate the activities of the lower centers; nevertheless, "as regards the mechanism of movement itself, it is the spinal marrow, perhaps the gray globular mass at its center which directs it, in the same way as the ganglion corresponding to each pair of legs directs movement in the insect."[130]

A number of lines of research and thought combined, therefore, in the mid-nineteenth century to alter radically the way in which the structure and function of the spinal cord was conceived. No longer was it seen as a process of the brain; instead it was viewed as an autonomous structure, or—to be more accurate—as a congeries of such structures. Edme Félix Alfred Vulpian (1826–1887) summarized this change when he wrote in 1866 that "we believe that the spinal cord is not only, as Galen believed, and as has been reiterated for a great many ages since him, a large nerve gathering together all the nerves of the body in order to conduct them to the brain; but that it is at the same time a true nervous center endowed with very remarkable functions."[131] Prominent among the movements in neuroscience that brought about this shift was the determination among many anatomists and physiologists after 1800 to attain concepts of the nervous system that would apply to all animals and unite the highest with the lowest neural organization.

The consequences of this endeavor extended still further. A new concept of the brain itself also emerged in parallel with that of the spinal cord we have described.

2.4. CONSEQUENCES FOR NOTIONS OF BRAIN STRUCTURE

Two aspects of romantic biology need to be recalled here. The first was its concern with origins and the "genetic" approach that followed from it. The second was the principle that the complex should be explained in the terms of the more simple. We have seen how these principles were applied to the elucidation of the structure of the spinal cord, notably by Gall. He had announced "as an axiom, that organs of an inferior order serve as preparatory apparatuses to organs which, in more perfect animals, are destined for more elevated functions."[132]

In accordance with this principle, Gall presented the ganglia of the vegetative nervous system as the "preparatory apparatus" for the spinal cord: it was by the accumulation of such centers along a central axis that the latter organ was formed. The next step in this account of the etiology of the nervous system seemed obvious: "after having treated the nervous systems of the viscera and the belly and of the chest, of the vertebral column and of the senses, the natural order leads us to consider the brain."[133] Moreover, consistent with his previous approach, Gall proposed to explicate this structure in the same terms as the spinal cord; the encephalon too was merely a collection of ganglia. Just as "the nervous system of the vegetative or automatic life, the spinal marrow or the instrument of the nervous system of voluntary movement, the nervous systems of the organs of sense, are each made up of discrete organs," so "the same law governs the form of the brain."[134]

In short, far from being the source of all other nervous organization, the brain was an elaboration of more basic structures. Specifically, it was the culmination of the spinal cord, the final development of the organs found lower in the cerebrospinal axis. Gall held this to be literally true. In embryogeny the spinal cord grew (like a tree) from below upward; the brain, because it was the uppermost, was also the last to appear.[135] Gall offered little evidence for this assertion; but in later years others, who possessed far greater embryological knowledge than he, made similar claims.[136] Richard Grainger summarized the state of knowledge in 1829: "Although there is some difference of opinion as to the exact order in which the various parts make their appearance, it seems to be ascertained that the ganglions of the great sympathetic [trunk] are formed before the spinal cord and brain; . . . that, next in order, the spinal cord is formed; and that lastly, the brain appears."[137]

This theory was, however, from the outset controversial. Other students of embryology maintained that the brain developed first, or that the spinal cord and brain appeared simultaneously in the embryo.[138] Those who were skeptical of Gall's general approach to the nervous system questioned the doctrine of the developmental primacy of the spinal cord.[139] But, increasingly, even those who sought a similar concept of nervous structure doubted its validity.[140] What Burdach and others maintained was that the developmental priority of the spinal cord was not crucial to the idea of the nervous system they promoted. Even if the brain did not, in fact, grow from the spinal cord, it remained conceptually derivative from the lower structures.

Reil took this stance in one of his discussions of the anatomy of the brain, published in 1809. He recognized that, to elucidate the organization of this organ, "one can go forwards from the spinal cord to the brain, or backwards from the brain to the spinal cord." What determined his choice between these two courses was his general biological philosophy, and specifically the belief that "out of nature's cornucopia the mosses are placed before the palms. The higher [plant] is the lower [one] elevated (*das potenzierte Niedere*)."[141] Therefore, although the brain and the spinal cord appeared simultaneously in the embryo, the former still "grew out of" the latter inasmuch as it was a higher form of the structural type embodied in the spinal cord.[142] As Friedrich Arnold (1803–1890) put it, "we have in the spinal cord the antetype (*Vorbild*) and the foundation for the entire structure of the brain."[143]

The homology between brain and spinal cord was manifested especially in their common ganglionic composition: indeed, together they formed the same series of ganglia. Reil wrote that the gray substance which had hitherto been the core of the spinal cord "now becomes the chain of ganglia which continues along the axis of the brain."[144] The exposition of this concept of cerebral composition was usually credited to Gall and was seen as one of his foremost contributions to neuroscience.[145] It received important corroboration from Blainville in an 1821 paper where the cerebellum, the quadrigeminal bodies, and the cerebral hemispheres were numbered among the gray matter accumulations, i.e., ganglia of the cerebrospinal axis.[146]

The ganglionic nature of the vertebrate brain was sustained by reference to three principal forms of evidence. The first and most important of these was comparative anatomy. Carpenter remarked in 1846 that it was by comparison of the human brain with that of lower animals that "we are enabled to trace the real analogies of the different parts of the Encephalon with the ganglionic masses which represent it among Invertebrated animals."[147] The identity that had been established between the ganglionic chain of invertebrates and the spinal cord was held to extend into the cranial portion of the cerebrospinal axis. As noted above, the origins of the human brain were discerned in the gradual augmentation of the most cephalad ganglion of the chain in the articulata. As Autenrieth put it in 1807, "the brain in these animals is hardly more than the biggest of the anterior pair of ganglia." In the lower vertebrates also the ganglionic character of the brain was quite evident. Only in mammals, and especially in humans, were the separate nervous centers effectively obscured by a process of concentration and augmentation.[148] In the words of Franz von Paula Gruithuisen (1774–1852), a well-known *Naturphilosoph,* along with the growth of the head, "the neural ganglionic form (*Nervenknotenform*) changes into the form of the brain."[149]

Similar statements were commonplace in the literature of the early decades of the nineteenth century.[150] Schönlein gave a particularly detailed exposition of this theory in 1816. The brain, he declared, arose out of an "assemblage of different parts," which were distinguishable in the lower animals, if not in human beings, by their structure, location, and period of development. A broad distinction could be drawn between those encephalic ganglia that were primary and those that were identified as secondary developments.[151] Among the primary ganglia were the medulla oblongata, the sensory ganglia, and the cerebral peduncles. All "other parts are the products of a secondary formation; not merely in respect of time and period, but also in the type of their formation and different origin." Thus, while the primary ganglia were vesicular in form, secondary formations, such as the cerebral hemispheres, took shape as membranes.[152] These primitive distinctions were most overt in fish and became gradually more obscure among the higher vertebrates.[153]

Schönlein's analysis of the constituent parts of the vertebrate brain was, with minor amendments and some elaboration, widely reproduced.

Carpenter took the process a stage further arguing that essentially the same ganglia that made up the brain of the fish were found in myriapoda. Carpenter also stressed that each of the separate encephalic divisions in the head of the fish, as of the invertebrate, were functionally distinct: each was related to a particular sensory apparatus. In contrast to these "basal ganglia," the cerebral hemispheres were either entirely absent or very rudimentary in invertebrates; in the lower fish, too, the cerebrum was but little developed. The higher vertebrates possessed the same fundamental parts, but with additions. Extra parts were superadded to the primitive ganglionic type; in consequence, "the increased complexity of the encephalic structure, in the higher vertebrates, is almost entirely due to the extraordinary development of the cerebral hemispheres, and of their commissural connexions with the other ganglionic masses."[154]

A second, corroborative source of evidence lay in embryology. It was argued that the embryogeny of the brain revealed it to be composed of discrete ganglia, some of which were primary and others secondary. Thus, Burdach argued that around the third month of development the distinct elements of the nervous system began to emerge. Of these, the gray "ganglionic" substance predominantly accumulated in a series of adjoining globular structures. The ganglia of the brain stem were the first to appear; in the early stages of development only a trace of the cerebral hemispheres was discernible.[155] The embryogeny of the human brain was therefore seen to parallel the stages by which the organ was elaborated among lower animals. Friedrich Tiedemann argued forcefully for this parallelism and made it central to his account of the anatomy of the fetal brain.[156] Tiedemann's claims were widely accepted. Indeed, when speaking of the general parallelism that was supposed to exist between the embryonic and zoological series, Fletcher asserted that "it is in the brain chiefly that this correspondence between the human embryo, in the different stages of its elaboration, and the lower tribes of animals displays itself."[157]

Lastly, the law of serial continuity was thought to confirm the proofs drawn from comparative anatomy and embryology. The invocation of this principle to sustain the theory that the spinal cord consisted of a number of independent segments has already been noted. Some anatomists extended this argument and proceeded to draw conclusions about encephalic structure from the supposed composition of its bony envelope. Indeed, Serres revealed that it was the possibility of constructing a theory of the anatomy of the brain analogous and parallel to that which transcendentalists like Geoffroy St. Hilaire had already achieved for the skull, that instigated his researches.[158] Bérard declared in 1823 that if, "according to the fruitful law of analogous organs," the cranium was merely "a vertebra adapted to particular uses," then one could infer, "by means of the same law that the human brain is only an extension of the spinal cord."[159] Because the brain stood in such close relation to the cord, it too shared its structural affinity with the osseous system. As Wilhelm Griesinger (1817–1868) stated:

> Just as the vertebral structure of the osseous spinal column recurs in the skull in a more elaborate way—in a more complicated plurality of bone-forms—so also proceeds the cranial portion of the central nervous system in a complex multiplicity of nerve masses, which at first sight seem to be constructed upon a different plan than the spinal cord but in which, despite many important differences, an analogy with the spinal cord and its immediate envelopes may be followed through.[160]

Gratiolet reaffirmed this principle in 1857, declaring that "the law of analogy which governs all the segments of the osseous axis, both in the vertebral column and in the cranium, equally dominates the parts . . . which it encloses." In the same way that it was possible to "comprehend under the same formula the head and the spine," so it was possible to infer that the brain and spinal cord must share the same—segmented—structure.[161]

2.5. CONCLUSION

This chapter began with a contrast between two concepts of the nervous system. On the one hand was the traditional "Galenic" notion of the brain as the sole origin and center of the system and of all other structures as its derivatives; on the other, the theory that replaced it. The chief features of the latter were an insistence on the need to understand the origins of the nervous system: on the importance of proceeding from the simple to the complex; on the plurality of nervous centers; and on the subordination of the brain, at least in "genetic" terms, to the lower of these centers, the spinal cord. The cord, in turn, was regarded as a collection of more primitive ganglionic elements, which were also found in the vegetative nervous system.

The preceding sections have shown how a comparative perspective underlay these changes. A comparative approach to problems of human anatomy and physiology led only to these results, however, when informed by certain heuristic principles. We have described how a "romantic" conception of living form and process channeled thought and research into certain avenues. It was the investigators who pursued these paths who produced the revolution in ideas of the cerebrospinal axis.

The new view of the brain and spinal cord that they instituted has proved remarkably durable. This can be illustrated by reference to a modern textbook, Ranson's *Anatomy of the nervous system*. There we find the doctrine of the unity of type—of the affinity between even widely separated organisms: "Despite the complexities of the reactions and morphology of the nervous system of vertebrates, certain fundamental patterns recognizable in the lowest forms of animals remain evident in it." Embryology, as well as comparative anatomy, is held to provide insights into the highly developed forms of the nervous system; the simple casts light on the more complex.[162]

Specifically, the nervous system of invertebrates, and above all of annelids, is relevant to understanding these structures in the higher animals: "the vertebrate nervous system has much in common with that of the earthworm"; there is a clear homology between the ventral ganglionic chain of these creatures and the spinal cord—both were segmented.[163] Moreover, in the gradual enlargement of the cephalad end of the worm, "the brain of higher forms is forecast."[164] Two general processes are discernible in the progress of the nervous system through the various animal classes. One is towards a greater concentration of the nervous system in a series of centrally placed ganglia. The other is that of "telencephalization;" that is, the augmentation and growing functional importance of the front end of the chain.[165]

The structure of the human brain is best understood by reference to that of the lower vertebrates. Such a comparison reveals that the encephalon is, in fact, a compound structure, made up of several more or less primitive segments. This type of organization is more apparent in the brain of a fish than of a human being; however, examination of the human embryo reveals that the same segmental organization is clearly visible in early development.[166] In general, "it is convenient to begin the study of the anatomy of the central nervous system with the spinal cord, which shows a segmental simplicity, and represents the pattern displayed in the original neural tube which, though recognizable in the brain, is there much modified."[167]

Insofar as any explanation is forthcoming for the homologies assumed in these remarks and for the "genetic" approach to nervous structure, it consists of some reference to the modern theory of evolution. This chapter has shown, however, that all of these principles were established long before the publication of Darwin's theory and were, in most cases, independent of any theory of physical descent. Their true roots lay in the romantic philosophy of biology we have considered. What can be said is that the Darwinian theory eventually offered a posteriori justification for the theory of unity of type that later morphologists found useful in justifying their commitment to this dogma.[168]

Two essential elements of modern notions of the structure and function of the nervous system are, however, lacking from the account of its origins so far given. They are the idea of the nerve cell as its ultimate unit and of the reflex as the basic mode of nervous action. The following chapter explores the way the first of these concepts arose and was developed. We shall see that many of the theoretical assumptions and goals that influenced the gross anatomy of the nervous system were also active in studies of its histology.

3

The Nerve Cell

3.1. MICROSCOPY OF THE NERVOUS SYSTEM BEFORE 1836

The microscope provoked an equivocal reaction among medical scientists in the first half of the nineteenth century. On the one hand, many of the leading anatomists of the period were deeply skeptical of microscopical observations. Bichat, for example, held that only observations obtained by the naked eye were to be trusted; all others were merely sources of fantastic error.[1] Gall shared this opinion.[2] They were probably led to this evaluation of the microscope by the abuse of the instrument by many eighteenth-century workers, who had used microscopy to support various speculative systems of the structure and workings of the body, and by deception due to primitive instruments and the absence of histological techniques.

Other scientists of the early nineteenth century set aside such doubts and made extensive use of microscopes in their efforts to understand the basic organization of tissues. Even professed disciples of Bichat such as P. A. Béclard joined the movement.[3] The nervous system received much attention in this as in other fields of biological research. Notably, one group of investigators adopted a theory first proposed by Antoni van Leeuwenhoek (1632–1723) in 1684 and which had enjoyed occasional revivals during the eighteenth century. According to this hypothesis all animal tissues were ultimately composed of minute "globules."[4] In the nineteenth century J. F. Meckel, the Younger, in Germany, Everard Home (1756–1832) in England, and Henri Milne-Edwards (1800–1885) in France, among others, applied the globule theory to the nervous system arguing that it, like the rest of the body, was made up of spherical globules variously arranged.[5]

Home's writings may be taken to illustrate this theory. Home was at one time among those skeptical of microscopy; he wrote in 1798:

> It is scarcely necessary to mention, that parts of an animal body are not fitted for being examined by glasses of a great magnifying power; and, wherever they are shown one hundred times larger than their natural size, no dependence can be placed upon their appearance.[6]

But Home came to revise this view largely it seems through the influence of Francis [Franz Andreas] Bauer (1758–1840), a scientific illustrator and microscopist who worked at Kew Gardens near London. In 1828 Home held that the microscope had suffered a decline "as a means of promoting anatomical and physiological enquiries" at the turn of the nineteenth century, partly because of the errors of earlier observers, and partly because "there was no individual expert in the use of the instrument, when high magnifying powers were employed" who was comparable to Leeuwenhoek. Now, however, "at the distance of time of a century and a half, there has risen up a person, whose knowledge of the microscope, and his experience of its use, has revived our confidence in the representations it produces." This person was Bauer; Home continued that it was "by his aid that I have been enabled to make out the more minute structure of the brain, and also that of the ganglion."[7]

In his 1823 lectures on comparative anatomy at the College of Surgeons in London, Home disclosed that it was after seeing the results of Bauer's microscopic analysis of the blood that he asked him to extend his investigations to the brain, "the most important organ of the human body."[8] The principal result of these investigations was to show both the medullary and the cortical substance of the brain to consist of globules. In the former component of the nervous system the globules were arranged into rows forming fibers; in the latter, the globules were separated by a fluid resembling blood serum and were interspersed by many minute blood vessels. The medullary and cortical substances differed also in the size of the globules they contained. Home, therefore, felt able to conclude that "the principal difference in the appearance of the different parts of the brain consists in the size of the globules and the proportions they bear to the other parts."[9]

The other components of the nervous system were subject to a similar analysis. The nerve fibers distributed throughout the body were, like those of the white matter of the brain, made up of lines of globules.[10] Home took pains to distinguish these by size from the globules found in muscle fiber.[11] The structure of the ganglia, Home declared, was "intermediate between that of the brain and nerves. The brain being composed of small globules, suspended in a transparent elastic jelly, nerves made up of single rows of globules, and ganglions consisting of a congeries of nervous fibres compacted together."[12]

Home believed that these observations upon the minute structure of the nervous system enabled him to make certain inferences about its operation. In particular, he held that the abundance of globules and gelatinous substance in the cerebral and cerebellar cortex together with the large number of fine blood vessels found in those tissues, revealed that "the cortical substance is a very important part of [the brain]." He drew on evidence from comparative anatomy to demonstrate that the cerebrum was intimately connected with intellectual faculties.[13]

Despite Home's confidence in his own and Bauer's ability to avoid the errors that had vitiated the efforts of earlier microscopists, within a few years of publication the structures that he had described and depicted with such confidence were shown to be for the most part illusory. The optical qualities of microscopes were improved in the late 1820s by Giovanni Battista Amici (1784–1863)[14] and Joseph Jackson Lister (1786–1869);[15] and workers using these new instruments dismissed the bulk of the "globules" detected by Home and others as artifacts or the result of spherical aberration inherent in the older microscopes when used at high powers of magnification.[16] By 1829, although Richard Grainger recorded the views of the globule theorists in his textbook of anatomy, he felt obliged to add that these observations had been largely discredited by the new achromatic microscope. In particular, Grainger drew attention to the refutation of globulism in a classic paper by Thomas Hodgkin (1798–1866) and Lister.[17]

The initial effect of the improved optical instruments of the late 1820s and early 1830s was therefore a negative one: the demolition of the globule hypothesis. It is sometimes supposed that these technical advances then led in an immediate and unproblematic way to novel, more adequate ideas of tissue structure. However, a number of recent studies of the microscopy of the mid-nineteenth century have stressed that no such easy progression took place.[18] Rather has noted the paradox that Hodgkin, despite his proficiency in the use of the achromatic microscope, did not until the end of his career use this instrument in his attempts to elucidate the structure of tumors. This example reveals "the limitations of a technical advance unaccompanied by an appropriate conceptual advance."[19] Conversely, those who did make extensive use of the achromatic microscope to investigate the fine texture of animal tissues were guided in their efforts by some theoretical framework. These conceptual influences structured the histological observations they produced.

One instance of this process is especially relevant to the present discussion. Christian Gottfried Ehrenberg (1795–1876) is generally credited with giving in 1833 and 1836 the first accurate account of cells in the gray matter of the brain and ganglia, although, as Andreoli remarks,

Ehrenberg did not (indeed could not) attach to these structures any of the significance they were later to receive.[20] Ehrenberg was unable to regard the *Körner* or *Kugeln* he described as cells, with all that implied, because the necessary conceptual resources for that inference had still to be formulated. In Ehrenberg's own terms, however, these "granules" did possess a definite theoretical significance: they helped to discredit a notion put forward by others, that the gray matter of the brain was a homogeneous, amorphous mass.

The idea that the brain was a *breiartige Masse,* or pulpy substance, in which globules floated had, according to Ehrenberg, been favored by Giovanni Maria della Torre (fl. 1760–1776) and Alexander Monro, *secundus* (1733–1817). It was revived in the nineteenth century when it became associated with a more wide-ranging system, namely, the theory that the brain was composed of an unorganized substance. This notion, Ehrenberg alleged, served "in particular the natural philosophical ideas, which presuppose the necessity of a material elementary primitive substance (*Grundsubstanz*)."[21] Ehrenberg expatiated on this point in his 1836 discussion. The hypothesis that "the brain is a pulpy mass, which consists of granules mutually united in rows, floating in a tough transparent fluid" was "very favorable to the philosophical ideas afterwards propagated, in which the great object of search was one material simple fundamental substance, of which the organic substances might be composed." This also was in keeping with the Hallerian concept of the brain's equipotentiality of function. It had been alleged that this substance was found in the embryo and in the simplest organisms, yet was also manifested in the human brain, the highest of all organs.[22] In short, those who adopted this hypothetical view of structure saw in the brain "a primary animal substance,"[23] and used this supposed fact to sustain a wider biological theory that stressed the affinities of the highest and lowest forms of life and the gradual stages of complication uniting apparently diverse organisms.

One author Ehrenberg may have had in mind when making these remarks is the *Naturphilosoph,* Gruithuisen, who argued for the existence of a primitive "polypous" matter from which all higher life forms developed. Embryonically, human beings began as an *Infusorien* or *polyenärtig* form; that is, in a condition similar to that of the lowest animals. Further, the special human organs and functions were gradually differentiated from this ground-stuff, which was initially capable of performing all bodily operations through its homogeneous substance. Specifically, at both the outset of human development and at the base of the zoological scale, there was no separate nervous system; originally the "polyp [i.e., the most primitive organic state] is wholly an organ of digestion, wholly an organ of touch, light, feeling, hearing, smell and movement."[24] Moreover, Gruithuisen insisted that, even when separate organ systems did emerge in the later stages of development and in more advanced animals, the higher retained an affinity with the lower. It did not cease to be "an infusorian in all its parts."[25] For this reason, even the human brain retained in its structure something of a "polypous" character.

Ehrenberg's own account of the microscopic appearances of the brain was in complete opposition to this system. He stressed the brain's complexity and its highly structured character: the layers of granules formed one part of this organized complexity.[26] While inimical to the ideas of the *Naturphilosophen,* this concept of cerebral structure accorded well with Ehrenberg's own philosophical schema. Throughout his career Ehrenberg was opposed to the idea that there was a graduated chain linking the lowest and the highest forms of life; he was also hostile to the notion that there was a primitive living *Urstoff* of which the simplest creatures were formed. Ehrenberg argued that all organisms were in fact complex: even the infusoria and polyps possessed, according to him, developed organ systems, including a complete nervous system.[27] By contradicting the theory that the brain was a "polypous mass," Ehrenberg denied a further alleged manifestation of the primitive, unorganized living substance. He showed that, on the contrary, the brain was composed of several discrete elements with distinct relations between them. Among these elements were the objects that were subsequently designated brain cells.

Others both before and after Ehrenberg remarked upon similar structures in the brain.[28] Indeed in 1830 the important textbook of physiology originally written by Georg Friedrich Hildebrandt (1764–1816) stated that "upon the existence of globules [in the brain] almost all microscopic observers agree, and different opinions exist only over their size and shape."[29] However, none of these observers ascribed to the globules they found in the brain any of the structural or functional importance they later possessed. Only after 1835 did they gain this significance, chiefly through the efforts of two scientists, J. E. Purkyně and G. G. Valentin.

Just as Ehrenberg's early account of these structures only attained its full meaning when viewed in the context of his general theoretical scheme and goals, so their elevation to physiologically and histologically crucial elements was intimately connected with Purkyně and Valentin's wide scientific and philosophical commitments. In particular, many of the notions derived from romantic thought, whose importance was stressed above (chaps. 1 and 2.2), exerted an influence upon these microscopic studies of the 1830s and 1840s also; indeed in many cases the achromatic microscope merely provided an opportunity to pursue the same research program by other means.

3.2. PURKYNĚ AND VALENTIN'S PHILOSOPHY OF NATURE

In 1828 Valentin went to the University of Breslau to study medicine; he soon came into contact with Purkyně, who supervised Valentin's doctoral dissertation and initiated him into microscopical studies. The relationship between the two quickly developed beyond that of pupil and master. Purkyně recognized Valentin's great talents and found in him a worthy collaborator.[30] The two worked together so closely in the mid-1830s that it is not always possible to distinguish their individual achievements. For example, in 1840 Robert Remak (1815–1865) noted that because in a paper on the histology of the nervous system published in 1836, Valentin had presented Purkyně's as well as his own observations, it was difficult to attribute individual credit for the discoveries recorded there.[31]

This intimate cooperation was predicated upon a correspondence in Purkyně and Valentin's general assumptions about nature and in their approach to science. Both were imbued with the romantic ideas that permeated the German-speaking world in the early decades of the nineteenth century. Thus, Toellner has remarked that Purkyně was a child of the romantic era; one who read and was deeply affected by Friedrich Leopold von Hardenberg (Novalis) (1772–1801), Johann Gottlieb Fichte (1762–1814), and F. W. J. Schelling, and who early in his career met Goethe.[32] Moreover, Teich has argued that Purkyně gained his appointment as professor of physiology at Breslau through the efforts of the influential circle around Hegel in Berlin, who "expected him to develop physiology in Breslau not only on a high scientific level but also in close relationship to philosophy."[33] Although never an orthodox Hegelian nor a dogmatic *Naturphilosoph,* Purkyně's thought does show the marked effect of certain aspects of the romantic philosophy of nature.

Above all, Purkyně was convinced of the unity of the cosmos, and this conviction had an important impact on his scientific conceptions.[34] In the first place Purkyně refused to accept any absolute demarcation between the organic and inorganic realms: both formed parts of a larger whole and were permeated by similar principles of organization and by analogous forces. It was necessary, Purkyně wrote in 1833, to try to grasp "the totality of natural phenomena"; specifically, physiology could not proceed as a wholly autonomous discipline, but must be closely connected with the physical sciences. Purkyně therefore called for a physiological physics, statics and mechanics, hydro- and aerodynamics, acoustics, and chemistry, that would reveal the pervasion of living bodies by phenomena found in the inorganic world.[35] Purkyně expanded this principle in 1852 when he held that because organisms arise out of inorganic matter, they retain an affinity with ordinary chemical and physical phenomena; as a result both the biological and physical sciences were "in essence but one science." However, Purkyně's argument was not, strictly speaking, reductionist. Instead, like many other scientists influenced by romanticism, he held that the separation of the study of nature into discrete departments must not be allowed to obscure the fundamental unity of nature and, therefore, of science.[36]

Second, Purkyně called for a unified synthetic approach within the science of life. The physiologist should not be concerned merely with the individual organism, with developmental investigations, or with studies of irritability and sensibility; instead physiology should treat all these and the other branches of biological research and seek to bring them into mutual relation and harmony.[37] This enterprise was founded upon the idea that underlying the evident diversity of living beings there were profound identities and analogies that bound together the different components of the organic realm.

For example, Purkyně "believed that the animal and vegetable kingdom [*sic*] had some fundamental properties in common, that a certain parallel is to be found in the development of both realms, and to comprehend the unity of life it is necessary to study the manifestations of development in both."[38] Purkyně and his students tried to demonstrate this developmental and structural affinity between plants and animals by microscopical studies carried out in the 1830s; these laid some essential foundations for the enunciation of the cell theory of animal life by Theodor Schwann (1810–1882) in 1839.[39]

The unity of life manifested itself not only between the two kingdoms, but also between different classes of animal. Purkyně's commitment to this axiom was evinced in his attitude to the studies on the early stages of development that were conducted in the later 1820s and in the 1830s. Purkyně had himself in 1825 detected the germinal vesicle in the avian egg; two years later Karl Ernst von Baer (1792–1876), stimulated by Purkyně's discovery, announced that he had found what seemed to him a homologous structure in mammals.[40] In the light of subsequent research von Baer's direct identification of the structure he observed with that described by Purkyně was mistaken. But for present purposes the significance of this episode lies in Purkyně's reaction to von Baer's announcement: he saw it as a vindication of the unity pervading the animal kingdom. In other words, von Baer's discovery was precisely what Purkyně's philosophical assumptions led him to expect. He wrote to von Baer in March, 1828 to express the "great joy" that the detection of a "germinal vesicle" in the mammal had brought him. He continued:

> It is true that I had the firm belief, that a like form must let itself be discovered in the entire animal kingdom, because it is a general law of nature, that organic formations, the nearer they are to their original state, so much the more show uniformity and analogy.[41]

Purkyně's belief in the unity of the developmental process among different animals was further displayed in 1834 when he noted the homologous parts found in the ova of all classes and asserted that human embryogeny could only be understood by reference to that of other animals. To justify such inferences about the character of one organism from phenomena found in another, seemingly distant animal, Purkyně cited the dictum of William Harvey (1578–1657): "Natura divina et perfecta semper sibi consona est."[42]

Unity was also evident between individuals. Although the outward form of organs like the brain might vary greatly, certain essential features (*Grundzüge*) were always observed. From these constant characteristics it was possible to construct the general "type" of that organ.[43] Moreover (as we shall presently see), certain organic forms were supposed to recur in diverse parts of the same individual.

Lastly, Purkyně denied that the occurrence of psychic phenomena constituted an exception to the rule of the unity of nature. The dualist contention that there was a spiritual realm over and above the physical was, he insisted, wrong. Purkyně claimed that the soul was only "a particular phenomenon of life (*Lebenserscheinung*)" intimately related to the nervous system. In consequence, psychology should be seen as a branch of physiology, not as a separate discipline. At first sight this might seem a reductionist or materialist position; but while he sought to materialize the mental, Purkyně also argued for the psychic quality of apparently purely material processes. In his view, "bodily life itself possesses a psychic character."[44] These complementary notions of the physiological nature of mind and of the psychic quality of corporeal phenomena, were to be central to the way Purkyně conceived the structure and function of the nervous system at the microscopic level.

Valentin too was exposed to the influence of romantic culture in his youth: Kisch notes the importance of these tendencies in the progressive Jewish community in which Valentin was raised.[45] His contact with Purkyně was no doubt also important in shaping Valentin's attitudes, for there was a remarkable correspondence in their basic ideas. Like Purkyně, Valentin was preoccupied with showing the unity of the biological world. In 1836, for example, he published an article that set out to show that the germinal spot (*Keimfleck*) recently identified by Rudolph

Wagner (1805–1864), was to be found throughout the animal kingdom.[46] Valentin was, moreover, much involved in the efforts made before 1839 to discern a common structural and developmental basis for all plant and animal tissues.[47] He was also committed to the notion of constant typical structures, or *Urformen,* that underlay living organization: "where," he wrote in 1836, "nature orders her parts according to a certain type, there this norm remains everywhere throughout the same," whatever changes in shape, composition, or relations the type might undergo.[48] We shall return to Valentin's typological reasoning when we consider his neurohistological work.

Valentin shared with Purkyně a particular conception of the relation of mind to matter and of the psychological to the physiological. Although he recognized some distinction between the sphere of philosophy, which comprised the study of purely psychic manifestation, Valentin in 1844 stressed the intimate relation between mental phenomena and the material conditions of the body, and especially of the nervous system. As a result, "physiology and psychology impinge upon each other in numerous ways."[49]

So far we have outlined the chief tenets of a worldview deriving from the romantic nature philosophy of the early nineteenth century to which both Purkyně and Valentin subscribed. In chapter 2 we argued that aspects of this philosophy were crucial to certain developments in gross anatomy; now we shall consider the way these same ideas structured microscopical observations and produced distinctive conceptions of the minute structure and function of living tissues.[50] This process is well illustrated in the most important piece of research jointly undertaken by Purkyně and Valentin—their study of the phenomenon of ciliary motion.[51]

Historians have noted that ciliary motion had long been known to occur, before Purkyně and Valentin's work, on the external surfaces of invertebrates. Purkyně and Valentin's originality and achievement lay in showing that the phenomenon was also to be found in vertebrate animals and in many different parts of the body, ranging from the genital organs to the ventricles of the brain.[52] The recognition that the various motions observed in all these cases were in fact instances of the same generic phenomenon was by no means obvious: it required an imaginative leap. Thus, when Valentin first noticed movement along the mucous membrane of the Eustachian tube, he did not at once associate it with phenomena found elsewhere in the animal kingdom. It was only when Purkyně drew a comparison with the vibratile motion of unicellular animals and other invertebrates that these analogies emerged.[53] Having once made the connection, Purkyně and Valentin proceeded systematically to seek examples of similar structures and movements in a wide range of animals and organs.

They were guided in this quest by their conviction of the unity of the living world. This idea served as a regulative principle that directed their investigations and, at least in some cases, made them presuppose certain findings. In their initial communication of 1835, for example, Purkyně and Valentin acknowledged their failure to detect ciliary motion in fish; nonetheless, they continued, "we do not deny it to exist, but maintain and conclude its existence to be supported, not so much by experimental knowledge, as by the unvarying analogy of the whole of nature and of all laws."[54] In the same year, after undertaking further investigations fraught with difficulties and frustrations, Purkyně and Valentin finally satisfied themselves that ciliary motion did indeed occur in the olfactory organs and in the female genital organs of fish.[55]

Throughout their studies of ciliary motion Purkyně and Valentin drew upon the conceptual resources afforded by romantic science. In particular, they borrowed and adapted a term used by Goethe, arguing that in ciliary motion they had discovered an instance of an *Urphänomen;* that is, a form of structure and action fundamental to a wide range of organisms.[56] This was the triumphant conclusion of their first 1835 publication. After listing the organisms in which ciliary motion had been detected, they asserted that it must be supposed to exist "from the infusoria to man."[57] Its status as an *Urphänomen* was further evinced by the number of sites where it occurred within a particular animal. All these instances were to be viewed as variations upon one original type (*idea primigena*).[58] In short, ciliary motion was an exemplary vindication of the romantic notion of basal types and of affinities and correspondences between different classes of animal and between different parts of the body.

It is likely that Purkyně would not have balked at the suggestion that his microscopic observations and scientific reasoning were affected by his philosophical preconceptions. Among his many interests was a keen concern with the part played by the self in perception and with the relationship between the mind and the material world in scientific discovery. In an 1834 article Purkyně repudiated the notion that the mind was the passive receptor of sensory information transmitted by the eye. In fact, he argued, the imagination (*Einbildungskraft*) played an active role and was actually a part of reality. Even in the

> simplest sights (*Anshauungen*), in mere lines or series of specific sensations, there resides an immanent imaginative power (*Einbildungsvermögen*)

> through which all perception is mediated, and without which the soul would act in the world of the senses, in sightless vacancy without spatial and temporal conception, merely in a chaos of immediate sensations, as is indeed the case in the higher forms of imbecility.[59]

There was, Purkyně declared, no distinction between the scientist and the artist in this respect; both were engaged in creative imaginative enterprises.[60]

He was not, however, espousing a form of subjective idealism by thus stressing the active role of the intellect in all cognition of the world. Purkyně avoided this stance by adopting a form of absolute idealism common to *Naturphilosophen:* according to this doctrine mind and world were not separate entities, but aspects of a unitary reality. In consequence, the mind did not impose arbitrary schema upon a mindless nature; rather, the ideas generated by the imagination corresponded to concepts that were realized in the material world. In Purkyně's own words, "the essence of the soul is one with that of nature in general; from which issues the harmony of our sensory knowledge with nature, the identity of the subjective and the objective, and the unity of all antitheses between the psychic and the physical."[61] For this reason *Dichtung und Wahrheit* (the imaginative and the scientific aspects of human intellectual activity) were, in truth, indistinguishable.[62]

When in 1844 Purkyně contributed the article "*Mikroskop*" to Wagner's *Handwörterbuch der Physiologie* he mentioned that the active constitutive role of the imagination was perhaps still more evident in the realm of microscopic observation. As well as technical accomplishment, a microscopist needed "the skill and art, yes the talent to see"; and the exercise of this talent did not consist merely in using a single sense but was a function of the combined capacities of the mind. Microscopic observations were therefore influenced by the qualities and characteristics of the observer, be these good or bad.[63]

Among the characteristics of such observers as Purkyně and Valentin was a particular conception of the natural world that inclined them to expect certain occurrences and to structure their perceptions by the conceptual apparatus they brought to the microscope. We have tried to show the importance of ideas derived from romantic *Naturphilosophie* to Purkyně and Valentin's research on ciliary motion and to describe how their explication of this phenomenon was a confirmation and exemplification of axioms about nature to which they subscribed. We turn now to their work in neurohistology to demonstrate that similar concerns and resources were active in this field of research also. For purposes of exposition Purkyně and Valentin's work will be treated separately; however, this arrangement should not obscure the extent to which they were expounding essentially the same concepts.

3.3. VALENTIN AND THE TYPE OF NERVOUS STRUCTURE

Several historians have remarked upon a marked tendency in Valentin's histological writings. Erich Hintzsche has commented upon Valentin's persistent determination to seek general laws in his microscopical research; and Hendrik Van der Loos has described the quest for "generalization and simplification" that characterizes Valentin's neurohistology.[64] More specifically, a definite and enduring goal dominated Valentin's microscopical studies: the discovery of simple common structural elements from which the complex and diverse parts of the body could be seen to derive.[65]

In this endeavor Valentin's adherence to typological forms of reasoning and to romantic ideas of the unity of nature are evident. His research can be considered as a direct extension of the efforts detailed in chapter 2.2 to discover the type of the nervous system at the gross anatomical level; only now the microscope supplied the means of pursuing these goals among the fine texture of the gray matter and nerves. Valentin was not alone in thus preserving the theoretical ends of earlier investigators while expanding upon their technical means. François Leuret (1797–1851) had in 1839 approved Gall's attempt to find a common structural element that would unite the central parts of invertebrate and vertebrate nervous systems. He held, however, that Gall's concept of the ganglionic type was deficient because it was based solely on observation of the outward forms of nervous organization; as a result, Gall had been obliged to resort to such spurious assertions as the claim that distinct swellings were visible along the human spinal cord, in order to establish the affinity of that organ with the ganglionic chain of articulate animals. The truth of Gall's basic contention was, Leuret maintained, far better sustained by considering the structure rather than the form of the nervous system. Whereas "the form of ganglions is very variable," the microscopic composition of the central parts of the nervous system was uniform and constant, both within the individual and among different organisms. In vertebrates and invertebrates alike every ganglion was composed of "globulous matter."[66]

Valentin expounded his concept of typical organic forms and placed it in the context of his wider philosophical scheme in his *Handbuch der Entwickelungsgeschichte des Menschen* (1835). Natural objects, he wrote, were apparently independent and discrete, but from a loftier viewpoint a network of complex connections between them emerged, and they appeared as the parts of a unified whole. It was, on this reasoning, of particular scientific importance to establish "the relation of the higher whole to individual beings," as well as the relations between these individuals.[67]

The mind abstracted certain characteristics common to a group of individuals and so subsumed their particularity within a larger concept. This concept represented the *Uridee* underlying a given group; and although the *Uridee* was not fully realized in any particular individual, it was inherent in the distinctive features of every member of the group. Each individual constituted a special realization of the fundamental group concept "and these various types of realizations are called metamorphoses of the *Uridee*."[68]

The concept of the *Uridee* had special relevance to understanding the arrangement of organisms into taxonomic classes; but Valentin gave it a wider application. Just as the taxa of the animal world could be regarded as metamorphoses of the *Uridee*, so could organs and the parts of organs also be viewed in a similar fashion; they too were modifications of some original model.

Valentin's terminology and his stress upon the role of the mind in constructing the *Uridee* might suggest that he considered the concept to be a useful but purely subjective instrument for ordering complex anatomical data. But for Valentin as for Purkyně, "ideas" were not merely mental constructs of a greater or lesser pragmatic value; they also possessed a concrete embodiment in nature. Valentin wrote that "for the realization of the *Uridee* in the animal kingdom in general the term "type" is used. We will, however, only employ this expression for the elaboration of the *Uridee* in the individual organs."[69] One instance of the application of this approach in a piece of research has been noted already: Purkyně and Valentin's theory that all tissues exhibiting ciliary motion were derived from one *idea primigena*.

An example of a greater significance is to be found in Valentin's discussion of the ovum in the different classes of animal. Valentin held the *Cardinalfrage* here to be "whether the egg of mammals is or is not analogous to that of birds before fertilization." Drawing upon his own and upon von Baer's observations, Valentin answered this question in the affirmative; there was an exact correspondence in the initial structure of the ovum in both classes. Valentin therefore concluded that "Nature in the formation of both the forms of ovum has followed that above described *Uridee*."[70]

The form in question—a vesicle enclosing a nucleus and perhaps a nucleolus—was, moreover, not found in this case alone. Long before

Schwann enunciated his cell theory in 1839, Valentin had argued that the vesicular structure was fundamental to a wide range of tissues in both plants and animals.[71] After 1839 Valentin gave a still more extensive significance to this structure, maintaining that "the general *Urform* of all tissues is . . . the cell."[72] The cell was conceived by Valentin as a triple organ formed by the superimposition or encapsulation of three elements: cell (i.e., membrane), nucleus, and nucleolus. This characteristic arrangement constituted the *Uridee* of the basic vesicular type.[73]

In 1836 Valentin published a long paper on the course and termination of the nerves, which amounted to a general theory of the minute structure of the nervous system. This theory was permeated by the general morphological ideas outlined above. His stated aim was to discover the *Urtypus* of ganglionic organization that was applicable to all parts of the nervous system in humans and that also formed a link between nervous organization in vertebrate and invertebrate animals. In effect, he pursued with the microscope the same goal that had guided Gall's anatomical reasoning. Valentin identified the microscopic type of the nervous system as a particular combination of terminal nerve fibers and globules (*Kugeln*), the latter in this case being true cells. The fibers did not communicate directly with the corpuscular elements but looped around them. Valentin described the typical form of the *Ganglienkugel* as consisting of an "outer, more or less delicate areolar (*Zellgewebe*) integument, a *nucleus,* and on the periphery of the same a smaller secondary *nucleolus.*"[74]

Such globules permeated by fine fibers were found in the ganglia of the vegetative nervous system and also in the brain and spinal cord. Valentin therefore concluded that the entire nervous system was composed of two *Urmassen:* globules and fibers. There was, he held, an "extraordinary analogy" at the level of microscopic organization between the "central" (cerebrospinal) and the "peripheral" (vegetative) nervous systems.[75] The "*Uridee* of the formation of both is to the smallest detail throughout the same." In short, Valentin asserted that he had discerned the "*Urtypus* of the whole nervous system."[76]

Having established the identity of the structural elements of the two chief divisions of the nervous system, Valentin proceeded to investigate whether there were any discernible analogies with other organ systems. There was, he maintained, little to be learned from a comparison between the nervous and the vascular systems; only slight and unimportant resemblances existed between the two. However, the reproductive system did offer significant analogies. Specifically, Valentin held that "in a remarkable manner, the *Uridee* of the form of the unfertilized ovum agrees with the *Uridee* of the constituent globules [of the nervous system, i.e., cells]." Both structures possessed an analogous membrane, contents, and nucleus. This insistence on the close analogy between nerve cell and ovum was one of the points of direct agreement between Valentin and Purkyně; and the comparison was to have major consequences for the way both men conceived the functional role of the corpuscles they discovered in the brain, spinal cord, and ganglia. This point shall be discussed below; at this stage it is sufficient to note that Valentin contended that the reason why there was such a striking resemblance between nerve globules and the ovum was that "the organs of generation possess the same rank of ideal efficacy (*Wirksamkeit*) (in part an even higher one) as the nervous system."[77]

At the conclusion of this discussion Valentin felt confident that he had established "the type of the nervous system of vertebrate animals"; that is, he had described a "very simple archetype (*Urbild*)" to which all the complex structures of the vertebrate nervous organization could ultimately be reduced. He was not, however, content to rest with this achievement: it was, he insisted, necessary to go on and to ask whether "the nervous system of the invertebrate animals, in respect of its finer organization, does or does not show analogies and correspondences with the vertebrates."[78]

Valentin did not approach this question with an open mind. His prior theoretical commitments—his belief in the general "law of uniformity" that prevailed in nature—predisposed him to hold from the outset to a presumption (*Vermuthung*) that a correspondence between the vertebrate and invertebrate nervous systems would be found.[79] Valentin first argued that a unity in nervous organization within the invertebrate subkingdom was apparent. Whether the nervous system took the form of a ventral chain of ganglia or of scattered visceral ganglia and nerves, "here also it is again clear how Nature always remains true to her originally chosen *Urtypen*"; whatever special modifications of nervous organization did appear among the invertebrates the law of uniformity was never violated.[80] Moreover, this "undreamed of conformity in structure of the individual parts of the ganglionic cord is not . . . confined to the external boundary of the particular parts of each ganglion, but also reveals itself in their inner organization." This histological uniformity consisted in the existence in all invertebrate ganglia of nucleated corpuscles (or cells). The universality of these structures incited Valentin to exclaim upon the "profound astonishment" provoked in "weak mortals" by the "masterly regularity of Nature in her smallest formations."[81]

Ubiquity of the corpuscular type of ganglionic organization also enabled Valentin to bring together the vertebrate and invertebrate nervous systems. Both in respect of the composition and deployment of the nerves and of the central parts of the nervous system vertebrates and invertebrates possessed homologous parts. It followed, Valentin maintained, that "the *Urtypus* of the nervous system, which we have depicted in the vertebrate animals, also occurs among the invertebrates extending to the smallest detail." Only the different arrangement of the same elementary parts distinguished the nervous system of the two subkingdoms.[82]

If now we review Valentin's argument, a certain pattern emerges. He set out to find a typical histological structure that would unify the two departments of the vertebrate nervous system: the cerebrospinal and the vegetative. A plexus of fibers enclosing distinctive globules constituted this *Urtypus*. Valentin then drew attention to the analogies between the nerve corpuscles and an apparently unrelated structure, the ovum. Lastly, he showed how the invertebrate nervous system was constructed upon essentially the same plan as that of vertebrates. Valentin's procedure thus conformed to the principles of romantic biology outlined above: he sought to unify the parts, first, of one organ system; then to detect analogies between organs; and, lastly, to draw together the organization of widely separated classes of animal.

More particularly, Valentin's argument bears a clear resemblance to those of some of the authors discussed in chapter 2. Like Gall and Burdach, Valentin took the idea of the ganglion conceived as a mass of gray matter communicating with nerves, as the structural unit that unified all forms of nervous organization. He shared with these earlier scientists a concern to show that the ventral cord of invertebrates was homologous with the spinal cord, and that the most cephalad ganglion of this chain corresponded to the vertebrate brain.[83] He also agreed with previous proponents of romantic science on such doctrines as the vertebral composition of the skull and that the brain of vertebrates was constructed on a common plan whose form was most obvious early in human embryogenesis and was most striking among the more primitive vertebrate animals.[84] But Valentin went beyond his predecessors in this tradition by seeking at the microscopic level the correspondences and analogies that others had detected in the gross structure of the nervous system.

Schwann took up Valentin's observations and incorporated them into his cell theory of animal life. Schwann placed special emphasis upon the analogy between the ganglion-globule and the ovum that Valentin had noted, using it to corroborate his own view that all tissues developed out of originally similar bodies. Schwann, however, placed more stress upon the membrane of these corpuscles than had Valentin; this was in keeping with the former's larger strategy of highlighting the similarities between the elementary components of plant and animal tissue.[85]

After the promulgation of the cell theory, Valentin modified his terminology somewhat, substituting "*Zelle*" for "*Kugeln*" in his writings. However, his basic concept of these structures remained unchanged. They were triple formations made up of nucleolus, nucleus, and membrane, which, together with the nerve fibers, made up the *Grundtypus* of both the cerebrospinal and the vegetative nervous systems.[86]

Valentin's 1836 paper is generally recognized as a milestone in the histology of the nervous system. In particular, Valentin deserves credit for indicating the basic ground elements that underlay the great variety of forms of nervous organization both within the human body and in the animal kingdom as a whole. We have argued that a knowledge of the philosophy of nature to which Valentin adhered is necessary for a proper understanding of his achievement. He sought by his microscopical investigations to vindicate the notion of ubiquitous typical structures that bound together the most diverse parts of the organic world into a unity. From these efforts emerged the first recognition that the nerve cell body (or globule) in conjunction with the fiber was fundamental to all forms of central nervous organization. We proceed now to show how Purkyně's ideas of the nature of the living world determined his view of the significance of these central parts to the functions of the nervous system.

3.4. PURKYNĚ AND THE PHYSIOLOGICAL NATURE OF NERVE CELLS

Purkyně occupies a well-defined place in most accounts of the early development of the nerve cell concept. Whereas Ehrenberg may have been the first to describe the corpuscles of the gray matter, it was Purkyně who recognized that these structures must be of great importance in the workings of the nervous system.[87] This claim is based upon remarkably slight evidence: the brief report of Purkyně's address on 23 September 1837 to the *Versammlung deutscher Naturforscher und Aerzte*. In this paper Purkyně set out to expand upon an account he had given earlier in 1837 of the microscopic structure of the brain.[88] Purkyně gave Ehrenberg the credit for first showing the existence of "ganglionic granules" (*Körner*) in the ganglia; this discovery had instigated the investigations by Purkyně himself to ascertain the complete topography of these structures in the nervous system. He was struck by the *Analogie* between Ehrenberg's granules and those found in the cerebral hemispheres as well as in other parts of the brain, such as the cerebellar cortex, where he discovered what was later to be known as "Purkyně's cell."[89] After describing the morphology and distribution of these granules Purkyně proceeded to make the statement upon which historians have laid such emphasis. In its entirety it reads:

> In respect of the significance of the ganglionic granules it should be noted, that they are probably central structures, for which their entire, triple concentric organization speaks, and which might stand to the elementary brain and nerve fibers as centers of energy to energy conductors, as ganglia to ganglion nerves, as the brain substance to the spinal cord and cranial nerves. They are collectors, generators and distributors of the neural organs.[90]

This passage shows that Purkyně held the ganglionic granules to have a functional importance of a quite definite kind. What is not immediately clear is why he assigned them this role. In this case a knowledge of subsequent developments hinders an understanding of the text. In later neuroscience, because the nerve cell was identified as a junction point where sensory signals were translated into motor impulses, the historian is tempted to assume that Purkyně was striving to articulate a protean version of this theory. In fact, Purkyně stated that nothing was established about the relations of the ganglionic granules to the fibers;[91] and the connections (if any) between these two elements were not central to the importance he attached to the ganglionic granule.

Purkyně's 1837 address therefore raises questions that cannot be answered by reference to it alone. At least one historian has recognized how puzzling it is that Purkyně should have assigned the significance he did to the ganglionic granules at a time when cell theory (let alone neuron theory) had not yet been articulated. The same historian also suggests that a proper appreciation of Purkyně's work can be reached only by an examination of how he approached this and related problems.[92] Purkyně's approach was, in turn, structured by his philosophical preconceptions and by the explanatory strategies these generated.

Purkyně's account of the nature and properties of the histological elements of the nervous system comprise several interconnected statements; each is connected with aspects of his own and others' work, and is only intelligible when placed in a wider context. In the first place, Purkyně was employing a form of inference from the macroscopic to the microscopic. This procedure was by no means novel; it had been recommended by Herman Boerhaave (1668–1738) in the first half of the eighteenth century when he wrote that the structure and function of the blood vessels could be discovered either by the use of the microscope and injections, "or by following the Rule of Analogy, *viz.* that in the human Body you may judge of the invisible Parts by those which appear visible."[93] Employing an analogy of this kind Purkyně suggested that the ganglionic corpuscles might stand in something of the same relationship to the fibers as the ganglion stood to the ganglion's nerves.

The idea that the nervous system consisted essentially of two elements, one that generated the "nervous energy" and one that conducted it throughout the body, had wide currency in the first third of the nineteenth century. In particular, the gray matter of the brain, spinal cord, and ganglia was assigned the former active function, whereas the nerves were allotted a purely internuncial role. Concerning the ganglia, Alexander Monro, *secundus* in 1783 had already proposed that they were additional sources of energy due to their supposed constituent gray matter, and that they provided extra energy to nerves passing through them (see chap. 7 n. 100). Following Gall, who extended this concept, many authors saw the gray matter as the nutritional matrix from which nerves sprang and in which they were augmented. Some went on to argue that it was from this source too that the fibers derived the impulses that they carried through the body. Thus Gruithuisen (an author with whose works Purkyně was acquainted) wrote in 1810: "the medullary fibers are nourished from the cortical substance, from which the nervous energy is also generated." The cerebral hemispheres, Gruithuisen declared, were an "inexhaustible source of nervous power."[94] Tiedemann denied Gall's contention that the olivary bodies were the ganglia from which nervous fascicles emerged; but he added, "I do not however pretend to deny, that the cortical substance, so richly provided with vessels . . . does not contribute to increase their energy and activity."[95] Blainville had a more specific notion of the function of the masses of gray matter. Having distinguished between the central parts of the nervous system and the nerves, he went on to define the ganglia as those parts of the nervous system that appeared to be "the points of departure and of arrival of the irritations that occur in the organism, and which are, for that very reason, the culminations or the origins of the cordons of transmission—the nerves."[96] Antoine Dugès went so far as to suggest that it is "the gray globular mass" at the center of the spinal cord, the analogue of the discrete ganglia running the length of insects, that directed movements.[97]

In part, therefore, Purkyně was transposing a commonly held contrast between active and commissural elements of the nervous system from the gross to the microscopic level. Histologically, the granules or cells of the gray matter took the role of generators of the nervous energy that was performed macroscopically by the gray matter of the ganglion en masse. Later authors followed Purkyně's lead in this matter. Thus Alfred Wilhelm Volkmann (1800–1877) in 1842 took a stance similar to Blainville's, maintaining that the masses of gray matter played "the principal role in the generation of nervous activity"; not only did they give rise to centrifugal stimuli but also received and assimilated stimuli transmitted from the peripheral parts of the body. The nerves merely conducted these impulses to and from the ganglia. Volkmann went on to seek the foundations of these differences of function in the intimate texture of ganglia and nerves. In particular, the physiological properties of the ganglia could be ascribed to their possession of cells—of "those small organs, which in their isolation produce from within the marvellous activity." The regulative activity of other cells, both in plants and animals, was according to Volkmann sufficient proof of this assertion.[98]

But whereas Volkmann wrote after the promulgation of Schwann's theory, which made such comparisons plausible and which focused attention upon the functional prominence of cells, Purkyně had come to similar conclusions before the cell theory. It remains to inquire, therefore, why he thought it likely that the granular structures he discerned in ganglia should be seen as generators of nervous energy. Purkyně's 1837 address makes it clear that he believed the peculiar structure of these globules to be a strong indication of their physiological importance: specifically, "their entire, triple concentric organization" suggested that they were the central organs from which the nerves obtained their energy. In effect what Purkyně was doing was to point out the correspondence in the structure of ganglionic granules and other histological elements in the body that were known to be physiologically active; he went on to assume that this similarity gave sufficient grounds for supposing that the ganglionic granules performed comparable functions. Underlying this confident leap from the known to the unknown was the romantic doctrine that analogous parts, acting in accordance with analogous principles, were distributed in even the most remote and apparently dissimilar organs. Purkyně laid particular stress on two such analogies, that between the ganglionic granules and the granules found in glands, and that with the ovum.[99]

The idea that the brain was a kind of gland was venerable; it had been advanced by Marcello Malphighi (1628–1694) and Thomas Wharton (1614–1673) in the seventeenth century and, despite criticisms from Haller and others, retained some credibility in the first half of the nineteenth century[100] (see chap. 5.2.2). In 1811 Gruithuisen wrote of the brain and spinal cord as "secretory organs" directly comparable to glands.[101] As late as 1849 the distinguished author of a textbook of microscopic anatomy, Arthur Hill Hassall (1817–1894), could still speak of the "secreting substance or grey matter of the brain"; by this time, however, the secreting agent of this as of the other "glands" was identified not as the cortical substance as a whole, but as its constituent cells. The "nerve or ganglionary cells," Hassall declared, "present essentially the same structure as all other glandular cells, and are doubtless continually passing through the same phases of development and destruction during the processes of nutrition and secretion."[102]

Malpighi had used analogy to support his view that the cerebral cortex had a secretory function, and a similarity between the histological elements of glands and ganglia had been casually remarked by Ehrenberg in 1833.[103] Valentin in 1835 had also described the structure of glandular and nervous tissue in similar terms.[104] It was Purkyně, however, who first placed great emphasis upon this and related histological correspondences and drew major physiological conclusions from the analogy.

On September 19, 1837, four days before he delivered his paper on the nervous system, Purkyně addressed the *Versammlung deutscher Naturforscher und Aerzte* on the "Structure of the stomach glands and on the processes of digestion." He noted the existence in these glands of granules (*Körner*) containing smaller corpuscles (in modern terms, cells and their nuclei). Purkyně asserted that these granules were the active elements of the gland; from them came the secretion. He went on to extend this conclusion to a progressively wider range of organs. The epithelial part of mucous membranes of the respiratory, digestive, and uterine organs were also made up of "discrete granules of different shape and size"; this analogy in the parenchyma of the glands and membranes indicated the existence of a new type of organic operation. Moreover, a similar analogy could be drawn between the structure and function of other organs and their products. In fact, the body could ultimately be reduced to three ubiquitous elements: fluids, fibers, and granules. Of these the last appeared as functionally the most important.[105]

Purkyně drew a comparison between the granular basal form and the cells of plants. He also anticipated Schwann by maintaining that just as each vegetable cell "has its *vita propria,* and prepares its own specific content out of the general fluids, . . . so one can conceive the secretory and formative (*Entbildungs*) process in the same way."[106]

It seems plausible to suggest that when a few days later Purkyně came to discuss the microscopical structure of the ganglion he was inclined to identify its globules as the active element because of the analogy with the ultimate secreting and nutritive organs he had previously discussed. Whether or not he conceived the nervous agent as an actual fluid, he did see it as something that was elaborated within the ganglionic granules just as the various secretions originated in the granules of glands.

This instance of analogical reasoning may seem farfetched but precedents for it existed in contemporary physiological thought. Apart from the persistence of general comparisons of the brain and a gland, authors of the *Naturphilosophie* school had developed a special rationale for such an analogy. Although organic properties such as secretion, sensation, and movement might seem to be quite separate and unlike, "philosophically" viewed these distinctions disappeared. All organic activity, asserted Gruithuisen, including nerve force was derived from a primitive unitary power (*Einkraft*); and even in animals where this power had become apparently highly departmentalized, an intimate connection existed between all the functions.[107]

Fortunately we do not have to remain content with conjecture about the influence of such notions upon Purkyně's thinking. In the course of an 1850 commentary on a late work of *Naturphilosophie,* Purkyně volunteered to recount the "history of my own train of thought in the exploration and conceptualization[?] (*Vorstellung*) of the physiological conditions of thought."[108] He revealed that Gruithuisen's doctrines had exerted an influence on his early thinking that had persisted despite subsequent advances in neuroscience.[109]

Purkyně did not refer specifically to Gruithuisen's having molded his ideas on the relations of the nervous to the other bodily functions. It is apparent, however, that whether from this or from another source, Purkyně had absorbed the notion of a close relation between the various physiological powers. He held that the concept of the ganglionic globules as the "energy centers" of the nervous system gained credence when the "other structures of the animal body" were taken into consideration; in particular, such a survey should take special note that "all glands and membranes of the animal body are constructed out of cells and granules." A wider set of analogies drove home the same point: in the embryo and in vegetables the same type of structure was repeatedly seen to perform the physiologically active role.[110] By viewing the granules of the ganglia as generators of nervous energy Purkyně was merely including this organ in what seemed to be the universal rule of nature. But his readiness to accept—and indeed to expect—the existence of such a rule was premised upon Purkyně's adherence to the principle of organic unity.

The tenets of the romantic philosophy of nature inclined him to search for analogical structures within the human body and to extend the quest for corresponding phenomena to other animals and even to vegetables. However, the search for unity and analogy did not cease at the limits of the organic world. The distinction between animate and inanimate was only relative, not absolute; in consequence, correspondences between physiological and physical phenomena should also be sought by the scientist.

Schelling, the founder of *Naturphilosophie,* had himself declared that "Nature cannot withdraw the material principle of life from the general laws which she herself originally impressed upon matter."[111] On the contrary, the laws of life must be seen merely as special manifestations of the *potentia* inherent in all matter. Thus, a later exponent of *Naturphilosophie* insisted that there was only one *Urkraft* in nature to which all its phenomena could ultimately be attributed. This force manifested itself in different forms: in the inanimate world, for example, it appeared as electricity; the vegetable kingdom thrived upon it; and in a heightened form it was present in the oxygen that made animal life possible; it was, moreover, what underlay the various vital powers of the body. Thus in the muscles the *Urkraft* expressed itself as irritability, whereas in the nerves it appeared as sensibility, and "in the human brain it thinks."[112]

Purkyně's commitment to the unity of life with other natural phenomena and his inclusion of the operations of the nervous system, including mind, within this totality have already been noted. He stated this principle emphatically in the course of an 1828 review of Burdach's *Vom Baue und Leben des Gehirns,* and he drew special attention to the claim of Burdach and of many other *Naturphilosophen* that there was "an analogy between the soul and the dynamic natural phenomena, light, electricity, etc."[113] Indeed, Burdach had gone further and maintained that the nervous force was a transformation of such physical forces as electricity, magnetism, and light and that it retained a close affinity with them.[114]

Although many of his contemporaries did believe that the nervous agent was identical with electricity or magnetism (see chap. 5.3.2), it is unlikely that Purkyně was of this opinion. He does, however, seem to have taken the view voiced by Valentin that "the working of both the nervous agent and of physical agents, rests upon analogous laws."[115] An analogy of this kind is evident in Purkyně's description of the ganglionic granules. They were generators, collectors, and distributors of nervous power. The reference to electricity becomes even more obvious when we recall that the German word *Sammler* can also mean an electrical battery. Whereas the granules thus created, stored, and released the nervous agent (analogously to an electrical pile), the nerves were merely the medium along which this energy was transmitted.[116]

This emphasis upon the similarities between nervous and physical force gives Purkyně's argument a distinctly reductionist aspect. It is true that he did seek to bring together as far as possible the concepts of physical science, biology, and psychology. However, Purkyně's insistence that the working of the nervous system, the organ of mind, must be understood by reference to the other forces of nature was complemented by his claim that even purely physical phenomena were in a sense psychic in character. Again, the root of this idea lay in the romantic philosophy of nature: the conscious human mind was, according to Schelling, only one aspect of the *Intelligenz* that pervaded the entire universe and that was immanent in all natural processes.[117] We have already noted the presence in Purkyně's thought of a similar doctrine. He stated it perhaps most explicitly in an 1846 discussion, the language of which bears the strong imprint of Schelling's writings. The human understanding observed an apparent opposition in nature between the spiritual and the material. But this antithesis was only apparent: its mediation was most obvious in organic life. In the organism even when no trace of consciousness appeared, "everything has a mental (*gedankgemassen*), spiritual character." Such unconscious intelligence was, Purkyně held, to be seen in plants, the lower animals, and in the human embryo.[118]

The analogy that Purkyně discerned between the ovum and the ganglionic granule was another major reason why he attributed such special importance to the latter structure. We have seen that Valentin pointed to the similarity between the ovum and the ganglionic corpuscle, both of which were, he said, built upon the type of a triple concentric structure. In 1841 he also argued that their mode of development was identical.[119] Valentin hinted that underlying this structural analogy was a similarity of function: the egg and the ganglionic granule were alike the seats of an intelligent—but not necessarily conscious—force.[120] Purkyně, too, maintained that there was a "striking analogy" between the ovum and the ganglionic granule and thought it justifiable to proceed to seek "correspondences (*Gleichungen*) in their vital functions."[121]

The significance of the ovum was, Purkyně held, fairly clear; it was the organ of specific reproduction. In order to perform this function it needed to embody a psychic element. It was through the ovum that "the living idea of a complete individual" was transmitted from one generation to the next; by its agency the specific type of an organism was preserved. The ovum contained the idea of this prototype (*Urbild*) as a kind of memory which it had the power to recreate substantially in the course of the developmental process.[122]

When these conceptions were transferred to the granular (cellular) components of ganglia, Purkyně held that "one can ascribe to them likewise an ideal in addition to a material content, which is partly intrinsic, partly, under appropriate conditions, disseminates effects outwards, and can receive such effects into itself." Thus, each ganglionic granule was a kind of thinking entity: an organic monad that possessed a particular energy appropriate to the execution of a range of bodily operations. This nervous energy was, according to Purkyně, directly analogous to that possessed by the ovum for the reproduction of the organism. Human consciousness was merely one mode or moment of the energy inherent in the ganglionic granules. There were as many "little souls" as there were granules in the brain; but these individual conscious entities were somehow bound together into the general soul of the entire body. The corpuscles of the ganglia of the vegetative nervous system differed from those of the brain only in that the quality of their consciousness was of a lower order than that of the histological components of the brain and spinal cord (see chap. 7.7.4).[123]

From this analysis it is evident that Purkyně's concept of the nerve cell or granule was not so much an anticipation of the neuron theory as a reiteration of philosophical speculations that were ancient even in the 1840s. The doctrine that the world was composed of thinking monads can be traced back as far as Gottfried Wilhelm Leibniz (1646–1716); but the panpsychist presumption that underlies this and similar ideas is far older. There was a resurgence of such notions in the first half of the nineteenth century chiefly in the work of the followers of Schelling. It was central to their system to assert that in the universe there was no absolute distinction between the material and the spiritual: mind was immanent in all matter and particular natural objects could be regarded as thinking beings.[124]

This philosophy of nature found expression as late as 1847 in the work of Benjamin Gottlob Ernst (fl. 1847). The universe, he maintained, was created by God's thought; there was, however, no distinction between the thinking creator and the material creation. On the contrary, the universe was identical and imbued with psychic characteristics: "we perceive his [God's] thoughts, feelings, and sensations as the starry heaven, and his substance as space."[125] Such speculations may seem merely bizarre to the modern reader; but Ernst's work deserves our attention for two reasons. First, in accordance with the common practice of romantic authors he drew an analogy between the macrocosm of the universe and the microcosm of man. Just as every divine thought had its material embodiment among the "starry hosts" so "every human thought gives rise to a microscopic corporeal being in the brain." Since the invention of the achromatic microscope these entities had become visible to the eye; they appeared as points in the brain surrounded by a "double ring." These separate beings were joined together by the multitude of nerve fibers.[126]

The second reason why Ernst's work warrants attention is that in 1850 Purkyně wrote a commentary on the second edition of Ernst's *Neues Planetenbuch*. We have already referred several times to this document because it was here that Purkyně provided the fullest statement of the philosophical assumptions underlying his ideas on the structure and function of the nervous system. It is significant that not only did he take Ernst's hypothesis seriously but he elaborated a similar panpsychist cosmology that saw intimate interrelations and correspondences between the living body and the universe in general. Having established the ubiquity of cellular monads in the brain and other organs, and having concluded that all vital processes including the nervous and intellectual, were performed by congeries of these entities, Purkyně claimed that the gaze turned naturally to "the infinite stellar space, where a similar more vast process of formation and action, pertaining to higher monads, the stars, excites in us the idea of an unending cosmic life, of which to us in our limited organisms and microcosms are given models for human contemplation and examination."[127]

Purkyně's concept of the organization and action of the brain and ganglia needs, therefore, to be seen in the context of his wider natural philosophy. This predisposed him to look for collections of monads in the nervous system that could be identified as the loci of conscious and unconscious mental activity; he found this *desideratum* in the "granules" that he and Valentin found in such abundance in the gray matter. More generally, we have argued that Purkyně and Valentin's other major achievements in the field of neurohistology can also be referred to the assumptions and goals derived from their immersion in romantic ideas of nature and science. Valentin sought to reduce the nervous organization to a simple type; in consequence he identified the nerve cell and fiber as the constantly recurring elements of the nervous system. After invoking the principle that analogies existed between diverse parts of the body, Purkyně concluded that ganglionic granules, which so resembled structures like the ovum that were known to be functionally important, must play the active role in the performance of the nervous function. The theory that the nervous system was composed of many individual units, each endowed with a limited psychic quality, also conformed with the ideas of mind and its relation to nature that Purkyně and Valentin derived from contemporary *Naturphilosophie.*

Because later in the nineteenth century *Naturphilosophie* fell into disrepute, much of its constructive influence upon science has until recently been overlooked. In the case of Purkyně and Valentin there is no question that it provided the framework that guided their microscopical research and within which their concepts of the minute structure and operation of the nervous system were reached. In particular, through their research, they established two axioms of lasting importance: (1) that the nerve cell together with the fiber were the principal components of the central parts of the nervous system, and (2) that these together cooperated to produce all forms of nervous function.

In two respects, however, their thinking was deficient. Until a relatively late date Purkyně and Valentin refused to accept that there was an anatomical connection between nerve cell and fiber. Second, the concept of how cell and fiber interacted put forward by Purkyně remained chiefly at the level of analogy and metaphor without supplying any convincing mechanism for nerve function at the microscopic level. By 1850 Purkyně had begun to remedy both these deficiencies. He recognized that "most ganglionic granules project themselves at one or more points into elementary nerve fibers and that probably the entire fiber system of the nerves takes its origin in the ganglionic granules of the brain and of the other ganglia of the body." He also saw that this anatomical fact was potentially of great importance to an understanding of the functions of the nervous system: the nerve cells were revealed as the points to which centripetal impulses were transmitted and from which centrifugal impulses arose.[128]

The contention that nerve cell and fiber were connected is found in the writings of a third major figure in the neurohistology of the mid-nineteenth century, Robert Remak. The attempt to apply the concepts of sensorimotor physiology to microscopic studies was also a prominent theme of Remak's work. However, in neither of these fields can Remak's achievements be understood in isolation; the following section attempts to place Remak's research in its historical setting.

3.5. THE CELL FIBER CONNECTION AND SENSORIMOTOR REASONING

3.5.1. Cell and Fiber

In 1842 Benedikt Stilling summarized the current state of knowledge of the structure of the nervous system. Only in recent times, he said, had the subject been investigated with any success; but, even so,

> despite more important discoveries, we stand at the threshold of knowledge of the texture and structure [of the nervous system]. That globules [cells] and cylinders [fibers] with semifluid contents form its mass—that is the result of our science.—However the arrangement of those parts in relation to each other is still completely unknown.[129]

Friedrich Heinrich Bidder (1810–1894) in a historical survey published in 1847 agreed: although Ehrenberg, Purkyně, and Valentin had identified the essential elements of the nervous system—cell and fiber—they had left their relationship undetermined. Whereas Purkyně had expressed an open mind on the subject, Valentin had adhered tenaciously to the view that fibers arose in the ganglia from terminal loops, a view that proved finally to be mistaken. It was Remak, Bidder held, who had first maintained that fibers did originate from cells.[130]

Bidder went on, however, to cast doubt on the accuracy and worth of Remak's observations despite their apparent vindication by later research. Such depreciation of Remak's efforts was, as Bruno Kisch has shown, common in the 1840s and later. Kisch has endeavored to remedy the injustice Remak suffered at the hands of his contemporaries and has argued that Remak anticipated all other researchers of the period in describing the true relation of cell to fiber.[131]

Kisch's judgment was shared by at least some of Remak's contemporaries. Notably, Stilling in 1856 declared that "to have pointed out the origin of the nerve fiber from the nerve cell (1837) . . . remains Remak's incontestable contribution."[132] Remak enunciated this doctrine in his doctoral dissertation of 1838, where he maintained that "the organic [autonomic] fibers come forth from those nucleated corpuscles" found in the autonomic ganglia.[133] But the qualification Stilling immediately made to his tribute to Remak is also significant. Remak "stated in fact only the origin of the organic and not of the dark-edged nerve fibers [from cells] at that time."[134] In modern terms, Remak held only that the unmyelinated but not the myelinated fibers arose from cells.

It is true that in one passage of his 1838 dissertation Remak does speak of fibers originating from cells in the spinal marrow as well as in the ganglia of the vegetative nervous system; and it is not clear whether he regarded these fibers as "organic" (unmyelinated) or as "primitive cylinders" (myelinated) of the cerebrospinal nervous system.[135] Remak's later writings show, however, that for several years after this publication he remained undecided on the relation of cells and fibers in the brain and spinal cord; certainly he did not believe that the relationship he had discerned in the ganglia must be replicated in the central parts of the cerebrospinal axis. At most Remak was prepared before 1846 to declare only that the myelinated fibers probably passed into the cells of the brain and spinal cord.[136]

The contributions of several other individuals need to be recognized if the process whereby this probability became an accepted axiom of neuroscience is to be grasped. The first of these is Adolph Hannover (1814–1894), who at Remak's instigation, undertook research on the course of the fibers in the cortical substance of the brain. In these investigations Hannover employed chromic acid, one of the first tissue fixation techniques. He declared in 1840 that "the origin of the brain fibers from the brain cells and their persisting connection with those central structures throughout the whole of life, is at the moment more than probable to me; I have made this observation so many times, that for me scarcely any doubt of the correctness of this interesting phenomenon prevails." In general, Hannover held, each cell produced two fibers, although some cells produced none.[137]

In 1842 Hermann Ludwig Ferdinand Helmholtz (1821–1894) conducted research on the ganglia of various invertebrates. These revealed certain cells possessing processes which, at their distal ends, resembled fibers.[138] Johann Georg Friedrich Will (1815–1868) in 1844 also showed a cell-fiber continuity in invertebrates.[139] Such workers as Emil Harless (1820–1862) and Rudolph Wagner produced similar conclusions for the relation of cell and fiber in vertebrate animals.[140] It should be noted, however, that all this research was characterized by much equivocation and confusion; the one point upon which observers were able to agree were the practical obstacles to determining the relation of fiber to cell in vertebrates. In particular, Bidder complained, it was extremely difficult to distinguish nervous elements from other structures, especially the connective tissue, under the microscope.[141] Wagner remarked upon his surprise at finding the cell-fiber connection in certain fish "so extremely clear and easily depictable"—a circumstance brought about by the paucity of areolar tissue in the ganglia of these animals.[142]

In contrast to these guarded and often contradictory statements was the clear assertion made by Rudolph Albert von Koelliker (1817–1905) who in 1844 held that

> *the fine fibers arise in the ganglia not from terminal loops [a reference to Valentin's theory] or free terminations, but as simple continuations of the processes of the ganglion-globules. In other words, the continuations of the ganglion-globules are the beginnings of these nerve fibers:* this is the unquestionable result of long and far from easy researches, specially directed on this subject.[143]

Koelliker claimed that what had previously been merely suspected by Hannover, Helmoltz, and Will (Remak is deliberately excluded from the list)—namely, that fibers arose from cells—was now established as a general law.[144] He later distanced himself further from these others by asserting that no one before him had demonstrated the transition and connection of cells with myelinated fibers; all that Hannover and the rest had done was to describe the long pale processes of cells and to infer that these united with fibers at some point.[145]

Whatever the justice of Koelliker's claims to originality, his 1844 publication does seem to have had a decisive influence on contemporary opinion. Thus, when in 1844 Volkmann wrote the article "*Nervenphysiologie*" for Wagner's *Handwörterbuch der Physiologie,* he held initially that the question of the origin of nerve fibers remained open. Volkmann noted the opinions of Remak, Hannover, Will, and Helmholtz, but did not consider them convincing.[146] After the text of the article was completed, however, Koelliker's research appeared and Volkmann felt it necessary to revise his earlier view. In the light of Koelliker's discoveries, as well as of his "predecessors," Volkmann held, it was probable "that the fibers take their origin from ganglion-globules. *Koelliker* saw this formation even in the spinal cord." Volkmann added an observation of his own made on the nerves of a frog's heart, which revealed the origin from a cell of a fiber and traced its progress for a considerable distance.[147]

The summary of the course of events in this field of science published by J. F. B. Polaillon (fl. 1865) in 1865 captures the relative significance of the various contributions to the doctrine of the unity of cell and fiber. Remak in 1838 had maintained only that the organic (unmyelinated) fibers arose from cells. The "labors of Helmholtz and of Will upon the invertebrates, had already done much to demonstrate the existence of nervous fibers in connection with the ganglion-globules. Hannover (1840) corroborated them for vertebrates, and Koelliker (1844) rendered this fact classic."[148]

A number of later investigations may also be mentioned. In particular, Remak himself maintained that Stilling's 1846 discovery of the nucleus of the pons (i.e., the red nucleus) supplied the first demonstration of the connection of multipolar cells with motor fibers. Gratiolet made a similar observation for the spinal cord in 1852.[149]

3.5.2. Microscopic Anatomy and Sensorimotor Physiology

It took time for these discoveries to attain the status of textbook orthodoxy. Moreover, even when the origin of some fibers from a cell was acknowledged, many workers were reluctant to accept that all fibers arose in this way.[150] Other questions such as the number of processes to a cell, the mode of union between cell and fiber, and the fine structure of each also remained contentious. Nonetheless, by 1856 the essence of the modern doctrine that cell and fiber form parts of an anatomical whole was established.[151] Polaillon in 1865 saw no need to equivocate: "at the present epoch, it is demonstrated anatomically that the ganglia contain cells as nervous centers, and that these cells give rise to [nerve] tubes." What is also important is that he attached major physiological implications to this anatomical fact, seeing it as vindication of Bichat's doctrine of the fundamental autonomy of the vegetative nervous system (see chap. 7.4).[152] This tendency to bring physiological reasoning to bear on anatomical facts and to seek to elucidate function by a study of form, was a widespread feature of the histology of the mid-nineteenth century.

The existence of a tradition of "physiological anatomy" in the nineteenth century has been recognized by historians (see chap. 1.2.1). But they have tended to regard this school as a peculiarly British phenomenon (e.g., Charles Bell), and to speak of it in deprecatory terms, suggesting that this approach to problems of function was archaic and unproductive.[153] Even those who take this view recognize that in the case of studies of the nervous system the anatomical approach was the source of many valuable insights.[154] An appreciation of the potential of anatomy to contribute to physiological knowledge was, moreover, not confined to

Britain but was widespread on the Continent, and especially in Germany.

Thus, in 1842, Stilling and Joseph Wallach (1813–1878) wrote that "in recent times anatomical researches have shown the way to physiological discoveries"; the "most dazzling" instance of this was Charles Bell's work on the nerve roots. (In view of Bell's dishonest behavior in his research reports [chap. 4.3], this was an unfortunate example to select. Magendie would have been more appropriate.) But the interaction between anatomy and physiology was not unidirectional: knowledge of function could suggest the existence of structural arrangements in the nervous system. For example, in his experimental investigations of the functions of the spinal cord, Stilling had shown that individual segments of the cord could operate independently of the brain or the remainder of the cord (thus confirming previous research, such as Whytt's [see chap. 4.2–3]). This physiological fact made it highly probable that a degree of autonomous segmentation was to be found in the anatomical structure of the cord.[155]

When he came to describe his microscopic observations Stilling made it clear that he had conducted this research with regard to the explanatory framework supplied by anatomical physiology. In his view, the gray matter of the spinal cord was not merely the anatomical but also the "physiological core" of the organ. He undertook to explore the relations between its various elements paying special attention to the passage of fibers from the spinal roots into the gray substance in order to elucidate the structural basis of the spinal function.[156]

Koelliker, too, insisted that anatomical investigations must be undertaken with an eye to their physiological importance.[157] As late as 1892 he maintained that the prosecutors of the anatomical sciences must "from the outset lay great weight on *physiology,* which is rigorously (*streng*) connected with morphology."[158] An example of Koelliker seeking to realize this principle in practice is found in the use he made of anatomical evidence in attempting to determine the functional properties of ganglia.[159]

Remak on one occasion cautioned against a too confident use of microscopical observations to establish physiological principles; such inference was a very difficult matter which must be approached with caution.[160] But from his earliest publications, Remak himself sought to infuse histology with physiological notions and to elucidate function by means of microscopical structure. Thus, in his first paper he tried to show that sensory and motor fibers were structurally distinct and so to provide "a new, anatomical confirmation of Bell's theory."[161] Two years later Remak settled the physiological question of whether the nervous system had an influence upon the purely vegetative (autonomic) functions of absorption and exudation chiefly by reference to the anatomical fact of the extensive supply of nerve fibers to the glands and other viscera.[162] Such examples in Remak's output could be multiplied.

In Remak's case this emphasis upon the anatomical as the principal route to physiological knowledge seems to have derived at least in part from a deep-rooted distrust of experimental results, and in this regard he can be likened to Gall and Charles Bell (see chap. 1.2.1), who, however, worked only at the macroscopic level. On occasion Remak held that anatomical findings were clearly superior to those derived from vivisection;[163] elsewhere he merely stated that facts drawn from anatomy were of equal validity to those uncovered by experiment.[164] Such a prejudice against experimental methods was not, however, universal among proponents of the anatomical method. Stilling himself undertook many experiments and regarded the results derived from this source and those from anatomy as complementary.[165]

As we have pointed out above, the relations of the anatomical to other methods of physiological research during the nineteenth century deserve fuller investigation. Here we wish only to point out the existence of this tradition and to show its importance for developments in neurohistology. The anatomical-physiological approach had a special significance in one particular area: results from microscopy were recruited to corroborate and to expand Bichat's notion that the ganglia of the vegetative nervous system were "small brains" or nervous centers capable of autonomous action. We shall discuss the histology of this system again in chapter 7.7.5. In Polaillon's words, during the early nineteenth century "physiological anticipations had outstripped anatomy." During the late 1830s and the 1840s histology seemed to catch up with and to confirm the ideas of the physiologists.[166]

Remak wrote in 1840 that the observations recorded in his doctoral dissertation had been undertaken with the aim of deriving "physiological significance" from the anatomical facts of the vegetative nervous system.[167] Although previous investigators had suspected that the ganglionic nerves were independent of the brain and spinal cord as we shall see in chapter 7, they had been unaware of the evidence that (in Remak's view) convincingly established this autonomy: the existence of a distinct class of "organic" nerve fibers.[168] Moreover, Remak had shown that, whereas the primitive cylinders (myelinated fibers) passed through the ganglia unaltered, new fibers did spring from the cells of ganglia and became the organic fibers of the ganglionic nerves. Even if this origin of fibers from cells remained controversial, Remak held that, on the basis of microscopical information, it was irrefutable that the organic fibers increased their quantity in the ganglia and must therefore originate partly from them.

The ganglia had to be regarded as centers (*Mittelpunkte*) and points of origin of the organic fibers; and this circumstance, Remak added, was significant for their physiological role.[169]

The fact that microscopic evidence revealed ganglia to be anatomical centers where fibers were concentrated and augmented was taken by Remak and his contemporaries as proof that they were also centers in the physiological sense for the regulation of the organs to which the gray organic fibers proceeded.[170] In this way the old doctrine of the ganglia as "small brains," or sources of nervous energy (see chap. 7.5) and the latest findings of microscopical anatomy were harmonized. Taken in isolation, Remak admitted, microscopical research revealed no more about the physiological importance of the ganglia than that they were sites where nervous fibers were augmented.[171] But when viewed in the light of prevalent theories of the functions of the ganglia, these observations took on a richer meaning and produced the basis for further speculation on the physiology of the vegetative nervous system.

We have noted above the notion that the gray matter of the nervous system generated the energy upon which nervous function depended. This idea remained among the assumptions with which many investigators approached the results supplied by the microscope. Thus, Remak in 1840 expressed the familiar contrast between the central, ganglionic parts of the nervous system that generated nervous energy and the nerves that merely conducted it.[172] He was more specific on another occasion when he maintained that it was the ganglion-globules of the central parts of the nervous system that must be regarded as "points of departure or of reinforcement" where the nervous energy was stored.[173] Similar references to the ganglionic gray matter as the "central part" of the nervous system, where the power that passed to the various parts of the body was generated and discharged, can be found in the writings of other histologists of the period, often in close relation to the anatomical facts that were supposed to confirm the hypothesis.[174] That cells were the true physiologically active parts of the nervous system was also widely accepted. Bidder, for example, wrote in 1847 that "the globules contained in the ganglion exert an influence on the performance of the cerebrospinal fibers passing through the same." Bidder added that a closer determination of the nature of this influence remained to be achieved.[175]

This rider of Bidder's is important because it indicates a widespread sentiment among mid-nineteenth-century workers who tried to combine histology with physiological concepts. It was insufficient, in their view, to assert that the ganglia were "centers of energy" that regulated the workings of the nervous system. Although the statement that cells were the active elements in this process was more precise it remained inadequate. What was needed was a dynamic theory of how the nervous function was mediated by the histological structures revealed by the microscope. Histologists saw the attainment of this goal as dependent on the incorporation into their science of the resources offered by sensorimotor physiology.

This determination was predicated upon a keen awareness among histologists, especially in Germany, of the importance of the development of sensorimotor physiology in the early decades of the nineteenth century. Valentin held that Marshall Hall's account of reflex action (chap. 4.4), together with Bell's distinction of the motor and sensory spinal root functions (chap. 4.3; Magendie's contribution was overlooked), were among the most important discoveries in the history of science.[176] Specifically, Hall had demonstrated the essential type of nervous event: the passage of a sensory impulse to a central point where it was reflected into a motor response.[177] This insight supplied a simple model of the workings of the nervous system to which all its actions, however complex, could ultimately be resolved. Thus Stilling in 1842 was able to declare that there were but two classes of activity embodied in the nervous system: the sensory and the motor.[178]

Remak, too, was firmly committed to this principle of simplification and sought to apply it, especially in his work on the vegetative nervous system. In his 1841 article on neurophysiology, he described the reflex type of action as that which distinguished animals from vegetables. Whereas the latter might be able to respond to immediate local stimuli, only in animals were sensory impulses reflected into movement by a central organ.[179] As we shall discover in Chapters 4 and 7, others before him had postulated reflex activity in the vegetative nervous system, usually acting by way of its ganglia. But in his writings on the physiology of this system, Remak strove to show, first, that the purely "organic" (autonomic) functions were subject to nervous regulation and, second, that this regulation conformed to the same sensorimotor pattern found in the functioning of the cerebrospinal axis.

Remak had argued the former point as early as 1838 when he defined the "organic" functions as all those independent of voluntary control. This comprehended both involuntary movement of every kind and the metabolic functions. Remak foresaw objections to the contention that the latter were subject to nervous control. These functions were by long-established usage "plantlike," i.e., vegetative processes. Moreover, Schwann had in 1839 given a new significance to this notion by arguing that nutrition and secretion were essentially cellular operations, which proceeded in animals as in plants independently of the nervous system. Remak in 1838 advanced various experimental and anatomical facts to show that the nervous system did influence at least the quantity if not the quality of the materials generated during these operations. Two years later he took account of the cell theory, but continued to insist upon nervous regulation.[180]

The problem of how the nervous system could affect what were apparently autonomous cellular processes could be resolved, Remak held, if the mode of nervous operation was grasped. It was difficult to conceive how both involuntary movement and secretion could be subject to the same regulatory mechanism; however, the actions of the nervous system in both cases not only could but, Remak insisted, must be understood in sensorimotor terms. The nervous principle possessed only two modalities: the centripetal and the centrifugal. The former produced stimuli (*Reizungen*) that might or might not be accompanied by consciousness. Conversely, centrifugal impulses must result in movements.[181] The way in which the nervous system influenced the vegetative functions must be accommodated within this general framework.

Nervous influence could only take the form of a kind of movement: either a contraction of the cell body itself or of the blood vessels that supplied them with nutrient. Remak thought it was more likely that the influence of the nervous system was immediately exerted upon the capillaries and only indirectly on the cells themselves. By varying the amount of nutritive material supplied to cells the nervous system could modify not only the quantity, but also the quality of the product. He thought it likely that such regulative movements were reflex in character; that is, they were instigated by an initial centripetal impulse. Remak concluded that, Schwann's doctrine notwithstanding, a *sensorium commune,* albeit an unconscious one, existed to centralize the vegetative activity of the body, just as the animal life was regulated by the conscious sensorium.[182]

Remak recognized that if this physiological schema was to carry conviction an anatomical grounding for its postulates must be provided. On occasion he acknowledged that histology was still unable to meet this need; but he believed that the basic elements that mediated the operations of the nervous system were known. Although sensory and motor fibers were the conductors of the two classes of nervous impulse, the ganglia of the brain, spinal cord, and probably of the vegetative nervous system, were the "central points" that generated and coordinated activity.[183]

He discussed the anatomical substratum of reflex action in more detail in 1841. Remak stressed that the existence of "central points" was crucial to the reflex theory, and argued that accumulations of gray matter not only in the brain and spinal cord but also in the viscera must be assigned this function. He went on to specify more closely the anatomical units that served as central points of reflex action: the ganglion-globules served as the "communication points" where centripetal were translated into centrifugal impulses. He did not, however, exclude the possibility that other parts of the nervous apparatus might perform the same function.[184]

In giving the ganglion-globules the role of mediators of reflex action, Remak expressed a view that received ready assent from mid-nineteenth-century scientists. Prior to the cell theory the ganglion en masse had already been identified as the central point of the reflex arc. Thus William Carpenter wrote in 1839 that for the performance of a reflex action, "a nervous circle is requisite, consisting of an *afferent* nerve on the peripheral extremities of which an impression is made; a ganglionic centre, where the white fibres of which that nerve consists terminate in grey matter, and those of the efferent nerve originate in like manner; and in an *efferent* trunk conducting to the contractile structure the motor impulse, which originates in some distant change in the relation between the grey and white matter."[185] By 1846 Carpenter had refined this definition, stating that a ganglionic center "essentially consists of a collection of nerve-vesicles or ganglion-globules," interspersed among the nerve fibers and maintaining that these vesicles served as "centres of nervous power."[186] R. B. Todd in 1845 asserted that it was the stimulation of the "vesicular matter" by afferent fibers that resulted in reflex action.[187]

Koelliker in Germany argued that the ganglia of the vegetative nervous system were the sites of both "simple and reflected movements" and were served by both sensory and motor fibers. To justify this claim he pointed to their cellular composition, maintaining that the "gray substance or the *ganglion-globules* [our italics] partly maintain the energy of the nerves connected with them, partly mediate the various reflexes from one fiber to another, and also by themselves stimulate the motor fibers immediately." These facts led physiologists to acknowledge, with a few exceptions, that the ganglion-globules were to be treated as the "central organs" of the nervous system.[188]

The demonstration of an anatomical connection between cell and fiber might appear an important corroboration of this doctrine. Surprisingly, however, Remak himself placed little emphasis upon this point. In 1840 he wrote that what was of importance for determining the physiological significance of the ganglia was the anatomical evidence that showed them to be the points of concentration and reinforcement of fibers. Remak went on "the question whether the organic nerve fibers originate and increase themselves immediately from the substance of ganglion-globules, or in their vicinity" was "for the time being of lesser importance."[189] In the following year he modified his position somewhat; the determination of whether fibers did originate from cells had relevance to the issue of whether "influence" could be communicated in the nervous system by mere contiguity, that is, "crossover transmission," to be described in chapter 4.6. Remak added that, in any case, the ganglia were to be seen as the central points of the organic nervous system.[190]

In contrast, other scientists made the cell-fiber connection central to their conception of the working of the nervous system at the microscopical level. Bidder in 1847 held that the achievement of recent neuroscience had been to provide fresh support for the venerable doctrine that the ganglia were "central organs." It was now established that the impulses for certain nervous actions proceeded from them and that the conduction from centripetal to centrifugal fibers also took place in ganglia. Bidder held that "the anatomical basis for this physiological significance of the ganglia must be sought in the presence of the globules." In order to gain even the most superficial insight into the processes occurring in ganglia, Bidder insisted that it was "above all necessary to attain knowledge of the type and mode of how fiber and globule stand in relation to each other." This need had been met, at least in part, through recent developments in neurohistology: "so that [the idea that] the impulses proceeding from the ganglion-globule were transmitted into the path of the nerve fibers, could henceforth be more easily understandable than formerly (*sonst*), when the embedment (*Einlagerung*) of the globules in the nervous cylinders was itself still unknown."[191]

Bidder's peculiar notion of the relation of cell to fiber needs to be recalled here; he thought of cells as embedded in fibers rather than of fibers issuing from cells. Nonetheless, his remarks show an awareness that the fact of the anatomical union of cell and fiber—a doctrine that was only just receiving general acceptance—made it easier to conceptualize the sensorimotor operations of the nervous system at the microscopic level. However, the passage of ideas between anatomy and physiology was not all one way. Whereas the doctrine of the cell-fiber connection contributed to theories of function, anatomical facts assumed a new meaning and aspect when viewed in the light of sensorimotor concepts. As Koelliker wrote in 1848, in purely anatomical terms fibers could be considered indifferently as either originating or terminating in cells. But, physiologically speaking, the motor fibers must issue from cells whereas sensory fibers ended in them.[192] Physiological thinking therefore imposed new significance upon the structures revealed by the microscope. The assignment of directionality to fibers specified their role within the animal economy; moreover, the position of the cell as the junction point between these two conductors also allotted a function to the cellular component of the nervous system.

A reciprocal and mutually enriching interaction between physiological and anatomical reasoning therefore characterized the neurohistology of the mid-nineteenth century. Increasing exactitude in the microscopy of the nervous system supplied a lack many observers saw in current physiological notions. Sensorimotor physiology assumed the existence of what Stilling called a "specific organization for movement" in the structure of the spinal cord and of the other central parts of the nervous system; however, the "anatomical causes" of motion and coordination remained to be discovered.[193] During the 1840s Stilling drew upon his own and others' histological observations in an effort to provide this *desideratum*. In 1843 he remarked that the relation of the fibers to the cells found in the spinal cord was as yet undetermined (although he noted the similarity of these cells to the *Kugeln* described by Remak in the ganglia of the vegetative nervous system); nevertheless, Stilling held that it was clear that the cells of the anterior gray column of the spinal cord must be connected with movement, just as the *substantia gelatinosa Rolandi* of the posterior gray column was related to sensation.[194] In his subsequent work Stilling sought to trace the passage of fibers from the posterior roots toward the multipolar cells of the anterior gray column; and thereby, as Schiller remarks, he supplied "much of the anatomical basis for the spinal reflex mechanism first accurately postulated by Marshall Hall."[195]

By 1854 Remak had assimilated Stilling's research. Indeed Stilling provided him with a number of preparations of the human spinal cord on which to make his own observations. These clearly showed the passage of fibers from the spinal roots of the motor nerves into the multipolar ganglion cells of the anterior gray column. Moreover, Remak held that it was possible to detect the existence of fibers communicating between the anterior and posterior gray columns of the spinal cord. Proceeding from the point of entry of the anterior root into the anterior-horn gray matter, the fibers passed into the part of the *substantia gelatinosa* where the posterior root arose; there they united with the processes of ganglion cells. Conversely, the bulk of the fibers from the posterior root passed through the *substantia gelatinosa* to terminate in the vicinity of the large multipolar cells of the anterior gray column. Remak concluded that

> Those circular fiber-pathways (*Faserzüge*) may well mark one of the routes, upon which in decapitated animals the irritation of sensible nerves causes reflex movements. It is noteworthy in this regard, that the longitudinal axis of the largest ganglion-cells is oriented to the long axis of the spinal cord and that in addition to the lateral processes, by means of which they connect with nerve-root fibers, they send out at both poles ramified fibers towards the cranial and as far as the sacral ends of the spinal cord.[196]

If histology thus served to provide a foundation for known physiological phenomena, sensorimotor ideas were also imposed upon anatomical data to enrich the meaning of microscopical observations. Rudolph Wagner at the conclusion of his 1846 article on the vegetative nervous system declared: "it is permissible to erect out of my fragmentary anatomical and physiological observations provisionally as a hypothesis a theory of reflex movement." Wagner presented a series of schematic diagrams designed to show the pathways taken by afferent and efferent fibers and the role of cells as central points where one form of impulse was transformed into the other.[197]

Such interpretations of histological structures became commonplace in later years; and it was in this context that the doctrine of the anatomical unity of cell and fiber acquired its full physiological significance. Gratiolet in 1857 asserted that the cells portrayed by Hannover, Will, Koelliker and others "are the centers towards which sensory fibers converge, and from which certain motor fibers radiate." These cells could, therefore, be conceived as so many

> intermediaries completing the nervous arcs; but they [cells] are not mere conductors of stimulations: each of them is a center for the generation of impulses. In effect, the sensory fiber acts upon the central cell and modifies it in such a manner as to provide in the cell a particular activity—a hidden property that sleeps but which a stimulation renders manifest.

The cell was like the bell awaiting the stroke, or the cannon the fuse that would release its potential for action. But in order for this potential to be released the cell's connection with afferent fibers was required; and for the impulse to reach the different parts of the body the cell must communicate with efferent fibers.[198]

A more developed version of this type of reasoning is found in the 1863 *Grundriss der Physiologie des Menschen* of Ludimar Hermann (1838–1914), who was to introduce the rudiments of the modern concepts of nerve conduction (see chap. 5.5). In his treatise the various classes of nervous action were enumerated together with the "central organs" that mediated these functions. The defining characteristic of the central organ was its possession of "*ganglion-cells,* which stand in immediate union with nerve-fibers." It was, Hermann insisted, precisely because ganglia cells alone were in anatomical connection with fibers that they should, "in general . . . be described as the central end-organs of the nerve-fibers."[199]

Hermann regarded the reflex as the simplest manifestation of how cells and fibers interacted to produce nervous function. In reflex action the "potential energies" (*Spannkräfte*) of the cell were released by the impulse transmitted along a fiber; the released energy of the cell then went to stimulate another fiber. To nerve cells could therefore, at least hypothetically, be ascribed "the capacity of transmitting from one communicating (*eintretenden*) nerve-fiber on to another; the conduction takes place from a centripetal fiber through one or several ganglion-cells finally to a centrifugal [fiber]." Where the stimulation was capable of activating more than one centrifugal fiber, Hermann added, there must be several pathways away from a cell. Seen in this light "the anatomically-proven existence of multipolar ganglion-cells is also a physiological necessity."[200]

Part of the attraction of employing sensorimotor concepts to explicate anatomical arrangements seems to have lain in the simplification and ordering of complex histological structures this procedure permitted. Mid-nineteenth-century authors produced "schemata"—more or less idealized representations of the complex and sometimes chaotic appearances the microscope revealed.[201] The converse also applied. The cell theory in this as in other departments of physiology uncovered a unified histological foundation for apparently diverse organs. For scientists operating within the framework of anatomical physiology, the achievement of such simplicity in structural concepts suggested that questions of function might be reformulated in comparably elementary terms. Thomas Henry Huxley (1825–1895) wrote in 1854 of the reduction in current neurohistology of the components of the nervous system to fibers and ganglionic corpuscles. It was, he went on,

> impossible to overrate the value of these discoveries; for if they are truths, the problem of nervous action is limited to these inquiries: (a) What are the properties of ganglionic corpuscles? (b) What are the properties of their two, or three commissural processes? For we are already pretty well acquainted with the properties of the sensory and motor processes.[202]

With hindsight some of the simplifications of structure and function of the nervous system made during this period appear too bold; subsequent investigations revealed a degree of complexity that qualified and sometimes overturned the sweeping generalizations of the first generation of neurohistologists. Nonetheless, simplification was central to the achievement of the microscopists of the 1830s and 1840s: they established that cells and fibers were the elements that composed the nervous system, and revealed the intimate relation existing between them. They also began the process of trying to show how sensorimotor functions were mediated by these structures. In this way they laid the essential foundations of later neuron theory.

3.6. SEQUEL

The formidable task confronting the early microscopists of the nineteenth century who examined nervous tissue was to apply to it the cell theory of animal life and thereby determine the nature of its basic units. We have learned how the discovery that these were nerve cell bodies connected directly to nerve fibers was made by pioneers such as Purkyně (1837), Remak (1838), Hannover (1840), and Helmholtz (1842). Their findings were fully substantiated by Koelliker, who in 1849, looking back to 1844, declared: "I have stated that the ganglion cells are connected with nerve fibers by their processes and that these two are continuous with one another."[203] Although controversy continued, further verification came from others including Karl Georg Friedrich Rudolph Leuckart (1823–1898), when in the following year he reported seeing filaments passing from nerve cells into nerve fibers in various parts of the nervous system.[204] From this Rudolph Wagner inferred that the cell gave off a process that ran as a nerve fiber through the body, finally ramifying and terminating in peripheral tissues, and he could demonstrate this in the electric lobe of the *Torpedo*'s brain, where the cells might have more than one such process, and could thus be multipolar. Moreover, the cell also possessed prolongations that seemed to connect with its neighbors.[205] In 1854 Wagner made the following important statement:

> The brain and spinal cord are nothing but an enormous accumulation of primitive [nerve] fibers and multipolar ganglion cells. Union of the fibers takes place only by means of the cells. Thus, anatomically verifiable pathways are the basis for all transmission between the fibers. To speak of the gray matter and its actions on the nerve fibers is a hazy way of expressing something that is clear: multipolar ganglion cells are linked by means of primitive fibers.[206]

Not only was this a morphological principle of the greatest fundamental significance but from the functional point of view it was of equal consequence, as we have learned. Adding to the above, Wagner declared:

> All the phenomena of innervation are dependent on the connections of [nerve] cells with each other, and on connections of central and peripheral pathways with individual cells or collections of cells acting as special centers of innervation of varying physiological importance.[207]

The next step in understanding the anatomy and physiology of the nerve cell[208] was to find out precisely how these cells, fibers, and other processes made contact among themselves. The problem remains today, but since the middle of the nineteenth century all advances have been determined by improvements in research methods. Conceptual foundations having been provided, technology took over so that the history of neurohistology becomes the history of histological techniques.[209] Better fixation of tissues had begun with Reil's alcohol method of 1809,[210] and vastly improved by Hannover's use of chromic acid, introduced in 1840.[211] Of greater potential were the first procedures for the coloring of nervous tissue, which gave unassailable evidence of cell-fiber union.[212] The chance discovery made by Joseph von Gerlach (1820–1896) around 1865 of the staining properties of carmine for animal tissues,[213] and the use of other dyes, led in 1872 to the best depiction of the nerve cell and its processes that had yet been produced.[214] But now a difference of opinion arose concerning the way that the nerve units made contact with one another.

Gerlach proposed that the cell body's processes formed a network intimately connecting all nerve cells, and Camillo Golgi (1843–1926), who had revolutionized neurohistology in 1873 with his silver staining technique[215] which delineated for the first time the cell body and all its processes in their entirety, also proposed a network, although of a different kind, and described it in 1883.[216] Thus was created the school of "reticularists" led by Golgi and opposed by those who believed the nerve cell and its processes to be in contiguity, but not continuity, with its neighbors, the "neuronists."[217] The latter collected overwhelming evidence in their favor, resulting from new histological methods of research, for they drew upon the work of Wilhelm His (1831–1904) who watched the neuron (cell body plus processes) grow[218] and of August Henri Forel (1848–1931) who studied its decay,[219] together with the remarkable histological observations of Santiago Ramón y Cajal (1852–1934),[220] and those made by employing a new *intra vitam* staining procedure introduced by Paul Ehrlich (1854–1915).[221] In 1891, Wilhelm Waldeyer (1836–1921) brought all these and other data together, and announced that they warranted the establishment of a "neuron doctrine,"[222] based on the proposition that

> [T]he axis cylinders of all nerve fibers (motor, secretory, sensitive [*sensible*] and sensory, conducting centrifugally or centripetally) have been proved to proceed *directly* from the *cells*. A connection with a fiber network, or an origin from such a network, does not take place.[223]

Despite the certainty expressed at that time, the debate between neuronists and reticularists continued, and in 1933 Ramón y Cajal was still posing the question "Neuron theory or reticular theory?" in one of his last publications.[224] The problem first tackled by the early microscopists of nervous tissue and which led to the neuron-network controversy was solved eventually by advancing technology. After World War II electron microscopy provided magnifications far beyond the optical instrument's capabilities and revealed that the neurone was a distinct and separate entity and that there was indeed no network.

4

The Reflex

4.1. INTRODUCTION

The evolution of the concept of reflex activity, and its background of sensorimotor physiology dealt with in the previous chapter, have received more attention from writers than any other topic in the history of the neurosciences.[1] There are several reasons for this emphasis. The most important is that the reflex has become a central concept to several biological specialties; and its inception and development have, as a result, attracted much interest. Psychologists in particular, who have always been concerned with the history of their discipline, have recognized the status of the reflex as a basic aspect of physiological psychology. Moreover, the work of Charles Scott Sherrington (1857–1952) in this century has done much to focus attention on the reflex as a fundamental physiological phenomenon. To complement such an extensive secondary literature, we plan to trace briefly in this chapter the notions of the reflex up to 1832 when Marshall Hall began his research on it, to discuss Hall's pioneer studies in some detail, and to consider the extension of the spinal reflex concept to the brain, a topic that so far has not been dealt with adequately. Finally, we shall examine the opening phases of the search for the reflex's morphological basis, the outcome of which was directly dependent upon the contemporary cell-fiber debate we have just discussed in chapter 3.5. In fact, when considering reflex physiology, we shall find that many of the themes in nineteenth-century biological thinking already seen to play a central role in the development of the neurosciences are again prominent.

4.2. EARLY HISTORY OF THE REFLEX TO 1784

The idea of the reflex grew from speculations on the phenomena of "sympathy" and involuntary movements that originated with the ancient Greek writers and were extended by seventeenth- and eighteenth-century investigators. "Sympathy," or its Latin equivalent "consensus," was a rapport thought to exist between parts of the body, especially the organs, that were not anatomically connected; it will be discussed further in chapter 7.3 where its role in the history of the vegetative or "sympathetic" (autonomic) system will be described. As Galen had originally pointed out, this involuntary interrelationship of sympathetic harmony in the body was effected by way of nerves or blood vessels. Involuntary acts such as sneezing, yawning, coughing, and vomiting were included, and sympathy between organs was thought to be particularly active in the diseased state, when one of them could respond sympathetically to another's distress, with the production of otherwise inexplicable symptoms and signs. Many of the examples of so-called sympathy turned out later to be based on reflex action, especially those involving the autonomic system and the structures it innervates. Like sympathy, the distinction between voluntary and involuntary motion can be traced back to antiquity, where we find that both Aristotle and Galen had made this fundamental differentiation.[2] The vital participation of the will, consciousness, or soul (according to one's beliefs) that differentiated them was a source of discussion and controversy until almost the end of the nineteenth century. Many physiologists continued to rely on hypothetical immaterial agents to explain these phenomena, and this practice inhibited a mechanistic understanding of involuntary movement. In the mid-seventeenth century, René Descartes (1596–1650) did provide a purely mechanistic account of such movements; however, as we shall see, his hypothesis did not exorcise the metaphysical entities that were still invoked in discussions of the subject in the late 1800s with echoes reaching into the twentieth century. Descartes initiated the concept of reflex action in 1649, constructing a simple and admittedly theoretical, yet effective, explanation which in principle is still acceptable today.[3] A sensory impression traveled to the brain, from where it was reflected (*réfléchi*), as in the manner of light, into motor nerves to bring about coordinated muscular contraction. The event occurred unconsciously or in spite of the will. However, it seems likely that too much has been made of this notion, and that, in particular, Descartes's contribution was exaggerated by nineteenth-century materialists, such as Emil du Bois-Reymond (1818–1896) (see chap. 5.5) in order to support their reductionist approach to physiology.[4] Nevertheless, Descartes's dualistic doctrine, whereby man's material, machine-like body was governed by an immaterial, rational soul in the pineal gland, had an immense influence on subsequent physiological thought. One aspect of this, concerning Pierre Flourens's views of brain function, will be discussed in chapter 6.5.

Also in the seventeenth century, Thomas Willis conceived of a mechanical process involving the reflexion of sensory impressions to create mental as well as motor responses. As in the case of Descartes, however, we should not in retrospect overemphasize the significance of this notion. It was but a small aspect of Willis's important work on the ancient concept of sympathy,[5] and at the time he was attempting chiefly to provide a rational explanation for this phenomenon, but one that could also explain reflexion. Thus, Willis believed that somatic and autonomic nerves could communicate with each other in their plexuses, so that sympathy between various bodily structures could take place without involving pathways to the brain or spinal cord. These rudimentary concepts were derived from speculation based on clinical and anatomical observations, but rarely on experiment,[6] and the precise manner of contact was unknown. The nerve fiber was not to be isolated until more than a century later, and our synaptic communication not for over two centuries.

But if movement originated in the brain, what was the explanation for the disturbing enigma of the brainless fetus that could move and the fact that decapitation of an animal did not instantly destroy all motion? These occurrences had been known for a very long time, and experiments on headless animals carried out in the seventeenth century merely substantiated them, by revealing that stimuli to the trunk or limbs could still induce movements. A variety of explanations were advanced, the most important being the celebrated notion of irritability introduced by Haller in 1753,[7] which he believed could account for involuntary or unconscious motion, as in the decollated animal. But the problem could only be adequately resolved by ascribing to certain parts of the nervous system, such as the spinal cord or ganglia, a degree of independence of action.

Robert Whytt of Edinburgh was the first who endeavored to achieve this, and it was his ambition to provide physiology with the simplicity and uniformity with which Isaac Newton (1642–1727) had endowed physics.[8] Whytt was one of the many eighteenth-century animists who contested Descartes's mechanistic interpretations of physiology, especially of the nervous system, and he insisted that the soul controlled involuntary motion, which unconsciously defended the body from harmful stimuli. Whytt also believed in the neurogenic theory concerning involuntary muscular actions of vital organs, such as heart, lungs and gut, established by Willis's erroneous concept of cerebellar function (see chap. 6.6.2). He, therefore, passionately opposed Haller's doctrine of irritability. This stated that the power of contraction resided in the muscle itself, the so-called *vis insita* which was activated by a nerve force, the *vis nervosa*. From the results of many experiments, to which Whytt added astute clinical observations, the first faint glimmer of the simple spinal reflex took shape.[9] He could demonstrate easily that the involuntary movements of a decollated animal did not arise from Haller's *vis insita,* because destruction of the spinal cord arrested them, an observation already made by Stephen Hales (1677–1761).[10] In line with his animistic views, Whytt postulated instead an all-pervading immaterial soul or life-force, his "sentient principle." This was responsible for all the phenomena of life and made muscular motion possible, because it resided in the extremities of the nerves as well as in the brain and spinal cord. It also accounted for movements in the headless animal. Furthermore, on the basis of his spinal cord experiments, both normal and morbid actions, previously attributed to the old doctrine of sympathy, seemed not now dependent upon peripheral nerve anastomoses in plexuses, but upon their endings in the central nervous system. A stimulus applied at one point could produce movement in a distant part, and the necessary mechanism could be called "reflex" rather than "sympathetic," although the term "sympathetic response" remained in use and synonymous with "reflex" until the nineteenth century. Whytt included in it the reactions of the iris, later known as "Whytt's reflex," and of glands (e.g., those producing tears or saliva), as well as involuntary muscular movements of the trunk and limbs. Reflex motions produced by irritation were owing to particular sensations aroused in certain organs and from thence communicated to brain or spinal cord. Nevertheless, the soul, and therefore some degree of consciousness, was necessary to all movements, and for this mechanism the nerves were essential. Sensation, reason, and life itself were in Whytt's view dependent on the soul. Although the activities occurring in reflex action were not necessarily carried out in full consciousness, they were not entirely mechanical.

Whytt had clearly proved that the spinal cord was necessary for the simple spinal reflex; this was the *Fundamentalversuch* of reflex physiology.[11] Later he showed that only a portion of the cord was needed.[12] He had discovered in the central nervous system the true source of the so-called sympathy of the nerves. Despite his invocation of hypothetical agencies, such as vitalistic forces or his sentient principle, Whytt had focused attention on the spinal cord, and it was on his concept of the reflex that late eighteenth- and nineteenth-century physiologists were to build. One of the former was Johann August Unzer (1727–1799), who helped to clarify and consolidate Whytt's opinions, in his book of 1771,[13] which can best be described as a system of physiological metaphysics. He introduced the terms "afferent" and "efferent," popularized "reflected," and gave a more precise account of the spinal reflex's pathway. He was willing to accept the possibility of reflexion taking place in nerve plexuses, nerve bifurcations, the ganglia, and the brain, but only in the case of the brain could impressions be perceived.

4.3. THE REFLEX: 1784 TO 1832

Marshall Hall's work constituted a landmark in the history of the reflex concept. We shall now consider the state of knowledge at the time when Hall began his research in 1832.

Although Jiří Procháska (1749–1820) worked chiefly in the eighteenth century and his main publication on the reflex was in 1784,[14] his considerable influence, like that of Whytt, lasted well into the nineteenth century. In keeping with Whytt, he adopted the inductive approach and used the frog as his experimental animal. Casting out the Cartesian approach to physiology, Procháska modeled his principles on those of Newton. He condemned philosophical speculation and groundless assumptions and challenged some of the contemporary neural concepts. Thus, although he accepted Haller's theory of a nerve force or *vis nervosa,* Procháska did not think of it as a mysterious power originating in the brain and activating muscles, but rather as a force latent in the nerves that could be activated by a stimulus, either internal or external, physical or psychical. It was a provisional concept deriving from physics that would help scientists to classify the known data concerning the nervous system. He thereby avoided erecting a hypothesis that could not be tested at that time.

Procháska envisaged two kinds of nerves; centripetal, concerned with sensation and perception, and centrifugal, concerned with motor activity. He also believed that the actual reflexion of the sensory impression into a motor message that traveled to a muscle or other effector organ, took place in a central area, the *sensorium commune*. Unlike Haller, who considered this to occupy the white matter of the whole brain, Procháska confined it to all of the spinal cord, the brain stem, the cerebral and cerebellar peduncles, and parts of the thalamus, from which it appeared that all nerves arose. It was an area quite distinct from the seat of the will and the soul, which were also resident in the encephalon. From these considerations, he was able to give an account of the reflex pathway, which even though based on eighteenth-century notions is still in principle acceptable today:

> External sensory impressions are carried at great speed along the whole length of the sensory nerves to their origins, where they are reflected in accordance with a certain law and pass into certain corresponding motor nerves through which they are again transmitted very swiftly to the muscles where they produce certain definite movements. The place where the sensory and motor nerves meet, as in a center, and where sensory impressions are reflected into motor nerves is called the *sensorium commune,* a term now accepted by many physiologists.[15]

In addition to the *sensorium commune,* however, there also existed a mechanism whereby sensory impressions could be reflected or consensus achieved in nerve ganglia and plexuses by means of anastomosing and communicating branches. They need not reach the central *sensorium,* a notion similar to Willis's elucidation of reflexion and sympathy, and also upheld by Unzer. Thus, the autonomic ganglia could serve as reflex centers (see chap. 3.5.2 and chap. 7.8). According to Procháska, reflex action was automatic and independent of the will and of the soul in the brain, for it occurred in the headless frog and in the anencephalic human monster. The actual process of reflexion was not a mechanical one; it did not, for example, obey the principles of optics as Descartes and others had thought, but was under the direction of a special, but unknown law, written as it were by nature on the pulp of the *sensorium commune,* as Procháska expressed it. Despite this ignorance, he was in agreement with Whytt that the reflex served the animal organism as a means of defense, maintaining that "the general law by which the *sensorium commune* reflects sensory impressions into motor is that of our preservation."[16]

Nevertheless, these important clarifications of the reflex concept made little impact on Procháska's contemporaries, and even a prominent scientist such as Friedrich Heinrich Alexander von Humboldt (1769–1859) in 1797 still adhered to archaic principles in his attempt to explain sympathy between nerves, declaring that "a nerve fiber is in the sensible atmosphere [i.e., sphere of influence] of another, or merely by their contact with one another as in the case of the optic and ciliary nerves."[17] As we shall see later, these ideas, which are quite foreign to our present day concept of nervous transmission, emerged again in the late 1830s, when renewed efforts were made to ascertain how the reflex pathway functioned.

In retrospect, we can recognize that Procháska, together with other pioneers such as Whytt and Unzer, had established the spinal reflex as a distinct physiological entity comprising an in-going sensory stimulus that evoked in the spinal cord, brain, or ganglion an emergent motor response, which represented an instinctive defense mechanism. By the early nineteenth century, however, the supply of meaningful and experimentally verifiable facts derived from the methods and techniques then available had been exhausted and, in addition, there was virtually no knowledge of the possible morphological arrangements that might be responsible for the experimental observations already made on the reflex. Likewise, no new physiological concepts that might have been elucidatory had been established. Some had hoped that the notion of animal electricity (see chap. 5) might provide valuable insights. Procháska himself in 1820 reported his attempts to identify *vis nervosa* with it, and to apply this to his concept of reflexes, which, he concluded

> are based on the electrical attraction or repulsion of beneficial or injurious irritations to life, depending on whether the poles of the organ and the irritation are unlike or like.[18]

However, after 1810 Procháska was under the spell of *Naturphilosophie,* which explains his devotion to polarity, and in this instance his opinions proved to be futile.[19] Also at the beginning of the nineteenth century, the wide range of reflex mechanisms although suspected, had not yet been adequately revealed. In retrospect, another obstacle to progress was a failure to grasp the full scope of reflex action in animal life and, in particular, in the working of the nervous system. Thus, there was a total unawareness of the way in which the reflex contributed to the integrative function of the nervous system as a whole, and, therefore, to the achievement of integrated behavior in the organism.

There had, however, been an increasing interest in the gross anatomy of the spinal cord ever since Whytt had pointed out its importance for the reflex. Vicq d'Azyr's noteworthy studies published in 1781 had not been improved on at the turn of the century,[20] but soon the anatomical researches of Gall and Spurzheim and the interpretations they placed upon them (see chap. 2.1) were to change this picture, so that the spinal cord began to take on new structural and functional significance. As we have seen, it now had an independent existence, and was made up of units, represented by a ganglion of gray matter for each spinal segment with attached spinal roots (see chap. 2.3). Contact between the two sides of the cord was by sympathy, rather than fiber communication.

In the second decade of the nineteenth century, Whytt's and Procháska's basic principles of the reflex were widely accepted by physiologists, including J. J. C. Legallois, who carried out one of the first detailed studies of spinal cord function, mentioned above in chapter 1.2.2. His report, published in 1812, was a confirmation and extension of the experimental findings of Whytt and Procháska in the frog, his primary intent being to contest doctrines based on the existence of vital properties in the body. Using improved techniques, Legallois performed a large number of experiments, with the object of proving that the movements and sensation of the trunk had their seat in the spinal cord, and that its central gray matter was an independent center of innervation. The experiments involving cord destruction are of special interest to our present theme, and his conclusion from them was as follows:

> Not only does the life of the trunk depend upon the spinal cord, but each region of it, in particular, depends on the part of the cord from which it receives its nerves; so that by destroying a certain portion of the cord only those regions that receive their nerves from this destroyed area die. All those parts that receive their nerves from the undestroyed cord continue to survive for a more or less long time.[21]

In the presence of multiple cord transections, the part of the body corresponding to each segment of the cord retained its motor and sensory functions. Agreeing with Gall, Legallois declared: "In a word there are in this case as many quite distinct centers of sensation as there are segments of the cord."[22] Using warm-blooded animals, Legallois could also demonstrate that cutting off the blood supply to certain regions of the cord had the same effects. His conclusion, therefore, was that the life of each part of the body depended on the integrity of the corresponding segment of the spinal cord and on an uninterrupted supply of oxygenated (i.e., arterial) blood.

These findings all seemed to fit very conveniently into the concept of the spinal reflex as we recognize it. However, Legallois's interpretations were erroneous in that he thought that transecting the spinal cord produced two independent centers of innervation, with two centers of volition, one above and one below the cut. Moreover, he declared that the movements in a limb of a decapitated animal excited by stimulation were irregular and uncoordinated, because it was cut off from the control of the medulla oblongata, regarded by him as the center for coordination, rather than the cerebellum (chap. 6.4.3), as well as respiration (chap. 6.4.1). Obviously they were reflex responses, but Legallois thought them due to the persistence of conscious sensation and voluntary motion in the undamaged part of the animal's cord. He was in fact agreeing with Erasmus Darwin (1731–1802) who in 1794 referred to fetal movements, now known to be reflex, as voluntary and accompanied by consciousness.[23] Mainly because Legallois incautiously applied his experimental findings in lower animals in which the brain played a much smaller role, to higher species, he considered the spinal cord to be the independent and exclusive source of voluntary movements and sensation of the trunk, either as a whole or in isolated portions. He then extrapolated beyond his experimental data by denying that the brain was the center for all motion and sensation, so that he could place their seat in the cord. The brain was not the unique source of nervous power, although it regulated bodily movements, the immediate principle of which originated in the cord. He concluded that the latter and the arterial blood were the two sources of life. The brain acted on the cord as the cord acted on the muscles, and in the central gray matter of the cord resided the principle of nervous power and life.

In spite of Legallois's shortcomings he helped greatly to focus attention upon the spinal cord, and he complemented the anatomical studies of Gall and Spurzheim, whose concept of a segmented cord discussed in chapter 2.1 (and elsewhere) was at that time being hotly debated. He was adding to the mounting evidence that refuted the ancient notion of the cord being likened to a conducting cable with no inherent function. But, his observations were not accepted by all his contemporaries, and the renowned clinician and morbid anatomist Jean Cruveilhier (1791–1874) preferred the old concept. On the basis of clinicopathological evidence, he disputed the findings of Legallois and others, stating in 1829 that they appeared to be "a grave physiological error based on ingenious experiments."[24] Nevertheless, Legallois had a wide following in France, and his opinions were transmitted by men such as Desmoulins,[25] Charles Prosper Ollivier d'Angers (1796–1845),[26] and Louis Florentin Calmeil (1798–1895), who repeated his experiments in a variety of animals and obtained comparable results.[27] In Britain, Alexander Philips Wilson Philip (1770–?1851) agreed that Legallois's experiments proved "in the most satisfactory manner" that one of the cord's main functions was to excite the voluntary muscles.[28] He was not, however, in full agreement, especially concerning the proposed sensory functions of the cord: "It is evident from many observations, however, that the sensorial power chiefly resides in the brain, and the nervous [motor] power in the spinal marrow."[29] It is interesting to observe here that as late as 1872 the concept of the spinal cord as "a connected chain of ganglia, capable of receiving impressions through the sensory nerves, and of generating the nerve-force," which produced the motor response of the spinal reflex, was still current, although in modified form[30] (see also chap. 2.3).

We should also mention here a significant, but infrequently discussed contribution, albeit indirectly, to the reflex concept. Herbert Mayo, who referred to Legallois's work although not by name in his treatise on physiology,[31] described in 1823 how he had traced out the pathway for the reaction of the iris to light, and his conclusion was the same as Whytt's: . . . "an impression is conveyed to the brain along the optic nerve, which is followed by an affection of the third pair [oculomotor cranial nerve], causing the pupil to contract or to dilate."[32] But going further than Whytt, Mayo declared that in the pigeon the meeting point of the two limbs was "the fore part of the crura cerebri [cerebral peduncles], together with the [optic] tubercles,"[33] from which it was considered the optic and oculomotor nerves arose. These statements would seem to constitute a perceptive analysis of a reflex arc, and the following comment by Mayo might be thought to elaborate further the basic reflex mechanism described by Procháska by means of a specific example, the light reflex: "An influence may be propagated from the sentient nerves of a part, to their correspondent nerves of motion, through the intervention of that part alone of the nervous centre, to which they are mutually attached."[34]

Although Mayo also described this phenomenon in his much-respected textbook of physiology,[35] it was infrequently referred to and seems to have had little influence at the time, due presumably to the fact that he did not associate it with reflex action per se, and believed that the contraction and dilation of the iris was a volitional act that had become involuntary. Another factor responsible for the lack of impact made by Mayo's findings was, no doubt, Marshall Hall's denunciation of his interpretations and the bitter feud between the two men that followed.[36] Mayo's discovery, nevertheless, played a role in the evolution of brain localization theory, as we shall discover later (chap. 6.4.1).

We should also note that the possibility of the vegetative or "sympathetic" (autonomic) nervous system controlling the reflexes, considered as sympathetic actions, was favored by some. It had been put forward by Unzer and others, and on the basis of experimental and clinical observations, Jean Louis Brachet (1789–1858) gave it support in 1830.[37] He proposed a special neural arrangement whereby vegetative, in addition to somatic, nerves provided communications necessary for sympathetic responses, in the form of circles of nerves and by other means. It accounted for a wide variety of bodily functions, and to some degree Brachet was correct, for reflexes exclusive to the vegetative nervous system were shown later in the nineteenth century to be of crucial importance in the execution of autonomic activities (see chap. 7.8). But he erred when he extended his system to include in it reflex action involved with generation, excretion, and secretion, as Marshall Hall was soon to point out.[38]

Meantime, a very much more significant discovery had been made. In 1811, Charles Bell had related to a small number of individuals by means of a privately printed monograph how he had found that the anterior spinal cord roots and the cerebrum, with which he considered they were directly connected by fibers, possessed both motor and sensory functions. The posterior roots, however, were concerned with the "secret," that is, autonomic and involuntary, activities of the body. As it seemed to him possible to trace the posterior roots through the spinal cord to the cerebellum, it followed that the latter was the organ for vital and unconscious actions, as Thomas Willis had argued a century and a half earlier (chap. 6.6.2). It is important to realize that in 1811 Bell was not interested primarily in the properties of the spinal roots, but was using them in an attempt to prove that the cerebrum and cerebellum had specific but quite different, functions. Operatively they were easier to approach than intracranial structures, and the results of the two experiments he carried out on the spinal roots led him to believe that he had achieved his objective. Bell could now reason that: "The spinal nerves being double, and having their roots in the spinal marrow, of which a portion comes from the cerebrum and a portion from the cerebellum, they convey the attributes of both grand divisions of the brain to every part."[39] Of crucial importance in respect of his future references to the outcome of this investigation is the fact that although in 1811 Bell claimed the anterior roots had motor functions, he made no reference to the posterior roots having sensory attributes.

For eleven years this topic remained unexplored, until in 1822 Magendie, probably unaware of Bell's studies, proved conclusively that the anterior roots were indeed motor but the posterior were sensory.[40] Thus began the celebrated Bell-Magendie priority polemic, accounts of which are numerous.[41] It is now widely accepted that although Bell made the first experimental observations on spinal root properties, his claims for full priority cannot be allowed, for two reasons. First, his pioneer, but sole, investigation was incomplete and the results he obtained did not warrant the conclusions deduced, which in any case were mainly erroneous. Second, and of much more sinister significance, is the damning evidence against Bell that, in an attempt to establish his leadership, he dishonestly appropriated Magendie's correct opinions and in the light of them deceitfully emended his own earlier publications before reprinting them to support his case.[42] Not only did Bell now assert that it was he who had first differentiated correctly between the spinal roots, but he also changed his position concerning brain functions, as we shall discuss below (chap. 6.4.1 and 4). The cerebrum was now considered to be the seat of voluntary movements only and the cerebellum the center for sensation. Cerebellar control over "secret" bodily processes received little further mention by Bell.

This unsavory squabble, echoes of which exist today, need not detain us, and we should only note that Magendie's experimental findings were fully confirmed by Johannes Müller in 1831.[43] Magendie's revelation, backed by Bell and Müller, further elucidated the sensory and motor path traversed by reflex activity, and in addition the existence of motor and sensory tracts in the spinal cord, and their role in the reflex now became a possibility. Throughout the 1820s, however, no new studies of the reflex were undertaken, and Bell's notion of a "nervous circle," although suggestive by name, was concerned with the muscle's dual nerve supply, both motor and sensory, and not with the reflex.[44] The afferent and efferent routes for the spinal reflex had been identified, but the central mechanism, whereby the centripetal impression was transformed into a centrifugal impulse, remained a mystery. This was to continue for some time, and there were even some who were willing to accept the fact that nature could never be fully comprehended by man, and that the central transformation was probably conducted by an immaterial principle. Solly, who was very far from being a theorist given to wild speculation, declared, when commenting on the state of affairs in 1836, that in the spinal cord occurred "some phenomenon the intimate nature of which we can never know, as in all probability it does not depend on any physical change, but from which resulted the contraction of the muscles."[45]

The obscure and occult nature of the process had already been referred to by Magendie, and on the basis of Legallois's findings, as well as his own identification of the functions of spinal cord roots and columns, he conjectured that there should be a "most secret sanctuary" in the center of the spinal cord, where messages were converted from sensory to motor.[46] Characteristically, however, Magendie was unwilling to accept such a supposition, because irritating the center of the cord produced neither sensation nor motion and he was averse to advancing a hypothesis without experimental support. The problem, therefore, remained unsolved, by the only method then available to him.

There was, of course, considerable knowledge of the macroscopical anatomy of the spinal cord, but this area of research was as impotent as experimental physiology. A knowledge of the cord's microscopical structure was needed, but in the 1820s and 1830s this was negligible, the small amount available being mostly both contradictory and confusing. This topic, which is an extension of chapter 3, will be discussed later in the present chapter. It was not until the 1840s that investigators began to sort out the microscopical complexities of the cord, the most outstanding pioneer being Benedikt Stilling, whose research led him to the conclusion already noted, that the central gray matter was "not only the anatomical, but the actual physiological core of the spinal cord."[47] By means of Stilling's "anatomical physiology," these studies had an influence on notions of spinal cord function, particularly the spinal reflex (see chap. 3.5.2), as well as initiating a line of investigation that would lead eventually to the elucidation of Magendie's "secret sanctuary" (see 4.6 below).

So far, Legallois, Magendie, Bell, Mayo, and others had provided a gross morphologic basis for the spinal reflex, but although the weight of evidence seemed in their favor, opposition was soon apparent. Countering this mechanistic approach (the main proponent of which was Marshall Hall as we shall soon see) were individuals who insisted on a psychological, or even metaphysical, dimension. They contested the strict separation of motor and sensory functions in the cord, and they argued that if this were possible, it could only occur if there were two individual souls, rather than one. In 1842, an anonymous writer attacked this view, asserting: "Then clearly there are points in the nervous system where they [sensation and movements] pass over into each other . . . obviously it is the same soul that both feels and moves."[48] Nevertheless, in the first three decades of the nineteenth century the postulated phenomenon of sympathy as an explanation for reflex action was still very much in evidence. As Ruth Fried (neé Leys) has pointed out,[49] there were many at that time who preferred the doctrines of Whytt and other eighteenth-century scientists, founded as they were on the immaterial nature of the central governing process which in Whytt's case was the "sentient principle."

This attitude was adopted by William Pultney Alison (1790–1859), who held the chair in the University of Edinburgh previously occupied by Whytt, and Fried has discussed his arguments in detail.[50] He was a vitalist, humoralist, and antimaterialist, and in 1826 he was the main defender of Whytt's opinions. In opposition to the purely morphological approach of his opponents, Alison insisted that sympathetic responses, that is, reflexes, depended on the mind or sensation and could not be accounted for in terms of anatomical pathways in the nervous system. As already noted, the latter were thought to be anastomoses between peripheral nerves, an idea originating with Willis, and still widely accepted at the beginning of the nineteenth century, particularly on the Continent. In essence, Alison was perpetuating the vitalistic views of his predecessor and in so doing he disputed the mechanistic concepts of anatomists such as Charles Bell. But, unlike Whytt, he believed that sensation must be equated with consciousness. According to him and to others like him, sensation was the chief factor in the production of sympathetic, that is, reflex, activity. Alison also contested Bell's theory of respiratory nerves, which included all nerves associated with the instinctive or involuntary movements of respiration, including speaking, singing, coughing, and sneezing. He was unable to accept these mechanical explanations, and he preferred instead to postulate sympathetic responses.[51]

However, his notions, like Bell's doctrine of the respiratory nerves, did not survive.

Concerning Willis's sympathetic action by means of nerve anastomoses, Andrea Comparetti (1746–1801) in 1780 had devoted a whole monograph to an explanation of how morbid consensual phenomena could be produced by these connections,[52] which we should point out must not be compared with present day synaptic communications between nerve cells (for the cell-fiber debate, see chap. 3.5). Willis's opinions were accepted widely, and as late as 1825, Friedrich Tiedemann, an outstanding anatomist, revitalized Willis's original doctrine.[53] The revival was however, short-lived, because microscopists were soon to discover that the joining of nerve fibers by anastomoses appeared to be very rare.[54] Moreover, physiologists could demonstrate unequivocally that the excitation in nerve fibers passing through a supposed anastomosis remained confined to these fibers and did not pass over into others.[55] On the whole, the evidence they presented was not convincing, and further knowledge of the microscopical and electrophysiological aspects of nerve fibers soon led to the elimination forever of the Willisian concept. The focus of attention then turned fully to the central nervous system.

It was against this background of debates over the merits of explaining sympathetic (reflex) action on the basis of anatomical or mechanistic factors, or by means of theories involving immaterial principles and sensation that the next significant advance in the physiology of the reflex took place. From it evolved the modern concept of reflex action.

4.4. MARSHALL HALL: 1832 TO 1857

If Whytt and Procháska were the outstanding physiologists of the reflex in the second half of the eighteenth century, Marshall Hall deserves this epithet in the first half of the nineteenth.[56] His labors led to the evolution of the reflex concept from a physiological phenomenon to a biological principle, recognized as a fundamental and essential feature of nervous activity, and destined to become eventually a basic component of neurophysiological thought.

In order fully to comprehend Hall's relations with the medical and scientific community of early Victorian Britain and on the Continent, in order to assess the reception his work received, and to judge its merits, we must take note of his personality. He was a man of small stature but immense conceit.[57] He was aggressive, quarrelsome, and of a rebellious nature, and he demonstrated excessive possessiveness concerning his discoveries. Yet he lacked all insight into his failings and was never able to understand why, "from the very first moment he published his great discovery of the excito-motory [reflex] system to the last days of his life, he was engaged in controversy," as a contemporary commented.[58] His vanity and self-esteem were unbounded, and he made it known that in the field of physiology, his research on the reflex had been equaled only by William Harvey on the circulation of the blood.[59] Moreover, he even took the trouble to compute the time he had spent on his research in order, presumably, to provide evidence of his industry and devotion to physiology and medicine, which in any case had never been in question.[60] The biography by Hall's widow provides us with an excellent source of information concerning his professional relationships.[61] It is an unstinted eulogy, with not a word of criticism, but with no understanding whatever of the reasons for "the biting blast of calumny, and the pelting hailstorm of the critics"[62] that her husband continually suffered. They shared a *folie-à-deux* mental state.

Although Hall managed to alienate most of his contemporaries, he was not entirely without friends. Thomas Henry Wakley (1795–1862), the controversial editor of the *Lancet,* praised Hall's work forcibly and eloquently, and belabored his enemies mercilessly.[63] Being equally abrasive and polemical, Wakley no doubt recognized a kindred spirit, but the support he gave Hall, for example, in a controversy with the Royal Society was also part of an attack on the alleged corruption and backwardness of that institution and of the medical profession at the time. Others in Britain also praised Hall, and according to Mrs. Hall, they included John Hughes Bennett (1812–1875), William Budd (1811–1880), Frederick Le Gros Clark (1811–1892), Michael Faraday (1791–1867), Richard Grainger, and a certain "Dr. Watson."[64] Foreigners who had little or no contact with Hall, other than by way of his writings, could make a more objective assessment of his work, and eminent physiologists, such as Johannes Müller, Pierre Flourens, and Izaak van Deen (1804–1869) praised it. The way in which Hall repeated in his publications these and other laudatory comments, indicates his insecurity and a constant need for approbation. He likewise frequently reiterated his own evaluation of his labor, one example being the following: "this [reflex] system, as a system, I consider as having been entirely elicited by my own laborious and persevering researches."[65] Hall was continually on the defensive, and he evinced a paranoia that impelled him continually to establish and defend the merit and priority of his disclosures in the field of reflex physiology. Thus, his publications are voluminous, repetitive, and tediously vituperative. But they are also of great importance, for despite the unfortunate personality traits just enumerated, Hall possessed matchless ingenuity and a clarity and originality of thought.

The main advances made by Marshall Hall in the field of "reflex action," as he termed it, can be readily surveyed. On 27 November 1832 he presented a preliminary report to the Zoological Society of London,[66] and in it he explained that "there is a property of the sentient and motor system of nerves which is independent of sensation and volition;—a property of motor nerves independent of immediate irritation."[67] This property presided over reflex movements and those that were partly voluntary and partly involuntary, such as respiration, sneezing, vomiting, and tickling, as well as having a role in morbid states. The detailed account of his investigations was communicated to the Royal Society on 13 June 1833,[68] and in it he defined his aim. It was to investigate "a principle of action in the animal economy, which has not hitherto, I think, been distinguished with sufficient precision from the other vital and animal functions."[69] He claimed later, in 1841, that as the studies of Whytt, Procháska, and others had not led to the establishment of reflex activity as a basic biological precept, he had set himself the laudable task of achieving this objective.[70] However, Hall was writing with hindsight, because in 1833 he made no reference to Procháska, an omission that was to have serious consequences for him later.

But he did take into account the contributions of his other predecessors, who had investigated spinal cord function, such as Legallois and Flourens, and was also aware of certain reports on the motor activity of anencephalics. Hall was especially influenced by Legallois's findings, even though he pronounced them faulty, stating that reflex action had been wrongly confounded with sensation and voluntary movements, an interpretation in keeping with the components of his special reflex system, but one that we would reject. There were, he announced, three specific sources for muscle action: volition; the motor apparatus of respiration; and irritability. To these he added a fourth, distinct principle, "to which I have ventured to give the designation of *the reflex*."[71] This was the first use in English of the substantive, "the reflex," in a biological sense.[72] Another etymological innovation occurred in the same article. Hall explained how the reflex operated by way of the spinal cord, which he denied was a mere bundle of transmitting nerves, and how it pursued a reflected course through it from the peripheral part of the body that had been stimulated, to the part moved by "nerves, which constitute the arc of the reflex function."[73] The term "reflex arc" was particularly appropriate and proved to be immediately popular, unlike Bell's "nervous circle," which as noted was concerned not with reflex action, but with muscle sense, the existence of which Hall denied.

Despite his persistent claims of originality, which we would accept, some of his contemporaries thought that apart from introducing the useful epithet "arc" for the morphological basis of reflex action, and the presentation of better experimental evidence that allowed him to distinguish more clearly between reflex and other motor activities, he had not progressed much beyond Procháska. This was a forewarning of impending allegations against him of plagiarism by those who denounced his incessant efforts to promote as his own a phenomenon that had already been recognized by many.[74] This attitude was reflected by Sherrington in 1902, when he admitted: "But, altogether, I could not see any real difference between his [Marshall Hall's] views of movements of headless animal, &c., and those of many of his predecessors, Hales, Whytt, Prochaska, and even Descartes."[75] Hall, however, would have been quick to counter this criticism, by pointing out that the 1833 paper accounted for only a small part of his research on reflex action.

These censures, both contemporary and later, belittled Hall's reflex system, which, in 1833, was in its simplest form, but which he was to elaborate and extend over the next twenty-three years. In fact, his doctrine was of considerable importance, because it emphasized the purely mechanistic basis that had been hinted at by Legallois, Bell, Mayo, and others; and moreover because it vigorously contested the incorporation into the reflex concept of immaterial principles like the "sentient principle," *vis nervosa,* and *sensorium commune* of eighteenth-century physiologists, and the vitalistic processes of Alison and his followers. Hall is, therefore, to be commended for exorcising these deterrents to scientific research, so often employed as mere hypotheses to cloak ignorance. Also, Hall extended the role of reflexes by pointing out that they presided over and maintained the "tone" of the sphincters, as well as being concerned in acts such as swallowing, vomiting, and sneezing. He studied the action of drugs on the reflex and predicted correctly its use in the elucidation of pharmacological problems. Above all he insisted on the fundamental significance of reflex activity in the animal organism, by declaring that all muscular system function, other than that owing to volition, respiration, or irritability, and excluding cardiac action, were dependent on it. His attempts, however, to apply the reflex to disorders of the nervous system achieved little. But he, at least, had the idea of doing so, and this for the first time. Many of his proposals may seem to us archaic and patently erroneous, but unfortunately for Hall they were dependent upon clinical neurology and morbid anatomy, which at the time were still in a primitive state. The significant point here was his wish to expand further a scheme that, with reasonable justification, he judged to be of wide relevance in the diseased as well as the healthy nervous system of human beings.

This was the first presentation of Hall's doctrine, and after 1833 his mission was to substantiate and elaborate it. In doing so he exhibited his characteristic traits: a consummate pride in his achievement; exaggerated claims and pathological possessiveness; vituperative attacks on all who opposed him; and repeated accounts of his scheme, spread through many publications. In 1836 he developed his reflex system further, in a series of lectures, by first dividing the nervous system into three functional units: the cerebral, or the sentient and voluntary; the true spinal, or the excito-motory, that is reflex; and the ganglionic, or the nutrient, the secretory, and the like.[76] It is the second of these, the excito-motory system, that must now engage our attention. Hall considered this to be his main discovery, and he wrote about it for the rest of his life, defending it vigorously and repeatedly against many critics, and continuing jealously to guard his priority. We need not follow this tedious progression, because the basic nature of the scheme did not alter much over the years, although he continued to accumulate further evidence in support of it, and to invent outlandish terms to describe it.

The 1833 report was enlarged, and on the sixteenth and twenty-third of February and the second of March of the following year, Hall read another paper before the Royal Society.[77] On this occasion, however, publication in the *Philosophical Transactions* was refused, and thus began a conflict with the Society that was to continue for the remainder of his life.[78] Hall, a Fellow of five years' standing, was unable to comprehend how such an important piece of research could be denied its rights, and the manner in which he compulsively, vindictively, and relentlessly pursued what he considered to be a personal injustice is well illustrated by a letter he wrote to the President-elect of the Royal Society eleven years later.[79] In it he attacked the Society and certain individuals for their role in the affair,[80] but he could not resist extolling his own virtues by claiming that, "My labours have, I hesitate not to say, issued in a discovery, the extent and value of which is without parallel in modern physiological science."[81] The Society's action has never been fully explained, but it seems likely that Hall's paper was judged to be no longer an entirely original communication, because he had already included much of its new material in his lectures published in 1836. Hall would not have accepted this explanation, for his suspicions and paranoia led him to believe that malign forces were ranged against him in the form of certain individuals' hostility, and well there might have been among lesser men of petty and envious nature. The Royal Society in the 1830s was not, however, the respected body it is today, and further investigation of its administration at that time may reveal the background to Hall's conflict with it. Be this as it may, he was unable to publish any further papers in the *Transactions,* and was denied any of the several honors and awards of the Society, an outcome that must have embittered him even more.

In 1837, Hall suffered a further setback. This was the publication in January of Alison's anonymous and destructive review of Hall's *Lectures* of 1836.[82] It has been described as a turning point in Hall's career, for in it Alison supported Whytt's doctrine, and claimed that Hall's system had been anticipated by it.[83] As mentioned above, Alison had already defended Whytt in 1826, and now he became Hall's leading opponent, attempting to prevent his demolition of the theory of sympathetic actions and the overthrow of Whytt's teachings. The review incited great interest not only in whether Hall's notions were correct, but of more sinister import, whether they were entirely original.

Probably as a result of this reaction, Hall was now beset by his most serious adversity. Not to be outdone by the Royal Society's rebuff, in 1837 he published the declined paper, together with a reprint of his 1833 article, in a monograph entitled *Memoirs on the Nervous System.*[84] It was at this point that the allegation of plagiarism was made against him, an event that was to become one of the best known episodes in Hall's tempestuous career.[85] The possibility had probably existed since 1833 in the minds of those who disliked him and who hoped that an accusation of this nature aimed at his character and integrity would damage his reputation severely, perhaps irreparably. The claim was that Hall had plagiarized Procháska's book of 1784.[86] It was, of course, inevitable that some of Hall's statements made in 1833 would be similar to Procháska's, but the fact that he did not refer to him seemed to lend support to the charge. There were, however, many original statements in it, together with unique opinions quite unlike those of Procháska. We can, in retrospect, judge Hall's antagonists by suggesting that with the help of his research the work of Procháska could be viewed in a new light and thus came to appear as similar—even as an anticipation—of Hall's. We need not, however, be concerned with the details of this somewhat sordid controversy. Again with hindsight, it appears to have been characterized by personal enmities and rivalries, vindictiveness, pettiness, jealousy, and political undertones.[87] It helps mainly to highlight the personality traits of Hall, and the contemporary state of the medical profession.[88] It does not, however, alter our assessment of Marshall Hall's contribution to reflex physiology.

In his *Memoirs* of 1837 Hall described his doctrine of reflex action that was to remain unchanged, except for minor modifications, additional confirmatory experimental and clinical evidence, and a name, "the diastaltic nervous system," provided by him in the late 1840s to describe the physiological activity of the spinal cord.[89] His diastaltic system was made up of the "true spinal marrow," extending from the quadrigeminal bodies to the cauda equina and composed of "excito-motory," that is, afferent-efferent nerves that were concerned exclusively with reflex action. This diastaltic or excito-motory system was quite distinct from, and in no way concerned with, sensation and voluntary movements, muscle irritability, or with the operations of the mind or of any other activities of the brain. Hall had already concluded that the movements of decapitated animals and anencephalic monsters induced by noxious stimuli were responses dependent on a principle that was entirely different from either sensation or volition, and he therefore found it necessary to evolve an entirely separate nervous system mechanism to accommodate its unique properties. He objected to Unzer's "afferent" and "efferent," and preferred "incident" and "reflex," respectively, as in the optical sense,[90] but like the many other expressions Hall proposed, they have not survived in medical terminology. But he planned to make sure that his reflex system would endure, and that it was inseparably associated with his name, by describing it repeatedly. The following appeared in a lecture of 1842:

> The true-spinal system consists of a series of nerves passing principally from the cutaneous surface, and the surface of mucous membranes, to the spinal marrow; and other series of nerves passing from the spinal marrow to a series of muscles, destined to be moved simultaneously. The former, thence designated the *incident* nerves; the latter, *reflex* nerves: the spinal marrow is their common *centre*.[91]

The spinal "cord" contained the spinal "marrow," by virtue of which it possessed a nervous force, and the notion of the spinal cord as a conducting cable without inherent function was thereby eliminated.

Hall's diastaltic system of spinal marrow and peripheral spinal nerve pathways was thought to be morphologically, as well as functionally, distinct, but he had no anatomical evidence either gross or microscopical to substantiate this. He seems to have been dismissive of anatomical studies, and, declaring that he was concerned not with mere tissues but with organs and phenomena, with physiological experiments, not with the dissection and tracing of fibers, he preferred to leave to others the task of delineating the system's nervous pathways.[92] We shall discuss below the early phases of the search for the anatomical basis of Hall's reflex system (4.6 below). There is a parallel here with Bell's system of respiratory nerves, the existence of which was disputed by Hall. In each case, an hypothesis based more on function than on morphology had been projected, and each scheme provided a purely mechanistic explanation of the phenomenon under consideration.

Whether Hall was indebted in any way to Bell's notion is not known, but he could have employed in his arguments the law of specific nerve energies that had been established by Johannes Müller in 1826.[93] If it were true that there existed specific nerves for specific functions, could there not also be special nerves devoted only to reflex action? Further aspects of Hall's system, whereby he eschewed all psychical processes and avoided completely the complexities of sensation, thus eliminating problems that had bedeviled earlier investigations, made his doctrine attractive to those who, toward the middle of the nineteenth century preferred a mechanical and materialistic explanation for biological phenomena. This approach, however, incurred the criticisms of Alison and his fellow vitalists, but whereas their arguments are now forgotten, many of Hall's ideas have been absorbed into the reflex physiology accepted today.

The excito-motory system was also considered to control the body's orifices and, as mentioned above, the sphincters guarding them, "in *all* acts of ingestion and egestion."[94] Thus, it was on duty day and night, keeping the sphincteric muscles contracted. As noted, Hall had refuted Bell's "nervous circle" and the associated concept of muscle sense. In fact he denied that muscles had sensory nerves of any kind. It follows that his concept of muscle "tone" could not, therefore, have been the reflex tone that we accept today, and which is dependent upon the afferent fibers of a muscle acting on its efferent fibers. Hall's experiments gave no proof of tone as we understand it, but he conceived of sphincteric "tone" arising from reflex action, whereas we know that it is myogenic in origin. Respiration was also part of the excito-motory action and under the control of appropriate excitor nerves.

The overall view of reflex activity conceived by Marshall Hall was a significant landmark in the advancement of neurophysiology. He insisted that his system allowed a classification of a wide variety of experimental facts, as well as physiological, pathological, and pharmacological phenomena.[95] By means of this basic doctrine, he believed that he was in a position to reinterpret almost every aspect of the nervous system, in health and in disease, and this in part accounts for his voluminous writings.[96] Although these efforts mostly lacked success, Hall was at least broadening the concept of the reflex, and preparing the way for its acceptance as a fundamental principle of nervous system action. The full scope of the reflex concept was only realized when some of the rigid restrictions Hall had placed upon its application had been overcome.

Hall was careful to show preference to those physiologists who produced experimental data favoring his doctrine, and to applaud their findings.[97] Thus, Flourens, in opposition to Legallois, by placing the seat of sensation in the cerebral hemispheres[98] (see chap. 6.4) and by identifying the spinal cord as the center of excitability and the sympathies or reflexes,[99] received Hall's approval. In return he was awarded the sort of compliment he desperately sought: "Your beautiful system of excitatory nerves, incident and reflex, rightly belongs to you . . . a noble and novel harmony of phenomena."[100] A few individuals gave Hall unsolicited praise, such as Grainger, who was devoted to him: "I am convinced *you* have discovered a *grand principle,* the greatest, I believe, that has *ever yet* been announced; and so I have publicly stated."[101] Those who were at variance with him, however, were castigated mercilessly, and this was the case with Procháska, when Hall eventually made reference to his work. Concerning him, Hall in 1843 commented that "it is impossible to adduce specimens of more complete confusion."[102] However, this may have been part of his response to the plagiarism charge—an attempt to belittle his alleged source. The case of Herbert Mayo is also interesting in this regard, for while attacking him Hall did not refer, other than in a few words, to his significant account of the arc of the pupillary reflex,[103] presumably because Hall denied all possibility of reflexes operating by way of the brain.

4.4.1. Summary

We can set aside Marshall Hall's personality traits, which colored most contemporary attempts to assess his contribution to reflex theory, and judge him retrospectively. It is certain that his introduction of the noun "reflex," like Waldeyer's invention of "neuron" (see chap. 3.6), was itself a simple, but extremely important event. A concept thus became a tangible entity rather than a curious event obfuscated by archaic notions and terminology. His use of "reflex arc" also helped to identify and define a phenomenon that previously had lacked precise form.

One of the most appealing aspects of Hall's doctrine was undoubtedly his claim that it had application both to the normal and abnormal nervous system. Ever since the ancient Greeks, the creation of a system that would bring together disparate biological or medical facts had always been attractive. Every era has had its schemes, ranging from the theory of humors to the eighteenth-century nosologists, and each provided an apparent precision, and thus a spurious solace, in place of a chaos of data. If the system allowed a classification of information, as

Hall's did, it was even more acceptable. We now know that, like other classifiers, his claims were farfetched, and that some of his enthusiastic attempts to attribute certain bodily processes to reflex action were later shown to be incorrect, as in the case of activities now known to be biochemical in nature (e.g., those regulated by hormones). Understandably, others, too, fell into this error, especially when studying functions of the gastrointestinal tract, such as the outpouring of digestive juices or the coordination of visceral action. Hall's efforts to enunciate a general physiological and pathological principle was much to his credit, but the neurological system that he formulated was not his first attempt to provide one, because before his research on the reflex began, he endeavored, without success, to relate respiration to muscle irritability.[104] Nevertheless, despite Hall's misplaced fervor and his unwarranted extrapolations, his opinion concerning the fundamental significance of the reflex has been amply justified, for we now appreciate that it is probably the most salient component of the nervous system. Moreover, the twentieth century has seen the foundation of two schools of neurophysiology based on it: the Sherringtonian in the West, and the Pavlovian in Russia. In the field of clinical neurology, the reflex concept as interpreted and applied by Hall to diseases of the nervous system was also to be singularly valuable. Even though his deductions were often erroneous, they added a new dimension to neurological study, and contributed significantly to the advancement of the discipline. It seems, for example, that the demand for a special hospital in London, devoted to patients suffering from paralysis and epilepsy, eventually the National Hospital in Queen Square, was in part stimulated by Hall's labors and his active campaign promoting this cause.

The "diastaltic nervous system" is now long forgotten, but Marshall Hall, despite his many faults, has an honored place in the history of the reflex concept. He opened a new era in its evolution, not only by means of the intellect, industry, and persistence that he displayed in championing the reflex, but also by the animosity and polemics that he stirred up while doing so. He stimulated a new interest in the experimental elucidation of the reflex. He revealed a much wider application of reflex action than anyone before him had guessed possible, he illustrated his theories and observations by clinical examples with greater astuteness and clarity than even Whytt had displayed, and his insistence on the cerebrospinal axis as a segmental series confirmed and established previous notions, leading eventually to modern views. However, Marshall Hall always maintained that his greatest contribution to the field of neurophysiology, and the one of which he was proudest, was the proposal of a unique spinal cord subsystem, the excito-motory, anatomically and functionally distinct from the rest of the nervous system, and he repeated this claim tediously in his publications. It is, therefore, ironic that the most cherished part of his life's work did not survive.

A remarkable assessment of Marshall Hall will be cited here to sum up his achievements. It was made by David Ferrier (1843–1928), like Hall an eminent physiologist, clinician, and pathologist, and who was never guilty of bestowing false praise:

> I know no name in the ranks of scientific medical inquiry, in this or in any other country, which stands higher than that of Marshall Hall, and no work which has done more to advance physiology and pathology of the nervous system, and not this only, but medicine and surgery in general, than his investigations into the nature and conditions of reflex action. This he was undoubtedly the first to formulate and expound, and clear from the vagueness and confusion which prevailed before him. The importance of his researches can scarcely be overestimated.[105]

There is no doubt that Hall subscribed importantly to the movement away from the nebulous notions of soul and other immaterial principles and toward an explanation for reflex action based on anatomy and the unique functions of the spinal cord. This in essence was Marshall Hall's contribution to reflex physiology.

4.5. THE EXTENSION OF HALL'S WORK: CEREBRAL REFLEXES

4.5.1. Early German Contributions

Hall's writings excited great interest abroad, especially in Germany and France. As noted, Flourens acclaimed his system, and Hall was also gratified by the independent studies of Johannes Müller, who reached certain conclusions similar to his own. Like Hall's, they were reported in 1833,[106] but Müller later graciously awarded priority to Hall.[107] Although he was mostly in accord with Hall and claimed that their research showed "striking agreement,"[108] Müller differed on a number of important points, in particular, on the interpretation of his results.[109] Thus, he had a view similar to Hall of the components of the reflex arc: namely, sensation, volition (*Wille*), and motion, but volition, he thought, could be in the brain as well as in the spinal cord, whereas Hall permitted only the cord and medulla oblongata to take part in reflex action. Müller enunciated a law, that he contended was of the greatest importance to both physiology and pathology:

> When sensations produced by external stimuli acting on sensory nerves bring about movements in other parts this is never due to a reciprocal action between sensory and motor fibers, but by the sensory excitation acting on the brain and spinal cord and from these traveling back to the motor fibers.[110]

But Müller no doubt partially pleased Hall by stating: "The spinal marrow has the ability to reflect sensory irritations to the motor nerves. It is a reflector."[111] How this came about, he had no idea, but he believed that other parts of the cord some distance from the segment involved by the initial sensory impression could take part. In fact, he denied that the reflex took place through a single cord segment. Furthermore, in Hall's system, true sensation played no part, whereas Müller considered that in the intact animal it did, and by way of the brain or spinal cord. In the absence of the brain, a skin stimulus passed to the cord in the form of the nerve principle (see chap. 5.4.7), but it did not excite true sensation there. In Müller's view the events were as follows.

> According to my opinion, the stimulation of a sensory spinal nerve first of all brings about a centripetal action of the nerve principle, which goes to the spinal cord. If it can reach the sensorium commune it is a conscious sensation. If it cannot reach the sensorium commune because the spinal cord has been transected, it exerts its whole force as a centripetal action on the cord. In each case a centripetal action of a sensory nerve can bring about a reflex movement. In the first case, it produces at the same time sensation, but in the second it does not, but it is sufficient for the production of reflex movement, or centrifugal reflexion.[112]

Müller, therefore, could not agree that all reflex action occurred without true sensation, and moreover, reflexes like sneezing and coughing were actually invoked by it. Finally, he was unwilling to accept Hall's excito-motory system, and he did not exclude completely the possibility of a psychical component in reflex action, the exclusion of which was an essential feature of Hall's doctrines. The roots of Müller's divergence from Hall in his idea of the reflex will be discussed presently. But despite their differences in interpretation, Hall and Müller each helped to establish the reflex as a vital biological property, and they each advertised the other's opinions. For Hall, this was especially valuable in view of Müller's immense reputation as the most respected physiologist of his day.

Other Germans also entered the field of reflex physiology. Among them was A. W. Volkmann, who in 1838[113] found himself in agreement with Müller's conclusions, and like him disputed Hall's views that the mind and sensation were not involved in reflex action. He inclined to the opinion of Whytt that the motions consequent upon sensory impressions were the result of sensations carried to the *sensorium* giving rise to appropriate spontaneous reactions. Also in accordance with Müller, he rejected the existence of a special excito-motory system, and he insisted that the spinal cord had sensory functions. Volkmann's views upon the contentious psychical component of the reflex are discussed below. We may note here, however, that after originally embracing the notion of a "spinal cord soul" that presided (at least in lower vertebrates) over reflex action, Volkmann eventually took the view that:

> Despite the extraordinary appropriateness of the former [reflex movements], which not infrequently are apparently adapted to chance circumstances . . . the degree of regularity they possess is such that the assumption of psychical guidance does not arise.[114]

He, thus, had concluded that the evidence so far available did not constitute proof for the existence of a psychical spinal cord function, or spinal cord soul, that later in the century became a controversial issue.[115] In view of the numerous speculations abroad at that time and later concerning the possible role of the soul, consciousness, volition, attention, sensation, perception, and other mental elements of reflex action, Volkmann's statement exhibited admirable scientific reserve. At the same time, he refuted[116] a theory of reflex action advanced by Johann Wilhelm Arnold (1801–1873), that required the participation of an unconscious psychical property, or soul, in the spinal cord.[117]

A further aspect of Volkmann's research was summarized by his statement of 1838: "The extent of the reflex movement depends principally on the strength of the stimulus and on the degree of the excitability."[118] Thus, the less the irritability, the more limited would be the reflex movement, the intensity of the stimulus remaining the same. Müller had made analogous comments:

> excitation transmitted to the spinal cord affects the motor nerves which arise nearest to its root of entry, and the irritation of the cord and its motor nerves decreases in proportion to the distance from that point.[119]

Richard Grainger in Britain had also arrived at this conclusion. It was likewise noted by Arnold that the quality, intensity, and location of a stimulus were important factors in the type of reflex response elicited.[120] These and other observations indicate that once the basic concept of reflex action had been accepted, physiologists began to examine the various factors that influenced it, and with greater precision and improved techniques they were able to commence the task of carefully defining each of the reflex's characteristics, an assignment that continues today. At mid-nineteenth century, the German school of physiology was taking over the lead in research on the reflex and Germans were to dominate the field until the last two decades of the century, when British physiologists again became supreme owing to the remarkable studies of C. S. Sherrington and the school he founded.[121] The center of gravity of reflex physiology had returned to Britain.

4.5.2. The Development of the Concept of Cerebral Reflexes

Within a remarkably short time after the publication of Hall's theories, the reflex concept had become the subject of much investigation and speculation in Germany. In Britain, too, despite the hostility that Hall's writings elicited in some quarters, physiologists like William Carpenter and Richard Grainger took up his ideas in their own work. It would, however, be misleading to regard all of these early studies in reflex physiology as mere developments of Hall's ideas; in some instances they went beyond and explicitly opposed certain aspects of Hall's own version of the reflex concept. Indeed, Wilhelm Griesinger in 1843 declared that in the light of the research of German scientists, "the more recent work of M. Hall (On the diseases etc. 1841) certainly appears almost anachronistic."[122]

Hall was anachronistic, Griesinger alleged, because he clung to the notion of a separate excito-motory system independent of the cerebrospinal and the vegetative (autonomic) nerves; this absolute separation was as unjustified on anatomical as on physiological and pathological grounds.[123] Griesinger's remarks highlight the fact that even those contemporaries who appreciated the immense potential of the reflex concept believed that Hall's theory contained weaknesses as well as strengths. Indeed, what were from one viewpoint strengths were from another limitations. The following discussion considers how certain physiologists in Germany and Britain sought to overcome what they saw as the excessively restrictive nature of Hall's idea of the reflex and to extend the concept to a much wider range of physiological and psychological phenomena than Hall had contemplated.

We do not claim that these individuals formed a "school" in the usual sense of the word. Although certain of the men we shall discuss knew of one another's works (for example, Carpenter modified his ideas in the light of the findings of Thomas Laycock [1812–1876]), others worked independently and within divergent research traditions. What we do claim is that all these scientists drew upon similar conceptual resources in extending the scope of the reflex to the brain. The most striking instance of this is the way in which Laycock and Griesinger arrived at the same conclusion by parallel paths and yet independently. This suggests that the usual criteria for seeking cohesion in the activities of individual workers (shared teachers, a common institutional setting, personal contacts) are not always adequate for the understanding of shared strategies and goals. In addition, the possible existence of an apportioned philosophical and scientific culture transcending local differences must be taken into account if the common elements in the work of disparate individuals are to be understood.

We noted above that a distinguishing feature of Hall's thought was his purely mechanistic concept of the reflex. According to Fried, in Hall's view the reflex "was a purely mechanical phenomenon entirely distinct from mind."[124] This mechanistic idea dispensed with the host of psychic, or quasi-psychic, entities previously invoked to account for the phenomena of reflex action and made possible a far greater theoretical clarity and precision than had been attained by Hall's predecessors. However, this elucidation was achieved at a cost; namely, the restriction of the reflex to a limited and sharply circumscribed range of functions. Hall held that reflex action was confined to the "true spinal cord"; that it did not obtain in any part of the cerebrospinal axis higher than the quadrigeminal bodies, and was entirely distinct from the other modes of nervous activity; in particular, it bore no relation to sensation or to voluntary motion.[125]

In short, Hall insisted upon an absolute bifurcation of the structures and the functions of the nervous system. He stated this sharp dichotomy between the "cerebral" and the "excito-motory" nervous systems most clearly in his 1837 *Memoirs:*

> 105. The functions of the cerebral system are,—sensation, perception, judgement, volition, voluntary motion. The sensations are conveyed to the cerebrum by the sentient nerves . . . ; the cerebrum itself may be viewed as the organ of mind,—that organ on which the *psyche* [in Greek characters], sits, as it were, enthroned; the voluntary nerves convey the mandates of the volition to the muscles which are to be called into action. All these functions are strictly *psychical.* They imply consciousness. Sensation without consciousness appears to me to be a contradiction in terms; the idea and the phraseology should be banished from physiology. . . .
> 107. How different from those which I have thus enumerated, are the functions which belong to the true spinal marrow! In these there is no sensation, no volition, no consciousness, nothing psychical. . . .
> 108. The true spinal system is independent of the cerebrum, and subsists when the cerebral lobes are removed. . . .
> 109. The cerebral system is the seat of the intellect; the true spinal marrow is, in an especial manner, the organ of the emotions and passions. It is on this part of the nervous system that the preservation of the individual and the continuation of the species depend.
> 110. The cerebral system connects us with the external world in everything

> that relates to sensation and volition, or mind; the true spinal system, is everything that relates to the appropriation of its materials, or their expulsion,—in everything that, in those respects, relates to nutrition and reproduction.[126]

Underlying this view of the structure and function of the nervous system was an implicit metaphysical doctrine. Fried has remarked that Hall, together with most of his British contemporaries, adhered to conventional dualist assumptions of the relation of the immaterial mind or soul to the nervous system and so to the rest of the body. Hall continued to uphold the doctrine that the soul could act upon the cerebrum to produce actions, and he had no intention of superseding this spiritualist model with a theory of cerebral reflexes.[127] What he did attempt to prove was the existence of an additional form of nervous function: as he wrote in 1837, "The reflex function appears . . . to be the complement of the functions of the nervous system hitherto known."[128]

The same dualism applied to physiological issues is apparent in the first volume of Todd and Bowman's textbook of 1845. There the nervous system was portrayed as the link between the mental and physical worlds. The authors conceded, however, that "the nervous system . . . can act independently of mental influence," and here they referred to Hall's concept of excito-motory movement.[129] There was no relation between the two classes of actions:

> The phenomena of Mind, even in their simplest degree of development, are so distinct from anything which observation teaches us to be produced by material agency, that we are bound to refer them to a cause different from that to which we refer the phenomena of living bodies. Although associated with the body by some unknown connecting link, the mind works quite independently of it; and, on the other hand, a large proportion of the bodily acts are independent of the mind.[130]

The inhibitory effects of theological prejudices upon scientific thought are apparent in such utterances. Todd and Bowman deferred to the religious sensibilities of their age when they piously declared: "The nature of the connexion between the mind and nervous matter has ever been, and must continue to be, the deepest mystery in physiology; and they who study the laws of Nature, as ordinances of God, will regard it as one of those secrets of his counsels 'which Angels desire to look into.'"[131] Hall's own piety is attested to by his widow, who records that as a physician in Nottingham he always traveled with "a Bible at his side, together with divers medical periodicals." She also revealed that Hall took a keen interest in a devotional work by George Wilkins (1785–

1865) called *Body and Soul* where the autonomy of the spiritual principle and its ability to act upon the body were affirmed.[132]

Hall's tacit transfer of his dualist assumptions to physiology can be seen as contributing to certain of the most positive aspects of his work. He was able to achieve the degree of simplification and clarity that he did in his studies of spinal reflexes precisely because he assumed that these were purely mechanical phenomena that bore no relation to mind, and that mental functions were therefore outside the scope of reflex theory. But the modern concept of the reflex is (at least in its extension) radically different from the schema with which Hall was content to rest. The reflex is not seen as one mode of nervous action among several others, but as the basal unit from which all other modes of nervous function are evolved. On this view the reflex cannot be confined to one limited portion of the nervous system—let alone to an autonomous system of its own; it must have application throughout the cerebrospinal axis, up to and including the cerebrum. It follows that mental function cannot be excluded from the scope of reflex theory, but must be seen as a further mode of reflex action.

This extended view of the relevance of the reflex to an understanding of the workings of the nervous system reached its fullest expression in the present century with the work of Sherrington and his followers on the side of the neuroscientists, and of Ivan Petrovich Pavlov (1849–1936), John Broadus Watson (1878–1958), and Burrhus Frederick Skinner (1904–) in experimental psychology. However, the roots of this unitary concept of nervous function are to be found in the mid-nineteenth century and were already present while Hall was still writing.

We have argued that Hall and most of his British contemporaries transferred the assumptions of dualist metaphysics to their physiological reasoning. Conversely, the most active proponents of achieving a unified view of nervous function by extending the application of the reflex tended to hold more monistic conceptions of the relation of mind to body. In particular, the ramifications of trends in early nineteenth-century German philosophy extended into this as into other areas of neuroscience.

Gode-von Aesch has underlined a fundamental urge that pervaded the romantic conception of nature: "the metaphysical craving for a complete integration of man into the natural order of things."[133] As noted in chapter 2.1, at one level this goal was pursued by comparative anatomical studies designed to show the unity underlying apparent disparities between human and animal structure. However, "the most serious obstacle in the path of such an integration was the fact that man possessed an organ which had not been found in animals. This was his soul."[134] In particular, the strict Cartesian dualism between mind and body, which restricted a soul to humans and regarded animals as mere automata, posited a fundamental hiatus in the fabric of the universe. Such an exception to the general continuity of nature was intolerable for romantic philosophers who held that "the newly discovered anatomical identity of all animals, according so beautifully with the conception of continuity in nature, could not possibly correspond to an unbridgeable heterogeneity in the psychic realm."[135]

There were two possible methods of repairing the rupture that Cartesian dualism had opened up both in human nature and in the living world as a whole. The distinction between them cannot, however, be pressed too far as at the extreme they tended to collapse into one another. At the level of the human microcosm, dualism could be overcome by imputing psychic qualities to the "merely" mechanical bodily functions; on this view soul and body were coextensive. At the macrocosmic level, the possession of a soul could be extended to all animals which thereby ceased to be only machines and attained affinity with humans who differed from other beings solely in the greater development of their psychic properties. The same reconciliation might, von Aesch notes, have been achieved "by denying also to man the privilege of a soul instead of extending it to all his lower brethren"; this course would have led to "an extreme materialistic monism."[136] In the event, all these approaches were to have consequences for the reception and elaboration of the reflex concept in Germany and to a lesser extent in Britain.

We have seen already that, despite their recognition of the seminal nature of Hall's work, early German students of the reflex, such as Müller and Volkmann, differed from him in significant respects. Above all they would not agree with Hall that the reflex bore no relation to sensation or volition and was wholly nonpsychic in character. As Volkmann put it in his 1838 article: "all those experiments which disprove the participation of the soul in reflex movements are inadequate." To him the apparent purposiveness of these movements was enough to prove that "here also the psychic principle comes into play."[137] Johannes Müller also concluded from the evidence of reflex movements that the soul was not confined to the brain; the psychic principle apparently existed (at least in a latent state) in parts of the body entirely separated from the encephalon.[138]

Both these authors, therefore, adopted the first of the romantic strategies mentioned above; they saw "mind" as an intrinsic property of organic structures other than the brain. It was not merely the spinal cord that was so endowed with psychic characteristics; on the contrary, all organic phenomena possessed a "rational" quality, whether or not accompanied by conscious design.[139]

We have already described in chapter 2.2 how some of the themes of romantic biology were evident in Müller's early writings. Despite his overt repudiation of *Naturphilosophie* some of its key assumptions persisted in his approach to scientific problems. It is possible to detect the presence of similar influences on Volkmann. Thus, in his 1837 *Die Lehre von dem leiblichen Leben* appears a characteristically romantic conception of the relation of the human body to the world: "man is the microcosm; his body is not merely [the] human body, but animal body and plant body, he is at the same time earth, water and air, all appearances of the world in general recur in him."[140] Moreover, Volkmann rejected any form of dualism that neglected the intimacy of mind and body. "The soul," he wrote, "has her seat in organic structures," and had an obvious relation to them. This fact led Volkmann to an important methodological conclusion; because mind and body were inseparable "the physiologist has not only the authority, but even the obligation to examine the nature of the soul."[141] In other words, at least from a physiological standpoint, mind should not be conceived as "a being of a peculiar kind," which was merely conjoined to the organisms that served as its instrument. Instead the soul must be treated as an integral part of the vital energy (*Lebenskraft*) itself. From its outset and through its entire course, life and soul were united.[142]

Such background assumptions go far to explain why Hall's mechanistic understanding of the reflex was modified by German authors. In an intellectual setting where the rigid Cartesian mind-body dichotomy had been greatly eroded, it was less plausible to consider the reflex as something entirely divorced from mind; rather, it was seen as yet another modality by which the soul ensured the integrity and continuance of the organism. Taken to its extreme this type of reasoning led to the notion of a "spinal soul" to which the phenomena of reflex action should be ascribed—a theory which, despite its archaic character, attracted adherents until late in the nineteenth century, as we have already noted.[143]

By insisting upon a psychical interpretation of the spinal reflex, German physiologists such as Müller, Volkmann, and Edward Friedrich Wilhelm Pflüger (1829–1900) are open to the charge that they failed to grasp one of the most central aspects of Marshall Hall's achievement: the abolition of mystifying entities from this branch of science and their replacement by a purely mechanistic concept of the reflex phenomenon. There is much force to this criticism; but, at the same time it is important to recognize that the metaphysical assumptions of German workers encouraged the development of the reflex concept in more fruitful ways. In particular, because they were less inclined to draw a firm demarcation between the peculiarly mental functions of the nervous system and its "lower" offices, Müller and Volkmann from the outset rejected Hall's restrictive view of the range of phenomena to which the reflex concept applied.[144]

Thus Müller held that reflexes occurred in the brain, and like his pupil, Robert Remak, whose studies have been examined in chapter 3.5.2, believed that they operated in the ganglia of the vegetative nervous system as well as in the spinal cord.[145] Hall regarded this extended notion of the reflex as a grave error and, despite some minor shifts in his position, was never reconciled to Müller's scheme.[146] In contrast, Volkmann held that Müller's reflex theory was superior to Hall's precisely because "not only the spinal cord and *medulla oblongata* serve as [a] central organ of refected movements, but, as *Johannes Müller* more correctly than *M. Hall* maintained, also the brain, and as I will later show, the ganglia."[147]

In 1837, Volkmann had already stated a theory of cerebral reflexes. Sympathetic effects (i.e., reflexes) could, he argued, be distributed either by the agency of the spinal cord or in other cases be mediated by the brain. For example, the stimulation of vomiting supplied by a nauseating taste, or of sneezing caused by a bright light, were also "reflex movements," which only occurred when "the stimulation is conducted through the sensory nerves to the brain and from here is transmitted out on to other organs."[148] Volkmann developed this theory in 1838, when he claimed that to confine reflex action solely to the spinal cord would be to exclude a number of phenomena that possessed an "essential connection" with other reflexes. He went so far as to suggest that "fundamentally every voluntary movement is a reflected one, for it proceeds from an idea (*Vorstellung*) which was summoned through sensory impressions of some kind . . . and reaches levels at which the brain, as connecting link, changes the incident stimulus to the volitional stimulus and transmits [it] to the spontaneous-motor fibers."[149]

In these passages Volkmann came near to adopting the second of the methods of bringing mind and body closer together. He sought to effect a reconciliation by reinterpreting the highest mental functions in terms derived from the physiology of the lower nervous centers. This tendency, which was to be of great importance in the future development of the neurosciences and of psychology, was present in a much more marked way in the work of one of Volkmann's contemporaries, Wilhelm Griesinger.

Griesinger is best known as a proponent of a materialistic theory of mental diseases, and Otto M. Marx has described him as a "vehement anti-Romantic."[150] Similarly, Erwin Ackerknecht writes: "Although in his youth he was exposed to the influences of the romantic movement,

Griesinger, like the rest of his generation was an antiromantic."[151] Both these authors stress Griesinger's attempts to assimilate mental processes to the physiological functions of the nervous system. However, such a somaticist approach was not necessarily altogether "anti-romantic": we have seen that nomism and a naturalistic interpretation of mental phenomena had a place in the romantic philosophy of nature (see chap. 3). Moreover, the idiom in which Griesinger expressed his efforts to reconcile neurology and psychology and the argumentative strategies he adopted in the pursuit of his aim reveal that the influence of the romantic movement made a more lasting impression upon him than Ackerknecht suggests.

Thus Griesinger held that physiology must treat mental life as a "special form of organic life, inseparable from the body."[152] Mind, he insisted, was not something superimposed upon the living body; it arose by imperceptible stages from physiological processes and had to be understood by means of the same concepts and laws that physiology had developed for the elucidation of other "phenomena of organized matter." In particular, Griesinger declared that the physiological concept of "the reflex action of the nervous system" had a crucial role to play in a scientific understanding of mind.[153] Griesinger proposed to comprehend the highest mental functions by means of the same terms that served to describe the lower functions of the nervous system; in other words, he refused to accept the antinomies that Hall had set up between voluntary and reflex action and between psychical and mechanical causation of movement.[154]

In effect, Griesinger adopted a strong version of the second strategy for reconciling mind and body. Rather than trying to explicate physiological phenomena in psychic terms, he sought the foundations of mind in the mode of functioning found in the lower nervous centers. He held that the assumption of a "psychic principle"—of an unconscious but purposeful soul—in the spinal cord was an abstraction which could not mediate the antithesis between "passive reception or sensation-automatic reception or voluntary-mechanism or psychic freedom." What could achieve such a mediation was an extension of the reflex concept from the spinal cord to the encephalon. Griesinger argued that a comparison of the mode of action of these two organs revealed that "both are not subject to different laws, and that in respect of [the] transmission of centripetal into centrifugal stimulus a remarkable harmony exists between the more or less conscious actions of the brain itself, which one calls ideas or efforts (*Vorstellungen oder Strebungen*), and between the phenomena of sensation and movement of the central organs." Given this harmony it was, he claimed, possible "to study the reflexes within consciousness."[155]

There is a similarity between this extension of the characteristic functions of the spinal cord to the brain and some of the anatomical arguments we encountered in chapter 2.2. In that case the structure of the brain was conceived as derivative from the spinal cord; and we argued that this reversal of perspective arose from the assumptions and goals of romantic biology. The resemblance between the two cases is not accidental. Griesinger was wedded to the notion of typical structures that, in modified forms, were repeated along the axis of the body. He went from the idea of a typical vertebra, which was the basal structure of both the spinal column and skull, to argue that the brain and spinal cord were constructed upon one schema.[156] In this view, just as the skull was a collection of modified vertebrae, so the brain was a congeries of metamorphosed ganglia.

It is plausible to regard the strategy of Griesinger's 1843 paper "Ueber psychische Reflexactionen" as the physiological corollary of this morphological strategy. This view is confirmed by Griesinger's introduction to an article published in the following year. There he stated explicitly that he was extending to the elucidation of nervous function a strategy that had already cast much light on the structure of the cerebrospinal axis. Moreover, he placed this move firmly in the context of the romantic biological tradition:

> Just as Goethe's *Idee* and Oken's proof of the common laws of formation for the vertebral and cranial bones proved most highly fruitful for the understanding of the structure of the skull, so we may hope that out of the comparison between the vital activity of the spinal cord and brain certain clues needed for the correct conceptualization of psychic phenomena will also come to light.[157]

Should this proposition need further justification, Griesinger thought it only necessary to point to the evident homologies between the cranial and spinal portions of the cerebrospinal axis, and, in particular, to "the identity of their formal elements—fibers and ganglia."[158] Griesinger also claimed that brain and spinal cord were subject to the same kinds of anatomical aberration in disease. All these analogies indicated that both organs conformed to "the same schema of normal function and the same modes of morbid activity."[159]

Griesinger had already in 1843 attempted to show the parallels between the sensorimotor functions of the spinal cord and the psychical phenomena peculiar to the brain. He argued that, just as the brain (whether literally or figuratively) "grew out of" the spinal cord, so brain functions evolved gradually from the simpler forms of reflex. This course required a categorical rejection of Hall's restricted view of the scope of the reflex and of his separation of reflex from voluntary movements and from consciousness.[160] In place of this dualism Griesinger proposed a monistic approach to nervous function, which saw a fundamental continuity between the simplest and the most complex functions of the nervous system. This unity at the microcosmic level was paralleled in the animal kingdom as a whole where human consciousness and volition were seen to emerge gradually from more limited forms of mental and physiological phenomena.

Griesinger held that in the lower vertebrates, such as amphibia, only a very dim analogue of human consciousness existed. Centripetal stimuli could issue in movements without necessarily giving rise to actual sensation—let alone to ideas; and will, in the human sense, scarcely existed in such creatures. Even when these animals retained their brains, there was little to distinguish their normal movements from the reflex capability they exhibited when decollated. Griesinger concluded that "voluntary and reflex movements among these animals in normal states almost form a unity."[161]

Therefore, the actions of these lower vertebrates were effectively independent of any developed form of consciousness; they were, nevertheless, purposeful. The bases of this expediency (*Zweckmässigkeit*) lay, Griesinger insisted, "even in the unmutilated animal, not in the free determination of a will, which in the human sense the animal does not possess at all," but "in the organization itself." But even though the brain of the lower animal could not be considered as the seat of consciousness and volition, it did perform important functions. In the unmutilated animal, the brain provided a source of stimulation (*Anregung*) for the "tone" (*Stimmung*) of the spinal cord and regulated movements. It was by the brain, even in the absence of consciousness, that sensory impressions were translated into harmonious and purposive movements. For Griesinger, therefore, the brain was a center for coordinating sensorimotor impulses before it became the seat of consciousness; biologically the former function came first. Like Rudolph Hermann Lotze (1817–1881), Griesinger held that the apparent purposefulness of the reflexes of decerebrated amphibia was due to the persistence in these animals of certain "habitual" reactions that had been impressed by the brain upon the spinal cord during life.[162]

In the higher animals there was apparently a marked difference. In their normal state, movements did not issue from directly centripetal stimuli, but were increasingly mediated by mental states and by free will. The dominant role of the brain became more evident and should the animal lose the use of this organ, the reflex movements that persisted showed none of the purposive quality apparent in lower animals. Griesinger insisted, however, that this difference between the two extremes of the vertebrate subkingdom was not absolute. A very extensive group of intermediate actions existed, the proximate cause of which lay either in unmodified sensation or in mental states that were so "dim" that their intellectual character remained in doubt. This class approximated to the purposive movements of the lower vertebrates, standing "so to speak, in the middle between purely reflex and voluntary movements, and it is for the most part very difficult in some cases to decide where the voluntary begins." More generally, the process whereby consciousness emerged in the animal kingdom was one of gradual evolution, with many intermediate stages between the simplest and the most developed forms of mentality; at some point the quantitative difference in the strength of mental impressions was converted into a qualitative change with which the self-conscious soul came into existence.[163]

Continuity was further preserved by the fact that the fundamental pattern of reflex action occurred even in the operations of the conscious mind. The impressions that came to consciousness (*Vorstellungen*) stood in the same relationship to effort (*Strebung*) in the area of brain activity as sensation stood to movement in the spinal cord. Indeed, Griesinger held that mental endeavor (*Bestrebung*) was merely "psychical movement." In the healthy mind a balance existed between impressions and strivings; this equilibrium produced the "psychical tone" of the individual, which was also called disposition or character.[164]

It is important to note that Griesinger believed that something of the mechanical, determined character of the spinal reflex was also found in mental operations. "The transition of conscious impressions into efforts," he wrote, "rests, entirely like the reflex action in the spinal cord, upon organic compulsion (*Zwang*) and drive (*Drang*)." There was, he maintained, no absolute distinction between mechanically determined and voluntary movement: the will was only an elaboration of the other semiconscious "strivings" after a goal that were found in the animal kingdom.[165]

Griesinger therefore held that the health of the psyche depended upon a harmonious balance between the sensory and motor impulses mediated by the brain. It followed that a disturbance of this balance led to mental illness.[166] In his mental pathology Griesinger proposed to seek to illuminate psychological processes by an application of physiological principles—the same course he had adopted in constructing his theory of the sound mind. Specifically, he proposed "again to proceed upwards from the spinal cord to the brain." In other words, he sought to find the analogues of the sensorimotor disorders of the spinal cord in the disturbed mental processes of the insane.[167]

Griesinger concluded his paper by emphasizing the virtual eschewal of the notion of the "soul" in his account of healthy and diseased mental activity. He saw little heuristic value in the use of such an abstraction. In place of this metaphysical concept he had tried to build a bridge between psychical and organic processes. Specifically, he had emphasized "the detailed parallelism . . . which shows itself between the vital manifestations of the spinal cord—sensation and movement—and between those of the brain—conscious impressions and efforts." As well as spinal reflexes, in which sensory impressions were translated into motor impulses, Griesinger had posited the existence of "psychic reflex actions," which took place in the brain, and were characterized by the transduction of mental impressions into efforts. There were also intermediate classes of reflex that were neither conscious nor fully unconscious.[168]

Within this scheme it was wrong, Griesinger held, to regard the brain as the instrument, or even as the "material substratum" of the soul. Rather, it was the task of anatomy and physiology to identify the functionally crucial portions of the brain, as they had already shown what parts of the spinal cord were sensory and motor in their office, and to show how the brain was able to execute its dual sensorimotor and mental functions. Griesinger confessed himself to be enough of a materialist to believe that the "organic apparatus" for both these closely related operations was to be found in the "artfully complicated structure of the brain."[169]

We have described a broad contrast between British and German interpretations of the reflex, and have tried to show how these divergences arose from the different metaphysical notions prevalent in both countries. However, to some extent the romantic philosophy of nature that had such an impact on Müller, Volkmann, and Griesinger achieved international dissemination. Such notions as the unity of organization, the parallelism between the embryonic and biological series, and the continuity of nature, found several advocates in the British biomedical community; and these theoretical commitments were eventually to have an impact upon the development of reflex physiology in that country.[170]

Just as biologists throughout the first third of the nineteenth century had sought a type of nervous structure that would unite the most diverse forms of nervous organization, so a complementary quest for the type of nervous function had also arisen. Thus Grainger (in a work to be considered below) wrote in 1837 that:

> The investigations of comparative anatomy, and the laborious inquiries into the process of development, have led to the establishment of one grand principle in the science of organization,—the unity of structure. There is no truth, in any branch of human knowledge, fixed on a more firm basis than

> this,—that although nature displays immense fertility, in varying and modifying the form, and other physical characters of the several organs; yet, that there is, in no one instance, a departure from the first original type.[171]

Given this axiom, "it would be an unparalleled anomaly in the laws of creation, if such unity of organization as is displayed, not only in the nervous, osseous, glandular, and other systems, but in the formation of the entire frame, were not accompanied by *a corresponding simplicity in the laws which regulate the actions of this perfect machinery*."[172] In short, Grainger insisted, "where there is such wonderful uniformity of structure, there must be uniformity of function."[173]

Grainger devoted so much effort to providing a putative anatomical basis for Hall's excito-motory actions precisely because he saw the concept of the reflex as being capable of fulfilling this *desideratum* by supplying a type of nervous function sufficiently simple, and yet sufficiently comprehensive, to unite the mode of function in humans with that of lower animals.[174] Others expressed a similar view of the biological importance of the reflex concept. Richard Owen wrote in 1843 of the excito-motory act as the "primary function" of the nervous system, which appeared in its "most simple and essential condition" in the invertebrates, but which was also manifested in humans.[175] The implications of this notion of the reflex as a basal biological function were developed more fully by William Carpenter, who also extended the idea to the psychological realm.

Carpenter strongly maintained the principles of the continuity of nature and of the progressive elaboration of initially simple types in the upward course of the *scala naturae*. The operation of this law—so evident in matters of structure—was also seen in the emergence of increasingly complex functions in nature. Carpenter held that the first intimations of the reflex function were found in the vegetable kingdom; although it lacked any nervous organization, a vegetable did manifest what Carpenter held to be the basis of all later developments: "the adaptation of its organism to surrounding circumstances." This adaptation was achieved by means of the plant's response to external "stimuli fitted to excite it."[176]

Carpenter argued that the large class of animal actions termed "instinctive" could be "comprehended in the same general definition." This analogy extended to the exclusively "animal" functions as well as to those, such as nutrition, held in common with vegetables.[177] Animals gradually developed a separate mechanism to perform such adaptations to stimuli, and so the germs of the nervous system arose. Those actions where an impression led directly to a response, without the intervention of sensation, corresponded to Marshall Hall's excito-motory acts in human beings. There was a further class of action that needed to be distinguished which was intermediate between the true reflex and the voluntary act: namely, "those which are the direct result of sensations acting immediately on the motor nerves without the intervention of volition." These actions were still independent of the will, although consciousness was necessary to their performance.[178] Carpenter later named them "consensual" acts.

In his subsequent writings Carpenter elaborated this scheme while keeping to his original explanatory principle. The successively more complex nervous actions of animals were to be depicted as developments from a primitive functional type, just as the structures that mediated them were complicated versions of the simple ganglion. Throughout he maintained that the "reflex function . . . is the simplest application of the Nervous System in the animal body."[179] Even the human nervous system continued to perform basic excito-motory and consensual acts.

Carpenter's argument therefore conformed to a pattern we have noted previously: he sought to understand the more complex nervous functions as developments of the more simple. As one moved up the cerebrospinal axis, progressively more involved and "psychic" forms of reflex were encountered; but at the same time a fundamental continuity was preserved.

For some time, however, Carpenter made an exception to this rule of functional uniformity. Although he described the human cerebral hemispheres as ganglia and viewed them as complications of the other nervous centers of the brain, Carpenter was cautious in 1846 about ascribing to the cerebrum a version of the reflex function that he held to be common to other ganglia. He implied that at a certain stage in cerebral development a discontinuity had occurred in the workings of the nervous system: together with the "increase in Intelligence" had come "the predominance of *Will* over the involuntary impulses." The cerebrum was the instrument of the will and not subject to reflex action. Referring to the failure of Flourens and others to excite the cerebrum during experiments (see chap. 6.4.2), Carpenter concluded "that the changes which *mental* operations produce in the cerebral fibres cannot be imitated, as changes in other motor fibres may be, by physical impressions."[180]

Carpenter revised this opinion between 1846 and 1855 when the fourth edition of his *Principles of Human Physiology* appeared, partly because of his desire to find a naturalistic explanation for the phenomena of mesmerism, and partly in the light of Thomas Laycock's research on cerebral function (to be discussed below).[181] The principal change was the postulation of a third class of reflex action, analogous to excito-motory and consensual in that it was occasioned by afferent stimuli being reflected into efferent impulses through a ganglion, but distinct in being accompanied by intellectual states. The ganglion involved was the cerebrum, and Carpenter maintained that the resulting motions must be considered as manifestations of the "reflex power of the Cerebrum, and consequently as no less automatic in their character than those which result from the reflex power of the Cranio Spinal axis." Carpenter called such actions "ideo-motor" when they were accompanied by ideas, and "emotional" when by a feeling.[182]

Carpenter's work thus shows in a striking way a tension between the monistic notions of nervous function he shared with some Continental workers and the dualist assumptions whose influence on Hall has already been noted. Carpenter was for theological reasons anxious not to undermine the role of a discrete, causally effective soul in humans, and therefore refused to accept that all cerebral function could be understood in the same terms that served to explicate the operation of the lower nervous centers. Carpenter did, however, attempt to mediate to some extent the absolute distinction others had made between the cerebral hemispheres and the other ganglia; in this way, the idea of a gradual development of structure and function in the nervous system could be preserved. By drawing the hemispheres at least partially into the framework of reflex action, Carpenter remained to some extent true to his professed biological philosophy.

Thomas Laycock's role in convincing Carpenter that some cerebral reflexes did occur was noted above. Laycock's thought was, even more than Carpenter's, imbued with the principles of romantic nature-philosophy. Moreover, in his case, the countervailing theological motives that led Carpenter to retain a core of dualism in his system did not apply. In consequence, Laycock produced a thoroughly monistic concept of the functions of the nervous system, which made no exceptions even for the supposedly most "spiritual" aspects of human beings.

Various reasons can be adduced for why Laycock was less affected by dualist preconceptions than many of his British contemporaries. In his theology he tended toward the heresy of "mortalism"—the belief that immortality was secured not by the survival of a separate spiritual principle but only by the resurrection of the body. Laycock's diary records that during his student days in London he spent much time discussing and considering these theological ideas, which seemed to indicate the "materiality of what is called the soul"; and that "mind is the result of organization."[183] Laycock also credited the phrenologists for having arrived at essentially the same conclusion: "The principles of phrenology are as follows:-1. Phrenology maintains that the mind and the body are inseparable in this world, and cannot be investigated apart from each other. It is man as a 'concrete Ego' and not as an immaterial Ego, that it examines. This principle is controverted by the doctrine of 'spirits', and the views of speculative theologians and metaphysicans, but it is evidently in concurrence with the daily practice and common sense of mankind."[184] Laycock differed, however, from the phrenologists in some of their more specific doctrines, such as their organology, holding that the laws of nervous action developed by Hall and others provided a sounder foundation for the study of the intimate union of the mental and the organic.[185]

But more important than either of these influences was Laycock's commitment throughout his career to the principle of the continuity of nature, continuity that was not interrupted by the appearance of mind. It was on these grounds that Laycock rejected categorically the dogma of "the speculative philosophy of Europe, that no animal besides man is endowed with a soul or mind; and that, consequently, the phenomena of mind are not to be studied in the inferior animals, but in the phenomena of human consciousness exclusively." Because of this separation "Man has been taken from community with his fellow-creatures, and placed in a world of Life and Feeling altogether apart";[186] from the viewpoint of romantic nature-philosophy such a separation was insufferable.

In place of Cartesian dualism, and the view maintained by many British philosophers and scientists that mind must be studied *sui generis,* Laycock stressed the advantages of "a combined consideration of psychical and vital phenomena." This necessitated taking account of all living organisms, the lowest as well as the highest, on the grounds that a continuity existed between them all and that "no bio-molecular movements take place in animals of even the highest organization, which have not their counterpart in vegetables and animals of the lowest forms."[187] In 1876 Laycock revealed some of the sources of such ideas; they had arisen from a reading of the works of Caspar Friedrich Wolff (1733–1794), Goethe, von Baer, and Jean Baptiste Pierre Antoine de Monet de Lamarck (1744–1829). These writings had convinced him that, in the study of life, thought, and will, "the law of *continuous* evolution is the guiding principle."[188]

Laycock saw the reflex concept as of crucial importance in his scheme of the continuous evolution of mind in animate nature. Like Griesinger he proposed to go from below upward: to show the organic roots of mentality rather than to extend mind to physiological phenomena. Laycock also shared Griesinger's view that there was a parallelism between the progressive emergence of nervous structure and function in the animal kingdom.

Laycock subscribed to a theory of the origins of the nervous system that we have already encountered (chap. 2.1). Initially, the nervous function was held to be diffused throughout the homogeneous tissue of the simplest organisms. The first manifestation of a separate nervous structure, Laycock wrote, was a ganglion in connection with nervous fibers; these ganglia were variously distributed, and tended to be equal in size and functional importance. As a result "just as a plant, so may an individual animal be really a congeries of individuals; each segment or ganglion with its dependent tissues having a power of maintaining a continued and independent existence when separated from the others." Farther along the scale of development one or more ganglia assumed a superiority over the rest: this was the germ of the brain. Laycock held that each of these stages passed gradually into the next; in consequence, there was an underlying affinity between the lower and the higher manifestations of nervous structure and function. Laycock stressed, in particular, the importance of the research of Tiedemann, J. F. Meckel the Younger, Serres, Solly, and others, that had established "the identity of structure of the brain and spinal cord." The structural homology between the more primitive and more advanced centers of the cerebrospinal axis was reflected in their modes of action: "just as the diffused nervous system embodies the elements of the ganglionic; and the movements in connection with the former (the movements of irritability) are typical of those dependent on the latter—the reflex or excited; so are the ganglionic phenomena illustrative of the cerebral; and the mode of action of the brain itself as the organ of mind, may in some degree be ascertained by an analysis of the series of phenomena just reviewed."[189]

Laycock elaborated this argument in 1840 when he declared "that the cranial ganglia, although the organ of consciousness, are subject to the same laws as those which govern the other ganglia, the diffused nervous system of animals and the vital mechanism of vegetables."[190] In short, just as the spinal reflex bore a "genetic" affinity to the irritability of the simplest animals and of plants, so the operation of the highest nervous centers in humans retained the fundamental reflex character of the lower.

Laycock acknowledged that this was a controversial doctrine to propound. There were "many who will consider it dangerous to concede, that apparently pure mental acts are only the results of vital machinery excited into action by physical agencies."[191] The notion that reflexes occurred above the brain stem was, moreover, utterly opposed to the views of Marshall Hall. In his public utterances Laycock treated Hall with respect. In private, however, he maintained that "Dr Hall really is a most obscure writer"; and asked the phrenologist George Combe

(1788–1858) for "his opinion of Dr Hall's craniological development. His forehead struck me as very peculiar."[192] Whatever his real view of the value of Hall's work, Laycock clearly regarded the former's concept of reflex action as too restricted; in his own account of the scope of the reflex, Laycock approximated much more closely to the views of German authors.

The title of Laycock's 1844 address to the Medical Section of the British Association for the Advancement of Science—"On the reflex function of the brain"—was, in Hall's terms, nonsense. But, as we have seen, the notion of cerebral reflexes had from the first been entertained by German scientists. In this address Laycock again stressed the anatomical bases of his theory of cerebral function: he was led to his concept of brain reflexes "by the general principle, that the ganglia within the cranium being a continuation of the spinal cord, must necessarily be regulated as to their reaction on external agencies by laws identical with those governing the functions of the spinal ganglia and their analogues in the lower animals." He also made clear the assumption of organic unity that underlay this chain of reasoning. Laycock alluded to recent advances "in comparative physiology, which shows us that the structure and functions of the nervous system in all animals are subject to the same laws of development and action . . . and that varied and dissimilar as they appear, each [part of the nervous system] may be made to illustrate the other."[193]

Laycock's frequent use of the notion of "analogy" presupposed that a corresponding unity occurred within the human body. He wrote in a letter to George Combe that, even with the aid of the microscope, the true structure of the brain would probably always escape the investigator; nevertheless, "We may do something by analogy and this I have attempted."[194] Laycock referred to a passage in his 1844 address where he had written of "The cerebral nerves being analogous to the posterior spinal nerves, and the encephalic ganglia analogous to the spinal ganglia." This analogy, he claimed, made plausible the suggestion that just as afferent stimulation of the spinal cord led to reflex movement, so a sensory impression in the brain could, when transmitted to the "analogue of the anterior gray matter," lead to movements no less automatic in their character. "If," he argued, "the cerebral ganglia be but a higher development of the spinal, the medullary, and cortical substance must correspond to the white and gray matter of the cord, and if it be acknowledged (as has indeed been proved beyond question), that a combined action of sets of muscles, exhibiting a design of conservation may be developed in the spinal cord without the aid of volition, how can we deny the same qualities to the encephalic ganglia, or in other words, to the cerebral hemispheres and their connexions?"[195]

Laycock's theory of the functional uniformity of the cerebrospinal axis therefore rested on the claim that the cerebral hemispheres possessed a "connate structure" to that of the ganglia of the spinal cord. We have seen that Griesinger referred to the doctrines of transcendental anatomy to enforce a similar inference. Laycock too in his discussion of the histological "substrata" of various nervous acts held that: "Just as in man certain organs are rudimentary, so also certain of these substrata are rudimentary; just as the osteology of man is formed on one general type, varied only to suit his mode of existence, so also these substrata are based on a fundamental type varied in like manner."[196] In short, Laycock had attempted to apply "The law of unity of type and function in animals . . . to the function of the cerebro-spinal axis in man";[197] this exercise had "shown (what is necessarily deduced from the law itself) that the transition of structure and function is gradual, and consequently, no strong line of demarcation can be drawn between the manifestations of its various functions. The automatic acts pass insensibly into the reflex, the reflex into the instinctive, the instinctive are *quasi* emotional, the emotional are intellectual. This gradation of structure and function observed in the nervous system, is observed also with reference to all other structures of his body."[198] The principle of reflex action throughout the nervous system was, therefore, merely an instance of the wider law of unity of type that governed all organic structures.

Griesinger and Laycock thus arrived at almost the same time at the idea of cerebral reflexes by closely analogous routes. Yet, so far as we can tell, they did so independently, each unaware of the other's work. The similarities between their ideas derived not from direct influence, but from a set of shared background assumptions about the unity of organic form and action that both men derived from their cultural milieu. The romantic nature-philosophy and its role in the development of other branches of neuroscience, which has been discussed elsewhere (chap. 1; chap. 2.2), played a major part in the overcoming of the structural and functional dualisms erected by Marshall Hall and in establishing the reflex as the ubiquitous element of nervous action throughout the cerebrospinal axis.

Historians have noted how Griesinger's and Laycock's writings prefigured certain key concepts of later experimental psychology. For example, Mette holds that Griesinger's parallel between the reflex processes of the brain and spinal cord anticipated the ideas employed by Pavlov and his school in the study of conditioned reflexes.[199] However, Ivan Mikhailovich Sechenov (1829–1905), who in 1863 published the best known early exposition of the theory that the reflex was the basis of all nervous function,[200] was apparently unacquainted with the work of either of his predecessors. Griesinger's and Laycock's importance seems to have lain in breaking down the rigid dichotomies between "mental" and "physiological" nervous functions, and so preparing later scientists to accept Sechenov's arguments. In Laycock's case, moreover, one can go beyond such general influence upon the prevailing climate of opinion and show a quite specific impact upon a distinguished follower, John Hughlings Jackson (1835–1911).

We have noted that by extending the reflex concept to the higher nervous centers and trying to apply it to the phenomena of mind, authors like Griesinger and Laycock to some extent vitiated the degree of simplification and clarity Marshall Hall had achieved by insisting on the purely mechanical nature of excito-motory acts and on their irrelevance to psychology. In Laycock's case at least, this move was undertaken because of a dissatisfaction with the existing systems of psychology. He wrote that his experience at York County Hospital of morbid conditions of the nervous system led him to appreciate "the imperfect nature of the views then current as to cerebral physiology, and their inadequacy to explain or elucidate functional diseases of the brain." Current mental philosophy was still more useless; in fact, "not a few metaphysicians hardly concede so much as the fundamental proposition, that the brain is the organ of mind, and necessary to the manifestation of its phenomena; for they practically ignore the science of cerebral physiology, and investigate the operations of mind as if the brain took no part in them."[201] Laycock's later work was chiefly directed to remedying this deficiency by making psychology a branch of physiology.

The extension of the reflex to the cerebrum played a central role in this strategy; thereby, the relevance of organic processes to the highest, apparently purely mental operations, was assured. Specifically, the sensorimotor nature of cerebral function (which Flourens and many after him had so strenuously denied)[202] became an established axiom of Laycock and his followers. This reversal of previous views of cerebral function was rich in consequences. Perhaps the most important was the elimination of consciousness as the defining characteristic of mind and as the condition of cerebral action. As Laycock wrote in 1855, in his system:

> the brain being a congeries of ganglia, did not differ in its laws of action from the other ganglia of the nervous system; and in particular, that like the spinal ganglia, it was subject to the laws of *reflex* action. It followed, therefore, that although, as the organ of conscious mind, its functions were carried on *with* consciousness, yet as being a series of ganglia analogous to the spinal, its functions might be, and often were, carried on *without* consciousness, or at least independently of the will, and of the accompanying sensations, if consciousness existed.[203]

Cerebral functions could therefore be actuated by the application of the appropriate stimuli without the necessary accompaniment of consciousness or volition. What had traditionally been regarded as "mind" ceased to be a causally potent entity and became a parallel, almost incidental, series of phenomena to the mechanical reflexes of the cerebral hemispheres.[204]

As is well known, John Hughlings Jackson began his medical career as a student of Laycock, and the latter's thinking had a lasting influence upon him.[205] On several occasions Jackson acknowledged this influence, pointing in particular to the importance of Laycock's claim that "the *brain,* although the organ of consciousness, *is subject to the laws of reflex action, and that, in this respect, it does not differ from the other ganglia of the nervous system.*"[206] The corollary of this principle in Jackson's own work was that, not only could cerebral functions be conceived in sensorimotor terms but that they must be so regarded by the neurologist to the exclusion of the categories of traditional psychology. H. T. Engelhardt has stressed the immense heuristic value of this decision to consider the nervous system in its entirety no longer "as the organ of the soul, but as the organ of sensory-motor integration," with states of consciousness delegated to an incidental status. Indeed, Engelhardt maintains that Jackson's application of this principle in his work on cortical localization can be regarded as marking "the real beginning of neurology proper."[207]

Such a view of the uniformity of nervous function became possible only when the traditional dualist assumptions that had established an absolute distinction between the "mental" and the purely physical functions of the nervous system were overcome. In this section we have discussed the principal means by which this barrier was eroded and the limits Hall had placed upon the concept of the reflex broken down. In particular, we have argued that the notion of a unity of function, as of structure, in the nervous system found in the writings of Griesinger and Laycock derived from the tenets of the romantic philosophy of nature. Whereas later authors such as Jackson justified their conviction in this uniformity by reference to the theory of evolution, it is important to remember that the roots of the initial breakdown of the barrier between spinal and cerebral action lay in an older biological system.

As well as the process whereby the reflex was extended to the higher centers of the cerebrospinal axis, Hall's reflex concept received numerous other revisions and elaborations in the twenty years following its promulgation. Other workers sought to remedy Hall's disdain for anatomy and to discover an anatomical basis for the physiological phenomena he had described. We have already discussed this problem in chapter 3.5.2, but we will now examine other aspects of it.

4.6. THE ANATOMY OF THE SPINAL REFLEX

We have noted earlier in this chapter that one of the early explanations for "sympathetic" (i.e., reflex) action was advanced by Thomas Willis in 1664. He speculated that peripheral nerve anastomoses were responsible, and the idea was corroborated and extended by Andrea Comparetti in 1780, although neither had any sound anatomical evidence. Despite its espousal in the early nineteenth century, as, for example, by Tiedemann in 1825, it did not survive thereafter, and attention turned instead to possible mechanisms in the central nervous system. The morphological basis of one of these, the pupillary reflex, was described accurately by Herbert Mayo in 1823, but as already mentioned, little notice seems to have been taken of it (4.3, above). Marshall Hall was well aware of the need to identify the actual procedure whereby the "excito" impression was reflected into a "motory" response, but he made no efforts himself to do so, and he referred to the problem as a *quaestio maximè vexata,*[208] or as a "*mystery.*"[209] He seemed content freely to confess that there were no anatomical grounds for his system,[210] but he hoped that others would be able to provide this missing link and thereby substantiate his established doctrine. Hall's loyal supporter, Richard Grainger (who held Hall in high regard), was able to identify it for he had accepted the excito-motory system, not in slavish imitation of its creator, but in the light of his own experiments and careful deduction. Like Carpenter and others, Grainger adapted a comparative approach to the spinal reflex, and he believed that the "reflex power" of the spinal cord as demonstrated by Hall was regulated by simple and precise laws, just as in the case of gravity. The word "power," therefore, signified a physical analogy, or a circumstance "which seems to indicate the existence of an universal principle in the movement of organized bodies."[211] Grainger also believed, correctly as it transpired, that the extent of reflex action depended in all cases on the intensity of the stimulus,[212] a relationship that had already been deduced by Johannes Müller, and it was substantiated by Volkmann a year later.

Following faithfully the functional features of the excito-motory system as set out by Hall, Grainger proceeded to trace out the supposed special pathway of the spinal reflex. He eschewed the increasingly popular microscope because of the known deceptions it could invoke and relied on the naked-eye examination of alcohol-hardened specimens. He reported thus:

> I am, myself, convinced that a peculiar order of nerves, called the excito-motory, not only exist in the cerebro-spinal, but, likewise, in the ganglionic [autonomic] system.[213]

We should recall that at this time, 1836–1837, almost nothing of the spinal cord's intricate microstructure was known. All that could so far be admitted was that it comprised nerve fibers arranged in columns that surrounded the central gray matter, and that these fibers were presumably continuous with those of the spinal roots and nerves. The examination of nervous tissue with the new compound microscope had only just begun and spinal cord cells had not yet been identified. Nor had the possible relationships between fiber and cell been contemplated (see chap. 3). In fact, Stilling's pioneer studies of spinal cord anatomy did not commence until January of 1842, and those relevant to the afferent-efferent pathway through the cord have been discussed already (chap. 3.5.2). Nevertheless, Grainger was seeking the incident or afferent and the reflex or efferent components of the spinal reflex, and the way in which reflection from the former to the latter came about. He reported: "After repeated examinations, I satisfied myself that each [spinal cord root] was connected both with the external fibrous part of the cord [white matter], and the internal grey substance."[214] It seemed to him that the reflex arc was now complete, and that the gray matter of the cord was the central organ of the excito-motory system. He admitted that Gall had first reported that the spinal nerves were connected with the central gray matter, also on the basis of macroscopical techniques alone. However, Grainger doubted whether he or Gall or any other observer had so far seen the junction between the root and cord fibers, if indeed there was one.

Others in Britain who accepted Hall's system, also believed, like Grainger, that they had isolated its specific nerve fibers. These included Carpenter, and the entomologist, George Newport (1803–1854), who both claimed that they had seen the two sets of nerves in the *Articulata*.[215] They affirmed that the longitudinal fibers of the ganglionic chain of these primitive creatures passed up to the cerebral ganglion (i.e., brain) and constituted sensory-volitional connections, whereas the transverse or commissural fibers that passed through the ganglionic chain were excito-motory and concerned with reflexes. Carpenter, having asserted that his comparative anatomical studies supported the existence of Hall's excito-motory system,[216] went on to conclude that in animals in general it existed for the introduction of food into the digestive cavity and for similar actions:

> a nervous circle is requisite, consisting of an *afferent* nerve on the peripheral extremities of which an impression is made;—a ganglionic center, where the white fibers of which that nerve consists terminate in grey matter, and those of the efferent nerve originate in like manner;—and an *efferent* trunk conducting to the contractile structure the motor impulse, which originates in some change in the relation between the grey and white matter.[217]

Like Grainger he too believed that Hall's doctrine had been proved correct.[218] Concerning the transverse fibers of the ganglionic chain, he agreed that they were reflex in function, in accordance with the theory of reflex movements as promulgated by Marshall Hall.[219]

R. B. Todd, however, in his utter refutation of Hall's system including the "true spinal cord" and the excito-motory fibers, denounced and rejected these interpretations.[220] We can but agree with him because, as in the case of Gall, it was not difficult to hypothesize a structural basis for a function at a time when so little was known of the microscopical elements of nervous tissue and their complex alignments. The immediate effect of this ignorance was to allow numerous speculations on the possible morphology of reflex arcs and concerning the anatomy of the spinal cord. Hall himself declared that this organ "is the elysio of the critic by profession, and of the guesser in physiology."[221] Todd included morphological considerations in his attack on Hall for he claimed that if Hall's spinal reflex fibers existed, they should be more numerous in the lumbar part of the spinal cord, because of the large excitor surfaces of the legs and the presence of the sphincters in its sphere of innervation. In fact, he pointed out, the lumbar enlargement was smaller than the cervical, and this cogent criticism, together with other facts both physiological and pathological, induced Todd to assert that concerning Hall's doctrine "such a supposition would involve the most palpable contra-indications, and is wholly inadmissable."[222] Obviously, further advances awaited the emergence and development of histological concepts (see chap. 3).

Like Marshall Hall, Johannes Müller had no idea how the central mechanism of reflex action might operate, and he did not postulate one. The majority of his countrymen, however, doubted the existence of special excito-motory fibers,[223] and in 1838 Volkmann advanced compelling objections.[224] He argued that if the foot of a recently decapitated frog were pricked with a fine needle, there ensued reflex movements in seemingly all the muscles of the body. But the needle point could not have irritated more than one or two nerve fibers, and if it was accepted that a stimulus traveled along only the fibers to which it had been communicated, it must follow that the excito-motory system allowed direct connections of the irritated filaments with the innumerable fibers to every muscle in the body in order to account for the mass action observed. It seemed to Volkmann that this invoked much too complex a mechanism, and he therefore advanced the hypothesis that "the nervous action may pass from one spinal cord fiber to another";[225] Remak, as we noted above (chap. 3.5.2), subscribed to this idea of nerve influence by contiguity. The notion was comparable to F. H. A. von Humboldt's report in 1797, whereby a nerve could be influenced by another, because it was in its sphere of influence, or by means of contact. We can term this process "crossover transmission," but as in the case of the speculative anastomoses of Thomas Willis, our present day notion of synaptic transmission must not be applied to it. A similar explanation was provided by Jakob Henle who had been stimulated by the work of Hall and Müller to explore the problem of the "nervous sympathies," and he discussed them at length in 1840.[226] On the basis of the limited knowledge of spinal cord anatomy, he stated that reflex activity took place mainly in its gray and white matter and in that of the brain, with the ganglia of the vegetative nervous system being concerned with certain reflexes that involved that system. He announced that:

> It is a matter of experience, that nerves transfer their states of excitement from one to another, and it is proved that, in the case of animals at least, this occurs only within the central [nervous system] organs. Communication of excitement in the central organs is the basis of all nervous sympathies [reflexes]. The laws that govern the spread of excitement in the central organs are also the laws of sympathy.[227]

It is interesting that as late as 1840 Henle was still using "sympathy" as a synonym for reflex activity, but Brown-Séquard in 1858 continued this practice, as we shall see shortly.

Henle maintained that excitation in the spinal cord could travel in three directions: in its breadth, its length, and antero-posteriorly. These various ways of communicating were, therefore, basic to "sympathetic" or reflex action, and in support of this Henle provided a lot of new evidence, mostly clinical. But in the case of "morbid sympathies," his arguments were much less effective,[228] and in this regard he can be compared with Marshall Hall, who also attempted to apply his doctrine to disorders of the nervous system with little success, as we would judge. Although some of Henle's comments on the role of the cord in the spinal reflex had been made already, as for example by Volkmann, he nevertheless provided one of the most rational accounts of reflex activity that had appeared so far. His conclusions were echoed by A. Dupré (fl. 1843) in 1843, when he declared that the reflex was dependent upon crossover transmission between communicating fibers in the spinal cord.[229] Like Henle, however, his proposal was vague and lacked the support of adequate histological data.

During the following year Volkmann elaborated further his opinions of 1838, and he agreed with Henle when he contended that although the law of isolated conductivity whereby impulses remained within one nerve fiber was true for the peripheral nerves, crossover transmission between fibers must take place in nerve plexuses, ganglia, the spinal cord, and the brain. He adduced evidence in favor of this from the healthy and diseased states in humans.[230] When applied to the spinal cord this idea meant that the conduction across it could take place by a stimulus leaping from a sensory to a motor nerve. As mentioned elsewhere, Volkmann and Henle at first did not accept that nerve-cell bodies and fibers were connected, thus forming the element to be known later as the neuron (see chap. 3). Nevertheless, they must be credited with having provided one of the first steps in the evolution of our notions of spinal reflex pathways.

Also, in his article of 1844, which received widespread praise, Volkmann extended his attack on Hall's excito-motory system of fibers.[231] He now pointed out that if it existed, it must follow that every piece of skin the size of a needle point had two fibers of specifically different function: one for reflex action and the other for sensation. The current information on the histology of peripheral nerve terminations made this an improbable arrangement, he argued, although as we now know in this instance his criticism cannot be sustained.

G. Kirschner (fl. 1840), one of Hall's several German translators, also invoked histological data to support his opposition to the excito-motory system.[232] He felt that if it were accepted, then special fibers must exist for voluntary motion and emotions and for the sensations of heat and cold as Stilling had suggested. But this, he reasoned, would mean that the number of specific pathways would be too great for minute nerves to hold them all, an argument that was acceptable at that time, but not entirely to modern scientists. Others, in the absence of correct and detailed microscopical data, advanced similar speculative objections which need not concern us here. It is interesting to note, however, that in place of Hall's system Kirschner proposed that every spot of skin corresponded to certain muscle movements, an arrangement that was coordinated in the spinal cord, and which perhaps faintly foreshadows the dermatome and myotome relationships that were discovered later in the nineteenth century.

We now come to a most significant advance in the elucidation of the spinal reflex's morphology, for it forecast the modern position. In chapter 3.5.2, we discussed Remak's opinions of 1841 on the anatomical substratum of reflex action and the basic elements that mediate nervous system operations; also how he proposed that the "central points" linking the afferent and efferent limbs of the reflex were the nerve cells. His evidence, however, was still limited, and others were more cautious. Thus, in 1846, Rudolph Wagner put forward the notion that instead of excitation jumping from fiber to fiber (by means of crossover transmission), nerve fibers were connected together by the cells of the spinal cord's gray matter, and that by this arrangement nervous irritation could be conveyed from the sensory to motor spinal root.[233] The reflex pathway was therefore based on what was much later to be termed "synaptic" rather than crossover transmission, but Wagner was careful to point out that he was presenting only a hypothesis: "It is permitted from my fragmentary anatomical and physiological observations to erect a theory for the mechanism of reflex movement, which for the time being is only an hypothesis."[234] As we now know, his supposition eventually turned out to be correct, but although it was denied by many subsequent writers, men like Carpenter, Todd, and Koelliker arrived at a similar conclusion (see chap. 3.5.2). Moreover, by means of Wagner's suggestion Remak's original proposal was fully justified. We have already discussed other controversies over the cell-fiber connection (see chap. 3.5.2).

Meanwhile, there were still those who accepted Hall's hypothesis of an excito-motory fiber system, and one of his few Continental supporters was Gustav Adolf Spiess (1802–1875).[235] His support of neural pathology that led to a fierce confrontation with Rudolf Virchow, who advocated cellular pathology, has already been related (see chap. 1 n. 38). In 1844, Spiess maintained that isolated conductivity was to be found in all parts of the nervous system, not alone in peripheral nerves as Volkmann had postulated. For him this was a fundamental law of animal organization. He believed that there could not be any crossover transference from sensory to motor nerves by way of the spinal cord, but instead he assumed the existence in the central nervous system of a special set of anastomosing fibers for reflex movements. This network seems to have corresponded to the central part of Hall's assumed system, and, like Hall, Spiess believed that the anatomists had not yet discovered it. As it turned out, each conjecture shared the same fate.

Obviously, the history of the spinal reflex's morphology was closely associated with the efforts of those who were exploring the form and function of the spinal cord's cells and fibers, and in chapter 3.5.2, we have discussed the work of Remak, Stilling, Wagner, Koelliker, Gratiolet, Hermann, and others in this field. Koelliker in 1850 supported Volkmann's conjecture that central nerve fibers could communicate by means of crossover transmission, and he therefore argued that unions between spinal fibers and cells were not exclusively responsible for reflex action.[236] However, he did maintain, as we have observed (chap. 3 n. 188), that vegetative ganglia could be sites for reflected movements; he was, in fact, agreeing with Remak that their cells were "central organs" of the nervous system. Another eminent anatomist, Johann Ludwig Conrad Schroeder van der Kolk (1797–1862), also made many references to the anatomy of the reflex in his book of 1859.[237] He did not accept Hall's excito-motory system, for he correctly judged it to be a hypothesis without any certain foundations. His opinion was that some of the nerve fibers in the posterior spinal root had reflex function, and that they probably took their route by way of groups of cells midway between the anterior and posterior horns of the spinal cord's gray matter to the anterior horn cells, which initiated voluntary and reflex movements. This was a purely morphological distinction, but as all the fibers seems to look the same, it was conditioned by the need for a sensorimotor reflex link in the cord. The two motor functions, volitional and reflex, were, however, served by the same fibers. Some of the posterior root reflex fibers ascended in the posterior horns of the spinal gray matter, and at different levels they passed from the posterior to the anterior horns, thus accounting for the diversity and multiplicity of reflex phenomena. Although opposing Hall's nerve fiber system, Schroeder van der Kolk made reference to special cells with reflex function. The following statement incorporating these into his proposed reflex anatomy is, in general, acceptable today:

> I think, therefore, that the difficult phenomena of reflex action can be satisfactorily explained by the theory of special groups of motor cells and of reflex cells, and the varying degrees of connexion in which these are placed with one another by means of their communicating filaments.[238]

In 1854, Rudolph Wagner still favored Hall's scheme, and he gave it support on the basis of the reflex fibers that Schroeder van der Kolk had claimed existed in the posterior spinal roots.[239] His further defense of it revealed that he was still not certain of direct connections between these fibers and the anterior horn cells, and that he could not exclude prior contacts with other spinal gray matter cells.[240]

Thus, by midcentury only a bare outline of the morphological characteristics of the spinal reflex had been revealed, owing to the crude nature of the microscopes, techniques, and neurohistological concepts that had been available so far to investigators. Nevertheless, there was mounting evidence confuting Marshall Hall's hypothesis of a separate excito-motory mechanism that functioned in the spinal cord by means of a special system of nerve fibers. It was becoming increasingly likely that the latter belonged to "Imaginary Anatomy," as George Henry Lewes (1817–1878) expressed it in 1877, when decrying both Hall's physiology and his "distinct system of excito-motor nerves."[241] But until nerve fiber-tracing methods in particular were developed much of spinal reflex anatomy was to be based to a great extent on hypothesis. We should at this point refer back to chapter 3.5.2 where we dealt with sensorimotor concepts and gave an account of Hermann's statements made in 1863, which represent a prelude to irrefutable and substantial advances in the morphology of the reflex later in the nineteenth century.

4.7. SUMMARY AND SEQUEL

In the first fifty years of the nineteenth century, the concept of the spinal reflex was established. At the beginning of the century it was in an embryonic state, being based on the ancient notions of sympathy and involuntary movements, on the speculations of Descartes and Willis advanced in the seventeenth century, and on experimental work chiefly by Whytt and Procháska in the eighteenth. By the middle of the nineteenth century, the idea had been greatly expanded and clarified, owing principally to the labors and the abrasive personality of Marshall Hall. It was being studied widely, and its properties in the healthy and diseased states were under investigation. Moreover, the potential of the reflex to become the key to achieving a unified conception of nervous function both within the human body and throughout the animal kingdom had been grasped; and the first steps to realize this potential had already been taken. However, the excito-motory reflex system that Hall sought to establish was under attack and was soon to disappear as contrary evidence, both physiological and morphological, was marshaled against it. But, despite the fact that some of its central tenets were to be demolished, many important aspects of it were to remain and are incorporated in present day knowledge. Without doubt it had stimulated a certain amount of valuable research, although on the whole the theory of reflex action remained relatively neglected among the neurophysiological topics then being investigated. One of the reasons for this was the question of its relevance to clinical medicine. Despite the efforts of Hall, Henle, and others to relate the spinal reflex to diseased states, and even though the notion of sympathy that it replaced had been applied extensively to them, its practical uses seemed, on the whole, to be limited. Thus, we find the renowned physiologist and neurologist Brown-Séquard making the following statement in 1858:

> Although Robert Whytt and several other writers, amongst whom I will name Tissot, Prochaska, Barthez, J. Mueller, Henle, and Prof. Martyn Paine, have published so many interesting facts concerning the sympathy between various parts of the body, physiologists and practitioners have not paid sufficient attention to this most important subject.[242]

But in the second half of the century, this neglect was remedied, as the physiology of the nervous system expanded rapidly, especially in

Germany, and during the last two decades in Britain under the guidance of C. S. Sherrington.[243] Spinal reflex activity was greatly clarified, the discovery of the neuron permitted the delineation of its precise pathway, and a host of pathological reflex responses provided the clinician with increasing diagnostic acumen. The study of brain reflexes—a concept pioneered, as we have seen, by Griesinger and Laycock—led by way of I. M. Sechenov's experiments eventually to the conditioned reflex of Pavlov.[244] Thus at the end of the nineteenth century, the research that had been carried out in the preceding one hundred years or so was being directed chiefly along two channels: the spinal reflex physiology of Sherrington and the conditioned reflex physiology of Pavlov.[245]

5

Nerve Function

5.1. INTRODUCTION

The way in which messages are carried through the body by way of the nerves has intrigued physicians since the earliest times. Precisely how muscles can be made to contract on demand and how sensory signals are conveyed to the brain has provided an enigma, first confronted by the ancient Greeks, and still with us today. The history of concepts of nerve function is, therefore, one of the longest in the evolution of the neurosciences.[1] It falls naturally into three periods of time: the first was before the publication in 1791 of an account by Luigi Galvani (1737–1798) of his remarkable experiments on animal electricity, or as it was later appropriately known, galvanism.[2] The second period dates from 1791 to the 1840s. The third period was opened by the German physiologist Emil du Bois-Reymond in the 1840s who established the discipline of electrophysiology of nerve and muscle on a firm scientific basis; it extends to the present day. The discussion that follows will be concerned principally with the second of these historical periods, during which the unequivocal demonstration of animal electricity was witnessed, and attempts were made to elucidate its nature and its role in the physiology of nerve conduction and muscle contraction. We shall, however, examine first the experiments of Galvani, and the interpretations he placed upon them, at the end of the eighteenth century so that we can appreciate the issues facing the early nineteenth-century investigators. At the end of the period, we shall observe how du Bois-Reymond was revolutionizing electrophysiological research and concepts and preparing for the third and modern era.

Today, we speak of the nerve impulse as the basic feature of a functioning nerve.[3] It is an event that lasts less than a thousandth of a second, and nerve conduction is achieved by a series of these events passing along the nerve fiber. Each event consists basically of a change in the permeability to ions of a minute section of the membrane covering the fiber or cell. This transient, and rapidly reversible, change allows positive sodium ions on the outside to pass through the membrane to the inside of the fiber, and negative potassium ions on the inside to move out. The exchange of ions that takes place is the immediate source of energy for the electrical current that accompanies the propagation of the nerve impulse. The internal potential or voltage of the inactive fiber or cell is negative to its exterior, and this is its resting potential (−70 thousandths of a volt). The resting nerve cell can thus be likened to a fully charged electrical battery, and in this state is said to be polarized. During the ionic exchanges just described, the charge becomes a plus quantity (+40 thousandths of a volt), a process known as depolarization. It is followed immediately by the potassium ions that have entered the cell or fiber leaving it, so that the resting potential is restored. This sudden increase and decrease in voltage produced by the alteration in the membrane's permeability and the ions traversing it is the nerve impulse, and the electrical changes thus brought about represent the action potential, which can be recorded on a suitable instrument such as the oscillograph as a spike (and known as the spike potential). The alteration in the electrical state of one piece of the membrane, that is, the nerve impulse, is passed to the next section of the fiber and so on, so that ionic intrusion and extrusion take place in sequence along its whole length. The nerve impulse can, therefore, be defined as a self-propagating chain reaction consisting of depolarization of the nerve fiber's membrane, or as a wave of negativity that travels along the fiber. This flow of current is the action current of the nerve, which is, therefore, a physicochemical event based on the differential permeability of the membrane to sodium and potassium regulated by the voltage difference across the membrane, and which is followed by a return to the resting state. The electric charge, or action potential, that can be detected by instruments in a functioning nerve, accompanies this physicochemical episode, but is secondary to it. Thus, the nerve impulse can also be described as an electrical signal fired along a nerve fiber, and seen on a tracing as a series of spikes, the action potentials. The immediate source of energy for the impulse, therefore, derives from the nerve itself, and not from the initial stimulus that sets off the sequence of events.

During the period to be reviewed, investigators were faced with three possible ways by which nerve conduction could be achieved. First, it seemed likely to some that it was due entirely to electricity, so that the nerve functioned like a wire conducting current electricity. Second, there was the possibility that the nerves possessed an inherent force, as yet unidentified but thought by some to be akin to electricity, and that electrical stimulation of a nerve, along with other varieties of excitation, merely activated it. Finally, perhaps the electricity that was eventually detected in nerves was the external manifestation of an underlying, unknown process. Our discussions below will concern the proponents of each of these possibilities, and we shall see that it was not until the middle of the nineteenth century that the third of them was established by du Bois-Reymond and his fellow physiologist, Helmholtz, but in particular by Ludimar Hermann, as the explanation that is basic to the modern concept of nerve function. It should be noted that we shall be dealing as much with the physiology of muscle contraction as with nerve function, because in the earlier stages of research the two were inseparable.

The investigation of nerve function in the nineteenth century stands apart from all other studies of the physiology of the nervous system. It is a rare example of a purely physiological problem that in the first half of the century required little or no anatomical support, once the nerve and muscle fibers had been accepted as morphological entities. Unlike most other parts of neurophysiology, a detailed knowledge of gross, comparative, developmental, or microscopical anatomy was not necessary in order to tackle the enigma of nerve function. As we learned in chap. 3.5.2, although research on the microscopical elements of the nervous system helped to elucidate the concept of the nerve cell and its fibers as the basic unit of nervous transmission, it did not contribute significantly to explaining the actual mechanism of nerve conduction, even though it did help to advance the sensorimotor physiology basic to reflex action (see chap. 4.6). In addition, the subject of nerve action had very little relevance to contemporary clinical medicine, except that electrotherapy, practiced since the eighteenth century, seemed to gain justification from the basic tenet that electricity was in some way concerned with the activity of nervous and muscular tissue. Moreover, those who carried out research on nerve and muscle were a race apart, for they were mostly pure medical scientists or physicists, who had little or no interest in, or contact with, the practice of medicine. We shall, however, be able only to glimpse the emergence in Germany at midcentury of a new type of physiologist, the organic physicist, devoted to the practice and propagation of mechanical reductionism, whereby all physiological phenomena were interpreted by means of the laws of physics and chemistry. Their aim was to unify the sciences in contemporary German philosophy (see chap. 3 n. 36). The main representatives of this school, so far as concerns the present discussion, were du Bois-Reymond, Helmholtz, and Hermann, three of the founders of modern biophysics.

5.2. GALVANI AND ANIMAL ELECTRICITY

5.2.1. Nerve Function Before Galvani

It is a remarkable fact that a concept of how a nerve functioned should have survived almost intact from Greco-Roman antiquity to the nineteenth century, but this was the case with the doctrine of the hollow nerve.[4] It was introduced by Erasistratus (fl. c. 260 B.C.) in the third century B.C., and accepted by Galen four centuries later, who stated that "according to Erasistratus, it [the nerve] contains within itself a cavity of sorts."[5] The basic supposition was that messages could travel along the lumen of the hollow nerve, and although subjected to various modifications, the theory was still alive in the early 1800s. Because it was universally accepted for so many centuries, owing chiefly to the authority of Galen, we can conclude that it must have satisfied the majority of scientists and physicians. This was the theory finally overthrown by the research on animal electricity first reported by Galvani in 1791.[6]

The agent responsible for the transmission of messages in the nerve postulated by the doctrine of the hollow nerve had varied from time to time, ranging from the "animal spirits" of the Greeks to the nervous force, power, or energy proposed in the eighteenth century.[7] A popular idea in the pre-Galvanic period inherited from earlier centuries was that the nerve contained a fluid, and that this mediated voluntary movement and sensation. Most accepted this view, including the most outstanding physiologist of the eighteenth century, Albrecht von Haller. However, he associated it with a motor force originating from the brain that resided in the nerve, the *vis nervosa,* and brought about muscle contraction.[8] It was regarded by Procháska as the biological analogue of Newton's *vis attractiva,* the force of gravity. In each case the expression did not commit its author to a concept of form or function, and thus to a hypothesis that could not be tested at that time (see chap. 4.3).

There had also been suggestions that muscle contraction and nerve action could be brought about by effervescence, ethereal oscillations, or by an explosion. Thus, when electricity was accepted as a biological property, it is understandable that it too should be proposed as the underlying phenomenon accounting for nerve and muscle function.[9] This seemed particularly appropriate in view of the fact that electricity at first was thought to be a subtle, imponderable fluid, a description that was also applied to nerve fluid. The first to write about the identity of the two was Stephen Hales, who in 1733 admitted that it was difficult to determine whether the "force" said to be generated by the blood, acted by way of the canal within the hollow nerve, or like electricity, along its surface.[10] Nevertheless, experiments, he declared, had shown "that a vibrating electrical Virtue can be conveyed and fully act with considerable Energy along the surface of animal Fibres, and therefore on the Nerves."[11]

As soon as Michel Adanson (1727–1806) in 1759 had proposed that the electric fish was the organic analogue of the Leyden jar,[12] it was also possible to make a comparison between the fish's shock and nerve action.[13] It had been known since antiquity that these creatures emitted a shock that stunned their victims, and the ancient Greeks had used them in the treatment of headache and other disorders, thus employing electrotherapy for the first time, although unknowingly.[14] Naturally, electric fish also intrigued scientists in the eighteenth century and have continued to do so ever since, and have contributed notably to the advancement of nerve physiology. Toward the end of the eighteenth century and early in the nineteenth, a number of distinguished men investigated the anatomy and physiology of the animal's electrical organ, which produces the shock they inflict. These men included John Walsh (1725–1795) in 1774, John Hunter in 1774 and 1775, Henry Cavendish (1731–1810) in 1796, von Humboldt in 1806, Humphry Davy (1778–1829) in 1829, and his brother John (1790–1868) in 1832 and 1834.[15] Their work and that of others helped further to popularize the notion that identified the active nerve agent with electricity, and because at the same time a shift in opinion against animal spirits, nerve fluid, and other speculative substances[16] occurred, this identification received wide attention. A number of prominent individuals espoused the identity of the two fluids and believed that nerve action was exclusively electrical in nature, and this was to remain acceptable until the middle of the nineteenth century.[17] A further development of the electrical hypothesis, whereby the brain was likened to the fish's electrical organ will be discussed below.

The comparison made between nerve and electrical fluids seemed a very natural one in the light of current biological knowledge, in particular the new data concerning the electric fishes. Yet there were many who were doubtful, and some, like Hales's contemporary, Robert Whytt, rejected all forms of physical and chemical energy as an explanation for nerve and muscle function. In 1751 he asserted that "we may fairly conclude that the contraction of an irritated muscle cannot be owing to effervescence, explosion, ethereal oscillation, or electrical energy."[18] The opinion was in keeping with his vitalistic creed, which led him to refute Haller's doctrine of irritability and to initiate one of the most renowned polemics of eighteenth-century medicine.[19] It is, therefore, of interest to note that the two agreed on the equally contentious issue of nerve action, because Haller also expressed doubt on the popular thesis of equating it with electricity. We have just mentioned his belief in a nonspecific nerve force, his *vis nervosa,* and in 1747 he expressed his doubts concerning an analogy with electricity.[20] For the next fifteen years this opinion, recorded in his introduction to physiology, did not change,[21] and in 1762 he reaffirmed his unwillingness to adopt the idea, although he did not reject it out of hand. Like the excellent scientist he was, he concluded that the evidence in its favor was not conclusive: "The possibility of a fiery, ethereal, electrical, or magnetic matter is not without suspicion."[22]

Haller's attitude to this enigma, as with many of the other problems he investigated, was of the utmost significance in view of his widespread and powerful following, and the decline of interest in the possibility of the nerve principle being electricity was in part due to it. But, in addition, no certain evidence for the association was forthcoming, so that opinion began gradually to move away from the hypothesis. Alexander Monro, *secundus* of Edinburgh and also an influential figure, assessed the position in 1783 as follows: "We seem, therefore, far from possessing positive arguments that the nerves operate by the medium of an electrical fluid."[23] He concluded thus: "That the matter on which the [nerve] energy depends is a secreted fluid, we are indeed far from being able to prove."[24] There were, however, at the end of the eighteenth century some who were not willing to accept this pessimism, and in the absence of adequate experimental evidence bolstered their inadequacies with speculation. J. A. Unzer in his theoretical system of nervous action had postulated several varieties of nerve force, and he used Haller's term *vis nervosa* in a more general way to describe all types of nerve activity, not the motor alone.[25] His contemporary, Prochàska, by his inductive approach, in 1784 extended the concept of *vis nervosa* so that it became the property of all nervous substance, and might be derived from "electricity, or phlogiston, or some species of air, or the matter of light, or something compounded of these."[26] On the whole, he eventually favored electricity, and he conjectured an analogy between it and his *vis nervosa,* although he had no experimental evidence to offer.[27] His mind, however, was not closed to other possibilities. We have already discussed Prochàska's concept of nerve conduction, when we dealt with his imporant contribution to reflex physiology (chap. 4.3), and we mentioned there how his interpretation of the term *vis nervosa* differed from that of its originator, Haller. In effect, Prochàska was using it, not to signify a mysterious force that traveled in the nerves from brain to effector organ, but as a provisional concept applied to the capacity of the nerve to receive external stimuli and transmit them very rapidly in either direction. This force or power remained latent in the nerve until it was evoked by a stimulus, rather like the spark from a rock struck with a hammer. The excitation could be internal or external, physical or psychical. Procháska's original approach to a very old problem is worthy of special note, because unlike all of his predecessors he was not proposing a nerve force, fluid, spirit, or whatever as an untestable hypothesis that obstructed progress, but instead a notion that would help to evaluate data on nervous system function already collected and to be collected in the future. As we have learned, his influence on one aspect of this, the reflex, lasted well into the nineteenth century. Concerning our three basic notions of nerve function, it seems, in retrospect, that Procháska was subscribing mainly to the second, whereby an unknown process inherent in the nerve, perhaps akin to electricity, could be triggered off by stimuli, including electricity. In addition, it has been suggested that his proposal fits quite well our third type, the one we accept today. However, the immense conceptual and practical differences between the two notions condemns this unhistorical interpretation. Later in life, Procháska seems to have inclined to our first kind of nerve function, for, as already noted, he subsequently made an analogy between his variety of *vis nervosa* and electricity.

There were also a few investigators, who, toward the end of the eighteenth century, were grappling with the general problem of biological electricity. The Dutchman, Martinius van Marum (1750–1837) was representative of this group, and he studied the electricity of plants as well as animals, together with its effect upon them.[28] Their enthusiasm and industry were commendable, but their achievements were negligible. However, in 1780 or earlier, Luigi Galvani of Bologna had begun the research that led eventually to his theory of animal electricity, enunciated in 1791.[29] It was this notion, crude and inaccurate as it appears to us, that would eventually sweep away the theories of nerve action postulating animal spirits, nerve fluid, and so forth, and would introduce the three possible explanations for nerve function that were associated with electricity.

5.2.2 Galvani's Research, 1780–1798

Galvani was by no means the first to recognize or to investigate the phenomenon of animal electricity, as some have supposed. Indeed, it can be said that the electrophysiology of nerve and muscle began as early as 1745, when the Leyden jar or condenser was invented.[30] Before this date, electricity could only be produced artificially by friction, mainly from the frictional machine, which had been invented by Otto von Guericke (1602–1686), Burgomeister of Magdeberg.[31] This was "vitreous" or "resinous" electricity, and the term "animal" electricity had been applied to the static electricity observed, for example, when cat's fur or human hair were rubbed, preferably on a dry day. The other source of "animal" electricity was thought to be the remarkable "natural" electricity produced by the electric fish, the Leyden jar's biological equivalent. However, the physiological effects of electricity could not be studied effectively until a method of condensing a large amount of "artificial" electrical energy into a small volume, together with a simple way of dispensing it, was available, and electrical principles vaguely understood. The Leyden jar answered this need in 1745. Despite the many experiments that made use of it, the indisputable demonstration of the ability of an electrical discharge to incite contraction of skeletal muscle was not achieved until eleven years later, in 1756 by Leopoldo Marco Antonio Caldani (1725–1813) of Padua, who was a fervent proponent of Hallerian irritability.[32] Another pioneer in this field was Giambattista Beccaria (1716–1781), who seems to have preceded Caldani, but with only a single experiment on the electrical stimulation of muscle, said to have been carried out in 1753.[33]

Not only was animal electricity well known before Galvani's studies began but the experimental preparation that he used so frequently, and often named after him, was likewise far from novel. It consisted of the skinned muscles of the frog's legs with the nerve and a piece of the spinal cord attached, similar to that first used by Jan Swammerdam (1637–1680) in 1666–1667, when he revealed that mechanical stimulation of the nerve produced contraction of the muscles.[34]

Thus, Galvani's research into electrophysiology of nerve and muscle was in no way unusual, for he was, in fact, repeating some of the experiments that others before him had carried out. However, the results he arrived at and the interpretations he placed upon them were entirely original, even though he may have been guided by "indefatigable, though blind, endeavour and a naive thirst for knowledge,"[35] as du Bois-Reymond uncharitably suggested. As we shall see, the latter made similar comments concerning the pioneer endeavors of other Italian electrophysiologists, carried out in a perplexing area of research with necessarily crude techniques and instruments. As in this case, his remarks were arrogant, derogatory, and colored by retrospective inferences, so that they provide a judgment of their perpetrator rather than of the individuals at whom they were aimed. A more accurate assessment of Galvani would recognize that he was the foremost precursor in the investigation of the electrical aspects of nerve-muscle physiology; and that he was the first to demonstrate current electricity, although unaware of the significance of this achievement. As we shall see, his studies on animal electricity are an excellent example of why the investigation of natural phenomena, whether encountered by design or by chance, is warranted, however trifling they may seem to be when first noticed.

B. I. Williams has explored the philosophical and empirical background to Galvani's experiments, but she was primarily concerned with muscular motion, rather than with nerve conduction.[36] She has discussed mechanical, electrical, and chemical aspects of muscle contraction and has identified and examined in detail the influences upon Galvani of Newtonian concepts of muscular motion and the Hallerian doctrine of irritability. As far as the general topic of nerve and muscle physiology, she concluded that:

> Galvani's position in the history of science has been found to be significant in as much as his work, begun in an era of philosophical speculation as to the identity of the forces responsible for muscular motion, initiated an era of experimental physiology.[37]

We can add that his studies on nerve action were equally significant and fertile.

A great deal has been written on Galvani and on the field of neuromuscular electrophysiology that he inspired.[38] Essentially, he carried out three sets of experiments. The results of the first two were published in his celebrated treatise of 1791,[39] and the third, which will be discussed later, anonymously in 1794. Although it seems certain that he had previously been experimenting on animal electricity, his important work began in 1780. It was in this year that he was greatly stimulated by a chance observation which both puzzled and intrigued him. When an uninsulated scalpel touched the nerve of a nerve-muscle frog preparation near to, but not in connection with, a discharging electric frictional machine, the muscles contracted. This only took place when the machine emitted a spark, and only when the metal screws of the lancet's handle were touched. Although Galvani did not recognize it, he was observing the effect of electrostatic induction from the machine, that is, the biological effects of artificial electricity. Rather than dismissing the fortuitous episode as curious, but inexplicable and therefore of little interest or significance, he embarked upon a series of experiments that he hoped would offer an elucidation of it. Ignoring du Bois-Reymond's unfair accusation, we can say that Galvani's originality lies in the fact that he accepted the challenge presented by a puzzling observation and pursued the problem relentlessly and enthusiastically. This event, encountered by accident, represents Galvani's first experiment, and he repeated it many times, substituting a long insulated wire for the scalpel and his assistant, and atmospheric electricity for that produced by the electrostatic machine. In each instance muscle contraction occurred.

Galvani's second experiment was performed early in September 1786, and it led to effects that were to be even more consequential. Again, there was an element of chance in his results as they were not the exclusive outcome of a carefully planned exercise to test a hypothesis. The fortuitous approximation of dissimilar metals with his frog preparation attached to one of the metals led to the same response obtained with frictional electricity or with "natural" electricity, that is, atmospheric lighting. Thus, when contact between copper and iron, for example, was made, nerve conduction and muscular contraction could be demonstrated. He had, in fact, proved that dissimilar metals in contact with fluid, in this case from the frog's tissues, were capable of generating an electric current.

These two fundamental discoveries in his first two sets of experiments, which were to prove revolutionary, provided the basis for Galvani's book of 1791, and from these discoveries he elaborated a theory of animal electricity. From the second experiment it seemed clear to him that nerve and muscle action was due either to electrical fluid inherent in the frog preparation, or to the contact made between the two metals. In the light of contemporary knowledge of bioelectricity and in view of the fact that he was a biologist not a physicist, it is understandable that he selected the first of the possibilities. He contended that the animal body possessed an electrical fluid peculiar to itself, the well-known "animal electricity," and he insisted that he had decisively proved its existence for the first time. He postulated that it was secreted by the cortex of the brain and distributed throughout the body by way of the nerves, which were suitable for its conduction. Thus, it could accumulate inside the nerves because the outer coverings prevented its escape, and it could then bring about contractions of the muscles. The latter were reservoirs of electricity, and they functioned in the same way as the Leyden jar for they were negative on their external surface and positive on their inside where the electricity accumulated. Muscular contraction took place when the irritable muscle fibers were stimulated by the electricity that had migrated along the nerve to the muscle's external surface, as in the manner of a Leyden jar discharging itself.[40]

Galvani's confidence in his experimental data allowed him to reject Haller's authoritative opposition to the role of electricity in the functions of the nervous system, and also those Hallerians such as Caldani and Felice Gaspar Ferdinand Fontana (1730–1805) who shared this opinion. Haller's main objection to the identification of nervous with electrical action had been that in the animal electricity could not be confined to the nerves, and therefore it spread widely owing to its all-pervasive nature. Galvani countered this criticism by postulating the existence of oily coverings to the nerves, but he was not referring here to the myelin sheath, which was not identified until nearly forty-five years later and named after Schwann.[41] Galvani asserted: "that externally they are oily, or have some other similar substance which prohibits the dissipation and effusion of this electric fluid out of the nerves."[42] Thus, the nerve's coverings acted as an insulator, but they were thin enough to allow the electrical fluid to escape at appropriate places in order to activate the muscles. Next, Galvani formulated a general theory of the production and utilization of animal electricity based entirely on ancient notions, current conjectures, and on his own findings and speculations. He concluded thus:

> Therefore, we believe it most likely that the electrical fluid is prepared by the force of the brain, being extracted from the blood, that it enters the nerves, and that it runs through them internally, whether they are hollow and empty or whether, as seems more probable, they carry a very tenuous lymph or another similar, special, very tenuous fluid, as it seems to many, secreted from the cortical substance of the brain. If this is so, the obscure, and for so long vainly-sought, nature of the animal spirits will perhaps finally be explicable. But however this may be, I believe that because of our experiments there will be no doubt in the future as to their electrical nature.[43]

This revealing passage tells us about Galvani as well as his work. He was utterly convinced that his many experiments had at last confirmed what had been suspected by a number of investigators for many years; that the animal spirits of the ancient Greeks were, in fact, the electrical fluid, animal electricity.[44] He was unable to break away from the traditional concepts of nerve functions that had been handed down from classical antiquity, and like so many other physiologists of the seventeenth and eighteenth centuries, Galvani was dressing an ancient concept in up-to-date garb, and was in fact merely exchanging one unproven hypothesis for another. Claude Bernard made reference many years later to this common method of "solving" scientific problems:

> If I recall to you these ideas that have not been current for a long time, it is in order to demonstrate that it was possible to change the terms and so replace animal spirits with an imponderable fluid, but without making any real progress. So long as one only substitutes one theory for another, in the absence of direct proof, science gains nothing; one old theory deserves another.[45]

No advance, in fact, was possible until eighteenth-century notions were abandoned completely. Galvani thus represents a midpoint figure, using what was to become a nineteenth-century concept to reinterpret one belonging to earlier centuries. He was, however, by no means the last to do so as we shall see. We can readily appreciate that Galvani felt that his studies had broken with the past, and although he could not participate fully in this liberation, we can savor in his writings the feeling of moving away from ancient ideas into a new and exciting field of research that awaited those who were willing to tread a new path in defiance of tradition, and were able even to challenge the all-powerful Hallerian doctrines that dominated contemporary physiological thought. Galvani was the instigator of the revolution, but the complete overthrow of ancient concepts was left to his successors; even during the seven years between the appearance of his classic treatise and his death, he took little part in the debate he had incited.

Before discussing the reception of Galvani's book, we should consider briefly the origins of his notion of the nervous system as a generator of animal electricity. He was, in fact, accepting as a basis for his assumptions the time-honored Greek doctrine of nerve spirits or fluid, which were produced in the brain and distributed to the body by way of the nerves.[46] As we observed in chapter 3.4, it had been elaborated by Malpighi and Wharton in the seventeenth century who claimed that the fluid was produced by the cerebral cortex, which acted like a gland, and so manufactured the principle that allowed the nerves to function.[47] In 1786 some still listed the brain as a gland, because it secreted a substance that was conveyed by the nerves to the periphery where it assisted in nutrition; the motor and sensory functions of the nerves were also dependent upon this mechanism, or on some other fluid or matter.[48] Furthermore, in 1827 there appeared the following statement in a posthumous edition of the highly esteemed writings of William Cullen: "The most common opinion is, that the brain is a secreting organ, which secretes a fluid necessary to the functions of the nervous system."[49] We have surveyed the way in which prominent early nineteenth-century scientists, such as Ehrenberg, Valentin, and Purkyně, refined this crude concept, and at the microscopical level made analogies between gray matter and glandular cells (chap. 3.4). It was also noted that even in 1849 an outstanding histologist, A. H. Hassall, continued to compare nerve cells with "all other glandular cells" (chap. 3 n. 102). Thus, during Galvani's lifetime, the idea was widely held, and he could further argue that if the brain produced a subtle nerve fluid that carried messages along the nerves, it seemed not unreasonable to equate this substance with another imponderable fluid, electricity. The brain could, therefore, be thought of as a device that generated and dispensed the electrical force, or a nervous power closely akin to it and possessing very comparable properties. We shall trace later the fate of this interesting conception, which was still under discussion in the middle of the nineteenth century (chap. 5.3.2).

5.2.3. Reception of Galvani's Opinions

Galvani's first announcement of the two series of experiments that have been described above appeared in the proceedings of the Academy of

Science and Arts at Bologna in March of 1791, and in book form later that year with the same title, *De viribus electricitatis in motu musculari. Commentarius.*[50] Its reception was best described by du Bois-Reymond, if somewhat sarcastically:

> The storm among physicists, physiologists and physicians, which the appearance of the commentary [*De viribus electricitatis,* 1791] created, can only be compared to the one that appeared on the political horizon of Europe at that time (1791). It can be said that wherever frogs were to be found, and where two different kinds of metal could be procured, everyone wished to see the mutilated limbs of frogs re-animated in this remarkable manner; the physiologists believed that at last the dream handed down from their ancestors of a vital power was within their grasp; the physicians, whom Galvani somewhat thoughtlessly encouraged to attempt the treatment of all manner of nervous disorders, such as sciatica, tetanus, and epilepsy, began to believe that no cure was impossible, and it was considered certain that in the future no one in a trance could be buried alive, provided only that he were galvanized![51]

To appreciate the impact made by the *De viribus electricitatis* it should be noted that after a period of immensely productive research on physical electricity (which culminated in the demonstrations of Benjamin Franklin [1706–1790] in 1752 that lightning, as had long been suspected,[52] was identical with electricity), there followed a relative lull for nearly forty years. Thus, the appearance of Galvani's publications, which would have caused a stir at any time, had an intensified effect, just when the science of electricity was in decline and when the belief that the electrical and nervous fluids were identical had come under attack from the Hallerians, Alexander Monro, and others.

As has been the case with many other revolutionary advances, the enthusiasm and speculations of some of Galvani's followers and successors outran the experimental evidence that was available in the late eighteenth and early nineteenth century. As du Bois-Reymond commented, some of the great excitement stirred up by the *De viribus electricitatis* stemmed from the conviction that here at last was a tool capable of penetrating the mysteries of life, namely electricity. The possibility that electricity was, in fact, life was frequently raised during the eighteenth century,[53] and it found support well into the nineteenth. Some of the Germans who submitted to the romantic philosophy of *Naturphilosophie* and sought analogies in nature believed this as we have already noted (chap. 3.4 nn. 113, 114), and reference will be made later to one of them below. John Abernethy (1764–1831) in 1817 also came close to this position, when he conceded that he did not necessarily believe that "electricity is life." He was postulating "that a subtile substance of a quickly and powerfully mobile nature, seems to pervade every thing, and appears to be the life of the world,"[54] and that it was, therefore, the life of organic bodies. However, the "powers of life regulated electrical actions,"[55] which could, for example, bring about changes of body temperature, so that electricity was not in overall control. The notion that animal electricity equated with life fired the popular imagination as well as the enthusiasm of certain members of the medical profession, and we find Thomas Skinner Surr (fl. 1806) of London, commenting in 1806 that a certain individual "expects by learning Galvanism, to be able to bring his dead horses to life again."[56]

Others, however, were unimpressed by the proposed association of electricity with vital processes, and among them was William Lawrence.[57] James Cowles Prichard (1786–1848) also protested forcefully that "it must be confessed that this analogy is so vague and indefinite, as to afford scarcely a shadow of probable evidence."[58] And as late as 1836, it was still necessary for John Fletcher to pour scorn upon the whole idea: "Anything more vague and visionary has never hitherto obstructed the progress of physiological science."[59] Negative responses to the extravagant claims made for Galvani's animal electricity, resulted in part from the contemporary, violent debate on the animal magnetism of Franz Anton Mesmer (1734–1815) and the unscientific charlatanry associated with it. To some, an association between animal electricity and magnetism seemed obvious, because they both appeared to depend for their operation upon a subtle fluid. Thus, in 1766 Mesmer had asserted that, on the basis of an analogy with the effects of the planets, the sun, and the moon upon one another and upon the earth, these bodies also exerted:

> a direct effect on all the consecutive parts of the animal body, expecially on the nervous system, by means of a fluid that penetrates everything; I ascertain this action by the INTENSITY AND REMISSION of the properties, such as gravity, cohesion, elasticity, irritability, electricity.[60]

The controversy had led to a denial of Mesmer's claims by the Académie des Sciences of Paris in 1784,[61] but despite the lack of scientific support, animal magnetism continued to flourish. As a consequence, the stigma associated with it spread to animal electricity, and there developed at the end of the eighteenth century a widespread feeling that galvanism, like mesmerism, should be viewed with caution until Galvani's results had been analyzed carefully, and his elucidations of them examined critically.

But the main opposition to Galvani's new theory of nerve and muscle action came from his scientific contemporaries, not on account of his experimental findings, because they were mostly confirmed on a number of occasions, but owing to the way in which he interpreted his results. It was this that sparked off one of the most celebrated controversies in the history of science.[62] Galvani's main adversary was Alessandro Volta (1745–1827), professor of physics in the neighboring university of Pavia, who was already involved in research on electricity and able therefore to repeat and confirm Galvani's discoveries. At first he complimented his countryman on a unique revelation, but on the basis of further experiments he launched a vigorous offensive, which began in 1792 and continued until 1800, two years after Galvani's death. He was only one of several scientists and physicians who disputed Galvani's conclusions, and the outcome of the debate they provoked had momentous results. From it derived two remarkable advances: the establishment of galvanism or animal electricity as a biological phenomenon; and in the field of physical electricity, the discovery of the electric cell or battery.

Briefly, Volta denied Galvani's notion of inherent electricity in the animal body, and instead maintained that the contraction of a muscle that was in circuit with dissimilar metals, as in Galvani's second experiment, occurred because it was excited by an electrical stimulus resulting from the contacts between the metals and not from the frog's tissues.[63] He thus introduced the concept of "metallic" electricity, the existence of which Galvani promptly denied. However, Volta was by far the better scientist, and he was able to establish it experimentally, at the same time refusing to accept the existence of animal electricity. In 1793 he declared:

> But I repeat, I must renounce not without regret, all these attractive ideas [of animal electricity], by means of which it seems to us possible to explain things admirably. Yes, it is necessary greatly to limit the action of electricity in animals, and to look upon it from another point of view, knowing that it is capable only of exciting the nerves as I have already indicated and as I am now going to prove.[64]

"Animal" electricity was merely artificially produced electricity, excited by the connection of two unlike metals made possible through a damp interface. Although the animal's nerves, muscles, and organs were readily thrown into action, they played but a passive role in the sequence of events. Volta's further contributions to the polemic were based first on these passive qualities of the animal system, second on his assumption that the arc of metal was the only source of electricity. But as A. Mauro has pointed out, he made little reference to the electric fish,[65] presumably realizing that he could not deny their remarkable ability to generate animal electricity, for to admit this would have confuted one of his fundamental tenets.

Clearly, the only way for Galvani to mount a defense against Volta, in order to uphold his theory of electricity produced solely by an animal and to counter the claims concerning metallic electricity, was to devise a method whereby muscle contraction in a frog could be induced in the absence of heterogeneous metals and of frictional electricity. It had to demonstrate the indisputable existence of a genuinely "internal" or endogenous animal electricity. He eventually succeeded in doing so, and the procedure he adopted represents his third experiment: the *contrazione senza metallo,* or "contraction without metals." In 1794 there appeared an anonymous tract, which has been ascribed with confidence to Galvani,[66] and in it is an account of what has been called "the fundamental experiment on the electricity of muscles and nerves."[67] Whereas some of his earlier experiments had been open to objections, this one was not. The sciatic nerve of a frog nerve-muscle preparation was brought into contact with the exterior surface of the thigh, and the muscle contracted immediately. The arc was made up only of nerve and muscle, and although Galvani did not realize it, he was demonstrating the effects of the frog's "injury current of the nerve," a term introduced by Hermann. There is also an injury current of muscle, and we now know that each can be detected when the injured area of a nerve or muscle is connected in circuit with its intact surface through a galvanometer. Another term for the injury current of nerve or muscle is the "demarcation current," also proposed by Hermann and applied in the same circumstances, that is, to the electrical current produced in an injured nerve or muscle at the point of demarcation between healthy and traumatized tissue.

In the present instance, the muscle twitch that Galvani had observed in his crucial experiment was due to the sciatic nerve of the preparation being excited by the demarcation potential or current of another nerve. However, in 1794, it was not recognized that the irritability of an injured nerve produced electricity, and Galvani claimed that the muscular contraction observed was due to animal electricity latent in the nerve. A significant aspect of this and other frog experiments has recently been discussed by Williams, for she has raised the possibility that the saline solution in which specimens were preserved had some influence on the results obtained by the early investigators of nerve and muscle physiology.[68] It might, in fact, help to account for the disparities that led to so much confusion, but from our point of view it is not always possible to discover whether a particular experimenter was using fresh or preserved frog material.

Volta's reply to Galvani's seemingly conclusive proof of endogenous animal electricity was that the muscle and nerve were dissimilar tissues, and the circuit they formed was completed by the tissue moisture between them, thus acting just as in the production of metallic electricity by dissimilar metals. From these preliminary skirmishes grew the Galvani-Volta polemic, but hereafter Galvani, who was a modest and retiring person, took less and less part in the controversy. His nephew, Giovanni Aldini (1762–1834), who had helped him in the experiment without metals and in the preparation of the anonymous pamphlet of 1794, now became the main defender of the concept of Galvanic animal electricity and spokesman for his uncle's beliefs. Little of his work was original, for he was but repeating, modifying, and publicizing Galvani's original research.[69] Looking back over fifty years, du Bois-Reymond dismissed his experiments with another biting comment: "His investigations are completely worthless."[70] In this instance there may have been some truth in his remark, owing to Aldini's mediocrity and lack of originality. It is generally thought that Aldini's motives stemmed from a desire to advance his own academic status as much as to promote and extend the doctrine of galvanism.

In the meantime, support for Galvani came from another quarter. The renowned German naturalist, von Humboldt, in a noteworthy treatise on galvanism published in 1797, reported a series of simple procedures that confirmed the experiment without metals of Galvani and Aldini.[71] He pointed out that muscle contraction in a nerve-muscle preparation took place when the circuit consisted solely of connected organic parts, the sciatic nerve, and the thigh muscles. In retrospect, it can be said that whereas Galvani had observed the injury current of nerve, von Humboldt was demonstrating the injury current of muscle because he had established a contact between the surface of the muscle at two points by means of a small piece of nerve. However, the evidence he gathered was sufficiently convincing for him to believe that he had refuted Volta's theory:

> The most important, and at the same time the most striking, result . . . is that the stimulus of the galvanic phenomena is present in the excitable organs themselves, and that metal as well as other substances that make up part of the circuit play only a secondary role.[72]

Humboldt, therefore, styled himself an "adversary of Herr Volta."[73] Volta, however, responded by rejecting this evidence, pointing out that as with Galvani, Aldini, and others, von Humboldt's evidence had been derived from experimenting only with isolated preparations removed from the living organism. It was surely impossible to attribute muscle contraction in a piece of dead tissue to "animal" electricity. Again, he argued that the manifestations of electricity were due to the linking together of moist, dissimilar tissues.

We can observe here that up to the early nineteenth century it was generally admitted that the immediate agent that produced the effects of galvanizing was the electrical fluid, either from the brain as Galvani had postulated, or according to Volta from the juxtaposition of dissimilar tissues. The actions exhibited by the animal body depended merely upon its extreme sensitivity to small quantities of this subtle fluid, and the experiments being carried out consisted chiefly of different combinations of conducting substances with parts of the animal's body, thus creating what was called the galvanic arc or circle. So far, animal electricity had been regarded entirely from a physical and biological point of view, but the emergence of research in chemistry at the end of the eighteenth century occasioned some discussion of its possible role in chemical processes. Probably the first to do so was Giovanni Valentino Fabbroni (1752–1822), professor of chemistry at Florence. In 1792 he proposed that Galvani's results with metals had been due not to an electrical fluid but to the reciprocal chemical interaction of dissimilar metals making contact by means of moisture. Perhaps basically galvanism was owing solely to chemical affinities, electricity being one of the concomitant effects. Therefore, the convulsions induced experimentally in the frog were the result of chemical charges produced by metal contacts made with liquid in the animal's body, whereby the fluid decomposed and its oxygen combined with the metal. New chemical substances, "oxide and saline crystals," declared Fabbroni, were thus formed by the contacts made between the metals:

> It, therefore, seems probable to me that these new compounds, or their elements, are responsible for the mysterious *stimulus* that produces the convulsive movements of the animal fiber in a large part at least of the phenomena of galvanism.[74]

Fabbroni was a forerunner of those like Sir Humphry Davy and Antoine César Becquerel (1788–1878), who revealed that chemical reactions produced electricity and that electricity could be generated only by the contact of dissimilar bodies when they reacted together chemically, or differed in temperature, or were rubbed together. There is no doubt that Fabbroni influenced ideas concerning the chemical theory of the electrical battery in the early nineteenth century. His suggestion of a "chemical operation" as the basic mechanism of bioelectrical processes in tissues has, in general, been proved correct as far as nerve conduction is concerned, but in a way quite unlike the one he envisaged. Thus, other than introducing a chemical dimension into a problem being investigated exclusively by physical and biological scientists, his contribution to our theme was small indeed, although provocative. He nevertheless deserves some recognition for others were to follow his lead as we shall see. John Bostock (1773–1846) appraised his work in 1818 as follows:

> Fabroni's [*sic*] paper did not appear to excite much attention at the time when it was published, as it directly opposed the current of popular opinion. But many of the statements have been since verified by succeeding philosophers; and when we consider that it was written before the discovery of the [Voltaic] pile, it must be regarded as displaying much sagacity and nice observation.[75]

As noted, von Humboldt in 1797 opposed Volta's denial of animal electricity, but, like Fabbroni, he was also deeply concerned with the possible role of chemical factors in its production. In fact, he pondered their relationship to life itself: "By this work, my experiments seem to have succeeded in bringing nearer the elucidation of the chemical processes of life."[76] He raised the possibility of chemical reactions producing electricity and thus muscle contractions:

> The phenomenon of turgescence (or the shortening of long fibers [muscle contraction]) can be considered as a result of a change in chemical composition, as a consequence of an unhindered external power of attraction.[77]

Von Humboldt's name must, therefore, be linked with that of Fabbroni as a pioneer in the investigation of the electrochemical aspects of nerve and muscle function, which resulted eventually in the recognition of the existence of a close relationship and interdependence between electrical and chemical processes.

But as the eighteenth century drew to a close, interest in the precise origin of animal electricity declined. Galvani had receded into the background, for he and his followers had no new evidence to support his theories, and furthermore he had suffered personal, domestic, and academic misfortunes. When he died in 1798 there was no one of comparable stature to defend and advance his doctrine even from a backstage position, although Aldini continued his efforts to do so, and, whatever his motivation, he certainly helped to prevent it becoming totally moribund. But, like his uncle, he had reached an impasse in his experimental work, and his exaggerated claims of the therapeutic value of galvanism had not raised his status in the eyes of contemporary scientists. Despite some spectacular and ghoulish experiments involving the use of oxen's heads and hanged criminals, he had nothing new to offer. Meantime, the attacks made by Volta and others continued, and, in the absence of any adequate defense or counterattack, they dominated the debate. Most of their research concerned metallic electricity, and the enigma of nerve and muscle action was being tackled almost exclusively by physicists. It was their leader, Volta, who made the next momentous contribution.

5.3. ANIMAL ELECTRICITY, 1800–1838

5.3.1. Decline of the Concept

In 1800 a letter from Volta to the Royal Society of London was read at one of its meetings, on 26 June. It reported his remarkable invention of an "artificial electric organ," directly analogous to the "natural" electric organ of the electric fish.[78] Its construction was based on his exploitation of metallic electricity, for it was made up of alternating plates of unlike metals, such as silver and zinc or copper and zinc, with pieces of moistened pasteboard between them. It was the first man-made electrical battery, and it symbolized the establishment of the electric current as a direct byproduct of Galvani's electricity produced by unlike metals that he had reported in 1791. Now, for the first time, there was available a method of providing a powerful yet stable flow of constant current electricity by means of chemical reactions, as was later to be revealed, in accordance with Fabbroni's crude hypothesis of 1792. It was entirely appropriate that this current became known as "galvanism," a term already in use, or as "Voltaic electricity," and the device that produced it was called the Voltaic "pile" or "cell." Today we describe this revolutionary appliance as a primitive wet-cell battery, while identifying it as one of the most fertile advances in the history of physics, chemistry, and technology,[79] and the electric current as "one of the outstanding landmarks in the history of science."[80] The benefits accruing from this simple apparatus have been described tersely: "With this new force, water was decomposed, metal was electro-deposited, the electro-magnet was created, and the electrical age was begun."[81]

It might be thought that nine years of experimentation for the creation of the pile was a long time, but the reasons for this do not concern us here.[82] What, however, is obvious is that Volta's invention presents two paradoxes. First, as already noted, despite his impassioned and effective attacks on Galvani's animal electricity, Volta was now admitting that electricity could be derived from an organic source, that is, the electric fish, even though previously he had utterly denied the existence of animal electricity. The second paradox is of great significance to our present theme, because although Volta's mechanical model of the electric organ of the electric fish stimulated a great deal of research into the physical nature of electricity,[83] little of this seemed applicable to physiology. Its exploitation in clinical medicine as electrotherapy need not be discussed here for, as in the eighteenth century, it contributed little or nothing at this time to the knowledge of nerve function.[84] In fact, the pile proved to be Volta's most significant counterstroke to animal electricity for it could now be argued with greater cogency that Galvani all along had not been observing the effects of the special electrical fluid emanating from the brain that he had postulated in 1791. The crucial experiment without metals could be explained on the grounds of experimental error or, as already noted, by the juxtaposition of dissimilar animal substances. Even though Volta took no further part in the debate after 1800, the tide was still flowing against Galvani's notion of animal electricity and more vigorously now than at the end of the eighteenth century. Although Aldini and others continued to defend it vigorously, they still lacked effective data and ideas. In 1803 Aldini published a book that contained an account of Galvani's 1794 experiment without metals,[85] but he also included reports on a number of inconsequential demonstrations that earned for him du Bois-Reymond's scorn and did nothing to provide the scientific basis that was so desperately needed for animal electricity. Aldini was merely reiterating Galvani's words when he stated that "Galvanism is excited in the animal machine without any intermediate body, and merely by the application of the nerves to the muscles."[86]

We now know that in spite of the strength and ingenuity of Volta's opposition to Galvani, he was wrong in his primary premise that animal electricity did not exist, and that everything could be explained on the basis of metallic electricity, or its biological analogue of unlike tissues. On the other hand, his lengthy study of the electrical phenomena discovered by Galvani led to the invention of the Voltaic pile, with its multitude of technological applications. But for the time being, in the first decade of the nineteenth century, it seemed to many that animal electricity was just another eighteenth-century concept that had not survived and was being consigned to oblivion.

This was not, however, universally so, for there remained in Germany an interest in electrophysiological research, stimulated and encouraged by the work of von Humboldt and by certain basic tenets of *Naturphilosophie*. The effects of the latter are best seen in the work of one of its advocates, Johann Wilhelm Ritter (1776–1810). Although his studies on electricity were relatively short-lived and covered the years 1792–1810, during this period his literary output dealing with its physiological, physical, chemical, and botanical aspects was prodigious.[87] His scientific method was empirical and experimental, but he interpreted his data in the light of *Naturphilosophie*[88] and, following the lead of others before him, he postulated that life could be equated with galvanism.[89] Proceeding further, Ritter became increasingly involved with the occult and asserted that the interdependence of inorganic nature and human physiological processes was determined by a subterranean electrical force.

His research on electrophysiology was only part of a larger program aimed at revealing that animal and metallic electricity were identical, thus substantiating one of the basic principles of *Naturphilosophie,* which was that there was a unity throughout nature.[90] Thus, animals and plants contained electrical cells connected in a "galvanic chain," and he used this to account for his various findings: for example, the phenomenon now known as the "creeping-in" of electricity at low currents into desensitized muscle; and the damping of responses from nerves treated with certain chemicals. Ritter described for the first time the so-called opening tetanus of muscle, and by observing the effects of chemicals on nerve and muscle excitation, he believed that he had disproved von Humboldt's results favoring Galvani's crucial, third experiment, the one without metals. Some have claimed that Ritter noticed polarization at physiological electrodes,[91] a complication that was to cause widespread confusion until du Bois-Reymond abolished it in 1859 by means of nonpolarizable electrodes. It also seems, by his own admission, that he was close to discovering the electric cell before Volta: "The way in which Volta succeeded in arriving at his discovery is still unknown. But, it has always seemed unpardonable of me to have been so near to it, without making use of what I had daily to hand."[92]

Despite these unquestionably noteworthy achievements, it is difficult to place Ritter historically. In retrospect it would appear that his pioneer discoveries and inventions were of considerable importance, but the fact that many of them had to be made again independently indicates that his voluminous writings were largely neglected, presumably owing to their bulk and to their philosophical overtones that later workers, who were endeavoring to free themselves from the influence of romantic biology, found distasteful. Thus, although there seems little doubt that Ritter won recognition and respect in Europe during his lifetime, these responses were apparently tinged with skepticism, owing to his adherence to *Naturphilosophie.*[93] This probably explains why his discoveries had no lasting effect, as judged by the paucity of reference to him by his successors, and why his continuing influence on the study of electricity was slight, especially outside Germany.[94]

Ritter's essay, *Darstellung des Gegensatzes* of 1805, is a good example of his approach to scientific problems. First of all he reported many experiments with numerous valuable observations, but in succeeding paragraphs, as one critic put it:

> in which he treats of the presence of antagonist excitabilities in inorganic nature—of magnetism and electricity as antagonists—of the relation of organized to unorganized matter—and of the relations of the earth to the sun, or of the cause of the periods of life (*das Zeitbestimmende im Leben*), he soars far beyond our capacities, and bids defiance to our language to follow him in his flights.[95]

Nevertheless his ingenuity was judged to be admirable, and he was described by a British writer as, "perhaps one of the most remarkable philosophers of the present times."[96]

It is not surprising, therefore, that Ritter has been given credit for keeping alive an interest in animal electricity in the years following the death of Galvani in 1798 and Volta's invention of the pile in 1800.[97] Nonetheless, his findings were not adequately appreciated until later in the nineteenth century, when the excesses of the *Naturphilosophen* had been dissipated. One of those who helped to dispel them was du Bois-Reymond, and he seems to have been in part responsible for the rediscovery and rehabilitation of Ritter. He accepted most of Ritter's experimental findings and gave approbation to them, but he found many of his interpretations unacceptable.[98] However, du Bois-Reymond, as in the case of other pioneers in electrophysiology, gave a distorted, and unfortunately authoritative, assessment of Ritter's merits, so that the latter's studies were given more praise than they probably deserved, an approach that has also been practiced recently regarding Ritter's studies in electrochemistry.[99]

Another important outcome of his work has been to show that *Naturphilosophie* did not necessarily have a universally stultifying effect upon scientific research, as some have thought. We have already made this point elsewhere, and in the field of physics there were other examples of the scientific method being employed to make significant discoveries that were then interpreted in the light of, and in support of, the principles of the philosophy of nature.[100]

Although Ritter may have inspired some electrophysiological research in the first decade of the nineteenth century, there were equal forces suppressing it. We have noted the harmful influence of mesmerism in the eighteenth century, and it was still present in the early nineteenth. The stigma it had earned, mainly owing to the antics and excesses of Mesmer and the early practitioners of the cult, continued, and those who professed a belief in animal electricity were stigmatized by those who equated it with animal magnetism. The similarity of the two in some minds at that time is revealed by the term "electrobiology," which was applied to a form of animal magnetism, and not to animal electricity as might be expected and is the case today. "Bioelectricity" referred to animal electricity and "biomagnetism" to animal magnetism. Moreover scientists still received no encouragement from clinicians, who instead often provoked further opposition to galvanism by their bizarre theories, based on dubious or faulty clinical data.[101]

But the decline in popularity of Galvani's thesis at the beginning of the nineteenth century was due not to a lack of disciples but mainly to the lack of new ideas and of improved experimental techniques. In their absence the concept of galvanism was in decay and the distinguished Swedish chemist, Jons Jacob Berzelius (1779–1848), summed up the situation in 1810 thus: "Galvani, the discoverer of that modification of electricity, which now bears his name . . . although he had not wanted followers, the insufficiency of his hypothesis is now pretty generally acknowledged."[102]

5.3.2. Brain as Source of Animal Electricity

This atrophic process was, however, due mainly to the fact that electrophysiological research had outstripped the ingenuity of those who could devise appliances for the detection and measurement of electrical current. Before discussing how in the 1820s this defect began to be remedied, we must explore the outcome of Galvani's proposal that the brain produced the body's animal electricity. It will be recalled that in 1791 his unique concept of the brain as a generator of electrical fluid had been grafted on to an ancient idea of the brain as a secreting gland.

Thus, in the nineteenth century's first decade there existed the notion that the brain produced either electricity or a nervous power possessing very similar properties, and we have observed how Purkyně, for example, had made analogies between nervous and physical powers when considering the activity of nerve cells (chap. 3.4). The celebrated anatomist J. C. Reil surmised that there existed a substance in the nerves analogous to animal electricity, and that it could act over a short distance by means of a kind of electrical atmosphere.[103] But as Berzelius later commented: "The manner in which he explains his hypothesis, and the arguments he introduces in support of it constitute an entertaining essay, but does not increase the sum of our real information."[104] Reil considered that the cerebellum could be the source of the nerve electricity, and he based his conjecture on the arrangement in it whereby contacts were made between blood vessels, gray matter, and white matter (i.e., between dissimilar substances, in this case, tissues) as in a Voltaic cell. Volta had already given this explanation in the case of Galvani's crucial third experiment for he had argued that electricity had been produced by heterogeneous tissues and that it was not inherent in the animal itself as Galvani claimed. Reil explained that "the vessels and the cortical substance in contact with the white matter may perhaps be the organ that produces activity, or the life spirit, like electromotor [forces] from a closed circuit."[105] There also appeared to be a relationship between cerebellar size and function, allowing Reil to assert that the latter "grows proportionally with its extension and increase in size, in exactly the same way in which the effects of electricity change, according to the different degrees of its strength."[106]

A contemporary of Reil, Luigi Rolando, working at the University of Sassari on the island of Sardinia, also formulated the idea that the brain was the source of a fluid analogous to the galvanic variety. He was probably influenced by Galvani, but he preferred to place the site of production elsewhere than in the cerebral cortex, as Galvani had suggested. At first he thought the corpus striatum was the most likely location on account of its alternating layers of gray and white matter, but he then decided that the cerebellum seemed more to resemble a Voltaic pile, because its folia suggested to him the leaves of this appliance. His conclusion was: "What greater proof is needed to demonstrate that the organ prepared a fluid analogous to that developed by the instrument cited?"[107] Moreover, believing that the cerebellum was somehow involved in muscular activity, Rolando wished to compare this with the motor function of the cerebrum, that he had demonstrated (chap. 6.4.3). He therefore linked in circuit first the cerebellum and then the cerebrum, with a Voltaic pile and a muscle and observed that the resultant muscular contractions were stronger when the cerebellum was included.[108] He consequently decided that this part of the brain must be compared with the electric organ of the electric fish, *Torpedo:*[109]

> I arrived at the firm belief that it is nothing but a true electromotor in which the nerve fluid, like that of the electric and Galvanic kind, is prepared and conducted though the various nerves in order to stimulate the muscles that serve locomotion.[110]

Both Reil and Rolando were reputable scientists and each reported his hypothesis in the first decade of the nineteenth century when knowledge of animal electricity was limited and confusion abounded. However, they had not gone as far as Galvani and had argued that the material produced by the brain was not necessarily the electrical fluid itself, but probably one that was closely associated. In the climate of their time their speculations were not entirely inappropriate, but as information increased they became less acceptable, and Johannes Müller in 1835 described Rolando's proposal as an "unproven supposition."[111]

Karl August Weinhold (1782–1829) of Halle also considered the central nervous system to be a galvanic battery and believed he had proved this by means of a bizarre experiment with most unlikely results. In 1817 he removed the cerebrum, cerebellum, and spinal cord of a kitten, so that it was rendered lifeless. But when he filled the cranium and spinal canal with an amalgam of zinc and silver, the animal revived, thus convincing him that the metallic electricity so produced had replaced the natural electricity generated by the nervous system.[112] As Neuburger observed with sarcasm, Professor Weinhold was an extravagantly gifted fabricator.[113]

Despite Müller's weighty opinion of Rolando, just cited, Jules Gabriel François Baillarger (1809–1890), who in 1840 was the first to describe the layers of the cerebral cortex and connecting white matter fibers,[114] expressed in the same article his view that by analogy the six alternating layers of gray and white substance resembled a Voltaic pile. It was this, not the cerebellum, according to him that generated the nervous fluid, necessary for activating the muscles by way of the nerves.[115] In keeping with still prevalent concepts, he assumed the fluid to be akin to electricity, having similar properties. One of the conclusions to his important paper of 1840 was as follows:

> 15° This analogy between the structure of the cerebral surface [cortex] and the make-up of the galvanic [Voltaic] appliances perhaps can be invoked as an argument greatly in favor of these two propositions:
>
> Nervous action, like electrical action, is not actually from the mass [of the brain], but from the surfaces [cortex].
>
> The nervous influx, like that of electricity, transmits itself by way of the surfaces [cortex].[116]

Admittedly he was only implying an analogy, but it seemed to him that the electrical and nervous fluids were closely associated.

At about the same time, R. B. Todd and William Bowman in their popular textbook of physiology, which they began to write in 1843, were also willing to accept the fluids being identical, as we shall see later. Concerning the origin of the nervous fluid, they, like Baillarger, discussed the apparent similarities between the production of electricity from the moist contacts of dissimilar metals and the heterogeneous cortical layers, likewise bathed in fluid.[117] For them, however, the microscopical structure of the cortex was of prime importance, and they argued that if it were true that the cortical cells were connected to the white matter, then each cell together with its fibers and the blood vessels surrounding it represented "a distinct apparatus for the development of nervous polarity [or "electrical tension" in modern terms]."[118] This we should compare with Purkyně's concept of the nerve cell discussed elsewhere (chap. 3.4). Todd's and Bowman's faith in the anatomical rather than the physiological approach to their problem is especially interesting, because it illustrates the predominance in Britain of morphological over physiological studies. In the present case the former was, however, of no assistance at that time, and they cautioned:

> But it would be hazardous to speculate on such a subject until [microscopical] anatomical research has revealed to us more information respecting the exact disposition of the elements of the vescicular [gray] matter.[119]

We can also cite here the opinion of an eminent British scientist, who approached the problem of the proposed brain origin for animal electricity with a deep knowledge of the physical aspects of electricity. In a series of lectures delivered in 1831, Frederick William Herschel (1792–1871) asserted that the prevailing state of electrical science and what was known of the electric fish warranted the conjecture that the brain represented an electric organ that could be spontaneously discharged at brief intervals along the nerves to the heart, for example, to excite its pulsations. This occurred "when the tension of the electricity developed reaches a certain point,"[120] the comparison with a nerve fluid being close. Furthermore, Herschel thought it reasonable

> to look to the brain, a wonderfully constituted organ, for which no mode of action possessing the least plausibility had ever been devised, as the source of the required electrical power.[121]

But the most ingenious of all the schemes that featured the brain as an electrical generator was that put forward by Paul Traugott Meissner (1778–1864), professor of chemistry at the polytechnical institute at Vienna.[122] In his book of 1832, he was primarily concerned with the basic laws of animal life, and he included a discussion on the way in which the nervous system in humans and animals controlled the body by means of electricity. First of all, the blood in the lungs became charged with the electricity that had been produced during the chemical process of breathing. It immediately traveled through the nerves of the lungs, and then by way of other parts of the ganglionic (our autonomic) nervous system to the brain and spinal cord, which were then similarly charged with electricity. The brain was in control of the will, which also operated by means of electricity, and using the latter, the brain excited the various organs to activity by way of their respective nerves, along which the currents passed. Although contrived with such skill and resourcefulness, this hypothesis received neither extensive notice nor lengthy survival. Concerning the nervous system in general, Meissner explained: "This represents the controller of the electrical fluid, and consequently is equivalent to what in the plant preserves the electric current of the terrestrial globe."[123]

Meissner was a *Naturphilosoph,* seeking, like its earlier devotees, to uncover the laws and unity of nature. Emil Huschke (1797–1858), professor of anatomy and embryology at Jena, was another, as will be clear from his thesis that "each man is a psychical as well as a physical formula, a physical and psychical member of the infinite world of body and soul."[124] It is interesting to observe that a follower of *Naturphilo-*

sophie was still to be found in 1854, and Huschke's adherence to it is reflected in his important treatise on the skull, brain, and soul of humans and animals published in that year. It is particularly noteworthy for its section on the pattern of the cerebral convolutions and sulci, but, there is also a section entitled "The brain, an electrical organ," where he discussed the problem that had intrigued Galvani, Reil, Rolando, Meissner, and others.[125] He studied, in particular, the convolutions of the cerebral hemispheres, and he proposed electrical analogies based on their alignment. These and the cerebellar folia acted, together with other parts of the brain, as an electrical machine, each portion having a specific role to play:

> Especially after the researches of Dubois-Reymond, does it not seem that the important relationship, if not identity, between nerve force and electricity has found increasing application to the bulk of the nervous system? Likewise it should be accepted as the elementary source of an electric current."[126]

On the whole, he chose the cerebrum as the main electrical apparatus, rather than the cerebellum favored by Reil and Rolando. The results of his research indicated to him that "the [term] brain describes a compound electrical apparatus."[127] But, as we have noted above, Claude Bernard later pointed out the futility of substituting one theory with another, in the absence of any real proof for either. All those we have mentioned here were, like Galvani, merely grafting new concepts and terms on to ancient notions, and their efforts brought about no progress in the understanding of nerve function. Thus, the analogy of the Voltaic cell with the brain led nowhere, but another analogy was more rewarding.

5.3.3. The Role of the Electric Fish

We have already discussed the important part played by the electric fish in the history of animal electricity during the eighteenth century. In the early nineteenth century it also helped to popularize the notion that the active nerve principle was identical with electricity.[128] A galaxy of distinguished scientists explored the anatomy and physiology of the electric fish in the late eighteenth century and throughout the nineteenth, including such men as Benjamin Franklin, John Hunter, Henry Cavendish, Geoffroy St. Hilaire, Galvani, Volta, von Humboldt, John Davy, Faraday, and Carlo Matteucci (1811–1868). At the end of the nineteenth century du Bois-Reymond was still studying them, and these fish have continued to receive attention up to the present day.

In the first decades of the nineteenth century, they appeared to offer a useful clue for the elucidation of nerve and muscle function for here was an example of what seemed to be an electrical force being produced in an animal's body without any assistance from an external agency, that is, true "animal" electricity. It could be argued that if this occurred naturally in one part of nature, why should it not be a basic biological principle of life in human beings, animals, and also plants. Having examined the opinions of those like Rolando who equated the animal brain with the electrical organ of the fish, we must now discover the arguments used by others, who, although not necessarily accepting this notion, nevertheless sought an equation between fish, electricity, and nerve force, the most important function of the latter being to travel along the nerves and bring about muscular contraction.

Although an identity between the shock of the electric fish and the shock received from a Leyden jar, known to store electricity, had first been proposed by Adanson in 1759,[129] and despite the similarities that seemed to exist between their electric organs and the Voltaic cell, as Volta himself begrudgingly accepted, some were still doubtful whether the electrical and nerve forces were identical. In 1834 C. G. Carus, referring to the study of electrical fish by von Humboldt,[130] commented:

> The true nature of this active power in the Electric Eel, for instance, as described by HUMBOLDT, still leaves much to be wished for, particularly as regards its relationship with electricity.[131]

Opinion was divided until the following year when A. C. Becquerel and Gilbert Breschet (1784–1845) in Venice, established beyond all doubt that the shock of one of the electrical fish, the *Torpedo,* was the result of an electrical discharge: "We began by confirming a property [of the Torpedo] that has been recognized for a long time, of giving a shock absolutely the same as that from the Leyden bottle."[132]

We can commence this brief survey of the role of the electrical fish in the shaping of early nineteenth century concepts of nerve action by the hypothesis formulated by Wollaston in 1809.[133] His belief was that bodily secretion in general was dependent upon electricity, which was conveyed by the nerves to the secretory gland, where it induced a flow of the organ's product. This idea, which he supported by citing the activities of the electrical fish, received wide approval. The concept of G. R. Treviranus was, however, much more ambitious, because he was attempting to equate electricity with life as others had already tried. He was an eminent follower of *Naturphilosophie,* and his aim in biology, a word he invented, was to discover and then to study the underlying laws of nature (see chap. 2.2). As with other *Naturphilosophen* already cited, he was especially concerned with the role of electricity, and he propounded the notion that the power concerned in the manifestations of electrical phenomena in animals could well be one of the forces on which the continuance of life in general depended. He added: "Perhaps it is the same power that through the [electric] organs produces the electric shocks, that is the immediate cause of the contraction [of muscle fibres]."[134]

Others did not go as far as this in their opinions on the nature of the nerve principle, and Wilson Philip, for example, was content to employ the electric fish as evidence in favor of animal electricity; "the phenomenon of electricity of electric animals" as he described it,[135] being the same as the common or Voltaic variety. On the other hand, he had more substantial support from ingenious experiments, carried out by colleagues under his direction, because of his dislike of vivisecting animals. These revealed that galvanic stimulation of the distal end of a sectioned nerve could reproduce the functions of that nerve, which to his mind allowed one to accept the equality of nervous and electrical fluid. For example, one of his experiments showed that gastric digestion could continue when galvanic electricity replaced the action of the vagus, and it was cited in the Continental literature for years thereafter.[136] In brief, Wilson Philip held that animal electricity was just common electricity modified in its properties by those of life, under the influence of which it operated in the living animal. Finally, we should again mention Carus, an active *Naturphilosoph,* who was on the whole more moderate in his views than some of his fellow devotees. But, like many of them, his major aim was to reveal the unity of the natural sciences, although he was not content to restrict his activities to speculation, for he was an acute observer and he evaluated carefully the empirical data he collected. Concerning the electricity generated by the electric fish, his opinion, despite his critical attitude toward von Humboldt, was the same as Treviranus's:

> it is not impossible that the nervous force collects in these cells [of the electric organ] (the same as in a condenser), and that it is discharged voluntarily, just as it accumulates in the substance of the muscles, so that contraction of their fibers can be brought about.[137]

There can be no doubt that in this early period, as in the eighteenth century, as well as later in the nineteenth and up to the present day, the electric fish acted as a potent stimulus to investigators of bioelectricity in the physical as well as the biological fields of research. But although it increased interest, it also had a deleterious effect for it encouraged the use of an analogy, since shown to be false. This was between the fish's electric organ and the muscle fibers. It was thought, correctly, that the latter could generate electricity in the same manner as the former. However, the fallacy was in assuming that the fibers produced electricity to a similar level of potential, or voltage, which we now know not to be the case. Yet another analogy should be mentioned here, because it also proved to be false and misleading. It is understandable that early workers in electrophysiology should make the mistake of comparing animal electricity in a nerve, with a current of Voltaic electricity flowing along a conducting wire. This was to remain a stumbling block until Helmholtz in 1850 measured the velocity of transmission in the nerve and revealed that whatever the nature of the process might be, it was not current electricity, because it traveled much too slowly. A serious error was, therefore, eliminated forever. But meantime, we must remember this false analogy and the one concerning the electric fish that faced the unsuspecting experimental electrician in the first few decades of the nineteenth century. There was also the erroneous assumption that the electric currents in resting frogs were of physiological significance, and the fact that scientists were unaware of the adverse effects of polarization on their experimental results. We can thus better appreciate the investigators' frequent bewilderment and sympathize with their despair provoked by a confused and chaotic field of research. To be aware of this state of affairs also helps us to understand the frequent misinterpretation made of experiments on animal electricity in the first few decades of the nineteenth century, and for the diminishing appeal of the subject as a field of experimental research. There was, however, another vital factor responsible for this decline of interest, and this was the grave technical inadequacies facing investigators, which for the moment were insurmountable.

5.3.4. Technical Advancement

The main problem facing those wishing further to explore the nature of Galvani's animal electricity was the purely practical one of detecting the presence and strength of the minute electrical current in a biological specimen.[138] Until instruments sensitive enough to provide this essential information existed, little or no advance could be made in the study of nerve and muscle function, beyond that already achieved by Galvani and his followers. The biologist, therefore, had to await the ingenuity of the physicist and technician, and until 1820 only crude electrostatic measuring devices were available.[139] We can now follow the stages in the development of a much more sensitive appliance, the galvanometer.

The possible relationship between the two physical forces, electricity and magnetism, excited interest, which was first manifested briefly in 1802 when Gian Domenico Romagnosi (1761–1835), an amateur scientist of Trento and of the University of Parma, reported "an experiment showing the action of the galvanic fluid on magnetism."[140] He had observed the influence of electricity from a Voltaic pile on a compass needle but, like others who also narrowly missed discovering the magnetic effect of the electric current, he did not investigate the phenomenon further. In any event, there was no further advance in this field until Hans Christian Oersted (1777–1851), professor of physics at the University of Copenhagen, took the next step. In 1812, Oersted formulated investigations involving both electricity and magnetism, but it was not until 1820 that he devised the decisive experiment, by means of which he revealed that a wire through which a current of electricity was flowing could induce a magnet to set itself at right angles to it.[141]

Oersted's discovery illustrates the scientist's reliance on the general analogies and parallels that exist between the various branches of science by means of which one strongly reminds him of another, although no direct connection is then apparent. In this instance the juxtaposing of electrical and magnetic forces has been described as an event "among the most memorable in the whole history of science."[142] Like his friend Ritter and other early electricians, Oersted was a devotee of *Naturphilosophie,* and its influence on his scientific work has been explored by historians.[143] It has been suggested that chance played a prominent role in his important discovery, but it seems that unwarranted emphasis has been laid on this factor, and instead it is now claimed that "it was *Naturphilosophie,* not chance, that led to the discovery of electromagnetism."[144] This episode, therefore, appears to be another example of the beneficial contributions of romantic biology to early nineteenth-century science. Also in 1820, the German physicist Johann Salomo Christoph Schweigger (1779–1857) extended Oersted's work, and was the first to note the way in which the magnetic effect was multiplied when a coil of wire carried a current instead of a straight piece. From this finding derived the first name given to the galvanometer, the electromagnetic "multiplier." Schweigger's device was based on the deviation of a copper-nickel bar in sal-ammoniac induced by weak currents of electricity,[145] and he demonstrated it to the Naturforschende Gesellschaft of Halle on 16 September and 4 November 1820.

Schweigger did not, however, make any attempts to refine his instrument nor did he discover precisely how it worked. Nevertheless, although it could not detect bioelectrical currents, it led the way to a succession of contrivances for the detection and recording of them, invented over the next century and a half, and ranging from the astatic galvanometer, to the reflecting-mirror galvanometer, the capillary electrometer, the string galvanometer, the cathode-ray oscilloscope, and eventually to the sophisticated apparatus used today.[146] Schweigger, like Ritter and Oersted, was an adherent of *Naturphilosophie* and in his studies always sought a higher synthesis in nature. This expressed itself in his theory of matter, which was offered as an alternative to the atomic theory of John Dalton (1766–1844), and was extended to involve the universe as a whole.[147] Simultaneously with Schweigger's research, but independent of it, Johann Christian Poggendorff (1796–1877) produced a similar apparatus.[148] Although these early multipliers, or galvanoscopes, could detect the presence of an electrical current, they could not measure it. Moreover, whereas they were of the greatest value in the investigation of current electricity, they were, as noted, too insensitive for experiments on animal electricity. But with the rapid advances being achieved in research on electricity and magnetism, improvements were soon forthcoming.

One of the first was introduced by the Italian physicist, Leopoldo Nobili (1784–1835) of Florence, who, in 1825, devised an ingenious instrument.[149] He made use of the astatic needle that had been invented in 1820 by André Marie Ampère (1775–1836), professor of mathematics at the École Polytechnique of Paris.[150] It neutralized, or greatly reduced, the effects of terrestrial magnetism, and with the addition of his own modifications, Nobili constructed an improved Schweigger astatic galvanometer that provided a sensitivity denied earlier workers. Nevertheless, it was still unable to register the presence of the brief and minute electrical signal produced in nerve conduction, that is, the current of action or our nervous impulse. But, after patient and persistent trial and error, Nobili detected the presence in the frog of an electric current on 3 November 1827. He was the first to provide instrumental proof of its existence.[151] Employing the skinned and decapitated frog (the preparation that had been used by Galvani and many others), he discovered a current on its body that passed cephalad from the legs, or, as we now know, from leg muscles, to nerves, to spinal cord. This was the current that had produced the effects witnessed by Galvani, and by those before and after him in their experiments on the frog. Nobili called it *la corrente propria della rana* and the French equivalents, *courant propre* or *courant de la grenouille,* became popular in the European literature. Unfortunately, in Britain it was known as the "proper current of the frog" instead of more appropriate renderings, such as "natural" or "intrinsic" current. We now know that this was the current of injury of muscle, or demarcation current, and Nobili's experiment revealed that, as would be expected, it resulted from decapitation. He was therefore, the first to demonstrate Galvani's animal electricity by means of a physical device, in particular the underlying event in his crucial experiment without metals of 1794. It should, however, be noted that Nobili's galvanometer was not more sensitive than a Galvani frog-preparation that twitched in the presence of a current that his instrument did not record.

Nobili's success derived mainly from his technical versatility, but he was unable to interpret his results correctly. Thus, he claimed, erroneously, that his *corrente propria della rana* was due to a thermoelectric effect, owing to the fact that the nerve was smaller in volume than the muscle and thus cooled more rapidly.[152] Nobili was not, of course, alone in his inability to discover the exact nature and origin of this phenomenon for no one else at that time could solve the problem. He was, nevertheless, a noteworthy pioneer, not only on account of his unique technical and experimental abilities but also because he initiated a revival of interest in electrophysiology after about thirty years relative inactivity. The next important steps were taken by Carlo Matteucci, who in 1838 began to investigate Nobili's frog current. But before discussing his work, we must look at studies being carried out in France in the 1820s and 1830s, and at the contemporary scene in Britain. They had this in common: the outcome of French and British endeavors was virtually nil. We should, however, find out why.

5.3.5. Research in France and Britain

In the 1830s, many experimenters were content to use the unmodified, and therefore inferior, multiplier of Schweigger and ignored Nobili's better model. Knowing as we do the minute dimension and the brief time span of the nervous impulse, and the fact that this instrument could not detect single action currents of nerve, it is not surprising that their results were either negative or contradictory, or both. It seems that most of this research was carried out by physiologists in France, but the outcome of their labors was greatly inferior to that of contemporary French physical electricians, who were achieving noteworthy results in their efforts to investigate electric current theory.[153] Naturally, the eminent physiologist F. A. Longet, in his treatise on the anatomy and physiology of the nervous system published in 1842, gave prominence to French biological research, although on the whole the contributions made were slender.[154]

It is curious that these studies of electrophysiology should be so inferior to those of the Italians and later, the Germans, at a time when in other parts of physiology, and especially of the nervous system, the French predominated. In the case of French and Germans working on the electrical aspects of nerve and muscle function, their differences, as in other aspects of the medical sciences, were to some extent due to opposing styles of research and guiding philosophical principles. We have noted how the *Naturphilosophie* of the Germans induced a number of individuals to explore the nature and significance of bioelectricity, and although their philosophical excesses may not have been helpful, some of their conclusions that were founded on empirical data were of significance for the history of nerve function.

In France, *Naturphilosophie* was virtually nonexistent and physiological research was guided by men such as Magendie and Flourens, who were inclined more to vivisections (as we have noted in chapter 1) and who preferred to accumulate experimental evidence piecemeal according to the philosophy of the ideologues, on the whole shunning theories and speculation (see chap. 6.5). Moreover, whereas the Germans were willing to carry out experiments on excised parts of animals *in vitro,* the French preferred to examine the whole living animal in which vital functions could be investigated.[155] In the case of electrophysiology, the German approach proved to be the more appropriate. Another difference was the Germans' seemingly greater technological ingenuity at this time in the field of electrophysiology, which the French could not match. Their poor performance was still apparent in the 1850s.

The nationalistic bias of French science in the 1830s may have been another factor that inhibited progress. Outmoded eighteenth-century concepts that had been sanctified by celebrated Frenchmen still exerted great influence. Cuvier, for example, in 1817 had made no reference to the possible role of electricity in nerve activity; his opinions might have derived from the seventeenth, let alone the eighteenth century. He declared that:

> It is very probable that the nerve acts on the [muscle] fiber by means of an imponderable fluid, more especially since it is adequately demonstrated that it does not act mechanically.[156]

P. A. Béclard had gone further and had attributed a "nervous force, nervous power, nervous influence"[157] to the brain, spinal cord, and nerves. These structures, he asserted in 1823, had a hierarchical control over the muscles, and thus removal of the brain greatly diminished the cord's activity; removal of the cord greatly diminished the nerve's activity; impairment of muscle contraction due to a loss of the nervous principle or force increased the closer to the muscle a nerve lesion was placed.[158]

In August of the same year, two distinguished French physiologists, Jean Louis Prévost (1790–1850) and Jean Baptiste André Dumas (1800–1884), presented a paper to the Académie des Sciences at Paris, in which they expounded a theory of muscle action based on electricity.[159] Although they could detect no true electrical activity in either functioning nerve or muscle by means of galvanometric studies, they postulated the presence of nerve currents and, like others before them, they wondered whether chemical stimuli produced their known effects on nerves by developing electricity. However, also in keeping with all the others who had done so, they offered only speculation. Prévost and Dumas are also remembered for their unique, but erroneous, theory of muscle contraction. They proposed that the nerves supplying a muscle did not have free terminations in them, as we know to be the case, but instead were arranged in loops parallel to each other and approaching the muscle fascicles at right angles. Where the fascicle was crossed by a nerve, it was thought to bend in a zigzag fashion due to a stimulus from the nerve, thereby bringing about muscle contraction. However, all their techniques were crude, and their hypotheses concerning nerve function were judged improbable and therefore rejected.

In view of the fact that Prévost and Dumas speculated concerning the possible role of chemical processes in nerve action, we should emphasize again the fact, frequently overlooked, that the relationship of these processes to bioelectricity, which was eventually to play such an important role in the elucidation of nervous transmission, was not entirely neglected at this time, despite the emphasis being placed on the presence of a purely physical phenomenon in nerve and muscle. We have referred already to Fabbroni's opinion of 1792, which raised the possibility of both chemical and physical factors, and that of von Humboldt. There were many more, but we should in particular note Cuvier's comment in 1817, when he declared that concerning operative influences, such as light, heat, odors, percussion, compression, and so forth: "It is very probable that these factors act on the nervous fluid in a chemical manner, thus altering its composition."[160] In the same year, Berzelius had described the discharge from the electric organ of the electric fish as "electricity elicited by an organic chemical process."[161] He based this assumption on the knowledge that the discharge was a voluntary act, as von Humboldt and other biologists had early realized, and therefore basically different from the physical process that took place in the Voltaic pile. A year later he reassessed the situation, and he had to admit that although the brain and nerves controlled the chemical processes of the body and could produce chemical effects

> yet we are constrained to confess, that the chemical operations therein are so far beyond our reach, that they entirely escape all our observations. Our deepest chemical researches, and the finest discoveries of later times, give us no information on this subject. Nothing of what chemistry has taught us so hitherto, has the smallest analogy to the operation of the nervous system, or affords us the least hint toward a knowledge of its occult nature.[162]

His praiseworthy restraint stands in stark contrast to the conjectures of some of his contemporaries.

Longet in 1842 also reported the experiments performed by Isidore Bernard David (fl. 1830).[163] Using a Schweigger multiplier, he claimed to have demonstrated electrical currents in the nerves of rabbits and hens, but it seems unlikely that he had done so. We should note that the object of his study was to confirm the identity of the nervous and electrical fluids. However, other investigators, including Charles Cléophas Person (fl. 1830) also of Paris, together with the celebrated scientists Johannes Müller and Carlo Matteucci, failed to verify David's findings. Müller, who repeated his experiments, considered that the Frenchman had been deceived.[164] Müller was combating the notion that nerve and electrical fluids were identical, which David had hoped to support. Like Müller, Person, who employed a sensitive galvanometer of his own design, could not detect any evidence of electricity in the nerves.[165]

Another Frenchman, Alfred Donné (1801–1878), the celebrated discoverer of the *Trichomonas vaginalis* organism (1836) and the blood platelet (1842), did detect the presence of electricity in various organs of the body, and even in fruit.[166] He also made a vague proposal concerning the possibility of a chemical component, for it seemed to him that there was an electrical action between the inner and outer surfaces of the skin, which he attributed to the alkaline and acid properties of its secretions. But again it was only a conjecture, with quite inadequate experimental evidence. It seems likely that, in keeping with many of his contemporaries, the chief reason why Donné misconstrued his results was because he was not aware of polarization and the secondary currents it induced, a stumbling block that was not to be removed for several decades. As mentioned above, this most serious hazard dogged the experimental labors of the pioneer electrophysiologists and led to untold confusion and contradiction.

In his survey of available data concerning nerve function, and paying special attention to those of French workers, Longet in 1842 concluded that

> despite the discovery of electromagnetism, that has made possible the most sensitive galvanometric instruments, there exists up to the present no direct proof in favor of the hypothesis that there are electric currents in the nerves.[167]

It was his considered opinion that "electricity is probably only a simple excitant of the permanent [intrinsic] nerve force, and its action must be equated with that of mechanical and chemical irritants."[168] He was, therefore, subscribing to the second of the three possible explanations for electricity's role in nerve action, which held that the nature of the underlying process was quite unknown, and that electricity was neither primary nor secondary, as in the other two explanations that had been offered, but merely one of several external excitants that could induce a nerve to function. Longet epitomized the situation succinctly in 1842:

> In order to explain in man and animals the phenomena of physical life, most authors are inclined to admit the presence of an imponderable agent known by different names such as *principle, agent or nervous fluid, nervous force, active principle of the nerves,* etc. . . . But if many physiologists see the nervous principle as an imponderable fluid, they differ in opinion when it comes to comparing it with another imponderable [fluid] that is already known; for some it is *identical* with the electrical fluid; for others, it is only *analogous* and can only be a simple modification like the magnetic fluid; for these last, the nervous force is a force *sui generis.*[169]

Once again we are reminded of Bernard's cogent comment that exchanging one theory for another without providing firm empirical evidence in either case is a recipe for stasis devoid of advancement. Judging by Longet's use of the archaic term "nerve force," by the results of the various studies he cited, and by his own conclusions, it seemed that little or no progress had been achieved so far in the nineteenth century. However, the pessimism he expressed was a reflection of an approach to the problem of nerve function that would never prove fruitful. As Bernard was implying, the time-honored notions of "nerve force," "nervous fluid," and the like had to be completely abandoned before any real progress could take place.

In 1850, we find that the situation in France had not changed appreciably. Emil du Bois-Reymond visited Paris at Easter of that year to demonstrate some of his experiments on electrophysiology to the Académie des Sciences, and in a letter to Carl Ludwig (1816–1895), he made these critical comments:

> The ignorance and restricted view of even the best men here is incredible. Longet, for example, who is an excellent fellow and has the best of intentions, makes not a single reference to [Ernst Wilhelm von] Brücke [1819–1892] in the section on vision in his new work on physiology; you, naturally, do not exist here any more than Brücke. They take Helmholtz for a lunatic. Your text book will be a couple of generations ahead of French ideas.[170]

It seemed, however, that the French were not alone in their inability to break with traditional theories. We have already referred to the opinions of R. B. Todd and W. Bowman in London concerning the brain as a possible source of animal electricity. But, in 1845, they also discussed at length whether "nervous force" was identical with current electricity.

However, the arguments they marshaled were mostly those used in the eighteenth century, updated by the application to them of the early nineteenth century crude observations on animal electricity.[171] With minor reservations they concluded, "Thus far we remark unquestionable analogy in the mode of development and of propagation of the electrical and nervous forces."[172] This was a reasonable judgment and shared by many at the time. However, it was not based on experimental evidence, and, in fact, at that time little or no physiological research of note was being carried out in Britain at all, let alone electrophysiological research.[173] The only scientist of stature who showed any interest in the practicalities of animal electricity was Michael Faraday, who in 1831 had opened up the immensely important field of electromagnetic induction.[174] He concerned himself to some extent with the biological as well as the physical aspects of electricity, and it is only natural that the electric fish should have engaged his attention.[175] In a paper read to the Royal Society on 6 December 1838 he evinced enthusiasm regarding the topic, and looked to the future with confidence:

> Wonderful as are the laws and phenomena of electricity when made evident to us in inorganic or dead matter, their interest can bear scarcely any comparison with that which attaches to the same force when connected with the nervous system and with life; and though the obscurity which for the present surrounds the subject may for the time also veil its importance, every advance in our knowledge of this mighty power in relation to inert things, helps to dissipate that obscurity, and to set forth more prominently the surpassing interest of this very high branch of Physical Philosophy. We are indeed but upon the threshold of what many, without presumption, believe man is permitted to know of this matter.[176]

Faraday was not entirely convinced that the nervous agent was only electricity, and he thought that the responsible agent in the nervous system might well be an unknown inorganic force. He argued that just as magnetism was a higher relation of force than electricity: "So it may well be imagined, that the nervous power may be of a still more exalted character, and yet within the reach of experiment."[177] Here Faraday was including bioelectricity in his attempt to correlate physical forces, such as electricity, magnetism, heat, light, chemical affinity, and other powers of nature.

These promising proposals and the influence that Faraday wielded had little effect on research into animal electricity in Britain. Here the medical profession seemed to be interested only in the possible therapeutic uses for electricity, without showing any concern about its physiology.[178] A comment from du Bois-Reymond is again valuable. He made it in 1852:

> Science can achieve but small gains there [Britain], but the more so for the general philosophical ideas of life (*Weltanschauung*). Physiology does not exist over there. They adopt the Hallerian point of view, but this will not hinder them from having the opportunity again of making some colossal discovery, the third after Harvey's and Bell's.[179]

However, in the case of the electrophysiology of nerve and muscle neither Faraday's nor du Bois-Reymond's hopes for the future were yet to be fulfilled. Even in 1887 the position had changed little because John Scott Burdon Sanderson (1828–1905), Waynflete Professor of Physiology at the University of Oxford, reported that accounts of the electrical aspects of nerve and muscle function were then new to the English scientific language.[180]

In contrast with the low quality of research into the physiology of nerve and muscle action being conducted in France during the 1830s and 1840s and the total absence of it in Britain, the traditional exploitation of this field by Italian scientists was fortunately revived after the lull that had taken place earlier in the century. Following the work of Nobili, a new phase of progress began dominated exclusively by Carlo Matteucci, and during it some of the fundamental principles and experimental techniques were established.

5.4. MATTEUCCI'S RESEARCH

5.4.1. Introduction

The stagnation in Italian research on electrophysiological topics that took place after 1800 ended in the late 1820s. Nobili in 1827 had reanimated studies in muscle and nerve function, and following him Matteucci in the late 1830s sustained and extended this new interest. He was a physicist and mathematician by training, who had already established a reputation by his writings on the physical aspects of electricity. In 1836 he began the investigation of animal electricity or galvanism, a study that he pursued actively until about 1850, although he continued thereafter to publish on the subject. During this period of only fourteen years, Matteucci made discoveries that were of great significance to the elucidation of muscle and nerve action; but unfortunately although he manifested praiseworthy experimental ingenuity, acute powers of observation, and inventive versatility, he lacked adequate insight and ability for logical reasoning with which to assess the mass of experimental data, often contradictory and confusing, that he assiduously collected. These defects eventually led him to the unusual course of denying certain observations and opinions that he had reported earlier. As we shall see, Matteucci's ability to contradict himself and to recant has tended to diminish the worth of his contributions in the eyes of his successors. There can be no doubt, however, that despite his intellectual shortcomings as a scientist his role as a pioneer was of considerable significance.[181] We should also applaud the fact that, whether he was right or wrong, he had the courage of his convictions and was able to change his mind publicly, a step that few have found easy to take and many impossible.

Early in his research on animal electricity, he gave credit to the past when he declared that:

> Forty years have elapsed without teaching us anything new on this topic; and it is to Nobili that we are indebted for ascertaining clearly that these [muscle] contractions are due to an electric current in the frog, directed from the muscles to the nerves.[182]

This was his point of departure.

5.4.2. Electric Fish and Frog Current

Like many before and after him, Matteucci was fascinated by the properties of the electric fish, and it was a study of them that led him into research on the electrical features of muscle and nerve function. In 1836, he began an extensive investigation of the *Torpedo* variety.[183] One of his discoveries was that the electrical discharge from the animal's electric organ originated in the fourth (*dernier*) lobe of its brain, "which I shall henceforth call the *electric lobe*."[184] But, more important for our present theme was the clear statement made by Matteucci that in *Torpedo* the nerve force was electrical in nature:

> The force that develops and circulates in the brain and system of nerves is transformed into electricity by the help of a special arrangement that nature has assigned to certain animals; and the electrical current is the only external agent that also has a most powerful action capable of producing a discharge, and in which an analogy with the nerve agent is consequently most likely.[185]

Matteucci then turned his attention to the frog current or *courant propre,* the effects of which had been observed by Galvani and many others, and which had been first detected instrumentally by Nobili. He was able to improve on the latter's techniques, and in 1838 published his first account of it.[186] Four years later a much more adequate demonstration of it was reported in mammals as well as in the frog.[187] Most significantly, however, Matteucci could always detect a current of electricity when an injured area of a voluntary muscle at rest was connected in circuit with a part of its intact surface through a galvanometer. Our interpretation of this finding is that he had revealed the existence of an electrical potential in the resting muscle (our "resting potential"), which was released when it was injured, and which represented the difference in potential between the inside and the outside of the muscle fiber. Matteucci had demonstrated and correctly detected the etiology of our demarcation potential or injury current of muscle. As Moruzzi has claimed, it represented "a fundamental step in the history of electrophysiology, since the present concept of the resting polarization of the membrane developed from it."[188] Matteucci discovered that the injured part was always negative with reference to the intact surface, and we now know that the current was induced to flow because of the difference in potential that existed between them, just as in any excitable tissue. This (our injury current of Hermann) was described by Matteucci, together with its experimental production, as follows:

> Furthermore, I have obtained a quite distinct current of 20 to 30 degrees by making a wound in the chest or thigh of a living animal (pigeon, rabbit, sheep) and by dipping into the inside of the wound one of the plates [galvanometer electrodes], while the other was put on the exposed [intact] surface of the injured muscles. The current in the animal was invariably directed from the inside of the wound to the external surface of the muscle. The constant direction of these currents and the quite distinct signs that I have obtained on my galvanometer have assured me that they cannot be attributed to any flaw in the experiment.[189]

He was also able to conclude that closing the circuit between the injured and uninjured muscle tissue was the factor directly responsible for the muscular contraction that ensued.

5.4.3. New Electrical Devices

A quality that has been common to all electrophysiologists up to the present day has been their capacity for inventing instruments and techniques necessary for their research. Matteucci possessed this faculty and he perfected two very simple devices, which proved to be of the greatest assistance to himself and to his successors. Essentially, his resourcefulness was directed to improve contemporary methods of detecting bioelectric currents.

Nobili had found that a Galvani-type muscle-nerve frog preparation was more sensitive than his multiplier, and Matteucci used this knowledge to devise a "galvanoscopic frog," which permitted him to study electrical currents in animals with increased precision.[190] It could not have been simpler for it consisted only of a frog-leg preparation placed in a glass cylinder with the nerve protruding at one end. Known also as the "rheoscopic frog," it could demonstrate the injury current of muscle, described above, for when an injured and an intact surface were placed in circuit by allowing the preparation's nerve to connect them, the muscle in the tube twitched. Matteucci believed that the nerve had completed the circuit, and that an arc, as in Galvani's experiment without metals, had thus been created: "This obviously proves that it is indeed an electric current that spreads in the nerve, since it is necessary to form an arc in which this same nerve [of the preparation] is included."[191] There could be no doubt that the response of the appliance was due to an electric current passing between the two parts of the muscle by way of a nerve in a living animal. Matteucci tested his device successfully in the fish, eel, and rabbit, and after many experiments, he concluded in 1844 that: "The frog used in this way, which I shall henceforth call the *galvanoscopic frog,* is certainly the most sensitive apparatus that we possess, provided it is renewed from time to time."[192]

Another simple and effective apparatus was Matteucci's electrophysiological pile. The principle had been introduced by Nobili, with a "frog-pile" made up of nerve-muscle preparations linked in series to produce an increased deflection of the galvanometer's needle. Matteucci wished to prove that the intrinsic, or *propre,* current of the muscle was truly endogenous and independent of all external factors that might be introduced by his experimental procedures, and he found this type of biological battery ideal for his purpose.[193] He constructed his model by arranging in series frogs' thighs cut in halves, with a cut (i.e., inner) surface of one in contact with the outer, intact surface of another. From this grouping of muscles, he could lead a current that flowed from the injured (i.e., negative) surface to the normal. This again was the current of injury produced by the potential difference of the two parts of the muscle, and Matteucci could show that his frog battery of muscle pieces in series could increase it, just as Nobili had done with his "frog pile." He noted that "at the moment that the deviation of the needle [of the galvanometer] takes place, it will be seen that this deviation is proportional to the number of half-thighs, that is, to the elements of the pile."[194] In modern terminology, we would explain that the raised intensity of the current is due to the multiplication of current, that is, an increase of the demarcation potential, and thus to summation of demarcation potentials.

5.4.4. The Induced Contraction

Another of Matteucci's basic contributions to electrophysiology was his discovery in September, 1841 that the contraction of a muscle was invariably accompanied by an electrical charge, which he could detect with his galvanoscopic frog. In retrospect we can recognize this as the first experimental demonstration of the muscle action potential or action current of the muscle. He found that when the nerve of one muscle-nerve preparation, for example, the nerve of a galvanoscopic frog, was placed on an actively contracting muscle of a second preparation, the galvanoscopic muscle twitched. This was Matteucci's *contrazione indotta,* or the "induced contraction" as du Bois-Reymond called it. As was then common and accepted practice, Matteucci, in order to establish priority for this discovery, sent an account of his experiment in a sealed package to the Académie des Sciences at Paris in 1841. At his request it was read by J. B. A. Dumas to the Académie on 24 October 1842,[195] and published in detail elsewhere.[196] The following is taken from the original communication:

> Prepare rapidly the thigh of a frog, leaving the nerve attached; place the latter on the thighs of another frog prepared in the usual way. If you then induce the [thigh] muscles of the second preparation to contract by means of an electrical stimulus, or by any other method, it will be observed that the leg muscles of the first frog also contract, at the moment that the contraction takes place in the second frog.[197]

Dumas's reaction to this finding was then given by the Académie reporter:

> If I do not deceive myself, added M. Dumas, it is the first time that muscle contraction in an animal has been seen to exercise any kind of influence upon the nerves of another animal and to bring about contraction.[198]

He also admitted that "to him the experiments seemed to open a new era of the most exquisite physiological researches,"[199] and in view of his personal knowledge of the subject, this was a significant comment.

Matteucci's remarkable observation was widely acclaimed and it has been justly regarded as the Italian's greatest discovery. However, it should be noted that S. T. Soemmerring had reported the phenomenon in 1811, for he had elicited twitch responses in the limbs of frogs, birds, and mammals, when they were placed on muscle being subjected to electrical stimulation.[200] As he had, however, no explanation to offer for it and did not investigate the matter further, it was soon forgotten. Matteucci's finding was confirmed by many, one of the most important being A. C. Becquerel, who proposed correctly that the nerve of the galvanoscopic frog had been excited by the electricity (action currents) of the contracting muscles of the other frog, and proved this by showing that interposed metal foil prevented the effect.[201] He concluded that if it were accepted that an electrical discharge occurred at the moment of muscle contraction, Matteucci "will have discovered one of the most important properties of muscles manifested during life, and sometimes even after death."[202] Becquerel must, therefore, be accepted as the first to offer the correct explanation for the induced twitch, and thus of the action current of muscle.

Despite the justifiably enthusiastic reception of Matteucci's *contrazione indotta,* three years later he denied its existence. As we have mentioned, his ability to renounce an opinion previously enunciated carefully and with conviction was one of Matteucci's regrettable failings. In a letter to Dumas in September 1845, he explained why he could no longer accept the induced twitch as an isolated and unique phenomenon:

> And after all, I have just demonstrated experimentally that the induced contraction can never be produced by electrical action, either direct or by induction. I repeat that the induced contraction is the first phase of an action at a distance, or, more correctly, of induction carried out by a contracting muscle on a nerve. I think that this principle will be of importance for the physics of the nervous system.[203]

By now Matteucci no longer accepted electrical currents in the nerves, and instead postulated some "nerve force" that determined nervous action:

> The phenomenon of induced contraction would seem to be a first fact [i.e., phase] of induction of that force which circulates in the nerves and which arouses muscular contraction . . . The induced contraction is only a new phenomenon of nervous force . . . *muscular induction.*[204]

In 1847 he denied an association between muscle action and electricity: "There is no experimental evidence in favour of the explanation of the phenomenon of induced contraction, by the assumption of the development of electricity during muscular contraction."[205] Matteucci thus rejected Becquerel's correct interpretation of the induced twitch. But three years later he had changed his mind again and now agreed that the twitch "is evidently an electrical phenomenon developed in the act of contraction."[206] His experiments had revealed that it was due to "the production of an electrical *disequilibrium* in the act of muscular equilibrium,"[207] whatever this might have meant. In the case of nerve conduction, he had returned to a belief in "the strict correlation existing between the electric current and nervous force."[208]

We need not follow Matteucci's vacillating and contradictory opinions because by 1850, when the above statements were made, he was no longer in a position to contribute further to the advance of electrophysiology. He was, therefore, unable to comprehend or interpret his experimental findings either past or present. As he asserted, also in 1850, "we await the light of new experiments to proceed safely further in this difficult field of science."[209] But the illumination he desired was not forthcoming. It was now emanating from Germany, soon leaving the Italian and French investigators in the shadows, never to emerge again as an effective force.

Despite his unusual behavior, which his fellow scientists (particularly du Bois-Reymond) found so infuriating, Matteucci had made a correct and valuable observation concerning the induced contraction of muscle. But his reasoning, and therefore his interpretations of it, were faulty, and it was left to du Bois-Reymond to confirm its occurrence and to assess fully its significance. As du Bois-Reymond stated when referring to Matteucci's denial of an electrical element: "By these remarks Matteucci has, without knowing it, done me a really kind service."[210] Thus, his credibility was exalted as Matteucci's was diminished, leaving the field to du Bois-Reymond. But with hindsight, we can observe that Matteucci pioneered the experimental demonstration of the induced twitch, Becquerel provided the correct explanation for it, whereas du Bois-Reymond consolidated and extended it.

5.4.5. The Negative Variation in Muscle

The final discovery made by Matteucci again illustrates not only his unique powers of observation, but, in addition, his inability correctly to interpret his experimental results and his unfortunate willingness to change his mind. In 1838 he had been the first to observe deflections of the galvanometer when a muscle contracted in strychnine tetanus,[211] but, paradoxically, the *courant propre* of Nobili was seen to diminish or disappear: "The influence of tetanus is such that the *courant propre* always decreases when the frog is stimulated. There are no longer any contractions nor any galvanometric signs."[212] In our terms, we would state that the resting potential (the difference in potential between the interior and exterior of a resting muscle) had decreased or terminated. This was the first demonstration of what we now call the negative variation of the demarcation potential or injury current, which is the action potential of muscle. Four years later Matteucci extended his account of the phenomenon, but his results were much the same.

> I have prepared frogs seized by convulsions due to an extract of *nux vomica* introduced into their stomachs. In these frogs there are indications of a current on the galvanometer, but weaker than usual; the contractions themselves are likewise less frequent and more difficult to obtain.[213]

When he varied the method of producing the tetanus the outcome was always the same: "The frog current becomes weaker when it is seized by a kind of tetanic state whatever the procedure by which this is aroused."[214] Once more Matteucci had made a precise and correct observation, but was unable to account for it. He was perplexed by this seemingly contradictory result, whereby an electric current had decreased and disappeared in the presence of tetanic muscular contraction, when the reverse might have been expected.

In 1843, du Bois-Reymond also described this phenomenon, but the explanation that he first advanced for it was untenable and was later shown to be erroneous.[215] This only helped to increase the confusion, especially in Matteucci's mind, and eventually in 1845 being unable to formulate a satisfactory interpretation, he concluded that his findings had been faulty and rejected them.[216] He did so at the same time as he recanted concerning the induced twitch. In addition, he was unable to discern a relationship between the two and a new elucidation of the twitch he proposed proved to be incorrect. Matteucci's behavior, manifesting a state of confusion, uncertainty, and fluctuation that led ultimately to the disavowal of his own experimental results, permitted his critics to attack him mercilessly. The foremost of them was du Bois-Reymond, who was able subsequently to reveal the true nature of the negative variation (*negativen Schwankung*), as he called it, and to offer the correct interpretation of it based on extensive experimentation.[217]

5.4.6. Chemical Factors

Like many others, Matteucci also considered the possible role of chemical factors in bioelectrical phenomena, and in 1840 he wondered if the muscle current was an electrochemical process. Thus, he had observed that an acidic or alkaline solution applied to a muscle could induce contraction with concomitant galvanometric evidence of an electrical discharge.[218] Two years later he was more certain when he declared:

> The cause of these [muscle] currents may well be a chemical action; but it must be admitted that this chemical action occurs between certain parts of an animal's organism such as those parts existing in a living animal.[219]

It, therefore, seemed that chemical processes could produce animal, as well as metallic, electricity, but did not necessarily take part in nerve action, even though "the development of electricity takes place in the muscles during life from the chemical action between the arterial blood and the muscle fiber."[220]

5.4.7. Nerve Currents

As Matteucci continued his research, his appraisal of the mass of puzzling experimental data that he had collected led him increasingly into error. This was especially the case with his attempt to demonstrate the presence of electrical currents in nerves. He was, of course, a victim of defective contemporary techniques and hypotheses, because the galvanometers available to him were still inadequate for the tasks to which he applied them and, furthermore, the false assumption that a nerve behaved in the same way as a metallic conductor of current electricity had an adverse effect upon his reasoning. Thus, one of Matteucci's greatest rebuffs and disappointments was that having demonstrated the frog current (current of injury or demarcation potentials) in muscles so clearly, he was never able to detect it in nerves.

In 1844 he began to collaborate with Longet, whose similar negative results have already been discussed above, in further attempts to identify a nerve current. They did not necessarily accept the presence of animal electricity in the nerves of the electric organ of *Torpedo,* which in any case was a special case and should not be compared with other animals.[221] They also argued that the larger the living animal they employed, the larger the nerves and, therefore, the more conspicuous the nerve current should be so that their chance of demonstrating it by means of a galvanometer should be enhanced, providing, of course, that such a phenomenon existed. But tests even on the horse's sciatic nerve proved fruitless. Their chagrin and frustration are understandable, because they had used the most delicate means of recognizing an electric current available to them, and they had observed all the known precautions in their experiments, particularly the avoidance of contaminated electrodes and, therefore, of polarization. However, they were honest enough to admit defeat on technical grounds:

> In view of the extreme sensitivity of our galvanometer, of the favorable conditions for the experiment, and of the precautions we have taken, we believe that we are permitted to conclude that no trace of electric currents exists in the nerves of living animals, detectable by the instruments we possess today.[222]

It is of interest to observe that this statement was made in 1844, one year after du Bois-Reymond had shown conclusively that electrical currents were present in nerves.[223] Matteucci and Longet made no reference to this historic report and presumably were not aware of German electrophysiological research.

Having professed instrumental inadequacy rather than awaiting technological improvements, they were, unfortunately, driven to the extreme position of denying altogether the existence of electricity in the nervous system. Matteucci now accepted Longet's hypothesis of 1842, to the effect that the nerve functioned by means of a special, but as yet unidentified nervous principle, agent, or force, and that electricity was but one of the several irritants that could excite and develop it. He, therefore, renounced the first of the three explanations given above for electricity's role in nerve action, whereby it was considered to be the primary agent in favor of the second, which accepted electricity only as an external and secondary etiological factor. "Galvanism," Longet had asserted, "thus seems to be only a simple excitor of the permanent [intrinsic] nerve force," the same as a mechanical or chemical stimulus.[224] Matteucci expressed himself similarly, espousing a specific sort of energy that so far had not been identified, although its properties closely resembled those of electricity. This was his final opinion on nerve function, and it was described in 1848 by du Bois-Reymond in the following terms:

> There are, according to him, no currents in the nerve. The muscle current circulates in the muscles only if they are prepared in a certain manner, and has no relation to their contraction. The so-called nerve principle is to him still a special hypothetical agent, which he prefers to explain on the basis of ethereal vibrations, and he declares that under all circumstances it cannot be distinguished from electricity.[225]

Johannes Müller also preferred this stance, and thus selected the second of the three hypotheses for the part played by electricity in nerve conduction. In his widely influential textbook of the mid-1830s, he had contested Matteucci's original proposal of an electrical basis for nerve action. His opinion regarding electricity was that "electrical reactions can be generated in nerves, but the way in which they act is quite different from that of [physical] electrical material."[226] He believed that "the nervous force in the nerve behaves like a reagent or an electrometer, because when it is irritated by the electrical current it brings about a [muscle] contraction."[227] As Matteucci, Longet, and others asserted, electricity instead of having a primary role was merely an excitant and played no part in natural nerve action.[228] Müller's conclusions, set out in 1835, were very similar to those of Matteucci. He declared:

> 1) That the vital actions of the nerves produce no electrical currents. 2) That the electrical force is quite different from nerve action (*Innervation*). 3) . . . we are as ignorant of the nature of the nervous principle as we are of light and electricity.[229]

However, in spite of this recorded opinion, Müller had not closed his mind entirely to the possibility of an electrical basis for nerve conduction, because in 1841 he had asked du Bois-Reymond to examine Matteucci's earlier work in an attempt to resolve the discord. His studies soon revealed that Müller, Longet, and Matteucci had been incorrect for he was able to identify and establish the phenomenon of nerve currents, a thesis that Matteucci had abandoned. Thereby, du Bois-Reymond opened the modern phase of nerve physiology. But meantime, even in 1861, Matteucci's views on nerve conduction and muscle contraction remained the same. The latter took place, he asserted, when "the excitation of a nerve by means of a current, as in the kindling of a mass of powder by a spark, gives rise in the muscle to chemical phenomena."[230] The comparison of this mechanism with that postulated by Procháska in 1784 is inescapable (see chaps. 4.3 and 5.2.1). In fact, the conclusions reached by Longet, Matteucci, and Müller have much in common with his conclusions. Despite the many conceptual and technological advances that had been achieved in the intervening years, the basic problem of nerve conduction remained, and as midcentury approached an acceptable solution did not seem to be in sight.

In this chapter we have been concerned only with the way in which a message could be carried along a nerve. An associated problem was to explain how the message in one fiber could find its way into a neighboring one. Long before the neuron had been identified and the synapses proposed, some investigators believed that communication between fibers was possible by means of "crossover transmission," as we have named it. In other words, messages could jump from fiber to fiber, and in chapters 3.5.2 and 4.6, we have discussed that mechanism when dealing with the nerve cell and the reflex. At a time when knowledge of the microscopic features of nervous tissue was very limited, it was thought by some that the reflex arc could be explained on the basis of this type of transmission. Thus, the ability of a sensory impression to initiate a motor signal, presumably in the spinal cord, could be accounted for. Moreover, it could also be responsible for the old notion of sympathy. However, the establishment of the true method of nerve conduction benefited, as we discovered in chapter 3.5.2, from the histological investigation of nerve cells and fibers and their role in sensorimotor physiology and the attendant reflex.

5.4.8. Summary

Because of Matteucci's varying and self-contradictory conclusions derived from identical data, and because of his speculations, his disorganized approach to admittedly very difficult problems, his confusion, and his muddled reasoning, he incurred the criticisms of many of his contemporaries. Regrettably, these have tended to diminish the positive aspects of his research and the worth of his overall achievement. Historians have been influenced, for example, by the comments of du Bois-Reymond who consistently criticized Matteucci, only some of his attack being fully justified. The reasons for this behavior toward Matteucci and other Italians, such as Galvani and Aldini, are not obvious, but they probably relate as much to du Bois-Reymond's personality as to theirs. Without doubt, du Bois-Reymond was a much better scientist than any of them, and he probably abhorred especially the way in which Matteucci interpreted some of his experimental findings, in particular, his proposal of a theoretical nerve principle rather than nerve electricity; and he must have found Matteucci's recantations inexcusable. He also protested that the Italian frequently republished reports that had appeared earlier, with little or no new material, or published the same paper in a variety of periodicals: "He can thus be appropriately described as plagiarizing himself."[231] There can be no argument, however, concerning the impact made by Matteucci's studies. Some measure of their merit is afforded by the action of the Académie des Sciences, which in 1842 awarded him the Montyon prize jointly with Longet. This was the coveted *Prix de Physiologie Expérimentale,* mainly in recognition of his *Essai sur les Phénomènes Électriques des Animaux* of 1840.[232]

In brief, Matteucci was responsible in the 1830s and 1840s for a resurgence of interest in nerve-muscle electrophysiology and for several major achievements in this field. He was the first adequately to detect galvanometrically in all animals tested the flow of electric current between the cut surface of a muscle and an undamaged part of it, the *courant propre* (our injury current or demarcation potential of muscle). He thus demonstrated the muscle's resting potential, and, even though he denied it later, he proved that muscle contraction always produced an electrical discharge, which could be led to a second preparation where it brought about the induced twitch. He thereby revealed the action current of muscle for the first time. He noted the decrease of muscle current during tetanus, but he could not interpret what we now recognize in both nerve and muscle as the negative variation of the demarcation potential (i.e., the action potential), which is the basic electrical accompaniment of the nerve impulse. By means of his bioelectrophysiological-pile, Matteucci demonstrated multiplication of current, and he could detect electrical currents with his galvanoscopic frog. These were his successes. But his failures must also be taken into account. We have discussed some of them already, in particular, his inability to detect electrical currents in nerves, but additionally Matteucci had the notion that muscle currents in animals increased in intensity with their higher ranking in the animal kingdom, which is not true. Also incorrect was a claim based on his experiments on injured muscle tissue that free electricity existed in animals. A further error was to suppose that dissimilar animal tissues arranged in series could act like a battery, as had been suggested in the case of the brain by earlier workers. Thus, in the case of the muscle, he complimented himself for what turned out to be a grave error. He felt that "it is sufficient for me to have well established that this contact of heterogeneous parts of the muscle generates electricity";[233] and "We must never forget the analogy between the muscular electromotor element and the Voltanian element."[234] Just as the cerebellum or cerebral cortex had been thought to represent an organic Voltaic pile, so with the muscle. The zinc of the pile was represented by discs of muscle fibers, the acid liquid by the blood, and the platinum by the sarcolemma. But, this analogy, like the other equating organic with physical forms of electricity, did not survive.

By examining all of Matteucci's work in electrophysiology, we can recognize the fundamental nature of his contribution to establishing the modern phase of nerve function research. In addition, by trying to understand du Bois-Reymond's biased opinions, a fairer judgment of his achievements should be possible. These two approaches will facilitate Matteucci's further rehabilitation. His numerous changes of heart and recantations, undoubtedly revealed faulty reasoning, but being honest to his experimental findings is a quality worthy of praise rather than abuse. The very fact that Matteucci acted as a gadfly to du Bois-Reymond, who was thereby stimulated to amass evidence in order to disprove and denounce an inferior scientist, was itself useful for the advancement of physiology. And although Matteucci was eclipsed by the German school of biophysics, much of his work has endured.

5.5. SUMMARY AND SEQUEL

Looking back from the middle of the nineteenth century, the course of animal electricity thus far must have seemed a checkered one. After feverish activity in the last two decades of the eighteenth century, due mainly to the research of Luigi Galvani and his followers and to the opposition of Volta who denied "animal" electricity, but established the "metallic" variety, there followed a period of stagnation. After Alessandro Volta's invention of the Voltaic pile in 1800, bioelectricity was neglected at a time when the physics of current electricity was advancing rapidly. But, the lull was due not only to telling criticisms of Galvani's doctrine of animal electricity but also to the lack of adequate laboratory instruments for the detection of the minute discharges of biological electricity responsible for the observation made by Galvani and all his successors.

As we pointed out at the beginning of this chapter, in the first half of the nineteenth century there were three ways in which electricity was thought to be involved in nerve transmission. First, electricity was said to be identical with the fluid thought to be the nerve's conducting agent, so that it was solely responsible for nerve action. Others claimed the reverse—that there were no electrical currents in nerves and that conduction took place by means of a nerve principle as yet unknown, electricity being merely a stimulus that set it in motion just as in the case of mechanical or chemical irritation. The third possibility was that there existed an underlying conducting process in the nerve, again unidentified, but which was accompanied by an electrical signal. The order in which these notions have been presented here also represents their chronological sequence. Thus, during the first three decades of the nineteenth century, the first was the most popular and analogies were made between the brain and the Voltaic pile or the electric organ of the electric fish. On the whole, little advancement was achieved.

The period of inertia that had commenced in 1800 ended when Leopoldo Nobili in 1827 and Carlo Matteucci in the late 1830s stimulated a resurrection of interest in the electrophysiological aspect of nerve and muscle action. This was brought about chiefly by improvements in electrical instruments and new experimental approaches. Nobili was the first to detect animal electricity by means of a galvanometer, and thus to demonstrate by instrumental means the current of injury of muscle that was responsible for the discoveries of Galvani and others. Matteucci went much farther for he was able to identify a number of phenomena fundamental to the electrophysiology of muscle and nerve. However, after at first accepting the existence of nerve currents of electricity per se, he was unable to reveal them with his galvanometers which were too insensitive. He, therefore, accepted the second type of nerve conduction, and in keeping with Johannes Müller and F. A. Longet denied the existence of electrical nerve currents so that the gains of earlier decades were put in jeopardy.

In 1841, however, a new phase of progress began with Emil du Bois-Reymond,[235] who belonged to a group of brilliant, young, German materialistic physiologists, the "organic physicists." In 1847 they swore to expunge from physiology all evidence of vitalism, present for example in the work of Müller, Matteucci, and Longet, and to reduce all biological phenomena to the principles of physics and chemistry.[236] From 1841 until his death in 1896, du Bois-Reymond labored exclusively in the field of electrophysiology and built on the work of his Italian predecessors to whom he was abusive and arrogant rather than grateful. By introducing ingenious physical methods and concepts, he established bioelectricity as a practical laboratory discipline. He invented many appliances for his experiments, such as the induction coil, Faradic stimulation equipment, but above all, more sensitive galvanometers. He was greatly influenced by Matteucci and began by repeating his work, but owing to his greater inventive genius and his precise and logical reasoning, he advanced far beyond Matteucci, although like his Italian counterpart he also fell into grievous error. He could demonstrate clearly the injury current or demarcation potential of nerve in animals, the existence of which Matteucci had eventually denied. This was his *Nervenstrom,* and he affirmed that as in the muscle the transverse cut surface of the nerve was negative to the longitudinal one. This negativity was increased when an external current of electricity was passed through the nerve so long as it proceeded in the same direction. When the current was reversed, however, the negativity decreased. To this du Bois-Reymond applied Michael Faraday's term "electrotonus," and he stimulated a great deal of research on it. He could also detect the presence of muscle currents in human beings, and he confirmed Matteucci's induced twitch, which occurred in a muscle stimulated by a nearby muscular contraction. The decreasing current in the tetanized muscle that had bewildered Matteucci and had led him into gross error was rediscovered, and du Bois-Reymond called it the negative variation of the muscle's injury current. It could be clearly distinguished from the negativity of electrotonus and was also present in nerve, our "action potential" of nerve. His explanation that it was due to a decreased demarcation potential was accepted until the 1930s. Unfortunately, du Bois-Reymond made two serious mistakes: the assumption that electrical currents preexisted in nerve or muscle at rest; and his hypothesis that all electrical events in nerve or muscle were owing to their electromotive molecules. To his everlasting annoyance and frustration, one of his students, Ludimar Hermann, proved both these notions to be erroneous. He pointed out conclusively that du Bois-Reymond's so-called resting current was in fact a current of injury, and this undermined his teacher's whole concept of nerve function.

At the middle of the nineteenth century the three possible explanations for nerve action still had their followers. Even du Bois-Reymond accepted the first, although with some reservation, and in 1848 made his well-known claim:

> If I have not completely deluded myself, I have succeeded in restoring to life in full reality that hundred-year-old dream of the physicist and physiologist, the identity of the nerve substance with electricity, if in somewhat modified form.[237]

Matteucci, Longet, and others were, however, still contesting the very existence of electrical nerve currents and adopted the second hypothesis, that electricity was merely an excitor of a nerve principle or force, the precise nature of which was unknown. In the second half of the nineteenth century these two concepts were disproved. The first was demolished by Hermann Helmholtz, one of the 1847 organic physicists, who in 1850 measured the speed of nerve conduction and found it to be much slower than that of a current of electricity flowing through a conducting wire.[238] The second survived longer, because we find Austin Flint (1812–1886) in 1872 still upholding the notion of a nerve force produced *sui generis* by the nerve centers and in no way related to electricity.[239] But du Bois-Reymond was already moving toward the third proposition, for he had suspected that the electrical signals he could so readily detect in a nerve were the external manifestations of the underlying, but unknown, conduction mechanism. To add further to his chagrin, however, it was Hermann who was the first to show that, unlike current electricity in a wire, the nerve's motive principle was a self-propagating wave of negativity that advanced in steps along it.[240] This was the beginning of our present notion of nerve function, but it was not until the present century that the electrical signal, the effects of which had been studied experimentally in muscles since the eighteenth century, was revealed to result from the transfer of ions across the membrane of the nerve fiber.[241] This we have already described as a physico-chemical event based on the differential permeability of the membrane to sodium and potassium.

We cannot do better than conclude with Galvani's optimistic and prophetic comment on nerve electricity made in 1791: "But as the matter stands, I believe that after these investigations of ours no one in the future will call in doubt the certainty of electricity."[242] Despite periods of despair occasioned by serious setbacks and consequent confusion, together with the disavowal by some of the most outstanding European physiologists of electricity in nerves, in the second half of the nineteenth century Galvani's prediction was realized, although in a form very different from the primitive concept of nerve function that he had entertained.

6

Brain Functions

6.1. INTRODUCTION

Perhaps the most important, and certainly one of the most contentious, episodes in the history of the neurosciences has been the attempts made to localize functions in the various parts of the brain.[1] Thus, in the case of the cerebral hemispheres, the distinguished neurologist, Sir Henry Head (1861–1940), declared: "The evolution of our knowledge of cerebral localisation is one of the most astonishing stories in the history of medicine."[2] It is also one of the longest, because it began in Alexandria during the fourth century B.C.

At the outset we should define the historical uses of the term *brain action,* and in so doing clarify *localization of brain function,* because in the past confusion has arisen from the loose usage of these terms. Historically, there have been three main concepts of how the brain acts. The first was that it performed as a whole, with all its parts possessing an equal functional significance, and thus no localization of specific function to individual regions was possible. This was the opinion of Albrecht von Haller in the eighteenth century and, as we shall see, it was his contention that motion and sensation were mediated by all the white matter of the brain: this was his doctrine of brain equipotentiality, or the unitary theory of brain action. Pierre Flourens, whose work will figure largely in this chapter, also accepted a somewhat similar unitary theory as part of his explanation of how the brain functioned. But unlike Haller, he claimed that each morphologically separate subdivision of the brain—i.e., the cerebral hemispheres, the cerebellum, the quadrigeminal bodies, and the medulla oblongata (probably our brain stem)—were functionally distinct and that each contributed to the brain's total energy, which he termed its *action commune.*

In addition, Flourens's theory included another type of brain action, and this represents the second concept of brain function. He endowed each of the brain's subdivisions with one or more specific functions, which were distributed uniformly throughout its substance and had no precise locations in it. These functions constituted each subdivision's *action propre* (or specific action), and it was the various *actions propres* that worked together to produce the brain's *action commune*.

The third idea of brain function was that, instead of various anatomical subdivisions of the brain having specific properties represented throughout their substance as Flourens demanded, they were made up of many discrete areas of particular functions. This we now know to be the case, for example, in the cerebral cortex. The regions or subdivisions were, therefore, functionally compound rather than unitary as in Flourens's scheme. We have called this the theory of compound, discrete, or punctate localization of brain function. It has in the past been best exemplified by Gall's system of hypothetical "organs" on the surface of the brain, and today it is generally accepted and is referred to occasionally as the "mosaic" or "parcellation" theory of cortical localization.

In the following pages we shall discuss the occurrence and interaction of these three doctrines. We begin with Galen's and Willis's *action propre,* and go on to Haller's brain equipotentality, to Gall's compound cortical localization, and finally to Flourens's combined *action propre* and *action commune,* which is the focus of our attention. But, in addition, during Haller's time as well as Flourens's, there were some who espoused compound localization, and as we now know this is the present day notion of brain action. Concerning the cerebral cortex, this was established experimentally in 1870, but there have been those in the present century such as Karl Spencer Lashley (1890–1958) who have returned to Flourens's concept and have applied to the cortex the terms "equipotentiality," "holistic," or "field" theory.[3]

We shall be concerned here primarily with the conflict that arose early in the nineteenth century between proponents of the second and third varieties of brain action, each of which proposed a localization of function. This resolved itself into a debate between Gall and his followers, who favored a compound type of brain localization, and Flourens who preferred an *action propre.*[4] It began in 1822 with the publication of Flourens's report on a series of remarkable brain experiments and continued until his death in 1867. The outcome was that Gall's organology was demolished as a scientific concept, and with it, unfortunately, the basic principle of compound localization in the cerebral cortex. Flourens was wrong, but his doctrine prevailed for forty-eight years, until three years after his death. In 1870, two young German physiologists, Gustav

Theodor Fritsch (1838–1927) and Eduard Hitzig (1838–1907) produced irrefutable experimental evidence that functional parcellation of the cortex existed and that in principle Gall had been correct.[5] In 6.5 we shall place the debate between proponents of Flourens's holistic and Gall's punctate or compound concept of brain function in its broader context. This physiological argument is fully intelligible only when certain salient features of the French intellectual context in the first half of the nineteenth century are taken into account. The issue of brain localization thus illustrates the point we have made elsewhere that developments in the neurosciences of this period cannot be divorced from movements and trends in nonscientific culture.

In the following pages we shall also discuss two other episodes in the history of the localization of brain function. They concern the discovery of the respiratory center in the medulla oblongata, another example of discrete localization; and the study of cerebellar function, which illustrates Flourens's notion of *action propre*. In fact, he played a prominent role in both these experimental investigations, where, unlike his notion of *action propre* in the cerebral hemispheres, his conclusions have proved to be entirely correct.

6.2. BRAIN LOCALIZATION BEFORE GALL

Gall evolved his unique doctrine of compound brain localization in Vienna during the 1780s and 1790s, but before discussing it we shall look briefly at earlier proposals concerning the three varieties of brain action.

Apparently Herophilus of Alexandria (fl. c. 300 B.C.) was the first to locate a specific function in an anatomical subdivision of the brain, for, according to Galen, he "seemed always to consider as the most important ventricle, not this [the third] ventricle, but the one in the cerebellum [the fourth]."[6] He placed the human soul therein, thus adopting a form of *action propre*. Galen himself also believed in the latter, because he claimed that whereas sensory nerves arose from all of the anterior and softer part of the brain (cerebrum), the motor ones came from the whole posterior and harder portion (cerebellum).[7] The medieval system of faculty psychology was another example of *action propre* brain function. Based on Galenic teaching, it was initiated by Nemesius of Emesa (fl. c. A.D. 390) as part of his attempt to interpret Greek scientific knowledge of the human body in the light of Christian philosophy.[8] By means of it individual mental faculties, such as *sensus communus* (common sense), reasoning, memory, and so forth were located in various parts of the brain's ventricular system, entirely on the basis of speculation.

It survived until the seventeenth century, when Willis replaced it and other conjectural theories with a new scheme, which he established on the basis of anatomical, experimental, and clinical observations bolstered with speculation.[9] It too belonged to the *action propre* type of brain localization, for he assigned mental functions to all of the cerebral cortex, involuntary movements and vital bodily functions to the whole cerebellum, and motor activity to the entire corpus striatum.

Willis's doctrine was widely adopted; but at the beginning of the eighteenth century we encounter the first example of compound or punctate brain localization. It was introduced by the remarkably perceptive French surgeon, Pourfour du Petit, who in 1710 described experiments suggesting that in the dog circumscribed areas of the cerebral hemispheres controlled motor activity on the opposite side of the body.[10] At the time, it represented a curious finding, but one that seemed of no relevance to contemporary brain physiology. It was soon forgotten, and in any case it would have been swept away along with Willis's notions, when Haller at midcentury established his doctrine of brain equipotentiality or a type of *action commune*. This theory was to prevail until the early decades of the nineteeth century.[11]

Haller's prime purpose in studying the nervous system was to determine which parts possessed sensitivity and which were essential for the continuation of life. He was, however, as Neuburger has pointed out,[12] investigating by experiment the basic physiological properties of the system's constituent tissues, such as nerve substance, white and gray matter, and so forth, and not its specific functions as an organ. Haller held that the medulla oblongata was the vital structure necessary for life, thus demolishing Willis's similar claims for the cerebellum. Concerning sensitivity of brain tissues his experiments revealed that the cerebral and cerebellar cortex was entirely inexcitable,[13] an error that survived for more than a century. Conversely, all the white matter of the brain was invariably highly irritable and therefore sensitive, and Haller's conclusion that this was the tissue representing the seat of all sensations, the *sensorium commune,* followed naturally. Although he conceded that the thalami, the cerebral peduncles, and the medulla oblongata were closely associated with motor activity, this, like sensation, was mediated by the brain's white matter, which acted in toto, for he denied absolutely any functional variations in the morphologically different subdivisions of the brain. He asserted that the white matter was functionally equivalent throughout the brain: "There is no difference between the white matter of the corpora striata, the [cerebral] peduncles, the medulla oblongata, the pons, and that of the cerebrum."[14] Therefore, all areas of the brain were integrated in their function, and each contributed to the common vital action of the organ, a phenomenon of particular importance in the presence of disease or injury of a brain component. In 1762 he declared that "when the cerebellum is injured, the vital force can be supplied by the cerebrum if it is unimpaired, or vice versa, when the cerebrum is destroyed, it can be provided by the intact cerebellum."[15] This was also to be Flourens's interpretation of *action commune,* but in addition it suggested the possibility of substitution within the nervous system, an idea that Flourens likewise condoned.

Such was Haller's doctrine of equal functional significance for all parts of the brain and of unitary brain action, a type of *action commune.* It was fully endorsed by his many followers, but in particular by his most outstanding student, Johann Gottfried Zinn (1727–1759), whose brilliant experimental researches were cut short by his untimely demise.[16] As we now recognize, Haller's teaching was a retrograde step, but it very soon received virtually universal approbation, so that Willis's concept of brain action and Pourfour du Petit's, together with others of minor significance, were suppressed. Gall's new system of compound or punctate localization was the first major attack on the Hallerian precept, as we shall see.

From a present day standpoint Haller's doctrines retarded the development of compound brain localization, which had been adumbrated by du Petit in 1710. However, Haller's work did help to lead physiologists away from the notion of a "rational soul" distributed throughout the entire body favored by eighteenth-century animists.[17] He insisted that the higher mental functions had a specific anatomical seat in the white matter of the brain, the so-called *sensorium commune,* already discussed above (chap. 4.2). The vegetative (i.e., autonomic) soul, however, resided in the ganglionic nervous system. Some, like Procháska in 1784, had attempted to localize the *sensorium commune* more precisely, although without experimental support. He proposed that it occupied only the brain stem, spinal cord, cerebellum, and thalamus.[18]

At the beginning of the nineteenth century the Hallerian doctrines still prevailed, and they seemed to linger longer in Britain than in other countries, as we have observed above (see chap. 5 n. 179). Concerning brain function, Haller's ideas were still held in Britain in 1811, as Bell reported:

> The prevailing doctrine of the anatomical schools is, that the whole brain is a common sensorium; that the extremities of the nerves are organized, so that each is fitted to receive a peculiar [i.e., specific] impression. . . .
>
> It is imagined that impressions, thus differing in kind, are carried along the nerves to the sensorium, and presented to the mind; and that the mind, by the same nerves which receive sensation, sends out the mandate of the will to the moving parts of the body.[19]

Nevertheless, elsewhere there had been a few dissenting voices, in the eighteenth and early nineteenth century. Both clinical and experimental evidence had convinced certain individuals that, in keeping with du Petit's earlier conclusions, the brain did in fact show evidence of a precise localization of function. However, this concerned sensorimotor localization and must be contrasted with Gall's parcellation of psychological activities. The next example after du Petit's of discrete localization of a specific function in the brain was the discovery by Anne Charles de Lorry (1726–1783) in 1760 of the so-called "ganglion of life." This, as we shall see later, turned out to be the respiratory center in the lower part of the medulla oblongata. Moreover, two years later Joseph Baader (fl. 1762), professor of materia medica, botany, and chemistry at Freiburg im Breisgau, employing clinico-pathological correlation, argued that the site of a brain lesion could be determined by observing the distribution of motor and sensory impairment in the patient.[20] Thus, on the basis of two cases he made a correct prediction:

> Perhaps, after similar comparisons involving many observations, we may at last be able to conclude with certainty that the part of the brain situated below the bregmatic [parietal] bone governs motion and sensation of the contralateral arm.[21]

Further experimental evidence for compound brain localization came from a group of French surgeons, and was claimed by Neuburger to be "one of the first achievements of modern brain physiology."[22] Louis Sebastian Saucerotte (1741–1814) in 1768 carried out ingenious experiments on the dog, which convinced him that the anterior part of the cerebrum innervated the lower limbs and the posterior the upper: "the origin of the nerves destined for the movements of the upper limbs is in the posterior part of the cerebrum, and, reciprocally, in the anterior for the lower limbs."[23] With modern knowledge of the dog's motor cortex, we can perhaps explain Saucerotte's findings by pointing out that the leg area lies far anteriorly, whereas those for the face and arm are placed laterally.[24] His contemporary, Jean Sabouraut (d. 1769) agreed and made the following prescient statement regarding compound brain localization:

> Without doubt each part of the body receives its nerves quite constantly from a certain part of the cerebral mass; and a lesion of this part of the cerebrum must necessarily disrupt, in particular, the functions of the parts of the body in which these nerves end; so that clinical observations, made with great care, will perhaps some day reveal the origins of the nerves of each organ.[25]

John Gregory (1724–1773) of Edinburgh was teaching in 1770 that with regard to intellectual processes:

> We have reason to suppose that each faculty of the mind is connected with a particular part of the Brain, as a stroke upon one part of the Head or Brain, will occasion a loss of Memory, etc.,—but what these Parts are, upon which the Faculties depend we know not.[26]

It might be argued that Gregory's statement could equally well refer to *action propre* rather than to compound localization, but it is, in fact, suggestive more of Gall's doctrine, which did not appear for about thirty years. It seems more likely, however, that part of this opinion originated in the writings of Galen, who argued that injury to different parts of the head brought about characteristic mental changes.[27] But unlike Gregory, Galen did not use this evidence to support a localization within the brain of mental faculties. It is important again to stress the difference between these attempts at the punctate localization of mental attributes, and the earlier ones directed at somatic functions. The former were leading the way to Gall.

One of the vital issues arising from the question whether compound localization occurred in the cerebral hemispheres, for example, centered on the response of their cortical mantle to irritating stimuli.[28] It arose first in the middle of the eighteenth century, when Haller concluded that it was inexcitable; as we have noted, this was an important element in his doctrine of brain action. It remained a problem until 1870 when Fritsch and Hitzig at last demonstrated the positive response of the cortex to excitation and that a mosaiclike compound localization of function existed beyond any doubt.[29] However, long before this date, Haller's assertion had been challenged by certain authors. One of the first to do so was the distinguished French physician and ideologue, Pierre Jean George Cabanis (1757–1808) in 1802. Like Haller he employed mechanical stimuli:

> If different points of the cerebral organ are pricked or irritated by whatever means, the convulsions that are usually produced in this way are observed to pass in turn from one muscle to another and often do not extend beyond those that correspond to [are connected with] the areas irritated.[30]

It would seem that he had observed a phenomenon that much later in the nineteenth century was called focal or Jacksonian convulsions. With the increase in knowledge of animal electricity towards the end of the eighteenth century, a new form of cortical stimulation had become available and L. M. A. Caldani, collaborating with Felice Fontana, was the first to exploit its possibilities.[31] He could produce convulsions by stimulating the brain, but his results, together with those of others, were probably due to the use of strong, nonphysiological currents, which stimulated deeper structures as well as the cerebral cortex, and also spread to the musculature by way of the nerves to produce their effects directly. However, von Humboldt's results were mainly negative, except in the case of an insect, which cannot be accepted as weighty evidence.[32]

We shall also mention here the experiments on electricity carried out by Luigi Rolando and reported in a book published in 1809, even though they followed the establishment of Gall's doctrine.[33] As we have already observed (chap. 5.3.2), Rolando thought the brain produced the electrical fluid that he argued was responsible for nerve function. Using a Voltaic pile, he stimulated different parts of the cerebral hemispheres in several quadrupeds and birds, and he obtained violent muscular contractions when the second electrode was placed on various parts of the body. Again, it seems likely that the currents used were too strong, and his results due to their abnormal spread beyond the cerebrum. Although we would judge his interpretations unwarranted, he concluded that the cerebral hemispheres were masses of fibers, the function of which was to produce specific movements. He was of the opinion that in the cerebrum "particular organs were destined to put the muscles in movement and others to produce sensation, and it was possible to destroy one of these faculties, whilst the other remained intact."[34] There were two reasons why Rolando's research had little or no effect. In the first place, his book was published at Sassari in Sardinia, during the Napoleonic wars, and this delayed the diffusion of his results to the rest of Europe for several years. Second, the Hallerian doctrine remained dominant, and on this account Rolando's opinions on compound localization would have had little effect upon it, even if they had received greater dissemination.

In fact none of these electrophysiological findings was conclusive enough to contest Haller's authority, and at the beginning of the nineteenth century there was ample evidence favoring his *action commune* interpretation of brain action, and very few experimental observations denying it. The longevity of his doctrine can be accounted for in part by the crudity of the experimental techniques then in use, by the brief period of postoperative observation or survival of the animals vivisected, and in part by ambiguous clinical and pathological data that still present diagnostic problems today. But there were other factors, such as the great difficulty of assessing sensory disturbances in mutilated, conscious animals, and the fact that no account was taken of changes in mental faculties, because it was thought that animals being mindless automata did not possess the latter. However, although this allusion to the Cartesian view of animals still survived, by 1800 it had been widely challenged.[35]

This then was the background to Gall's revolutionary suggestion made in the last decade of the eighteenth century that, in opposition to Hallerian teaching, the functions of the cerebral hemispheres and cerebellum were represented in discrete areas on their surfaces. He was establishing a special variety of compound or punctate brain localization, a type of faculty psychology.

6.3. GALL AND HIS ORGANOLOGY

6.3.1. Introduction

The functional areas of the cerebral cortex range in complexity from simple motor acts to intricate mental processes. Paradoxically, it was the latter that first received attention. In 1672 Thomas Willis conjectured that the cortex provided storage space for memories,[36] and at the beginning of the nineteenth century the first major advance in the theory of compound localization concerned psychological activity in the cortex. This was the well-known attempt by Gall in collaboration with Spurzheim to locate moral, character, and psychological propensities on the surface of the brain.

We do not today doubt that the brain is the seat of mental processes, and in 1806 most were of a like persuasion, as a British writer commented: "nobody has ever doubted, from the time of Epicurus down to the present day, that men think by means of their heads, as they walk by means of their heels."[37] The opinion was not, however, universal, as is clear from the statement of Francis, Lord Jeffrey (1773–1850) made in 1826 when attacking phrenology:

> The truth, we do not scruple to say it, is, that there is not the smallest reason for supposing that the mind ever operates through the agency of any material organs, except in its perception of material objects, or in the spontaneous movements of the body which it inhabits; and that this whole science [of phrenology] rests upon a postulate or assumption, for which there is neither any shadow of evidence, nor any show of reasoning.[38]

A comparable view was taken by John Bostock who argued that phenomena of the mind being immaterial could not be grouped with those ascribed to matter. Moreover, he asked, what evidence was there to indicate a necessary connection between the condition of the brain and the state of the intellect? He concluded: "I conceive myself warranted in drawing the inference, that mind is not a property of the brain, in the same way that contractility is a property of the muscle, or sensibility of the nerve."[39] There were also a number of important physicians, mainly at Paris, who followed the suggestion of Bichat and his predecessors and placed certain psychological influences in the ganglionic nervous system or in the viscera supplied by it. We shall discuss them later (chap. 7.7.3. See also 6.5).

A doctrine of punctate or compound brain localization was proposed by Gall in Vienna, toward the end of the eighteenth century. His first book was published in 1791 and it was concerned with medico-philosophical investigations into the nature and "culture" [*Kunst*] of the diseased and healthy state of man.[40] In it is found the first expression of Gall's fundamental beliefs that led him eventually to the establishment of a unique concept of psychology. This was his "organology" (better known by a later name, "phrenology"), which can be briefly defined as a theory based on the supposition that the mental powers of the individual consisted of separate psychical and moral faculties, each having its own "organ" precisely located on the surface of the brain. The connection of Gall's organology with his general concept of the nervous system as discussed in chapter 2 must be noted here. A further leap of faith allowed him to contend that an examination of the external contours of the skull by palpation provided a direct guide to the degree of development, or lack of development, of each underlying "organ." This in turn permitted an assessment of the state of the various faculties, so that a person's psychological makeup could thus be determined. There were, therefore, two parts to Gall's hypothesis: first, a physiological portion that proposed the localization of functions on the surface of the brain; and second, a psychological component, the composition of the mental state. It is with the first of these that we are mainly concerned.

Gall was joined in 1800 by Spurzheim and together they propagated Gall's doctrine and began dissecting the brain. However, they met with opposition from the church and state, so that they were forced to leave Vienna on 5 March 1805. For two years they traveled through Europe, visiting Germany, Denmark, Holland, Switzerland, and they eventually reached Paris in 1807. Here their partnership lasted until 1812 when Spurzheim left for Britain. He died twenty years later during a visit to America, while Gall remained in Paris for the rest of his life.[41] Their names are inseparably connected with the popularization of Gall's doctrine and with brain dissection. Concerning the former, it was entirely the creation of Gall, and Spurzheim's modifications of it helped to bring about the dissolution of their partnership, which we shall discuss later. In the case of brain anatomy, it is difficult to assign individual contributions to either partner, but despite the skills displayed by Spurzheim in dissecting and demonstrating, Gall initiated and directed his studies, and it seems reasonable therefore, to refer below only to Gall by name, although acknowledging here Spurzheim's role in their overall achievements.[42]

Because of phrenology's bizarre origins and principles and its wide influence in the nineteenth century, it has attracted a great deal of attention from historians, especially recently.[43] But, at the outset, a distinction must be made between the original doctrine of mind localization devised by Gall, and the modified form produced by Spurzheim and popularized by him and his followers. We can discuss this by first exploring the evolution of the various terms that were introduced to describe each.

6.3.2. Terminology

Although Gall's name is universally associated with "phrenology," he did not, in fact, invent the term or ever use it, or the popular phrase, "phrenology, or the doctrine of the mind." He preferred to call his doctrine "functions of the brain" or "brain physiology." However, the first term he used was *Schädellehre* ("craniology"),[44] which he eventually abandoned, because it suggested that his system was concerned primarily with the cranium and only secondarily with functions of the brain that it contained, whereas the reverse was the case. "Craniology" and "craniologie," however, persisted well into the nineteenth century. Gall's objection to "doctrine of the mind" or "mental science," and their Greek equivalent, "phrenology," was because of his desire not to equate the functions of the brain solely with mind. This seems to have been a small objection, and without doubt "phrenology" was the best available, for it closely expressed his basic precept. Why then did he reject it? The simple answer seems to be that "phrenology" was made popular by Spurzheim and applied to his modification of the original scheme, introduced contrary to Gall's wishes. It, therefore, did not refer to Gall's "functions of the brain," and to have accepted the term would have signified his approval of the altered system, and this he was not willing to do.

Several other terms were proposed, deriving from the system's two linked principles. First was the existence of cortical "organs" representing moral and mental faculties and "organology," therefore, seemed appropriate; Gall gave it sanction by using it (*organologie*) in the title of one of his books.[45] The second principle was the effect the surface "organs" had on the overlying cranium, and the technique of estimating their size was, therefore, called "organoscopy," or "cranioscopy." "Encephalonomy" or "cephalonomy" meaning "brain functions" were nearest of all to Gall's basic assumption, but they did not receive wide use. Another early, and for a time, popular phrase was "physiognomical system."[46]

It is usually stated that "phrenology" was introduced in 1815 by

Thomas Ignatius Maria Forster (1789–1860) in an article on the anatomy and physiology of the nervous system as described by Gall and Spurzheim.[47] However, it is also claimed that it was used as early as 1805 by the celebrated American physician, Benjamin Rush (1745–1813) of Philadelphia. Apparently it appeared in his lectures on "the state of phrenology, if I may be allowed to coin a word to designate the science of the mind."[48] In 1806 he defined it as "the history of the faculties and operations of the human mind,"[49] and he used it in the sense that "psychology" is employed today. However, a vociferous contender for the priority of having invented and popularized "phrenology" was Spurzheim, who was an acquaintance of Forster. In 1818, six years after parting from Gall, he used "phraenologie" for the first time, in the title of a book,[50] and in the following year, George Combe of Edinburgh, one of his most ardent followers, claimed that Spurzheim had been using the word "for some years."[51] Yet in 1817, an anonymous supporter of Spurzheim had already proposed "phrenology." His reason for doing so is reminiscent of Gall's arguments in favor of "organology":

> The word *craniology* is an invention of Spurzheim's enemies. It is not of the bone he treats, but of the manifestations of the mind as dependent on organization. Phrenology would be a more appropriate word.[52]

By 1820 Spurzheim had appropriated the word as his own, although still using it sparingly.[53] Thereafter, he blatantly asserted his priority, as for example in 1825:

> THE name PHRENOLOGY is derived from two Greek words: [*phrene*]—mind, and [*logos*]—discourse. I have chosen it to designate the doctrine of the special faculties of the mind, and of the relations between their manifestations and the body; particularly the brain.[54]

From all this, it is evident that the precise origin of "phrenology" is still obscure. Whether Forster plagiarized Rush, or whether Spurzheim took it from Rush or Forster, or created the term independently, as he claimed, is not known. Nor is Combe's role, if any, clear.

6.3.3. Organology versus Phrenology

It is of vital importance to differentiate between Gall's "organology" and Spurzheim's "phrenology." In 1812 when the two parted company forever these two psychophysiological schemes existed. Thereafter, Spurzheim continued to alter Gall's organology and, as noted, he applied the term "phrenology" to his new scheme in 1818.

Whereas Gall remained skeptical of a universal correlation between mental processes and cranial topography, and believed that an acceptable association could be found in only a small number of individuals, who possessed particularly well-developed "organs," Spurzheim had no such reservations. His phrenology could be successfully applied to all, an attitude reflected in his enthusiastic popularization of phrenology, which he mounted like a social crusade, rather than devoting himself more to the advancement of science as Gall, on the whole, preferred. Furthermore, although Gall accepted the existence of evil propensities in man, Spurzheim purposely omitted them from his categories, because he conceived that man was created potentially good. Eschewing Gall's pessimism, he argued that the human race could be perfected by the aid of phrenology.

Concerning the cerebral "organs" themselves, Gall was honest enough to admit that his system was incomplete and that additional "organs" might have to be added. Spurzheim obliged by increasing their number from twenty-seven to thirty-five. He added, for example, an "organ" for hope and ones for other propensities, but whereas Gall specified four types of memory, Spurzheim did not even recognize it as a faculty. All in all, he was advocating a primitive faculty psychology based on plausibility rather than proof that was ultimately shown to be untenable. His attempts to account for human actions had no relevance to scientific psychology, and they were never accepted by scientists. Unfortunately, the attacks against him were also leveled at Gall, who had to suffer on account of his erstwhile colleague's misrepresentation of the treasured doctrine that he had so carefully formulated and nurtured. There was a further charge against Spurzheim that undeservedly also affected Gall. When preparing his analysis of the mind into thirty-seven powers and propensities, it seems likely that Spurzheim borrowed from the Scottish faculty psychologists, and this possible influence upon his modification of Gall's "organology" will be discussed below. Again Gall had to suffer severe censures that were brought against him unjustly.

Another difference between Gall and Spurzheim was their general approaches to their individual psychophysiological system. To the end, Gall, its creator, maintained his empirical stance, and he came close to what we would call an experimental psychologist, savoring facts but, on the whole, disliking theories. Spurzheim, however, gradually increased his involvement with topics that had nothing to do with brain anatomy and physiology, such as metaphysics and speculation on educational, religious, sociological, and penological issues. In view of these dissimilarities, together with personality and perhaps other differences, it is little wonder that their partnership did not survive.

It is, therefore, necessary to consider the phrenology of Spurzheim and his many followers as a cult separate from Gall's organology, with its own history and impact upon human activity. It is to phrenology that most historians have turned their attention because of its fascinating and important social entanglements, as we shall learn later. It has, however, no relevance to our present theme. In view of this evidence, we intend below always to distinguish between the psychological system of Gall and that of Spurzheim, and to this end the term "phrenology" will be used only when referring to Spurzheim's system, and "organology" when Gall's is mentioned.[55]

6.3.4. Gall's Basic Principles

We have considered elsewhere (chaps. 1 n. 61 and 2 n. 26) some of Gall's important contributions to the anatomy of the nervous system, and we must now examine his fundamental attitude to the relationships that existed between form and function.[56] He considered the two inseparable and this was especially true of the brain:

> It is only when anatomists can know as much as possible concerning each phenomenon of the living animal, so that anatomy and physiology will in this way be blended together one with the other, that the knowledge of the nervous system will attain its highest degree of perfection.[57]

However, he did not employ anatomical findings directly to deduce physiological associations; he argued that, in fact, it was rare for anatomy to lead to the elucidation of function. Indeed, in the case of the brain, anatomy only served to confirm physiological discoveries, in the present instance his psychophysiological doctrine. As we have explained in chapter 1.2.1, he could claim that "it is thus without the help of any anatomical dissection that we have ourselves made most of our physiological discoveries."[58] Later he wrote:

> The physiology of the brain need not be contradictory to the anatomy of the brain; its anatomy must become the support of its physiology. But physiology has been found independently of anatomy. Nothing whatever in brain physiology has conflicted with an anatomical fact; nothing has been interpreted by structure or by the arrangement of parts of the brain; brain anatomy has served only to confirm physiological discoveries.[59]

When dealing with an integrated organ composed of many functional associations, the physiological approach was essential, according to Gall. In his opinion, the mechanical dissectors, such as Vicq d'Azyr,[60] who sliced the brain into pieces had achieved no physiological enlightenment. This strengthened his view that the procedure of elucidating function before structure was the correct one. Gall's method of dissecting has been discussed already (chap. 2.1), and we recall that by tracing fibers from the spinal cord upward to the brain he was demonstrating his primary concern with function which had no place in the activities of pure anatomists, whose techniques could not possibly reveal any functional continuity. His investigation of the comparative anatomy of the cerebral convolutions also helped to confirm his belief that the basic methodology he employed was correct. Thus, the gradation of convolutional patterns in the ascending scale of animals convinced him that his physiological precept concerning mental activities was correct:

> When we see that nature follows such a course, how can it still be doubted that each part of the brain has different functions to fulfill, and that as a consequence, the brain of man and animals must be composed of as many special organs as the man or animal has distinct moral or intellectual faculties, inclinations, and aptitudes for work.[61]

As Temkin has pointed out,[62] such statements are borne out by the fact that Gall had already established his concept of cerebral cortical organs in his book of 1791 and, therefore, before he began dissecting the brain.[63]

Gall's definition of the way in which the brain functioned provided him with a foundation upon which he could erect his new psychophysiological system. Thus, for him the physiology of the brain constituted principally a knowledge of man's elemental faculties and qualities and of the seat of their material representations. His preference for "functions of the brain" as the name for his system is understandable. The importance of brain function could not be overestimated for it was his belief "that researches to discover the organs of the moral and intellectual faculties of man are a most necessary study, and the most important in brain physiology."[64]

It was Gall's aim to provide empirical evidence in order to establish the brain as the undisputed organ of mind. In so doing he was continuing a line of investigation that was firmly established by the end of the eighteenth century. Recognizing his predecessors in this field of study, Gall predicted ultimate success:

> It will not be long before, vanquished by evidence, one will agree with [Charles] Bonnet [1720–1793], [Étienne Bonnot de] Condillac [1714–1780], Herder, Cabanis, Prochaska, Soemmerring, Reil, etc., that all the *phenomena* of animated nature are dependent upon the organism in general, and that all the *intellectual phenomena* are dependent upon the brain in particular.[65]

As noted, Gall created his theory of brain function and then searched the brain for a morphological basis. Contesting the currently popular theory of nonlimited or generalized cerebral function deriving from Haller and his followers, he espoused the contrary views. The following is Gall's description of the nervous system in general and of the brain in particular:

> Indeed, we believe that the whole collection of nerves [the nervous system] is made up of many specific systems; that these systems differ amongst themselves in their intimate structure as in their respective functions; that the functions or faculties are in direct proportion to the development of the organs appropriate to them; that there is more or less connection between the various apparatuses, and consequently reciprocal influence [pp. 228–229] . . . we find also that the brain is composed of as many specific systems as distinct functions it performs [p. 229] . . . But what definitely favors most of these ideas is anatomical facts by which we have established that the nerves arise in various places and from various masses of gray substance, and that the various specific systems of the brain are brought into being (*sont realisés*) in the plurality of the fascicles, layers, and convolutions [p. 230].[66]

As we observed above, there were still remnants of seventeenth-century concepts of the structure of the cerebral cortex current in Gall's time; Galvani's use of them is recalled particularly (see chap. 5.2.2). However, Gall, with noteworthy originality and persuasive tenacity, was the first to deviate from them and to offer an alternative view based on gross anatomical observations. He drew attention to the cortex by proposing that it was a peripheral elaboration of white matter fiber systems, especially those deriving from the pyramids. It was the *matrix nervorum* from which nerve fibers arose, and whereas the gray matter had a nutritive function, the white conducted messages. This was an improved form of Malpighi's erroneous concept of the cortex as a gland secreting into the nerve "tubules" of the white matter. Gall recognized two varieties of white-matter fibers in the cerebral hemispheres: the projection or association and the commissural variety, as they are now known. We should recall that Gall was working exclusively at the macroscopical level, and although he may have been aware of the few crude attempts to view brain tissue through the microscope, he carried out no studies with an instrument that he judged (in keeping with several of his contemporaries) to provide more confusion than enlightenment.

6.3.5. The Genesis of Gall's Brain Physiology

6.3.5.1. *Bonnet and Herder*. A good deal has been written on the roots of Gall's doctrine, but one of the most helpful studies is by Professor Erna Lesky of Vienna.[67] In his book of 1809, written in collaboration with Spurzheim, Gall replied to the criticisms brought against him by Cuvier and his fellow Commissioners of the Académie des Sciences at Paris in their assessment of Gall and Spurzheim's anatomical research. In so doing he made reference to two men who, in contrast to the mechanical anatomists, had come to what he considered to be a more correct view of brain structure, despite the fact that they were concerned more with physiology and philosophy than with anatomy.[68] These were the Swiss biologist, Bonnet, and the German philosopher, Herder, who together provided part of the ideological background, not only to Gall's psychophysiological system, but also to his basic biological and physiological beliefs. One can go further and state that Bonnet and Herder were indeed responsible for a whole new approach to mental processes that began to replace the mechanistic psychology of the Enlightenment in the last two decades of the eighteenth century and which was handed on to the nineteenth century by men such as Gall.

Bonnet's influence is of special interest, because in 1770 he gave a definition of the brain that closely resembled Gall's:

> Without being initiated into the Secrets of Anatomy, it is known, at least in general, that a *Brain* is an Organ of intricate composition, or rather really an Assemblage of different Organs, themselves formed by the combination and intertwining of a prodigious number of Fibers, Nerves, Vessels, etc.[69]

But the passage from Bonnet's writings that impressed Gall the most was the following:

> It follows from this, that an Intelligence [a rational being] that would understand thoroughly the Mechanisms of the Brain, and that would perceive in the greatest detail all that took place there, would read as from a Book. This prodigious number of infinitely small Organs appropriate for Sensation and for Thought would be to this Intelligence as Printed Characters are to us. We turn the leaves of Books and we study them; it would be sufficient for this Intelligence to gaze upon Brains.[70]

Gall cited it, for example, in his book of 1809[71] and in it can be discerned the relationship between brain organs and mental activity that underpinned his doctrine. However, although he made ample reference to Bonnet, by name, as well as to Herder, it was judged by some that his indebtedness to him had been inadequately acknowledged.[72] In 1825 Gall defended himself ably, refuting all allegations and dispelling any possible charge of plagiarism.[73] Bonnet's influence was nevertheless considerable.

In 1770, Bonnet had stressed that the "organs" of the brain were not only related functionally to mental processes, but in addition they were intended to handle sensations and concepts. We can now discern more clearly how much Gall depended upon him. To explicate the structure of the "organs," Bonnet conjectured a mechanistic explanation based on solidistic principles derived from Descartes. The quotation from Bonnet cited above is one of several allusions to this notion, and it was the same elsewhere in the body, which was itself a machine; the "organs" were composed of "fibers," that is, hypothetical and not microscopical structures. Concerning the nervous system, the elemental fiber was not recognized by means of the microscope until 1781 by Fontana.[74]

Although Bonnet in no way advanced the doctrine of cerebral localization, the plurality and specificity of his "organs" especially attracted Gall, even though he contested his sensationism, whereby the external world was projected upon the internal world by way of impressions registered by the senses. For this and other reasons Gall could not accept all of Bonnet's psychophysical scheme, but instead he selected parts appropriate to his own evolving system. In addition to the notion of "organs," Gall also absorbed the analogy Bonnet made between the functions of external and internal sense organs. It is of considerable importance because Lesky has discovered the following revealing statement in Gall's *Philosophisch-medizinische Untersuchungen* of 1791, which contains the earliest elements of his doctrine:

> Most philosophers, it is true, find it ridiculous that the various mental capacities and concepts should be thought to have their seat in different parts of the brain. But if this is ridiculous, then it is ridiculous also that the different senses are located in different parts of the body, that our several parts feel in different ways . . . : for sight and hearing are just as much mental talents as are the different kinds of ideas.[75]

Essential though Bonnet's ideas were to the establishment of Gall's doctrine, those of Herder were even more influential. It was his writings on natural philosophy and anthropology that proved to be most potent, and the years 1784 to 1791 during which Herder's great work *Ideen zur Philosophie der Geschichte der Menscheit* was published[76] was the very period when Gall was creating his own new system of psychology, and which culminated with his seminal book of 1791, mentioned above. Unlike Bonnet's sterile, mechanistic scheme of nature, Herder promoted a dynamic and vitalistic one, which was controlled by a single law of nature whereby unity of structure and function was a basic principle of both the inorganic and organic world. The impact on Gall was immediate and lasting for he learned from Herder the importance of a comparative approach to mental processes, and, of equal importance, the apparent value of establishing function before investigating structure.[77] These, as we have seen, were the fundamental principles that guided Gall throughout his life, and as Lesky has expressed it: "Herder's methodological mission and his comparative genetical concept was literally constitutive for Gall's cerebral anatomy."[78]

As mentioned elsewhere, Gall also had a theory of reinforcement of nerve fibers as they passed through gray matter, which could be applied to cerebral and cerebellar white-matter fibers, cranial nerves, spinal nerves, and the nerves of the vegetative nervous system. This process had its ultimate expression in the development of the cerebral convolutions as the true cortical "organs" of normal and intellectual powers.[79] The notion of reinforcement underlying Gall's principle of nerve function throughout the nervous system also may have been adopted from Herder, who had a concept of "reinforcing," with a consequent refinement of animal organizations by improvement. He described it thus:

> 3. The further the muscle powers enter the sphere of the nerves, the more they are imprisoned in this [higher animal] organization, and subdued to *the purposes of perception*. The more numerous and delicate the nerves an animal has, the more frequent their connections, the more artful their reinforcing (*Verstärken*), and allied to the vital parts and senses, and finally the larger and more subtle the meeting place of all sensations, the brain, the more rational and refined will be the kind of organization.[80]

However, this reference may seem slender evidence, and Herder did not elaborate on what he meant by "reinforcement."

A more striking similarity between the writings of Gall and Herder is the statement made by the latter: "The brain of every animal is fashioned according to the structure of its head, or rather the head according to the animal's brain, because Nature works from the inside outwards."[81] Herder was referring here to physical factors such as the way in which animals and humans held their heads, and the effect of the upright posture in humans and primates. The skull in humans was high, rounded, and boldly curved, thus forming "the uniquely beautiful apartment for the formation of rational ideas."[82] He was especially impressed by the position of the head because "here, I believe, lies the difference that produces this or that instinct, that elaborates an animal or human mind: for each creature is in all of its part one living and cooperating whole."[83] The front of the human skull was ample in volume to accommodate thought, and the posterior small, so that the cerebellum, an animal organ, would not predominate. He continued:

> It is the same with other parts of the face; as organs of sense they manifest the finest proportion of the sensory faculties of the brain and every deviation from this proportion is an approach to the animal. I am certain that on the agreement of these parts will be created a valuable science to which a

> physiognomy based on conjecture would not easily attain. The foundations of the external form are inside; for everything has been fashioned by the organic powers operating from within outwards; and Nature has made every creature such a complete form as though she had created nothing else.[84]

These and similar comments of Herder must surely have had a profound influence on Gall, and it seems possible that the "valuable science" predicted by Herder turned out to be organology.

Gall's book of 1791 made many contacts with Herder's philosophical propositions, particularly regarding the nervous system, and it appears to contain several of the basic elements of Gall's doctrine of "functions of the brain." As noted, it was after its publication that he began dissecting the brain in order to provide a morphological basis for his physiological hypotheses. His general views of the brain, however, continued to develop and, as Erna Lesky has revealed for the first time, Gall's idea of type derived from Herder. Thus, Gall proposed the existence of a general type of nervous system, observable by examining it in a variety of animals. This suggestion was in keeping with the contemporary attempts to discover a model for all plants and animals. He could make structural and functional analogies between plants and nervous systems, so that laws common to each of them were recognizable. His integration of concepts of structure and function, together with his model of an archetypal nervous system, had important by-products: the various anatomical discoveries in the nervous system with which he has been credited (see chaps. 1 n. 61 and 2 n. 26). Gall's plant analogy, also perhaps derived from Herder, suggested to him an organic and dynamic independence that could be attributed to the organs of the mind. Mental activity was perfected as the animal scale leading to humans was ascended, and these organs were interpreted as structural developments of nervous tissue and centers for the production of impulses. They were located in an internal human world organized by innate predispositions and emotions.

As Lesky has indicated, the evolution of Gall's thought is a fascinating study. It is of significance not only to the creation of his own doctrines, especially that of organology, but also, more generally, to a change of attitude toward mental activity that took place in the last twenty years or so of the eighteenth century. The mechanistic psychology of the Enlightenment was being undermined by Herder's philosophy, and it was Gall who helped to carry his revolution into the nineteenth century.

6.3.5.2. *Scottish Faculty Psychology.* The possibility that Gall had been influenced by representatives of Scottish faculty psychology has been suggested, and we must broach it briefly here. A resemblance between Gall and Spurzheim's lists of faculties residing in the various cerebral "organs" and those of earlier writers was mentioned first by Louis Francisque Lélut (1804–1877) in 1836; we shall encounter him later as a cogent critic of Gall.[85] The first of these writers was Francis Hutcheson (1694–1746), Professor of Moral Philosophy at the University of Glasgow, and remembered for his doctrine of moral sense, his book on the origins of ideas of beauty and virtue, and for his phrase "the greatest happiness for the greatest number," later utilized by Jeremy Bentham (1748–1832) in the development of utilitarianism.[86] The second was one of Hutcheson's successors at Glasgow, Thomas Reid (1710–1796),[87] and the third, Dugald Stewart (1753–1828),[88] Professor of Moral Philosophy at the University of Edinburgh. Each had tackled the problem of identifying the functional unities that were manifest in the conduct of individuals in their efforts as faculty psychologists to analyze the mind. However, as far as Gall's organology is concerned there appears to be no relationship with them. Although Gall was dependent upon predecessors like Bonnet, Herder, and others, there is no evidence to suggest that he was aware of the Scottish school.[89] Only Hutcheson or Reid could have influenced him when he was preparing his doctrine in the 1780s and 1790s, because Stewart's work, which stemmed from Reid's did not appear until 1827. But comparing the lists of Hutcheson and Reid with those of Gall reveals more differences than similarities.[90] Adolphe Garnier (1801–1864) in 1839 also exonerated Gall from the charge of plagiarism, but could not excuse Spurzheim and his British followers, in particular George Combe, who must all have been aware of the three illustrious Scots philosophers.[91] As noted, it seems likely that it was Spurzheim who borrowed, but the blame was unjustly shared by Gall.

6.3.5.3. *Physiognomy*. If some of the fundamental tenets of Gall's empirical psychology had been established by 1791, how were these used to create his system of organology? He now had to draw upon the data of physiognomy, upon his personal observations, and upon anecdotes, analogies, and conjectures.

At the end of the eighteenth century, physiognomy was a well established method of investigating the personality and psychological constitution of individuals, and in the 1790s, when Gall was formulating his system of primitive behavioristic psychology, it was enjoying great popularity.[92] It is usually accepted that the first attempt to assess human character by means of facial features was reported by Giovanni Battista della Porta (1536–1605) in 1586,[93] and from then until the present day a very large amount of literature on the subject has accumulated. One of the more influential contributions to it appeared in 1772, written by Johann Caspar Lavater (1741–1801), and republished in many editions and translations ever since.[94] He made shrewd appraisals of physical characteristics of individuals, such as stance, attitude, and stature, as well as facial and cranial delineations. By means of his writings and lectures, Lavater was responsible for the widespread approbation given to physiognomy at the end of the eighteenth century.[95] It was against this background that Gall, already much affected by the biological philosophies of Bonnet and Herder, began his search for a new classification of psychological attributes.[96] Although necessarily based on a considerable amount of unscientific material, it was at least an earnest inquiry into the possible functions of organic structures.

As Gall gradually pieced together his systems, he made use of at least one observation dating from his boyhood. Even at an early age he was an acute observer and he took note of objects and events around him that others overlooked. Thus, he was intrigued by what seemed to be two obvious characteristics of schoolboys: they varied in intellect and in cranial and facial configuration. Instead of being content to accept these mundane facts, he then attempted to correlate them, and his only success, based on one case, is well known. One of Gall's schoolmates had protruding eyes, "ox-eyes" as he called him, and also the ability to memorize long passages from books, a feat that Gall could not accomplish. When in medical school he believed that he had confirmed this association, for those with outstanding linguistic attainments had protruding eyes. He further established it by examining mental asylum and prison inmates, and from the same material he deduced a general correlation between mental traits and cranial contour. Now, proceeding step by step, he accumulated further observations, but unfortunately, he also accepted uncritically a variety of nonscientific data and so brought disrepute upon himself. He fancied that he could detect external manifestations for each separate human talent or propensity, and that he was able to discern the intellectual and moral character of an individual by the shape and irregularities of the cranium. In this way, Gall founded a doctrine formed of several strands from the concepts, observations, and speculations of his predecessors, yet based on his own material and interpretations and, therefore, highly original.

However, whereas the physiognomist maintained that the physical features of a person's face and body reflected character, disposition, ability, instincts, and so forth, all being expressive of the soul, Gall was primarily concerned with the brain, the functions of which were mirrored on the cranial vault where the effect represented a secondary part of his scheme. As he insisted: "The object of my researches is the brain; the skull is but a faithful impression of the external surface of the brain and consequently only a part of the main objective."[97] Gall had, in fact, reversed the principles of the physiognomists by adopting a purely materialistic approach. For him, character and intellect were simply the sum of the combined functions of his brain "organs," so that character was the brain. Instead of subscribing to the usual explanations for mental processes, which attributed them to extracorporeal forces or delegated them to various viscera of the body, Gall maintained that a "plurality of organs" on the surface of the brain, each with its own specific moral or mental faculty, functioned together to create the intellect and character. Mental processes had natural causes which could be identified and determined. The "organs" could increase or decrease in size, according to the amount of their specific faculties the individual possessed. The people with retentive memories, therefore, had bulging eyes because the "organ" in which language, including verbal memory, was represented was on the orbital surface of the frontal lobes. This lay on the posterior part of the superior orbital plate so that when the "organ" was hypertrophied, as in these individuals, the eyeballs were pushed forward. Similarly, Gall was able to account for a person's aggressive nature by discovering cranial protrusions behind the ears which he announced were the "organs" of combativeness.

Gall's method of reaching such conclusions, which were but hypotheses and then using them as the kingpin in the construction of a doctrine, brought him into obloquy. One can imagine experimentalists like Magendie and Flourens despising a man who approached a physiological problem in this way and who thought he had established a scientific truth, which was, however, based on little more than unverified, inspired guesses with no real experimental support.

Nevertheless, Gall's approach was entirely materialistic, and it is not surprising that he rejected *Naturphilosophie* although he shared some of the key assumptions of the proponents of this system (see chap. 2.2) and that its advocates, in their turn, rejected him.

6.3.6. The Early Reception of Gall's Doctrine

During 1796, Gall began lecturing privately in Vienna on his new doctrine of human psychology, then known as *Schädellehre* ("craniology"). His primary intention, which amounted to an exposure of the workshop of the human mind to secular inspection by means of a simple, nonmystical but tangible method, had two immediate, although contradictory, consequences. In the first place, his lectures were greeted with great interest and excitement by the laity, both fashionable and of lower rank, but they also incited consternation and antagonism among theologians, court officials, and idealistic natural philosophers. Their charge against Gall was the preaching of a materialistic doctrine, devoid of ecclesiastical overtones, and promoting a denial of moral liberty. In addition, whereas physiognomy accommodated the soul, *Schädellehre* was, in the eyes of some, blatantly atheistic.[98] The opposition to him gradually increased, and during 1801 and 1802 he was accused of corrupting morals and endangering religion. His subversive lectures were eventually banned by the Austrian government,[99] and in 1805 he left Vienna, with his disciple Spurzheim.

Gall's reception by the rest of Europe was also mixed. During his tour of the Continent from 1805 to 1807 and his twenty-one years' residence in Paris, he achieved both fame and infamy. Similar opposition founded on religious, moral, and philosophical objections soon became apparent and these will be discussed in chap. 6.5. Some physiologists and anatomists denounced his willingness to construct a doctrine on unsubstantiated hypotheses, and they accused him of quackery and, like Mesmer, of capitalizing financially on a gullible public. No doubt there was some truth in the last of these allegations. Other critics were derisory and ridiculed Gall's system; one of them was August Friedrich Ferdinand von Kotzbue (1761–1819), the German dramatist, who, in the manner of Aristophanes (c. 450– ? 385 B.C.), aimed to make Gall a laughingstock by means of a satirical comedy entitled *"Die Organe des Gehirns"*[100] published at Leipzig in 1806. It featured such characters as Herr Rückenmark, Herr von Hellstern, and Katzrabe. But although it mocked *Schädellehre,* it also provided useful publicity.

Nevertheless there was also favorable reaction, and the fame Gall achieved derived from the many who supported his system. A number of plaudits could be cited, but that of Christoph Wilhelm Hufeland (1762–1836) was especially significant, because he was one of the most outstanding German physicians of his time and did not subscribe wholeheartedly to *Schädellehre.*

> And I am fully persuaded that *he* [Gall] belongs to the most remarkable persons of our age, and his doctrine to the boldest and most important advances that have been made in the study of nature.
>
> It is necessary to see and hear him himself, in order to perceive how far removed he is from every kind of quackery, metaphysical enthusiasm, and the spirit of party. Endued with a rare spirit of observation, acuteness, and the talent of deduction; brought up in the bosom of nature, and by constant intercourse with her, became her favourite; he has detected a number of phenomena in the whole circle of organic beings, which have hitherto been not at all, or but superficially observed. He has ingeniously combined these observations, discovered their analogical relations and import, deduced influences from them, and established certain truths, which are particularly worthy of our notice, because they are the pure result of observation alone. It is thus that he has contemplated the properties, connections, and functions of the nervous system.[101]

In addition, Hufeland provided here a useful summary of how the system was created. Concerning Gall's qualities as a dissector of the brain, there was also praise from many (see chaps. 1 n. 61 and 2 n. 26).

6.3.7. Gall's Publications

For the first twelve years or so of its existence, Gall published little on his doctrine and relied on lectures given by himself, by Spurzheim, or by their followers together with their books to propagate his creed. He was, however, steadily accumulating data for a definitive treatise. On 14 March 1808, he submitted a memoir to the Acadèmie des Sciences at Paris in an unsuccessful attempt to gain membership, and in it gave details of his and Spurzheim's anatomical discoveries. The committee appointed to assess it consisted of Jaques René Tenon (1724–1816), Raphael Bienvenu Sabatier (1732–1811), Antoine Portal (1742–1832), and Philippe Pinel, under the chairmanship of Georges Cuvier. They completed their report one month later, on 15 April 1808, and it was read at the Académie *séance* of 25 April.[102] As we have seen, on the whole, their comments were more critical than complimentary, which caused Gall and Spurzheim great disappointment at a time when they were cultivating a wide following for their organology (see chap. 2.1).

Their first joint publication in book form appeared in the following year, and in it they quoted sections from the committee's report and challenged the criticisms leveled at them.[103] The definitive account of their new psychological system began publication in 1810, with the appearance of the first folio volume of a sumptuous and expensive five-volume work, including a splendid atlas of one hundred elegant plates.[104] It was completed in 1819, but in the meantime, Spurzheim had severed connections with Gall, and after volume one and 146 pages of volume two, the joint venture ended and the remainder of the work was from the pen of Gall alone. A second edition, with Gall as the sole author, was published 1822 to 1825, and in 1825; the atlas was not included, but a collection of Gall's replies to his critics was added. Its main title proclaimed that the whole purpose of his theory of psychology concerned "functions of the brain and its parts."[105] The term "organology" is used, but "phrenology" is nowhere to be found. Although Spurzheim continued to publish voluminously on phrenology and brain anatomy, this was Gall's last major work completed nine years before his death.

6.3.8. The Nature of Gall's Doctrine

Gall's and Spurzheim's systems evoked two basic principles: the doctrine of compound functional localization; and a primitive, behavioristic, and faculty psychology. In retrospect, we judge them to be unlikely bedfellows, for it was a strange association between a scientific hypothesis that had received the unwarranted dignity of being considered a doctrine, and a psychological system, which in the case of Spurzheim's version was a social philosophy disseminating a popular reform movement. Our interest lies primarily in the first of these, but we should remember that Gall and his contemporaries, together with the vast majority of his supporters up to 1870, were not directly concerned with it. It was the second that occupied their attention, and a brief and general account of it to amplify the definition given above is now necessary, and thereafter some account of the far-ranging influence it wielded. Only Gall's system of organology in its completed form will be described, without reference to its evolution in his mind. There were three underlying principles. First, the mind was not a single unit, but instead it comprised twenty-seven independent and specific mental faculties, aptitudes, or propensities, each of which could be defined and assessed. There were animal propensities such as amativeness, combativeness, alimentiveness, together with moral faculties like self-esteem, veneration, and conscientiousness. Second, these aptitudes were localized in twenty-seven distinct "organs" on the surface of the brain. Third, the organs varied in size in proportion to the amount of the particular faculty they contained, and this variation in volume was registered by the overlying skull in the form of an elevation or depression of the bone. Thus by examining the configuration of the cranium, the organologist could make an accurate analysis of character, personality, and mental makeup.

It can be argued that by parcellating the brain surface, Gall was reflecting the localistic theory of pathology that had begun in Paris at the beginning of the nineteenth century and was being enthusiastically pursued throughout his residence there. Previous concepts of disease causation had favored a disturbance or imbalance of the whole body, or system, whereas anatomical pathology, or morbid anatomy, was based on the existence of localized lesions. Gall was preaching a similar creed when instead of a diffuse or poorly localized arrangement of mental processes, he advocated the existence of a circumscribed region of the brain, that is, an "organ" for each of them.

A brain "organ" was referred to by Gall as "a nervous apparatus" or "cerebral region," and it was composed of gray and white matter, but without recognizable boundaries between it and its neighbors. They were not, however, contiguous, and the gaps between them made up about one third of the total brain surface. Gall confessed the incompleteness of his system, and pointed out that there was space for others to accommodate additional "organs" lacking from the original scheme. As noted, Spurzheim obligingly increased their number to thirty-five. Later in the century forty-three were accepted, but it was usually agreed that certain areas of brain surface, such as at the base and out of reach of the palpating fingers, were uncharted territory. The frontal sinuses, which vary considerably in size in different individuals, obviously presented a grave problem that was never satisfactorily resolved.

Gall's twenty-seven "organs" representing specific functions of the mind were as follows: 1. Instinct of reproduction, 2. Love of offspring, 3. Friendship, 4. Self-defense and courage, 5. Carnivorous instinct, tendency to murder, 6. Cunning, cleverness, 7. Ownership, covetousness, tendency to steal, 8. Pride, arrogance, haughtiness, love of authority, 9. Vanity, ambition, love of glory, 10. Caution, forethought, 11. Memory of things and facts, educability, 12. Sense of places and space, 13. Memory and sense of people, 14. Memory of words, 15. Sense of language and speech, 16. Sense of color, 17. Sense of sound, music, 18. Sense of numbers, mathematics, 19. Sense of mechanics, architecture, 20. Wisdom, 21. Sense of metaphysics, 22. Satire, witticisms, 23. Poetical talent, 24. Kindness, compassion, morality, 25. Mimicry, 26. Religion, 27. Firmness of purpose, obstinacy, constancy.

6.3.9. The Influence of Organology and Phrenology

The controversy aroused by the crusading endeavors of Gall and Spurzheim, and the interest it engendered in the nineteenth century, were greater in volume than the effects of Darwin's theory of evolution, because the latter had much less impact upon the layman. Organology and phrenology, on the other hand, could be more readily comprehended and their practical benefits were more apparent to the nonscientist. We shall discuss in more detail in 6.5 below the philosophical and cultural reactions to Gall's thesis, but meantime, we can observe that the debate waxed and waned throughout the century, mainly during two periods. The first was when the two cults were at their height of popularity, in the 1820s and 1830s, before the objections of Flourens (to be studied later), and others took full effect and brought about their decline in approbation. Controversial issues concerned the frontal sinuses and artificial and pathological cranial deformation. And there was also the question of the temperaments that had been overlooked and had to be included, although they related to the general shape of the head rather than to local variations in contour. The second period of controversy began in 1870, when the discovery of punctate localization in the cerebral cortex was proved experimentally for the first time.[106] Gall's doctrine was thus revived, for devotees claimed quite unjustifiably that at last he had been proven correct by means of scientific evidence. This phase is still in existence as a few phrenologists exist today.[107]

The popularity and spread of Gall's organology and Spurzheim's phrenology, but especially the latter, was phenomenal in each of these periods. As we have just noted, the main explanation for this lies in the fact that they provided a system of psychology for the masses, and supplied the only available complete science of man, whereby all aspects of human nature could be elucidated. Moreover, they professed to explain how humans were constituted, and did so in a relatively simple fashion and without reference to intangible, mystical, or incomprehensible concepts. They offered individuals not only an easy but also a practical method of finding out about themselves, and about those around them. An individual could thus discover how to create happiness for himself or herself and for others, how to choose a spouse or a career, and how to resolve domestic issues such as the way to bring up children. The two creeds were therefore the common man's "scientific" method of character analysis, aptitude testing, and vocational guidance, and it has been claimed that in the United States it "was one of the factors which brought science to the American mind and provided a rationalistic explanation of human life."[108]

After Gall's death in 1828, his organology was superseded by Spurzheim's phrenology, which remained in ascendancy to the present day, *phrenology* becoming the accepted term for both Gall's and Spurzheim's systems. Nevertheless, there have always been a few individuals who preferred the original doctrine of Gall, and among them was one of the last British phrenologists who died in the early 1970s.[109]

As early as 1815, Forster recognized the numerous uses that Gall's system could be put to.[110] He pointed out that it was of value in education by the cultivation of the appropriate faculties of the intellect, by the regulation of moral character, and by increasing application and aptitude. It helped to make the punishments fit the crimes of malefactors, it could be used in the treatment of the insane, and even in the interpretation of dreams, and could also assist in the selection of a profession. Thus, phrenology was of interest to the physician, especially the alienist (psychiatrist), to the scientist, the social thinker, the reformer, and educators of all types, as well as to those who savored its optimism and were attracted by naturalistic interpretation of life. It was a form of salvation offering universal hope and a vision of ultimate perfection that was within each individual's grasp.

According to Gall, the faculties in the "organs" were capable of growth by means of exercise, and this possibility opened a door to an immense area of influence. An individual could, therefore, cultivate and improve his socially desirable propensities and at the same time inhibit his vices, which was in step with the Victorian concept of progress and self-improvement. The appeal to reformers of a method of social betterment is obvious: if a person could achieve control over his or her mind and character, the potential role of self-education, educational schemes, and social reforms become readily apparent. A study of punishment in relation to crime could be made and the reform of the criminal and the management of prisons facilitated. A part of the field of health reform, in which health legislation was established and popularized, was also open to the phrenologist, and important issues associated with heredity came within his domain. Gall had disputed the Lockeian concept of the *tabula rasa,* whereby experience was thought to be recorded in order to formulate the individual's mental state. He favored the hereditary transmission of the mental and moral traits basic to his doctrine.[111] Here the influence upon him was probably that of Marie Jean Antoine Nicholas de Caritat, Marquis de Condorcet (1743–1794) and Cabanis, for each had believed that mental as well as physical characteristics could be transmitted, and this could occur owing to the properties of the mind being dependent upon the structural arrangement of the brain.[112]

The phrenologists, in fact, were among the first to formulate an attitude to human nature, which placed an emphasis on physical and mental qualities being inherited. They were also the most effective popularizers of hereditarian ideas before Darwinism and eugenics appeared, and in the case of the latter they influenced its development.[113] The applications and the further potentialities of phrenology seemed limitless, and its involvement with many of the sociointellectual revolutions of the nineteenth century indicates its importance as a trace element in Victorian society. We can enumerate at least twelve areas of knowledge and endeavor that it pervaded: brain physiology, psychology, psychiatry, biology, anthropology, penology, education, philosophy, social structure, literature, politics, and religion. It follows that the literature generated is immense.[114] This vast spectrum of influence and the depth of phrenology's penetration led R. Cooter to make the following claim:

> Recent scholarship thus comes to view phrenology as one of the most important intellectual manifestations of the nineteenth century—important not because of what it accomplished if measured by the yardsticks of orthodox political and social history, but because of the wide range of Victorian values, ideas and attitudes it appears to have mediated. As a bridge between traditional ideas and institutions and secularized reforms the doctrine played an instrumental role. . . .

And that "the background chapter on phrenology can no longer go unwritten if we are to arrive at a satisfactory analysis of nineteenth century thought viewed in its proper context."[115]

However, despite the influence that phrenology had in so many disciplines, it was rejected by the scientific world almost from the moment of its inception. The background to this rejection is considered in 6.5 below.

6.3.10. Summary and Sequel

There were three main beneficial results deriving from Gall's unique psychophysiological doctrine of organology. First, his teachings, his writings, and the controversies he generated directed considerable attention to the brain, the intimate study of which was lagging behind that of other parts of the nervous system as a result of Haller's holistic theory of brain function. Also the skilled dissections carried out by Gall and by Spurzheim themselves inspired many to study the complexities of brain morphology (see chap. 2 n. 26). Second, Gall revived the idea of brain localization which had also been suppressed by Haller's teachings. Admittedly, his concept of a brain-surface parcellation of moral and mental attributes is in no way comparable with the modern mosaic concept of functional localization in the cerebral cortex, but Gall nevertheless had resurrected and greatly extended Thomas Willis's conjecture on cortical function. Moreover, the notion of localization fundamental to Gall's organology survived the onslaughts upon his psychological system and, as we shall see, it can be traced through the nineteenth century to 1870, when it was confirmed experimentally, although for somatic and not psychological activity. The third benefit accruing from Gall's work was his insistence that all aspects of mind activity must be located in the brain. As noted below, there were a number of physicians in the early years of the nineteenth century who followed Cabanis's and Bichat's opinion of locating certain psychological processes in the vegetative nervous system; Gall's teaching helped to eradicate this notion, although not entirely (see chap. 7.7.3).

These points were emphasized by Hufeland in 1807, when he made one of the fairest judgments of Gall's organology:

> I adopt Gall's doctrine in as much as it assigns the energy of the mind to the brain as its organ, and in this organ assigns to particular and distinct energies a particular and appropriate organisation of the brain. But I deny that these individual organs are always intimated by elevations of the surface of the skull. Still more confidently do I deny that the elevations upon the

> skull arise solely from this cause, and that therefore a sure inference may be drawn from them to the dispositions and tendencies of the mind. The doctrine, therefore, is true in theory, but there are no means of applying it in particular cases. In other words, the *organology* is on the whole true, but the *organoscopy* cannot be relied upon.[116]

Thus the basic idea of parcellation of the brain's surface into Gall's "organs" was acceptable to some, but his further elaboration of the theory, that is, "organoscopy," was not. In retrospect, it appears that Gall's psychological system was compounded of two main parts: the basic assumption of discrete localization of function in the brain; and the doctrine of organology built upon it. As we have pointed out, the first of these is our main interest here, but to Gall and his followers, it did not have the significance we now place upon it, and they had no idea that they were purveying a notion that was eventually to become fundamental to modern ideas of brain function. In turn, the second is not our concern whereas it was the *raison d'être* for the whole organological and phrenological movement. There is, however, a connecting link between the two and this will lead us from the early decades of the nineteenth century to 1870.

Thus, while phrenology pursued its course into increasing scientific obscurity, events more important to our present theme—the evolution of the doctrine of brain localization—were taking place. These constitute the bridging link just mentioned, and were represented by the association Gall had made between the faculty of language and verbal memory, and the frontal lobes of the cerebral hemispheres. The way in which he first identified this "organ" has already been related, but owing to its outstanding significance in the further history of brain localization, we must examine it in more detail. Gall differentiated between verbal memory and the faculty of language, but he connected together the "organs" that represented these faculties, and he sited them in the frontal lobe convolutions:

> I consider as the organ of memory of words that part of the brain that rests on the posterior half of the vault of the orbit [the supra-orbital plate]. . . . We have considered the sense of words to be only a fragment of the sense of language, of speech.[117]

The precise position of these "organs" was in "the greater part of the middle portion of the inferior-anterior convolutions situated on the superior plate of the orbit or the vault,"[118] that is, equivalent to our orbital gyri. When enlarged, they pushed the eyes forward:

> Persons who have eyes like this [i.e., exophthalmic], possess not only an excellent memory for words, but they also have a special disposition for the study of languages, for criticism, and in general for everything relating to literature. They edit dictionaries, write history; they are very suited to the functions of librarian and conservator; they collect the treasures of all centuries; they compile learned volumes; they study antiquities thoroughly, and if at the same time they have certain additional faculties, they have the admiration of the world on account of their great erudition.[119]

These quotations not only detail the "organs" we are at present interested in but also provide a flavor of Gall's doctrine. His "organs" were all described in this way, introducing poorly or unsubstantiated associations that we can readily contest. It must, for example, have been apparent to him, or to one of his followers, that a degree of exophthalmos did not occur without exception in librarians and museum curators, despite the fact that the number available for inspection at that time must have been small.

Gall died in 1828, but while he still lived a decisive step in the history of brain localization had been made, and it had stemmed directly from his pioneer work. We have seen (chap. 1.2.4), that the renowned and respected French physician, Jean Baptiste Bouillaud, had noted that loss of speech in patients was frequently associated with a lesion of the anterior, that is frontal, lobe of the cerebral hemispheres; laterality was not discussed. On 21 February 1825, he read a paper to the Académie Royale de la Médicine at Paris, in which he concluded that "the coordinating organ of speech (*organe législateur de la parole*) resided in the anterior lobe of the brain."[120] However, this opinion, also expressed by others, received little recognition, mainly because there was an obvious link between it and the extravagant claims of phrenology that, as we shall learn shortly, had been totally discredited by Flourens. Bouillaud's suggestion of cortical "organs" for other muscular movements was also not accepted. It was not until the 1860s that the possibility of a localized area of the brain being responsible for speech functions was again raised, now by Simon Alexandre Ernest Aubertin (1825–?1893)[121] and Paul Broca (1824–1880),[122] also in Paris. Broca brought forward excellent evidence in support of the thesis that the faculty of speech was governed by a localized area of cerebral cortex in the frontal lobe, but on its convexity and not on its undersurface as Gall had postulated. At the same time, John Hughlings Jackson came to a similar conclusion when he argued on the basis of clinical observations only that muscular movements were controlled by specific areas of the cerebral cortex. However, so far there had been no experimental evidence, but when this was provided in 1870 by Fritsch and Hitzig,[123] Gall's theory of punctate brain localization was proved correct in principle. However, he was right for the wrong reasons, and only in retrospect can his doctrine be associated with the present day concept of cortical mosaic localization. Likewise, the specific example of Gall's "organs" of word-meaning and language located in the frontal lobe was but an inspired conjecture. We shall discuss further this fascinating sequence of events later in this chapter.

6.4. PIERRE FLOURENS: CEREBRUM

6.4.1. Introduction

In 1822 Pierre Flourens presented to the Académie des Sciences his well-known report that challenged Gall's basic premise of punctate localization of psychological functions on the surface of the brain. Although not primarily intended to dispute this doctrine, it represents the beginning of an antagonism that was to continue until his death forty-five years later. On the strength of experimental evidence, Flourens asserted that the cerebral hemispheres, like the other subdivisions of the brain, carried out specific functions, their *action propre,* but that these were distributed throughout their individual structures, with no precise localizations as Gall insisted. The cerebral hemispheres, along with the other subdivisions of the brain contributed by means of their *action propre* to the total energy of the nervous system, that is, its *action commune*. Before discussing the details of his unique scheme, we shall review some of the evidence favoring the various theories of brain action that were presented in the early nineteenth century before Flourens's paper appeared in 1822.

Although Cuvier in 1805 maintained of Haller's concept of equipotentiality of brain action that "each day seems to add to the probability of an opposite opinion,"[124] his system still claimed staunch supporters notably Charles Bell and Blainville. We have already recorded Bell's statement of 1811, when he reported current thought on brain function. His idea was a modified form of Haller's doctrine: instead of the entire brain acting as a whole (*action commune*), he preferred the notion of specific functions beings present in each of the brain's "grand divisions and sub-divisions,"[125] where they were distributed throughout their substance (*action propre*). This was the same as Galen's concept and was to be part of Flourens's, whose terms have been included above in parentheses.

As we have already noted (chap. 4.3), Bell, in his *Idea of a New Anatomy of the Brain* distributed privately in 1811 also aspired to create a new functional significance for the brain. This, in fact, was the purpose of his research, and not primarily to investigate the spinal roots as is usually assumed. The cerebrum (cerebral hemispheres), being attached to the anterior roots, must possess its motor and sensory attributes, and as the posterior roots, which looked after the "secret" (autonomic and involuntary) bodily activities were connected with the cerebellum according to his erroneous opinion, this organ must have their attributes:

> The cerebrum I consider as the grand organ by which the mind is united to the body. Into it all the nerves from the external organs of sense enter; and from it all the nerves which are agents of the will [that is, motion] pass out.

And:

> The secret [autonomic] operations of the bodily frame, and the connections which unite parts of the body into a system, are through the cerebellum and nerves proceeding from it.

He therefore concluded that "the cerebrum and the cerebellum were parts distinct in function."[126] It was only after the appearance of Magendie's report in 1822 that Bell dishonestly modified his original concept of cerebral, cerebellar, and spinal root properties. In conveniently-emended versions of his 1811 opinions, Bell now asserted that the cerebrum and anterior spinal roots were in charge of motor activity, and that the cerebellum and posterior roots controlled sensibility.

Thus, Bell pronounced against Gall's organology, and he advocated a return to the Galenic and modified Hallerian concept of equipotentiality. A similar conclusion was reached by Blainville. In 1821 he made a statement that has been thought to echo Gall's words, but seems to have been more in keeping with Flourens's *action propre* than compound brain localization: "We ought to consider the nervous system as divided into as many parts as there are grand functions performed by the animal body."[127]

As in the eighteenth century, we can in retrospect discern some evidence for punctate localization in the early nineteenth century. There was, for example, the cardinal discovery made by Legallois in 1812 of a small region of the medulla oblongata that controls respiration, our respiratory center.[128] This was the *noeud vital* or "vital node," a term used first in botany by Lamarck in 1802,[129] and transferred to animal physiology by Flourens in 1824. Flourens employed this term to designate all of the medulla oblongata, which contained not only the respiratory mechanisms, but, according to him, was the prime center for motion, and perhaps accommodated other essential functional areas. It "constitutes," he declared, "the central nucleus, the common bond, and as Lamarck has so happily said of the collar of plants [for example, of the mushroom], it is the *noeud vital* of this [nervous] system."[130] Only in 1851 did Flourens apply *noeud vital* to the respiratory center alone. For centuries it had been known that the integrity of the medulla oblongata was essential for the continuation of life, for Galen had shown experimentally that if it was transected "the animal perishes immediately."[131] In 1760, Lorry repeated these investigations, and, as we have noted, was the first to define an area at the upper end of the cervical spinal cord, damage to which resulted in instantaneous death. The animal, "suffered complete paralysis of its vital functions, that is to say, death, although the same events did not occur either at a higher or lower level."[132] He was, in fact, the pioneer of punctate brain localization, as well as the discoverer of the *noeud vital*. However, he had not located the respiratory center precisely, for the lesions he inflicted had damaged only its efferent pathways to the respiratory muscles.

The more accurate delimitation of the center itself was the work of Legallois, reported in 1812. He, too, carried out transections of the upper spinal cord, but noted that although they abolished respiratory movements of the trunk, those of the head persisted indicating that the controlling center was in the brain, not in the cord. He stated:

> Respiration is not dependent upon the whole brain, but on a quite circumscribed part of the medulla oblongata, which is situated a short distance from the occipital foramen and close to the origins of the eighth pair of nerves (or pneumogastics [vagi]).[133]

Here then was a significant pronouncement. For the first time, an area of brain substance within a major subdivision of the brain and having a specific function had been defined accurately by experiment. Although supporting the same doctrine, Legallois's location of an area of precise, somatic activity, like that of certain eighteenth century discoverers of punctate cortical function mentioned above, particularly Pourfour du Petit, stands in stark contrast to Gall's "organs" of psychic phenomena. But it was to be fifty-eight years before Fritsch and Hitzig could demonstrate the existence in the cerebral cortex of a comparable arrangement of discrete delimitations of somatic functions. Legallois also underlined the basic principle of functional brain localization, when he described how he was able to establish the precise locality of the *noeud vital*. It was his belief that this approach would eventually reveal the presence of other areas of special function in the brain:

> For, every time a certain portion is destroyed, be it of the brain or of the spinal cord, a function is compelled to cease suddenly, and before the time known beforehand when it would stop naturally, it is certain that this function depends upon the area destroyed. It is in this way that I have recognized that the prime motive power of respiration has its seat in that part of the medulla oblongata that gives rise to the nerves of the eighth pair [vagi]; and it is by this method that up to a certain point it will be possible to discover the use of certain parts of the brain.[134]

How right he was! This way of reasoning was adopted by Flourens in particular, with regard to his *action propre* type of brain action. It was also to be applied to the concept of compound localization, for example, in the cerebral cortex.

The contribution of Flourens to detecting the precise location of the respiratory center is of particular interest to us. In his experimental work on the brain, he admitted of no discrete locations of functions within the major brain subdivisions, for each part of them purveyed the same function or functions. And yet, we now learn that his research on the medulla oblongata, had as its goal the delineation within it of a circumscribed area that possessed a very special and vital action.[135] This did not conform to *action propre* which would have demanded that all of the medulla oblongata must be concerned with the control of respiration, as at first he proposed. From this we can perhaps infer that Flourens did not contest discrete localization per se, but only its application to the cerebral cortex in the way Gall had proposed. The real enemy was, therefore, to be Gall and his organology, as we shall learn later. Meantime, Flourens was concerned to extend the research of Lorry and Legallois, in order to determine the more exact situation and extent of "the primary motor point of the respiratory mechanism."[136] We need not follow the details of his studies, which he had begun in 1825 on the fish,[137] and ended in 1862,[138] but he not only achieved this objective within the limits of his capabilities and technical resources, he also found that the center was bilateral. Although Charles Bell could make little advance in the problem of how the center worked, Flourens had been able to initiate research into the way in which the respiratory muscles were controlled and coordinated in the *noeud vital*.[139] But the ultimate method of studying its morphological limits, by microscopy, was not yet available.

Further evidence of discrete areas of brain exercising specific functions came from Herbert Mayo, as we have learned above (chap. 4.3). In 1823 he found that the pupillary reflex in the pigeon depended upon the integrity of a small circumscript area of its brain: "the fore part of the crura cerebri [cerebral peduncles], together with the [optic] tubercles."[140] Again this was a somatic phenomenon, far removed from Gall's mythical "organs" and their assumed propensities. Further, in 1826, Serres suggested additional vital centers in various components of the brain stem:

> The olive is *excitor of movements of the heart;* the restiform body [inferior cerebellar peduncle], is *excitor of pulmonary respiration.* The funiculus that separates these two bundles is *the excitor of the stomach.*[141]

Although the evidence he presented for them was quite inadequate and his conclusions erroneous, Serres, nevertheless, was obviously accepting the possibility of discrete localization in one of the major subdivisions of the brain, and the same was true of Dugès, who in 1838 specified the olivary bodies in the brain stem as the seat of voice production in view of the fact that they were well developed in humans, but absent in most vertebrates.[142]

As well as these various proposals, mostly derived from experimental observations, there were a number made during the first two or three decades of the nineteenth century that lacked such origins. Thus, some of the followers of *Naturphilosophie* indulged in speculating on the discrete localization of functions in specific brain areas. Of these, the most active was Burdach who published in 1826.[143] The basal ganglia, he believed, were the site of sensory perception and consciousness, volition was in the corpora striata, and sensation, particularly visual, and consciousness in the thalami.[144] The corpora quadrigemina housed subjective cognition, sensation, and coenesthesia (the general feeling of well-being), and also had influences on digestion and appetite.[145] The corpus callosum acted as a center for mental activity,[146] the fornix for the bodily expression of fantasy, and the mammillary bodies for sensory perception. The pineal body influenced the general state of brain activity, and the medulla oblongata was in particular the seat of unconscious instincts and the basis of mental life.[147] Treviranus, another *Naturphilosoph,* localized functions to various parts of the cerebral hemispheres: vision in the posterior lobe, olfaction in the anterior, and hearing in the cerebellum.[148] Furthermore, he believed that the Ammon's horns were concerned with memory, because of their close association with structures devoted to olfaction,[149] and that the cerebellar vermis influenced respiratory movements.[150] According to Carus, the flocculi of the cerebellum were associated with mechanisms of hearing,[151] and to Schönlein the olivary bodies represented the point where all motor and sensory nerves met and associated.[152] Although the opinion of Adam Karl August Eschenmayer (1768–1852) concerning the functions of the pineal body is very reminiscent of that advanced by Descartes in the seventeenth century, and was mostly conjectural in nature,[153] this was not the case with all these suggestions for punctate brain localization. Usually anatomical similarities or physiological analogies had prompted their author's selection of a function for a specific region or structure of the brain, and it has since been revealed that they were not all erroneous or completely fanciful.

By the 1820s there seemed to be three groups of individuals who favored punctate brain localization and opposed Hallerian brain equipotentiality. By far the largest was made up of supporters of Gall's theory, and the other two were comprised of brain stem localizers and the *Naturphilosophen.* In 1822 all this changed because when Flourens introduced his new experimental evidence, which created a modified form of Haller's theory, the localizers were dispersed, almost without trace as far as the scientific community was concerned.

6.4.2. Flourens's Evidence

It was pointed out in 1840 that whereas Haller and Magendie and Bell had introduced revolutionary concepts concerning the functions of the nerve-muscle complex and the spinal roots, respectively, Flourens's studies had done the same for central nervous system centers by openng up vast new fields of research into the functions of the cerebral hemispheres, the cerebellum, and the medulla oblongata.[154] We have discussed his important contribution to the location of the respiratory center in the medulla oblongata, and must now examine why in 1840 he was thought to have greatly advanced the knowledge of cerebral function. In fact, we now know that this part of Flourens's work contained many errors, but such was his skill and authority that with it he was able to contest Gall's organology and eventually to demolish it forever as a scientific idea. However, at the same time he completely suppressed for more than forty years the correct physiological concept of compound or discrete brain localization. Flourens's experimental research on the cerebral hemispheres is well known, but we must explore now its origins and the general principles he deduced from it.[155] We have already referred to it in chapter 1.2.2, where we selected him as one of the outstanding exponents of experimental physiology in the first half of the nineteenth century.

In 1819, when twenty-five years old, Flourens began to investigate theories of sensation, and two years later he gave a course of lectures in Paris, in which he examined the relationships between the physiology of sensation and the sensationist philosophies of John Locke (1632–1704), Condillac, Cabanis, and the other French ideologues.[156] (See chap. 6.5.) Thereafter, he turned his main attention to the way in which the nervous system handled sensory impressions and brought about muscular contraction, and on the basis of this, he could classify the various parts of the nervous system. He described the main purpose of his research as follows:

> The localization of properties by the localization of organs is really the end-all and be-all of this work. It is by this double localization of organs and properties that I first succeeded in distinguishing two orders of parts in the nervous system: the parts capable of exciting muscular contraction directly; and those incapable of doing so.[157]

He presented the results of these studies to the Académie des Sciences in Paris during March and April of 1822.[158] In order to assess the possible significance and merit of Flourens's claims, a committee chaired by Cuvier was set up, and its findings were accepted by the Académie on 22 July 1822.[159] A full account of his investigations appeared in July of 1823,[160] and in a celebrated treatise on the properties and functions of the vertebrate nervous system published a year later.[161]

It is important to realize that in 1819 Flourens greeted organology enthusiastically,[162] but by 1822 he had come under the influence of Cuvier, and thereafter renounced Gall's teachings, and instead upheld the concepts of *action propre* and *commune.* He had accepted Cuvier's view of the whole brain as the material instrument of an indivisible soul, and he maintained this position for the rest of his life. We shall discuss below (6.5) the background to this remarkable philosophical shift, which is not referred to in his book of 1824 and must be inferred by comparing it with earlier and later writings.

Flourens began his research by dividing the nervous system into six morphologically distinct subdivisions: the cerebral hemispheres, the cerebellum, the quadrigeminal or optic bodies, the medulla oblongata, the spinal cord, and the nerves. And immediately he made a break with Hallerian tradition by declaring that they were also functionally distinct, and that Haller's concept of the brain as a homogeneous and equipotential organ was incorrect. These revolutionary notions were based on an extraordinary series of experiments that has been repeatedly applauded ever since they were first reported in 1822.[163] He employed both ablation and stimulation techniques, applying them to each of the subdivisions of the nervous system that he had listed. His general conclusion was as follows:

> Thus the different parts [subdivisions] of the nervous system all have distinct properties, special functions and fixed roles; none encroaches upon another. The nerve *excites;* the spinal cord *connects;* the cerebral hemispheres *will* and *feel.* From the independence of the organ derives the independence of the phenomena.[164]

The cerebrum was the seat of intelligence, volition, and sensation, the medulla oblongata, an excitant of motion, but the cerebellum was neither sensible nor irritable for it coordinated bodily movements. These represented the *action propre* type of brain action, whereby each brain region had one or more specific functions that were purveyed by all its substance, the exception being the *noeud vital* in the medulla oblongata. But independent of these particular actions, the subdivisions also contributed to the total energy of the brain, and this was their *action commune.* As Flourens phrased it: "that is, [an influence] from each on all, and all on each."[165]

In disease the reverse could take place and the loss of a region affected the entire system: "Thus, the cerebral hemispheres *will* and *feel;* this is their *action propre:* the suppression of these hemispheres weakens the energy of the whole nervous system; this is their *action commune.*"[166] Similarly, the cerebellum's *action propre* was to coordinate, but its *action commune* was to influence the energy of the whole system. But although the subdivisions were distinct, both anatomically and physiologically, they acted together in a closely integrated manner by means of their *action commune:*

> In the final analysis, the cerebral hemispheres, the cerebellum, the quadrigeminal bodies, the medulla oblongata, the spinal cord, and the nerves, all these essentially different parts of the nervous system have specific properties, appropriate functions, and clear effects; and in spite of this remarkable diversity of properties, functions, and effects, they form nothing less than a single system.[167]

The integrative action of the nervous system could be illustrated by the way in which bodily movements came about. They were willed by the cerebrum, coordinated by the cerebellum, and the necessary muscle contractions produced by the spinal cord and nerves. The effects of ablation were that removal of the cerebrum led to a weakness of movement, removal of the cerebellum increased this greatly, and the removal of the medulla oblongata, cord, or nerves abolished it.

The idea of unity and integral action was obviously of great importance to Flourens's system, because he repeated his views on it on several occasions. Regarding the nervous system he stated:

> 4. But it is a unitary system, all of its parts concur, conspire, and consent; what distinguishes them is an appropriate and specific manner of acting [*action propre*]; what unites them is a reciprocal action by means of their common energy [*action commune*].[168]

And again, he insisted that, "Unity is the outstanding principle that rules. It is everywhere, it dominates everything. The nervous system therefore, forms but a unitary system."[169]

We shall now examine more closely Flourens's experimental study of the cerebral hemispheres, and his similar work on the cerebellum will be described below (6.6). The techniques he introduced were mostly novel and ingenious (see chap. 1.2.2), for in his ablation procedures he carried out serial removals of slices of the cerebrum in a large number of animals, but mainly birds, and he was able to amass a welter of precise observations, as remarkable for their accuracy as for the terse and precise style he employed to describe them in his research protocols. He found that after bilateral cerebral hemispherectomy all signs of volition and sensory awareness were lost, although movement of each muscle of the body could be induced by external stimuli. Thus the animals could readily stand on their feet, they ran when struck, flew when tossed into the air, defended themselves when teased, swallowed food placed in their mouths, and even the pupillary muscles responded to light. But stimuli were always needed to elicit these movements, and if left alone they sat as though asleep and starved while sitting on a pile of food. Flourens reported on one of them as follows: "When I left it on its own it remained immobile and as though engrossed [in something]. In a word, an animal condemned to perpetual sleep."[170]

From this and other evidence, Flourens concluded that the cerebral hemispheres must be the seat of all volition, sensory perception (including the special senses), memory, instincts, judgment, and learning. But these properties were not localized to special parts of the cerebrum, for they each occupied all parts of it. He, therefore, argued that "the faculty of feeling, perceiving, and willing thus form an essentially unitary faculty."[171] As we shall see below, Flourens's physiology of the cerebral hemispheres thus assumed and defended a particular doctrine of the mind as (*pace* Gall) a unitary entity. Observing that considerable amounts of cerebral tissue could be removed without functions being lost, Flourens concluded that even a limited portion of the hemispheres sufficed for the exercise of their function.[172] It is perhaps remarkable that during the eighteen years between the first and second editions of his book, although he carried out further experiments, none of them induced him to change his original opinions, so that in 1842 he wrote:

> There are . . . no diverse seats, neither for the various faculties, nor for the different perceptions. The faculty of perceiving, of judging, or of willing one thing resides in the same locations as the faculty of perceiving, of judging, of willing another; and consequently this essentially unitary faculty resides essentially in a single organ.[173]

A number of noteworthy side issues arose from Flourens's astute powers of observation. He noted that although cerebral hemispherectomy abolished vision, the pupillary reflex was preserved[174] from which he deduced the important fact that sensory and motor functions could be completely separated. There is no evidence, however, that he took an active part in the Bell-Magendie debate on spinal root function that had begun in the summer of 1822, at the same time as he presented his communication to the Académie.[175] However, it was his belief that nerves conducted both properties. Another crucial neurological principle was substitution of function between parts of the cerebral hemispheres, which was a natural consequence of his notion of the distribution of function within them: "As the cerebral hemispheres contribute effectively in their entirety to the exercise of their functions, it is quite natural that one of their parts can take the place of another."[176] But Flourens was not unique, because, as noted, Haller had already made reference to a phenomenon that later in the nineteenth century was to claim considerable importance.[177]

The second experimental technique that found favor with Flourens was direct stimulation of the brain, which had been in practice for many years, as we learned above (chap. 1.2.2). He made use only of mechanical means by pricking (*piqûre*) or pinching,[178] and although he had experimented with galvanic stimulation, he does not seem to have published his results.[179] In rabbits, dogs, and pigeons, he stimulated most parts of the brain and found that the quadrigeminal bodies (or their homologues) were the most rostral structures, irritation of which produced contractions of muscles. The nerves, spinal cord, and medulla oblongata (at that time his *noeud vital*) all possessed irritability, and this could incite muscular contractions. The cerebellum, basal ganglia, and the cerebral hemispheres were, however, inexcitable. In particular, he agreed with Haller and his followers that irritation of the cerebral cortex produced no movements, and this evidence together with that gleaned from his ablation studies led Flourens to his most serious error. He concluded that "the cerebral hemispheres are not in any way capable of exciting muscular contractions directly."[180] The hemispheres could initiate them by means of the will that resided there, but they could not cause them directly. This was the role of the medulla oblongata.

It was this apparently authoritative opinion that contributed most to the delay in accepting a cerebral control of motor activity, despite the clinical evidence agreeing with it. It was to be a debate between experimental and clinicopathological observations, and by means of Flourens's dexterous use of both scalpel and pen, the former data seemed more precise and acceptable than the treacherous and unreliable manifestations of diseases or injuries of the human brain. A further experiment also supported Haller's concept of an inactive cerebral cortex, and also prevented the emergence of the concept of cortical functions, mainly by refuting Gall's organology. It was one of the most striking and significant of Flourens's procedures, because he claimed to have removed the entire cerebral cortex in three pigeons.[181] They suffered an immediate loss of "the use of all their senses and all their intellectual faculties,"[182] but gradually they recovered their sight, hearing, judgment, and volition, and soon returned to normal. Although not apparently directed at Gall's system, the evidence it provided was to prove lethal to it. However, we may justifiably wonder how Flourens could have performed a complete decortication in a pigeon, and furthermore how he evaluated its mental state. In retrospect, we would consider that the conclusions he arrived at were not warranted, but they nevertheless provided excellent ammunition against Gall and his followers.

In fact, all of Flourens's research on the cerebral hemispheres is open to objection, and the interpretations of brain actions he derived from them were, thus, erroneous. As was the case with many before him, his failure to excite the cerebral cortex was due to inadequate and inappropriate forms of stimulation. But it was shown many years later that the brain of the bird, Flourens's favorite experimental animal, is more difficult to stimulate than that of any other species, even with greatly improved and much more effective equipment.[183] Moreover, there is today agreement that the bird does not possess a cerebral cortex per se as in the mammal.[184] Nevertheless, it seems very likely that Flourens was aware of the statement made by Vicq d'Azyr in the 1790s: "The brain of birds is conceived on a different plan than that of man and quadrupeds."[185]

The problem of species variations, however, remained a mostly unrecognized factor affecting the outcome of animal experiments and the theories founded upon them. Thus, in 1841 Magendie had to call attention to the fact that the characteristics of various parts of animals' brains were not necessarily the same in different species: "a curious fact that anatomy alone has never discussed, and which now it is unable to explain"[186] (see chap. 1.2.2). Moritz Schiff (1823–1896), looking back at Flourens's work, criticized him for not extending his experiments, especially those involving decortication, to the brains of higher animals, in which the outcome would have been different.[187] At the same time, he called attention to the obvious differences in the form and function of different animals' brains. It can also be said that Flourens's ablations of the cerebral hemispheres had often been too extensive, because later investigators found that if they were less radical and confined themselves strictly to the hemispheres, animals did not suffer complete loss of sensation for they could still see, hear, and appreciate painful stimuli.

Concerning Flourens's research reasoning, one of his fundamental assumptions in all of his brain ablations was based on Legallois's statement of 1812. Thus, if a function disappeared after a certain area of brain was removed or destroyed, it was argued that this function must have resided in that area of the brain. For example: "Memory, vision, hearing, volition, in a word all sensations, disappear with the cerebral hemispheres. The cerebral hemispheres are, therefore, the unique organ of sensations."[188] Although philosophical constraints may be imposed on this proposition by warning that related ideas associated with the basic faculty being located elsewhere must be taken into account,[189] a more serious criticism derives from modern concepts of brain action. Flourens's reasoning was, in fact, an oversimplification, because later in the nineteenth century it was realized that an animal with a focal lesion or ablation had to be observed for days or weeks postoperatively before the true and permanent functional deficit could be assessed (see chap. 1.2.2). The effects of surgical shock, immediate neural shock, and of circulatory and functional disturbances of neighboring, and sometimes distant parts anatomically connected, had to be taken into account, as well as phenomena such as compensation and substitution. Other mechanisms were also in action in the immediate postoperative state, including active inhibition and feedback control, as elucidated by the modern concept of neuronal circuits rather than "centers." By these means it is possible for a local lesion to produce an imbalance in the rest of the brain's circuitry. Admittedly, Flourens had in some cases extended the period of observation following his experiment, so that his results were an advance on those of his contemporaries, but compared with the number of his observations in the acute stage, those in the chronic were relatively rare.[190] All of these factors, mostly unknown to these early experimentalists, had significant effects on their results and they account in part for the variations in reports on the sequelae of brain mutilation.

Although these legitimate criticisms have been leveled at Flourens's scientific method, his outstanding operative techniques have never been censured. We have questioned whether he carried out effectively some of the procedures he reported, but nevertheless, as Cuvier and his fellow Commissioners noted,[191] the success of Flourens's research was partly due to the considerable increase in knowledge of brain anatomy that had taken place at the end of the eighteenth century and the first two decades of the nineteenth century, thanks to the labors of men such as Vicq d'Azyr, Reil, Soemmerring, Cuvier, Burdach, Bell, but especially of Gall and Spurzheim, whose concept of compound brain localization he was, ironically, to destroy. In particular, his radically improved method of brain ablation was dependent upon anatomy, and this has been discussed in chapter 1.2.2. He had, of course, inherited techniques from Haller and his school, and also from the eighteenth-century surgeons, like Saucerotte and Sabouraut, referred to above, who had used their operative skills to refine the procedures they adopted. As far as method was concerned, Flourens was one of the first physiologists to discuss at length the physiological *modus operandi* he employed.[192] The following was his basic dogma and is a statement we have already cited, but is worthy of repetition:

> Everything in experimental researches depends upon the method; for it is the method that produces the results. A new method leads to new results; a rigorous method to precise results; an uncertain method can lead only to confused results.[193]

An important and unique contribution that Flourens made to method seems to us a very obvious step, but this was not so at the time. This, as we have already noted (chap. 1.2.2), was the introduction of visual control by exposing adequately the part of the brain to be ablated, damaged, or stimulated. He could, therefore, be anatomically precise and inspect carefully the extent, for example, of the slices he cut from the cerebral hemispheres or the cerebellum. Moreover, he could avoid damage to neighboring structures, the functions of which he was not concerned with, and, most importantly, he was less likely to rupture blood vessels unintentionally.

Neuburger, by reminding us that Flourens was by no means the only one in the 1820s who was working in this research area, provides us with a more accurate historical perspective. But he also points out that Flourens eclipsed both previous and contemporary experimentalists: "because of the fundamental reform in experimental physiology of the central nervous system that he brought about. He created a new method, he formulated problems in a new way, and he endeavored to substantiate his clearly defined ideas with plain facts."[194]

6.4.3. Luigi Rolando: Cerebrum

One of Flourens's contemporaries referred to by Neuburger was Rolando, who, as we have already learned, in 1809 reported the results of stimulating the cerebral hemispheres. On the basis of this research he was led to accept a compound type of brain localization, with "particular organs" responsible for motor activity. But he also carried out ablation experiments similar to those of Flourens's and thus represented his most significant forerunner. However, his work was unknown in France until 1822, when Flourens's research was reported.[195] In March of the following year, and four months before Flourens's Académie report was published,[196] one of Rolando's students in Paris, Jacques Coster (1795–1868), with great ostentation, claimed priority for his master's research on the brain, and he accused Flourens of plagiarism.[197] Thereafter, the part of Rolando's book of 1809 describing the experiments he had carried out was translated into French and was published by Magendie;[198] this was reprinted by Flourens in his treatise of 1824.[199] Coster's allegations, however, posed no threat to Flourens for he was able readily to refute the claims made against him and to testify that apart from being quite unaware of the Italian's prior studies, his own intentions, techniques, and interpretations were different.[200] In fact, it is obvious to us that it would not have detracted from the uniqueness and importance of his experimental results and the opinions to be derived from them had he been able liberally to cite Rolando's monograph in his publications of the early 1820s. But, in any case he received the full support of the influential Magendie,[201] and unlike the contemporaneous priority squabble between Bell and Magendie concerning the spinal cord root functions, the dispute never became a serious issue, and neither Rolando nor Coster persisted with their accusations.

In the case of Rolando's experiments on the electrical excitation of the cerebral hemispheres and the cerebellum, Flourens gave what was almost certainly the correct interpretation of the claim to have elicited muscular contractions: "it is because the galvanic fluid is *conducted* by them [cerebrum and cerebellum] to the *directly excitable parts of the contraction* [i.e., the muscles]."[202] Like Flourens, he had inflicted damage on the cerebral hemispheres of a variety of animals,[203] and one of his fundamental discoveries was that damage to the cerebrum produced a very different picture from similar experiments on the cerebellum. This represented a direct attack on Haller's concept of unitary brain action, or *action commune,* which held that the cerebrum and cerebellum had the same functions. In particular, Rolando could show that injury inflicted on the cerebellum affected control of voluntary motion, but that mental activity was preserved. Cerebral damage, on the other hand, could produce stupor of varying intensity and also led to a loss of precision in carrying out movements. Rolando was astute enough to observe, as Flourens did later, that these movements never occurred spontaneously, but invariably had to be provoked. Sensation, including the special senses, was also lost, together with mental functions, but the ability to maintain equilibrium was not affected. From these findings, it is clear that Rolando, like Flourens, was a remarkably acute observer, in particular by his recognition of psychological disturbances, which at that time were thought by some investigators not to occur in animals, because they claimed that beasts lacked all intellectual activity. In brief, Rolando could claim that the cerebrum was associated with spontaneity, consciousness, mental reactions, sensory perception, and voluntary movements.

Although there were striking resemblances between Rolando's and Flourens's research, there were also several differences. In his paper of 1822, Flourens stated that he had confirmed Rolando's findings, but a reporter added:

> However, we must add that M. Rolando, having only made holes in the skull and removed portions [of the brain] with a spoon, was not able to achieve the same precision as M. Flourens, who after having exposed the brain, removed parts of it serially by exact slices, always satisfying himself by immediately inspecting the extent of each of his procedures.[204]

The differences between the results of the two investigators were, therefore, thought to be due mainly to variations in techniques. Magendie considered correctly that Rolando had incurred postoperative intracranial bleeding, which would account for the stupor in some of his animals.[205] It is of interest to note that from his own experiments, Magendie conjectured that the thalami were in some way connected with the power of motion, and despite Flourens's attempts at exactness, he criticized him, as well as Rolando, for not maintaining adequate precision in the descriptions of the exact location of the serial cerebral removals they each had carried out.

In summary, it must be admitted that despite his crude techniques Rolando's experiments were worthy of great praise; and his interpretations, although likewise inferior to Flourens's did him great credit. As we shall see below (6.6), his views on cerebellar function were overshadowed by the more correct ones advanced by Flourens. But as regards the cerebral hemispheres, Rolando was nearer the truth, because he allocated motor activity to them and proposed a compound or discrete type of localization within them. We now know that Rolando was correct when he included motor activity in the functions of the cerebrum, and that Flourens was wrong to insist that the ablation experiments, like those devoted to stimulation, were negative; his erroneous dictum was that "[I]t has been shown by my experiments that neither the cerebral lobes nor the cerebellum produce *muscular contractions directly*."[206] Rolando's proposals concerning the vital role of electricity in the nervous system (see chap. 5.3.3) may have seemed bizarre to many, but when viewed against the background of the first decade of the nineteenth century they are no more curious than others advanced by illustrious contemporaries. The fact that his name is now known to most medical practitioners on account of the fissure on the surface of the cerebrum, whereas Flourens's goes unrecognized, is some compensation for the small amount of credit usually given him for his noteworthy and creditable explorations of brain action.

6.4.4. Reception of Flourens's Opinions

The most significant feature of Rolando's investigations of the cerebral hemispheres was his conclusion that they were concerned with voluntary motor activity. Like the French surgeons of the eighteenth century and others, he was contesting Haller's doctrine, but unfortunately his opinions were not widely known until 1822, when they were immediately and effectively suppressed by Flourens, whose views on the subject of cerebral and cerebellar function were preferred by a very large majority. The doctrine upon which Flourens's opinions inflicted most damage, however, was that of Gall, and we shall discuss in 6.5 below Gall's criticisms of it. But, Flourens's studies had received the wholehearted patronage of France's most distinguished life scientist, Baron Cuvier, so that his reputation as an experimental physiologist was established almost overnight. His stature was further increased when several physiologists of note confirmed many of his experimental findings. One of the first to do so was a research worker in Magendie's laboratory, Michel Foderà (1793–1848), who in 1822 verified Flourens's contention that the cerebrum was insensitive to various forms of stimulation, because he could detect neither convulsions nor pain appreciation in his animals.[207] However, both occurred with irritation of the medulla oblongata, which he described as "the most essential part of the brain," a comment that Flourens in his turn proved correct when later he was investigating the *noeud vital*. Foderà also introduced the concept of exhaustibility into neurophysiology, and he noted the important fact that the younger the experimental animal, the less the effects of nervous system lesions had on it, because functional impairment could be more readily compensated for in younger than in older animals. Both exhaustibility and compensation had caused confusion and contradictory experimental results previously.

Foderà's supervisor, Magendie, found himself in only partial accord with Flourens, for he believed that apart from vision, sensation was not localized to the cerebral hemispheres.[208] He made an interesting, but erroneous, comparison between the senile deterioration of intellect and of vision, in support of the latter being located in the cerebrum. "The cerebrum," he declared, "becomes insensible to the perception of light, as it becomes unable to exercise other intellectual activities."[209] He also discovered that direct stimulation of either the white or gray matter elicited no response, in the way of pain or convulsions.[210] Concerning motor activity, Magendie had earlier localized it to the fiber connections between brain stem and cerebral hemispheres, that is, probably in the internal capsule. Thus, in keeping with Flourens he denied its existence in the main body of the cerebrum. Trauma to deep brain structures in young rabbits had no effect on voluntary motion: "But I had not injured the white matter fibres radiating from the pyramids to the cerebral hemispheres [? pyramidal tract] at all. It would appear that the properties relating to movements reside chiefly in this part of the brain."[211]

Support for Flourens also came from Longet, working with dogs, rabbits, and kids in an attempt to evoke muscle contractions or convulsive twitchings by means of various forms of excitation applied to the cerebral white and gray matter. They were all negative because "the cerebral hemispheres can be irritated mechanically, chemically, galvanically in animals without giving rise to convulsive tremors."[212] At the same time, however, Longet was aware of the paradox imposed by the occurrence of convulsions in patients proven at autopsy to harbor a lesion in a cerebral hemisphere. He tried to circumvent it by proposing that unnatural stimuli were used in the experiments, or that in humans the medulla oblongata, known to excite convulsions, was affected sympathetically. His final opinion was based mainly on pathological data:

> In summary, and supposing that distinct and fixed regions of the cerebrum corresponding to various voluntary movements have to be acknowledged, it is by no means shown, least of all by us, that there has been anything positive in the proposed localizations concerning the active principles of these movements.[213]

Longet clearly was not entirely convinced that punctate localization did not exist for he was being torn between his and Flourens's experimental evidence and that arising from cerebral disease, whereas Flourens paid no heed to clinical phenomena in humans.

There were, however, others who were convinced that the cerebral hemispheres lacked excitability completely. Julius Ludwig Budge (1811–1884) was one of these, but he based his opinions mainly on the negative stimulation experiments of others. He ignored, or was not aware of, the experiments of Pourfour du Petit and others in the eighteenth century:

> If, in keeping with the present scientific point of view, we can conclude that a part of the nervous system that elicits no [muscle] contractions when stimulated contains no motor fibers, then we can state with the greatest

certainty that there is not a single fiber in the cerebral hemispheres that proceeds to voluntary muscle. Not a single observer has seen movements in the latter after stimulation of the cerebrum.[214]

Carlo Matteucci, who, as we have observed (chap. 5.4), was an important contributer to the understanding of the electrical aspects of muscle and nerve activity, could confirm Budge's statement, when in 1844 he reported his inability to excite the cerebral hemispheres with electricity, which he equated in potency with the various other stimulation methods used by previous workers.[215] Being basically a physicist, he had to admit that his knowledge of brain anatomy was limited, presumably to allay the criticisms of medical practitioners. Even Edward Friedrich Wilhelm Weber (1806–1871) in 1846, using his new magnetic rotational apparatus which had recently revealed the existence of vagal inhibition, could elicit no muscular contractions when he stimulated the brain of a frog.[216] But, as Ferrier pointed out thirty years later, experimentation on the frog brain aimed at motor localization "is scarcely possible."[217]

We need not cite the many authors who also denied sensitivity and motion to the cerebral hemispheres. But in 1858, Schiff was as forthright in his opinion as earlier investigators had been: "I confirm the statement based on the reports of many investigators that stimulation of the cerebral hemispheres, the corpus striatum, and of the cerebellum do not elicit a trace of twitching in any muscle of the body."[218] And as late as 1860, when the revelation of cerebral cortical excitability was but a decade away, van Deen went farther than anyone before him by claiming that not only was the cortex unresponsive to stimuli, but that the whole nervous system was inexcitable to electricity.[219] Such results can only be explained on the grounds of faulty experimental and instrumental techniques.

At a time when the experimental method in physiology was being adopted enthusiastically, Flourens won further honor for having exploited it so ingeniously, and French, German, and Italian scientists applauded him for his contributions to neurophysiology. Few comments, however, came from Britain, and one of these illustrates the isolation of at least one of its medical scientists. Richard Grainger made the following revealing comment in 1837:

> The enquiries of M. Flourens induced that excellent physiologist to conclude, that the cerebral lobes are the exclusive seat of perception, sensation, and volition; but so strong is the apparent testimony of an opposite nature, that, excepting Sir C. Bell and Dr. [Marshall] Hall, not a single physiologist has admitted this conclusion.[220]

Such an assessment is a judgment on Grainger's familiarity with European physiology rather than on Flourens's accomplishments. Nevertheless, there were eventually a few medical scientists in Britain who took up Flourens's view of the cerebral hemispheres, and among them was W. B. Carpenter who popularized it in his textbooks.[221]

Support for Florens's conclusions came from clinicians as well as physiologists and added to the widespread favorable reaction accorded them. They seemed to explain, for example, the puzzling observation that extensive disease or injury of one cerebral hemisphere could exist without somatic or psychological deficit, because the other hemisphere was still intact and functioning normally. But the clinical aspects of cerebral disease also brought opposition to Flourens's conclusions. Léon Louis Rostan (1790–1866) in 1823 correlated disturbances of function in various parts of the body with the localization of function in the brain. He explained that "the functions devolving on each part of this organ [the brain] being well-known, it is evident that it can be determined *a priori* according to the disorder of function [of the body parts], which part [of the brain] is damaged."[222] At first glance, this statement seems to support the punctate type of brain localization, but, in fact, Rostan was also including Haller's and Flourens's organ-equipotentiality type.

There was, however, no doubt concerning the opposition to the Hallerian and Flourentian doctrines mounted by Bouillaud in 1825. It was well known by physicians that a lesion of a cerebral hemisphere could produce symptoms in one contralateral limb only, albeit rarely, whereas if Flourens's conclusions were correct and functions were represented throughout a hemisphere, the whole contralateral half-body should be affected. It could be argued that in view of this significant clinical finding there must be several cerebral motor centers, for without them involvement of one part of the body would be impossible: "The plurality of the cerebral centers destined for movement, is, in fact, proven by the isolated occurrence of partial paralyses corresponding to a local change in the brain."[223]

As we have related and will discuss again below, Bouillaud was in favor of Gall's punctate localization, but not his organology. Thus, speech dysfunction occurred when disease invaded the frontal lobes; paralysis of the lower limbs arose from a lesion of the parietal lobe or the corpus striatum, and of the upper limbs from one of the occipital lobes, or of the thalamus. Similarly, he suggested (erroneously however), that palsies of ocular muscles indicated a lesion in a circumscribed area of the brain, but its site had not been determined. Employing clinical rather than experimental data, Bouillaud represented the chief opponent to Flourens's doctrine, but it was not until the early 1860s that sufficient evidence had been amassed to overthrow it.

In the meantime, this opposition had little effect, even though Bouillaud was joined by others, including the renowned clinicopathological correlator, Gabriel Andral (1797–1876), who carefully compared the symptoms and signs in a series of patients with the local cerebral lesions he found at autopsy. His attempt at localization necessarily lacked precision, but he believed that some of his findings would actually oppose the opinion of those who thought they had discovered special parts of the brain that presided over the movements of the upper and lower limbs. Nevertheless, he declared with confidence and caution that:

> It is very likely that these special parts exist, since each limb can be convulsed separately, paralyzed separately, etc.; but, it seems to us that these special parts have still to be discovered and we know nothing that would be as fatal to this attractive doctrine of the localization of cerebral functions than the premature localizations that one has wished to make of late.[224]

Andral's reference to focal limb convulsions as an indication of local motor areas in the cerebrum is an interesting anticipation of Hughling Jackson's use of the same clinical phenomenon in predicting the cortical representation of limb movements.[225] In the final part of the quotation Andral was refering to Gall and his supporters, who were suggesting a very different kind of punctate brain localization.

Another interesting development at this time was the reintroduction, in opposition to Flourens, of an eighteenth-century notion of punctate cerebral localization. We have discussed the experimental work of French surgeons, such as Saucerotte, who had proposed the existence in the dog's cerebral hemispheres of circumscribed areas that controlled limb movements. Now French physicians began to seek clinicopathological evidence, as well as experimental, in its support. In 1823, A. L. Foville and Félix Pinel-Grandchamp (b. 1798), having noted the fiber arrangements in the cerebral hemispheres, accepted the anterior (i.e., frontal) lobes as the source of motive power for the lower limbs, because of the influence on it by the corpora striata through the fibers that reached it. By a similar argument, they claimed that the anterior limbs were controlled by the middle and posterior (i.e., parietal and occipital) lobes on account of their fiber association with the thalami.[226] The hemispheres, therefore, possessed two "organs" of movement. Serres subscribed to the same view, declaring on clinical grounds that:

> Above all, one must conclude from all that precedes that the cerebral hemispheres exercise a very powerful action on voluntary movements; so that radiations of the corpus striatum influence the legs especially, and those of the thalamus the arms.[227]

Only by this mechanism could the various types of paralyses and convulsions in patients with cerebral disease be satisfactorily explained. He was able to provide experimental verification for this,[228] and he cited the work of J. B. Lacrampe-Loustau (fl. 1824) who had repeated Saucerotte's original experiments of 1768, and found that cutting the fibers radiating from the corpus striatum always paralyzed the hind legs.[229] He must, in fact, have sectioned part of the motor pathway spreading out from the internal capsule. Serres laid special emphasis on this localization of motor functions in the cerebrum, in view of Flourens's uncompromising edict that "My experiments establish that the *cerebral hemispheres* do not produce any movement directly."[230] On the basis of his studies of patients and experimental animals, Serres made a clinical pronouncement that was equally uncompromising, but in his case he was correct, whereas Flourens was ultimately shown to be wrong. "*The location,*" he asserted, "*of a given disease of the cerebrospinal axis is determined by the symptoms.* It is up to physicians and physiologists to judge to what degree I have provided a solution to this."[231] He also appended a list of localizing clinical features to assist practitioners,[232] which supplies us with an excellent summary of thought on the punctate localization of somatic, autonomic, and mental activities as it existed in the 1820s.

It is significant that Gall's doctrine of discrete "organs" was now extended by Serres to a scheme of punctate localization employing organs differing from those characteristic of organology. Thus, his "excitors of the intellectual faculties"[233] in the cerebral hemispheres were not organological in nature, and although they were multiple, isolated, discrete, and distinct, they acted in unison. Another hint of Gall's notions was that Serres believed the median lobe of the cerebellum to be the excitor of the generative organs.[234] However, his unique views received little attention at a time when a belief in punctate brain localization amounted to heresy, and the relegation of the individual professing it to the ranks of the disavowed, even though Serres was, in fact, not opposed to Gall's organology. Clinicians also rejected his conclusions, and they argued that if motor functions of the limbs were represented in two separate parts of the brain, a contralateral monoplegia resulting from a cerebral lesion should be relatively common, whereas it was rare. This was the monoplegia argument used to contest Flourens's type of brain localization, but in reverse. Thus, hemiplegia being the usual manifestation of hemisphere disease demanded that if a controlling motor center existed, then it should be in one and the same part of the brain.

Another French morbid anatomist, Claude François Lallemand, also joined the debate to oppose Flourens. His position was unique, because he was the only person to equate the localization of somatic with mental activity. It seemed to him that Gall's "organs" could look after both, so that the punctate localization of motor functions espoused, by the French surgeons of the eighteenth century, and by Foville, Serres, and others in the early nineteenth, could be combined with organology. The cerebral motor centers were not necessary and Lallemand first of all denied their existence:

> The idea of placing the upper and lower limbs under the exclusive control of the thalamus and the corpus striatum, has no doubt been inspired by Gall's system; but with a little reflexion, it is understandable that on the contrary nothing was more difficult to reconcile.[235]

He then developed his argument in favor of organological functions being combined with the motor:

> If, as I do not doubt, each instinct, intellectual or moral, has its seat in a part of the brain, it must be fully admitted that each of these parts has a direct and immediate influence on *all* the organs of movement; for each single one of these [organological] faculties is capable of provoking prompt, energetic, and complicated movements.[236]

He concluded thus:

> The supposition that the functions of the upper and lower limbs can reside exclusively in any part of the brain is, therefore, incompatible with Gall's system, although at first sight it seems a natural consequence. *A priori* it was easy to see that this hypothesis would turn out to be contradicted by the facts.[237]

Further use of morbid anatomical evidence was made by Louis Antoine Desmoulins, when he attempted to confirm Gall's system. He claimed that "pathological anatomy proves that the faculties of intellectual forces reside or decay on the surfaces of the cerebral hemispheres."[238] Thus various disorders could attack the cerebral cortex, especially those of an inflammatory nature. He also made a significant discovery that supported Gall's organology, but which in the future was to have an important role to play in establishing the doctrine of punctate cortical localization. Having mentioned patients, who obviously had a motor type of dysphasia, he remarked: "But, in all these cases, the anterior part of the cerebral hemisphere was altered."[239] As he stated, this was in keeping with the organological doctrine, and its significance will be discussed below in relation to Bouillaud's identical finding. On the basis of his experience with cases of apoplexy, Desmoulins also accepted the presence in the cerebral hemispheres of the sense of touch and of muscle movement for the opposite side of the body, and these faculties were probably located in or near the basal ganglia.

But, perhaps the most striking example of the method of deducing cerebral function from pathological states was the research of Jean Baptiste Maximilian Parchappe de Vinay (see chap. 1.2.5). He studied in particular the type of tertiary syphilis known as general paralysis of the insane, which is characterized by dementia, paralysis, and sensory loss.[240] The main pathological changes were found in the cerebral cortex, and Parchappe therefore assumed that intellectual, volitional, and sensory functions resided there. He did not, however, attempt to localize them further, even though he admitted he had been influenced by Gall's teachings. It seems that he was also in partial agreement with Flourens, who had placed mental, volitional, and sensory activity in the cerebral hemispheres. Parchappe's scheme, therefore, is a combination of both Gall's and Flourens's doctrines. Later, in 1856, he could describe the main clinical manifestations of general paralysis of the insane, and their dissociation in disease as follows:

> In the terminal stages of general paralysis, the defect of intelligence is more profound than that of movement, and the combined disorder of intelligence and movement is more profound than the defect of sensibility; sensibility is only abolished with voluntary movement when the whole thickness of the cortex is disorganized.[241]

Parchappe thus provided pathological proof for the physiological role of the cerebral cortex, a method that he considered superior to experimentation, and with greater potential. He claimed that "if Gall's doctrine is correct, the hope of verifying the seat of the disorders in the mentally alienated can be entertained, at the same time as explaining the different [features of] delirium."[242]

Flourens's concept of cerebral function was to reign supreme for another thirty years or more, but it was clinicopathological evidence of this nature that finally overturned it (aided by the experimental excitation of the cerebral cortex). Despite the variability and unreliability of such evidence and the very limited diagnostic methods and morbid anatomical techniques that were available, it eventually proved superior to Flourens's laboratory proof, and that provided by his many supporters. We must now examine the cultural background to the controversy evoked by Gall's doctrine of punctate localization of brain function and the etiology of Flourens's effective attack upon it.

6.5. THE CULTURAL CONTEXT OF THE LOCALIZATION DEBATES IN EARLY NINETEENTH-CENTURY FRANCE

We have described how at the beginning of the nineteenth century Gall mounted a formidable challenge to the Hallerian doctrine that the brain had functional equipotentiality. Gall held that the brain was composed of several discrete parts each with its peculiar properties and offices (see chap. 2.4). In particular, he argued that the cerebral cortex was a congeries of such "organs" representing the intellectual and moral faculties, emotions, and instincts and were located at determinate sites on its surface.

As we have seen, despite the widespread attention Gall's doctrine received, it never achieved general acceptance by his fellow scientists. In contrast, the theory of brain function promoted by Flourens attained almost immediate recognition, and his writings effectively destroyed the scientific respectability of Gall's view of cerebral localization. In its place Flourens substituted his notion that although the brain was composed of several functionally distinct subdivisions, these acted as wholes because the properties they possessed were distributed, and therefore represented, throughout their substance. This was his *action propre* concept. In the case of mental functions, the cerebral hemispheres were, as Gall proposed, the seat of intelligence, but Flourens insisted that it was impossible to assign discrete seats to particular psychological faculties within them. He also maintained that the cerebrum was not as irritable as the lower nervous centers, and the hemispheres were thus depicted to some extent as different from the rest of the nervous system, as well as being independent of the sensorimotor principles that applied to subcortical structures.

Flourens's concept of cerebral function enjoyed the status of orthodoxy until the 1870s and Gall's idea of precise sites on the cortex for particular faculties fell into abeyance. The few scientists mentioned above who tried to establish the possibility of localizing functions in the cerebrum realized that they had to combat the opinions of "the celebrated experimenter, M. Flourens," whose theories were shared by the great bulk of the scientific community and constituted a stumbling-block to attempts to treat the cerebral hemispheres in sensorimotor terms and to localize functions within them.[243]

It is apparent from the criticism that Bouillaud's attempt to identify an "organ of speech" in the anterior lobes of the cerebrum (see 6.3.10) attracted that such suggestions were not treated as isolated hypotheses to be judged on their individual merits. On the contrary they were set in the context of wider debates that agitated French intellectual life at the time. Thus Jean Cruveilhier declared that the issue Bouillaud had raised "is one of the gravest; it is not only of interest for a particular question; . . . phrenology as a whole is implicated in its solution."[244] In turn the claims of phrenology were viewed in relation to yet more general contentions about the nature of mind, human nature, and even of the nature of God. To understand the fate of Gall's doctrine of cortical localization, as well as Flourens's concept of the cerebral hemispheres, we must place these scientific theories against the background of early nineteenth-century French philosophy. Indeed, we must acknowledge that it is impossible to draw any firm line of demarcation between scientific, philosophical, religious, and political controversies. Considerations deriving from such seemingly remote provinces were decisive in shaping discussion of brain function during this period. We begin, therefore, with an outline of the state of philosophy in France at the time Gall and Flourens were developing and expounding their theories.

In his 1834 account of contemporary French philosophy Jean Philibert Damiron (1794–1862) distinguished three dominant schools: the sensualists, represented by such figures as Cabanis and Antoine Louis Claude, Comte Destutt de Tracy (1754–1836); the theological school, the most notable members of which were Joseph Marie de Maistre (1754–1821) and Louis Gabriel Ambroise de Bonald (1754–1840); and the eclectics, perhaps the most numerous of all the philosophical sects, whose leading spokesmen were Marie François Maine de Biran (1766–1824) and Victor Cousin (1792–1840).[245] What, at bottom, distinguished the view of these schools were the different theories of mind they espoused; but this difference over psychological questions had ramifications extending into virtually every department of intellectual life.

According to Bonald, physiology did not escape the effects of this philosophical dispute; scientists too were divided on their view of basic metaphysical questions. Although "all physiologists admit . . . the cooperation of the brain (*cerveau* [i.e., cerebrum]) in the production of thought," some held that "organization in general, and that of the brain in particular should be the productive cause of thought"; whereas others maintained that the brain was no more than the "means of operation of the soul." The soul used the brain as it used other organs, but was not dependent upon it.[246] The former concept of mind was characteristic of the sensualist school and lay at the heart of their attempts to construct a monistic philosophy of man and nature. The sensualist sought to achieve a unity within the human body by arguing that the phenomena of thought and feeling were not *sui generis,* but merely one form of organic function. In Bonald's words, they believed thought to be "the product of the brain which receives sensations, digests them, and makes of them thought by secretion, precisely as the stomach receives aliments, digests them, and makes of them chyle, blood and other humours," as Cabanis had maintained earlier. Complementing this physiological monism was a zoological naturalism that held there to be no fundamental hiatus between the human and the animal mind: the former was merely a developed version of traits apparent in lower organisms.[247]

Whatever differences may have divided them, both the theological and the eclectic schools agreed in rejecting this monistic anthropology and psychology. As Boas notes the sensationalists' attempt to assimilate the human to the animal was repugnant to orthodox Christian doctrine;[248] and after 1815 French Catholicism experienced a revival with several able advocates to press its own concept of human beings. The eclectics, although less tied to dogmas than the theological school, also found the naturalistic ideas of Cabanis and his supporters intolerable, chiefly on ethical grounds. Such a view of the human mind was held to be demeaning to man and destructive of morality. Thus Nicolas Massias (1764–1848) complained in 1821 that the "cold doctrine" of Claude Adrien Helvétius (1715–1771) and Cabanis saw "in the pleasures of love only need satisfied; in women only the instrument of lust; and they make no distinction . . . between the brutality of a sapajou [monkey] and the profound and delicate sentiments of an honest man. Justice for them is merely the sword which subdues the weak, and morality merely a speculation in which it is a matter of getting the greatest benefits with the least possible risk . . . finally nature appears to them to be only the chance movements of matter."[249]

In place of monism and its pernicious moral and theological consequences the theological and eclectic schools insisted that there were not one, but two substances in the universe: mind and matter; and that the interval between the two was "not less than between being and nonbeing." On one hand was extended, divisible and inert matter; on the other mind was "simple and indivisible, subjecting the organs to the will, being conscious of itself and of its relations." Although matter was "the image of death . . . intelligence is action and life."[250]

This revival of Cartesian dualism was, in particular, central to the eclectic program; Cousin argued that "the first task of the philosopher is a study of the Ego, a study . . . [that] began with Descartes."[251] Cousin and his numerous followers insisted that the Cartesian *Moi*—the self-conscious ego—must be regarded as prior to nature and as irreducible to matter.[252] From this axiom sound ethical and theological notions would, they maintained, follow naturally. All these *desiderata* were for the eclectics part of the same intellectual parcel. "We are," Cousin announced, "declared partisans of all systems favourable to the holy cause of the spirituality of the soul, of liberty and responsibility of actions, of the fundamental distinction between good and evil, of disinterested virtue, of a God [who is] the creator and regulator of worlds, support and refuge of humanity."[253]

After his arrival in Paris in 1807, Gall's writings and lectures were drawn inexorably into the controversies between the various philosophical schools over these issues. Despite Gall's own protests and disclaimers, his organology was either espoused as favorable or attacked as inimical to the competing philosophies of mind. Specifically, Gall's system was willy-nilly recruited to the cause of sensualism. At first glance this might seem an odd union: Gall was a strenuous opponent of the sensualist doctrine that all knowledge and intellectual qualities were obtained through the senses and an advocate of the innateness of ideas.[254] But in other fundamental respects there were strong analogies between Gall's doctrines and those of the sensualist, which all parties were swift to identify. Reactions to Gall tended, therefore, to depend on the author's stance vis-à-vis sensualism and all it entailed.

Damiron, for example, while fully aware of the differences between Gall and the followers of Condillac, classified Gall as a member of the sensualist school on the grounds that "he belongs there in effect because of a fundamental principle, the principle that all faculties derive from the organism."[255] Others assimilated Gall to the sensualists for the same reason. E. Frédéric Dubois d'Amiens (1799–1873) declared in 1845 that Gall's organicism "is only sensualism disguised"—not because Gall subscribed to the sensationalist account of the origin of knowledge, but because he seemed to share the view that mental properties were inseparable from the workings of the nervous system.[256] Thus L. F. Lélut drew a close comparison between Gall's ideas on this subject and those of the doyen of the sensualist school, Cabanis. Despite his emphasis upon the role of sensation in shaping the mind, Cabanis had, Lélut declared, held that each individual possessed certain inherent predispositions that had their basis in the inherent characteristics of the nervous centers. This was in essence also the conclusion Gall had drawn from "the new sensualism of his doctrines." Only whereas Cabanis had located these mental centers throughout the nervous system (including autonomic nerves of the viscera [see chap. 7.7.3]), Gall had concentrated them in the brain. He also laid more stress on the effect of inherent dispositions as opposed to circumstances on the human mind than had the sensualists. Both agreed, however, that mind was dependent upon organization and not fundamentally dissimilar from other bodily functions.[257] Gall was thus tainted with the physiological monism of Cabanis. In 1845 Flourens cited Cabanis's statement that the brain produces thought like the liver secretes bile; this he described as a "proposition far-fetched to the point of [being] ridiculous, but which ultimately is Gall's own proposition."[258]

Moreover, as several historians have noted, Gall's views on the relation of the human mind to that of animals were very similar to those of the sensualist school.[259] Gall's works abound with statements of the unity of man with other animals and of the need to study human nature in relation to *la nature entière*. It was indeed difficult to say "where animality ends and where humanity commences." This continuity extended into the realm of mind.[260]

Contemporaries pointed to this strong naturalistic tendency as further proof of the similarity between Gall and the sensualist school. Such an emphasis upon the affinity of human nature to that of animals was in complete accord with the opinions of the intellectual heirs of eighteenth-century sensualism, such as Maximilien Henri de Saint-Simon (1720–1799) and Isidore Auguste Marie François Xavier Comte (1798–1857). Whereas the former derived from the work of Cabanis the principle that "the human spirit is studied at its place in nature,"[261] the latter held that Gall had completed the task that the sensualists had merely essayed of making psychology a branch of zoology.[262]

As well as such favorable assessments, however, there were those who subjected Gall's writings to the same censure that they had reserved for previous efforts to "make of man an animal."[263] Again ethical and theological considerations were to the fore in such condemnations. Frédéric Joseph Bérard grouped together Gall and Cabanis when he decried all those who saw no moral objection to reducing humans to the status of animals;[264] while Lélut held that Gall had incurred the charge of atheism that had been leveled at the sensualists.[265]

Gall approximated the sensualists in another respect: he shared many of the social and political goals associated with the group. In the journal *La Décade Philosophique*, the official organ of the ideologue party, Jacques Louis Moreau de la Sarthe (1771–1826) claimed that it was necessary to invert the Hippocratic dictum that philosophy must be introduced into medicine; in current social conditions "it is necessary rather to introduce medicine into philosophy." The result of this marriage of physiology and metaphysics would be a new science of "anthropology" which would encompass all areas of human life, including questions of legislation and government.[266]

Clearly the implementation of such a program would involve a great augmentation of the power and prestige of the medical profession. Jean Burdin (?–1835) argued in 1803 that only medical men would provide satisfactory answers to the problems that had preoccupied metaphysicians for generations; the human mind could only be understood by those with a sound knowledge of the human organism. Burdin deployed the doctrines of sensationalism to demonstrate the close correlations between the physical and the moral in human beings.[267]

Saint-Simon took up these ideas in his *Mémoire sur la Science de l'Homme,* where he insisted that ethics and politics could only become "scientific" when they were viewed from a physiological perspective. Only medical men possessed the necessary qualifications for this task and Saint-Simon lamented the lack of acknowledgment and influence they enjoyed in France. He hoped that the labors of such as Cabanis, Bichat, and Vicq d'Azyr would begin to remedy this neglect and help to bring about the *révolution scientifique* that was the condition of social amelioration.[268]

Among the recipients of this memoir was Gall,[269] and there are traces of the same desire to aggrandize the medical profession in his writings. Gall recognized that professional considerations were involved in the definition of the relation of mind to body. After raising the question of whether mental faculties were dependent upon an autonomous entity or upon certain material conditions, he went on to expatiate upon the practical implications of the solution given to this apparently abstract question. If the mental principle acted independently of the bodily organs, "all its functions [are] beyond the sphere of the physiologist; the metaphysician and the theologian can alone pronounce on its nature." But Gall went on to insist on the numerous facts that established the dependence of the mental upon the physical.[270] Elsewhere he maintained that medical men were best equipped to pronounce upon matters of mental science, and that this competence extended to the discussion of administrative and legislative questions. His doctrines were, in consequence, relevant to "human affairs" in general—not merely to the psychology of the individual, but also to education and penal policy.[271]

It was therefore with some justification that a reviewer in 1819 stressed the importance of Gall's work to the perfection of the "science of man." His doctrines could contribute to a process outlined by the "savant Cabanis": the creation of a "rational philosophy by means of the physiology which should serve as [its] basis."[272]

But although calls for the medicalization of psychology and of social policy found favor in certain quarters (and especially among those who saw themselves as perpetuating the spirit of the French Revolution), such proposals raised hackles elsewhere. The spokesmen of both the theological and eclectic schools agreed in rejecting any incorporation of psychology and ethics into an extended natural science of human beings. Bonald, for example, did not deny that there were close links between the mental and the physical, but he insisted that there was a separate category of psychological fact that was irreducible to physiology. He connected the existence of this discrete psychological realm with the existence of a distinct spiritual principle in man: whereas the task of physiology was to study the human body, the psychologist was concerned with the properties of a separate and still more important entity.[273]

Defense of the autonomy of psychology against any efforts at physiological monism were also prominent in the writings of the eclectics. Maine de Biran took up this theme in 1808 during an address to the Société Médicale de Bergerac. His stated aim was to examine "the system of Dr Gall"; but Maine de Biran made it clear that he did not regard Gall's ideas in isolation, but as one instance of a wider movement to establish determinate connections between mental faculties and parts of the nervous system. In attempting this task, Maine de Biran insisted, they went beyond their own proper province and infringed "the domain of metaphysics"; the physiologists must therefore defer to the metaphysician when the issue of the validity of such attempts at localization was raised.[274]

Maine de Biran informed his medical audience that his aim was to secure the "rights" of the science of psychology over and against those of physiology. Man, he maintained, was an *être mixte;* and there were discrete sciences appropriate to the study of the different aspects of his nature. The properties of the human organism were certainly the province of the physiologist. But this study did not, could not, extend to an understanding of the human mind or to such "practical" subjects as ethics and economics; these belonged to the psychologist. Just as the lines dividing the material and spiritual aspects of human nature were *bien tranchée,* so the various sciences of human beings could never be reduced to one.[275] Systems like those of Cabanis and Gall that sought to elide these fundamental distinctions were *ab initio* unacceptable.

The affinities between Gall's doctrines and those of the sensualist become still stronger when we turn from the work of their author to that of his later interpreters and supporters. In particular, phrenology in France after 1836 was dominated by Joseph Victor Broussais (1772–1838). Although a relatively late convert to phrenology, Broussais was a longtime proponent of a physiological approach to psychological questions, who followed explicitly in the footsteps of Cabanis. Even after his espousal of the cause of phrenology Broussais continued, according to one of his obituarists, to owe more to Cabanis than to Gall.[276] Another remarked that "Cabanis is the true master of Broussais, because for him, the moral is only the physical considered under certain particular points of view."[277] A less complimentary reviewer, Pierre Flourens, declared that the first chapters of Broussais's *Cours de phrénologie* "are nothing but a confused mixture of ideas of Condillac, conveyed by Cabanis, and the ideas of the phrenologists."[278]

Broussais had already in 1828 praised the sensualist school as embodying the best elements of French philosophy: he singled out for special praise their "fine doctrine of the connections of the physical and the moral." Broussais maintained that the works of this school gave "to physiology and to medicine the exclusive right to dictate the laws of ideology." Conversely, he was a scathing critic of "spiritualist" philosophy, and especially of the eclectics.[279] In his later writings Broussais took up Gall's theories on cerebral structure and functions, but only to pursue the same polemical ends.

Partly because of tendencies in his own thought and partly because of the way he was used by others, Gall's work thus became inextricably involved in the complex and often heated controversies that agitated French intellectual life in the early nineteenth century. This involvement had a decisive effect on the reception of his system. An eloquent advocate like Broussais might seem a great asset to Gall's cause; but it must be remembered that Broussais and many like him were less concerned with the scientific merits of Gall's work than with harnessing his system to much older philosophical traditions. Because he was as a result associated with the intellectual, social, and political pretensions of the sensualist school, Gall became the target for criticism by all those who belonged to the other philosophical factions.

What most militated against a favorable reception of Gall was that his theories were seen as irreconcilable with and inimical to the "spiritualist" philosophy that came into vogue in France after 1815. The spirituality of the soul and its independence of the nervous system was the central dogma of the theological and eclectic schools. Upon it hinged, according to many philosophers, not only the immortality of the individual but the existence of God, personal morality, and social order. If, on the contrary, the soul was merely "a function of the body," then such terms as just and unjust, good and bad, would lose all meaning; egoism would triumph over social instincts, and the war of Thomas Hobbes (1588–1679) *omnium contra omnes* would become a reality. If there was a God, he was not interested in the fate of humanity, but was prepared to countenance the destruction of the personality along with the dissolution of the nervous system; there was therefore nothing to hope for beyond this life. In short, any materialist conception of mind brought with it "not only in metaphysics but in morals, in religion, [and] in all others, equally incomplete and exclusive solutions of the great questions that interest humanity."[280]

Gall's doctrine was judged in these terms. His system was, Lélut declared in 1843, "essentially materialist and fatalistic." Not only did it "deny the life to come but . . . it kills the present life, in chaining free will and destroying all morality." A theory with such pernicious consequences must rest on a false premise. Lélut proceeded to try to undermine the credibility of Gall's system by an examination of his organology.[281]

Lélut's strategy is typical inasmuch as others also saw Gall's doctrine of the plurality of cerebral organs as the most objectionable part of his theory, indeed, as the aspect of his thought that most clearly articulated what was wrong with the system as a whole. All the various schools of spiritualist philosophy agreed that indivisibility was the defining characteristic of the immaterial mental principle they postulated. Auguste Hilarion de Kératry (1769–1859) stated this fundamental axiom concisely in 1817: "there is," he wrote, "certainly unity in the sentient principle, for without this condition, the individual would be multiple. . . . Spirituality issues from unity."[282] Moreover, according to the doctrine of Cartesian dualism, this unity precluded the sentient principle from having any dimensions or location in space; if it could be said to occupy this or that position, then it would also be divisible.[283]

This concept of mind was for many a stumblingblock to all theories seeking to localize mental faculties in the brain. Maine de Biran held that whereas the subject matter of physiology was material, compound, and therefore subject to analysis, psychology had for its province "a subject essentially *one* and simple." It followed that "physiological analysis tends . . . always to decompose functions . . . and to localize them in locations or particular organs, in which and by which they can alone be conceived"; but "ideological or intellectual analysis never decomposes, properly speaking." The idea of a site or location for mental phenomena was entirely alien to psychological reasoning. Physiologists who ignored this distinction between the methodology appropriate to the science of the body and that of mind were (to use an anachronistic expression) guilty of a category error; and their attempted localizations were in principle invalid because they contradicted the essential nature of mind.[284] It was difficult enough to conceive of a single point in the brain that might be considered as the seat of the soul; but to suggest as Gall had done that there existed a *plurality* of such sites was, in Maine de Biran's view, beyond the bounds of serious discussion.[285]

Many other philosophers rejected Gall's theory of cerebral localization on the same grounds. Any attempt to divide and to localize mental functions within the nervous center, wrote Damiron in 1834, was vitiated by the "clear and certain idea that we have of the unity of our person."[286] Damiron also explained why it was so important to insist upon this principle: if the mind was capable of division and localization then it must in some sense be material and dependent on organization—and therefore mortal. If, however, the mind were shown to be "simple and identical," then it must also be "in consequence, indecomposable, imperishable by decomposition . . . for we see nothing die except by means of dissolution." If the mind was incapable of division it was, Damiron alleged, also incapable of death. The unity of the soul was therefore a guarantee of immortality.[287]

Nor were such prejudices confined to philosophers; certain scientists also allowed the metaphysical principles current in their culture to determine their attitude to the physiological question of cerebral localization. Thus Étienne Jean Georget (1795–1828) admitted in 1821 that "the difficulty [in accepting Gall's system] which appears to me the most strong and the least easy to resolve is this: how does it come about that there is *only one self* (*moi*)?" On Gall's theory there should surely be as many *mois* as there were intellectual organs.[288] Two years later Bérard similarly declared that "the system of the plurality of [cerebral] organs is shown to be false by the unity of consciousness of the most varied sensations." All mental operations were, he argued, located in "a principle which is *one,* and which is distinct from the organs."[289] Bérard repeated Damiron's argument that the immortality of the soul depended upon its indivisibility: "to die is to change form: now the *moi* is one, indivisible, and as a result imperishable. The moral principle therefore persists after death by its very nature." When a society ceased to believe in the dogma of immortality, he added, it was in great danger.[290]

Perhaps the most influential of the physiologists who rejected Gall's theory of the plurality of organs at least partly on metaphysical grounds was Cuvier. In the report that he and other members of the Académie des Sciences prepared on the writings of Gall and Spurzheim all analogy between the brain and other, purely material, organs were rejected: "the functions of the brain are of an entirely different order"—it acted as an intermediary between the nerves and the "spirit." Its intellectual faculties "supposed the mutual for ever incomprehensible influence of divisible matter and indivisible *moi,* [the] insuperable hiatus in the system of our ideas and [the] eternal stumbling-block of all philosophies."[291] This last statement is especially interesting because it is a close paraphrase of Maine de Biran's assertion that "the manner in which any organization, [which is] always conceived or imagined as extended, divisible and compound, can be connected to a thinking subject, to a reflecting *moi,* [which is] essentially one and simple, will be the eternal stumbling-block of all philosophical doctrines."[292] In effect, the Commission established by the Académie to judge Gall's theories was acknowledging as binding the kind of metaphysical restraints that Maine de Biran sought to impose upon physiological discourse, restraints which left no room for a theory of punctate cerebral localization.[293]

Gall's attempt to divide and localize mental faculties was therefore seen as an attempt "to materialize the soul,"[294] an exercise that was entirely incompatible with the prevailing metaphysics of the period. Broussais, for his part, made it a point to emphasize the conflict between Gall's assumptions and those of spiritualist philosophy. Now that phrenology had established that "there are particular organs for each of the cerebral functions, one recognizes how ridiculous it is to suppose that an intelligent entity resides inside the head." Although some (including medical men) had insisted on the metaphysical proposition that "the *moi does away with (tuait)* the plurality of organs, the absurdity of this assertion is demonstrated by the facts."[295] Although spiritualist philosophers and those physiologists who accepted their principles had regarded the materialistic implications of cerebral localization aghast, Broussais welcomed and dwelled upon these aspects of Gall's theory. Whereas volition and other mental faculties had been assigned to an immaterial entity by the whims of philosophers, "phrenological observation localizes them in the nervous system. . . . The facts of the intellect thus divided cease to be a simple fact, as the psychologist would have; it is not at all a substance independent of the brain that produces them; it is the brain itself, by means of its different regions, which serves as the medium of their manifestation."[296]

Gall himself recognized that the prevalence of such notions as the spirituality of mind and of its indivisibility were among the chief obstacles to the acceptance of his doctrines. The "metaphysicians" were committed to the concept of "the simplicity of thought, and consequently to a simple organ of the soul." In this view it was "impossible to occupy oneself with the functions of each part of the brain or with the examination of the organs of each faculty of the mind." These metaphysicians, he complained, were imposing their doctrines on physiology: "always the unity of the *moi* repels the idea of the plurality of [cerebral] organs."[297] In 1825 Gall took issue with such physiologists as Bérard who had submitted to the demands of the philosophers and were content to study "anatomy and physiology in the closets of metaphysicians." It was such who were unable to reconcile the plurality of cerebral organs with the unity of the *moi;* and who, "for this reason . . . make up their mind to reject this plurality."[298]

The philosophical context in which Gall's views were expounded goes far, therefore, toward explaining the hostile reception they met. This intellectual background is also essential to understanding the development of the views of the man who did most to destroy Gall's scientific credibility. We must repeat that Flourens in the course of his career passed from one to the other of the extremes of contemporary intellectual life. For several years after he came to Paris in 1815, Flourens was an advocate of physiological materialism and psychological monism. Nowhere are these commitments more evident than in the two- article review of Gall's *Anatomie et Physiologie du Système Nerveux* he published in 1819–1820.

In these two articles, which appeared in the *Révue Encyclopédique*, Flourens was copious in his praise of such leaders of the sensualist school as Destutt de Tracy, the "philosopher of genius" who had demonstrated that "*thinking* is nothing but *feeling*."[299] We have already learned that as late as 1821 Flourens gave a series of lectures at the Athenée Médicale de Paris on the "Physiological theory of sensations," which was imbued with the principles of de Tracy and Cabanis; still more surprisingly Flourens listed Gall among the other philosophers and scientists who had contributed to understanding "the real connections between philosophy and physiology."[300]

In the first part of his review Flourens described Gall as the direct successor and as the improver of the sensualist philosophy. What united Gall to Cabanis was their common belief that "the human understanding is . . . only a subject of natural history, and consequently it can only be studied as one of the functions of the organism." Whereas Cabanis was credited with the distinction of having grasped the *grande vérité incontestable* of the pervasive influence of the physical upon the moral, Gall was the first to have "determined rigorously the proper organs of the intelligence, and [to have] assigned the precise conditions of this faculty."[301] Flourens thus subscribed to the naturalism and monism of the sensualist school and welcomed Gall's system precisely because it confirmed and amplified the axiom that the human mind was a natural entity that could only be comprehended by an enhanced knowledge of the physiology of the nervous system. He favored an assimilation of psychology to physiology: the facts upon which Gall's doctrine of cerebral functions rested "embrace the most lofty considerations of metaphysics and of physiology. They prove that these two sciences, far from being in effect distinct, are, so to speak, complementary. Man, the common subject-matter of their researches, is one: the sciences that study him therefore will offer only half-formed mutilations, so long as they will not be brought by themselves to unity."[302]

Moreover, Flourens's approval of Gall was not confined to such broad principles; he also endorsed the detail of Gall's conception of cerebral function, including the doctrine of the plurality of cerebral organs. This theory was, he held, essential to the unified science of man for which he called. Psychologists must recognize that "the words *intellectual faculties* are not and cannot be other than synonyms of . . . *cerebral faculties*." Flourens made it clear that he believed that the intellectual faculties were no more than the "activity" (*jeu*) of the organs discerned by Gall on the brain. Given this principle, he continued, "it follows incontestably that each essentially distinct faculty demands a special organic modification: for it is impossible to suppose identity of cause where I see no identity of effect." There were, therefore, as many separate brain organs as there were mental faculties. Thirty years of research had, Flourens declared, enabled Gall to identify the seat of most of these organs.[303]

Flourens criticized Gall in these 1819–1820 articles for not being sufficiently rigorous in pursuing the implications of his physiological psychology. Occasionally, he complained, Gall deviated from sound interpretative rules and employed "vague and indefinite expressions," such as "soul" and "spirit," which "appear to me to have no meaning in his system." At most such abstract nouns connoted nothing more than "the collection or the sum of the intellectual faculties." "Intelligence" was merely "a generic and abstract word" denoting the plurality of mental faculties. It was a grave error to imagine that such terms referred to some real entity.[304]

In this early publication, therefore, Flourens praised Gall's theory for its naturalistic and monistic conception of the human mind; for its insistence that mental faculties must be viewed physiologically as functions of the brain; and, above all, for recognizing that "since these [mental] faculties are multiple, it is apparent that their organs must also be [multiple]." In effect, "M. Gall has reduced each particular faculty to a particular cerebral organ, and this double determination is precisely what constitutes the physiology of the cerebrum."[305] Philosophers who spoke of a substantive spiritual principle, on the other hand, were dismissed as guilty of a terminological confusion.

As Appel notes in her discussion of another strongly materialistic article by Flourens from this period, "that the writer of such a review should later become the defender of Cartesian dualism against Gall seems incredible."[306] Yet Flourens did make this transition, apparently within a few years of the remarks we have quoted. In the present state of scholarship it is impossible to offer more than a tentative explanation of this transformation; however, it appears that Flourens's growing dependence upon Cuvier for patronage played a crucial role in this process, as we have already mentioned above.

During his early years in Paris Flourens seems to have been drawn to the camp of Cuvier's great antagonist, Étienne Geoffroy St. Hilaire.

It was probably through Geoffroy's agency that Flourens was commissioned to write articles for the *Revue Encyclopédique;* and Flourens responded by writing in 1819 a highly flattering review of Geoffroy's *Philosophie anatomique.*[307] Geoffroy was a warm supporter of Gall, whose admission to the Académie des Sciences he unsuccessfully tried to secure in 1821.[308] Flourens's favorable reception of Gall's *Anatomie et Physiologie du Système Nerveux* was, therefore, in accordance with his initial mentor's views.

By 1822, however, Flourens had shifted his allegiances and was established as a protégé of Cuvier. It appears that he modified his opinions to comply with those of his patron. For example, in place of his earlier espousal of Geoffroy's doctrine of the unity of organic type, Flourens came to adopt Cuvier's position that several forms of organization existed in the animal kingdom, and that these were irreducible to any single plan. Thus Flourens insisted in 1845 that there was no single type of the nervous system uniting the nervous organization of the zoophyte to that of the mollusc or of the articulate.[309] As well as contradicting Geoffroy, this declaration was starkly opposed to Gall's contention that there was indeed a single type of the nervous system from which all the particular varieties of nervous organization derived (see chap. 2.4).

We have seen, moreover, that Cuvier subscribed to a metaphysical dualism that was irreconcilable with Gall's concept of cerebral structure and function. In the report of 1808 Cuvier and his fellow Commissioners insisted on the unbridgeable hiatus between "divisible matter and the indivisible *moi.*"[310] This strict dualism was a far cry from the dogmatic monism that Flourens had espoused in his articles of 1819–1820; and he modified his views on this subject also to bring them into line with those of Cuvier.

This philosophical shift is not stated explicitly in Flourens's *Recherches Expérimentales* of 1824; it has to be inferred by viewing this work in relation to his previous and subsequent writings. At first sight Flourens's experimental research on the nervous system seems to be a model of theory-free, nonphilosophical observation of facts. However, we should recognize that the ideology of "positive facts" and the eschewal of overt metaphysical speculation were central parts of the framework that Cuvier sought to impose upon science.[311] Further, Flourens's silences are as revealing of his change of opinion as what he does say. The references to Cabanis have disappeared, as has any mention of Gall's work, which Flourens had in 1819 held to be "destined to constitute at the same time an epoch in the loftiest portions of the physical and metaphysical [sciences]."[312]

Gall in his critique of Flourens's experiments had no doubt that underlying their apparent objectivity were tacit philosophical assumptions. Gall pointed in particular to Flourens's stress upon the fundamental unity of the nervous system as evidence of the theory-laden nature of his work. "Unity," he declared, "is the greatest day-dream, the *non plus ultra* of bombastic metaphysicians." He presented various proofs of the plurality of the cerebral organs, maintaining that these were "unchallengeable facts." Yet "M. Flourens is enough of a magician to reconcile them all with a unique organ, with unity." Here again, declared Gall, was evidence of "the principles of lofty metaphysics" that pervaded Flourens's account.[313] We should recall that in Flourens's articles of 1819–1820 this emphasis upon unity is completely absent. On the contrary, he placed great stress upon the plurality of the nervous system in general and of the cerebral hemispheres in particular, arguing that his axiom was essential to a rational concept of mind as a natural entity amenable to scientific study.

Cuvier made no reference to the metaphysical aspects of Flourens's work in his discussion of the *Recherches Expérimentales*. But he at least found nothing there to offend. We have noted that the support of Cuvier was largely responsible for the favorable reception of his work by the scientific community. It is also safe to assume that if Flourens had persisted in the philosophical views he had expressed between 1819 and 1820, Cuvier's reaction to his work would have been quite different.

Historians of science have seen in Flourens's experimental research evidence of tacit philosophical commitments that structure the physiological doctrines at which he arrived. Flourens took on the dualist assumptions favored by influential schools of French philosophy and carried them over into his scientific investigations. The effect of these presuppositions was, in part, a negative one: thus Young reports that "Flourens' belief in Cartesian dualism and the indivisibility of the mind appears to have made it easy for him to refrain from the sort of systematic, localized ablations which would have confirmed cerebral localization."[314] But Flourens's metaphysics also played a positive role in his thought: it provided a set of axioms about the nature of the mind and its relations to the brain which he proceeded to translate into physiological terms and to corroborate experimentally. In particular, to quote Young again,

> Flourens' view of the hemispheres is a consequence of his psychological assumptions. . . . If the understanding is a unit, its organ must also act in a unitary fashion. He repeats his experimental evidence in support of the thesis that "the cerebral hemispheres concur, by their whole mass, in the full and entire exercise of the intelligence." Any qualification of the unity of the soul or its organs is, as Flourens sees it, equivalent to denying the existence of the mind or soul. To divide the functions of the soul among different parts of the brain is equivalent to materialism.[315]

Once again we should recall that such materialization by means of division and localization was precisely what Flourens initially welcomed in Gall's system. In contrast, he wrote in the *Recherches Expérimentales,* and we have already drawn attention to this statement, that "there are . . . no diverse seats, neither for the various faculties, nor for the different sensations. The faculty of feeling, or judging, or of willing one thing resides in the same locations as that of feeling, of judging, of willing another; and consequently this essentially unitary faculty resides essentially in a single organ."[316]

Flourens was not alone in trying to render physiology agreeable to a spiritualist concept of mind. Dubois d'Amiens wrote in 1845 that such an exercise was a necessary complement to the efforts of philosophers of the eclectic school such as Cousin. They had sought to refute the pernicious doctrines of sensualism and materialism by philosophical means; but because these theories rested largely upon alleged scientific facts it was necessary to "examine and in particular to examine physiologically the foundations of this doctrine, to speak the same language, to appeal to the same facts, in order to show that spiritualism can show itself just as well in the amphitheatre of physiology as in the chair of philosophy."[317]

Damiron had in 1834 made much the same point. He noted that most physiologists tended to adopt a materialistic stance, but that a few had begun to introduce spiritualistic metaphysics into their physiological discussions. For example, Bérard admitted in his works the existence of an immaterial principle, independent of the material organization, which was the source of bodily movement.[318] Bérard attacked Gall's ideas from this standpoint, and his writings are of special interest because in certain respects they anticipate Flourens's arguments. In an article of 1813 that Bérard composed together with Horace de Montègre (1805–1864), Gall's doctrine of plurality was rejected in favor of a unitary concept of cerebral structure and function. Bérard and Montègre made explicit the metaphysical system that informed their physiological conclusion: they insisted on the existence of the *moi* as a substantial entity that interacted with, but was separate from the brain. The brain was therefore the instrument. Whereas Gall had seen the brain as a congeries of autonomous organs, Bérard and Montègre held that "the brain is characterized . . . by its unity; one cannot admit any sharp divisions in this organ; this disposition proves that it is impossible to find distinct organs in the brain." This anatomical unity was the necessary corollary of the unity of the *moi.*[319]

Moreover, according to Bérard and Montègre experimental studies also confirmed a unitary concept of the brain. After describing ablation experiments by Zinn, Lorry, and others, they drew conclusions almost identical with those at which Flourens was to arrive: "lesions of the brain . . . most often have a general effect. This effect bears on all the functions of the animal life at one and the same time; it degrades them all equally." Only occasionally did a specific lesion result in a specific dysfunction.[320] Bérard amplified these views in 1823: "there is," he wrote, "no part of the brain the lesion of which has brought as its consequence the suspension of all the intellectual faculties, just as there is none that could be destroyed, and the intellectual faculties retain their integrity; therefore the *moi* is present at all parts of the brain and is not, properly speaking, at any part; it makes use of all its parts to sustain its actions and it can dispense with them."[321]

By 1823 Bérard may have been aware of Flourens's research as further experimental evidence of the "absolute unity" of the *moi*. Dubois d'Amiens cited Flourens by name in his attempts to establish the equipotentiality of the cerebral hemispheres, and held him up as the scientist who, more than any other, had proved by his experiments that "the doctrine of Gall is absolutely without foundation, and that science today proceeds along other paths."[322] Flourens's "positive" observations thus served to corroborate the philosophy of the unity and independence of the soul, while at the same time refuting the materialistic views with which Gall's system had become associated and which had brought about his expulsion from Vienna.

In his later writings Flourens himself became quite explicit about the metaphysical implications of his science and held that extrascientific considerations were relevant in the evaluation of physiological doctrines. Thus in the history of studies on the human brain he published in 1862 Flourens criticized Gall's theory because "it gives the lie to the inner sense, which demands the unity and not the division of the soul." Moreover, he also thought it relevant to point to the alleged moral consequences of Gall's ideas: on phrenological principles, he held, sympathy passed from the victim to the perpetrator of a crime—"the poor man! he had been himself a victim of his organization."[323]

But the text in which Flourens's metaphysical commitments are most obvious is his *Examen de la Phrénologie* (1845). Here he set himself up as the spokesman of the "good" philosophy of Descartes against the "bad" philosophy of Gall.[324] In fact, it was the philosophy of Descartes as rehabilitated and modified by the eclectic school that Flourens defended; and it is as an aspect of the controversies between these spiritualist thinkers and their sensualist protagonists that we must view Flourens's book. We have already noted that, like so many of his contemporaries, Flourens saw a direct line of succession between Cabanis and Gall. In 1819 this was reason to recommend Gall's system; by 1845 it was a cause for reproach.[325] As for Gall's theory of the plurality of organs, Flourens now made overt and frequent use of the results of his *Recherches Expérimentales* to discredit Gall's claims and to establish the contrary doctrine that "intelligence is . . . unitary." Gall's views were, above all, unacceptable because they denied "the unity of the *moi.*"[326] Flourens thus took as his own the central dogma of eclecticism and made it a criterion by which to discriminate between scientific theories. Also like the eclectics, Flourens pointed to the danger a system such as Gall's posed to the concept of free will: Gall was to be condemned on moral as well as on physiological and psychological grounds.[327] Flourens recognized that Gall did not necessarily wish to undermine the key concepts of spiritualist philosophy; but here he was guilty of fudging the veritable consequences of his system. According to Flourens, Gall "suppresses the *moi,* and wishes that there is a soul. He suppresses free will, and wishes that there is morality." Flourens quoted the claim of Denis Diderot (1713–1784) that if free will were lost, then all moral and social order would collapse.[328]

For Flourens, therefore, as for many of his contempraries, metaphysical questions were not merely of noetic interest but crucial practical issues also depended upon their determination. When Gall violated the Cartesian categorical distinction between mind and matter by suggesting that mental faculties could be localized on the surface of the brain, he offended against a wide range of entrenched cultural prejudices. In the first instance, he denied the principle of the unity of the mind, which in Flourens's view was tantamount to denying the existence of the soul as a separate entity. This, in turn, led to a repudiation of the doctrine of free will with all the pernicious moral consequences that entailed.[329] Others, as we have seen, thought that personal immortality also hinged upon the doctrine of the unity of the *moi.* Given this background, Flourens's rejection of the doctrine of cerebral localization ceases to appear as an unproblematic inference from experimental results, but as an endorsement by him of a widely held and strongly supported view that any such localization was incompatible with the nature of mind.

What made Flourens's espousal of this view so important was that he was not only a speculative philosopher, but also an experimenter of genius with a power of expression that led most of his scientific contemporaries to accept, almost uncritically, that his conclusions on the nature of cerebral function must be correct. Although a few clinicians disputed them, as has been related above, such was Flourens's authority that "no new experiments fundamentally affecting the role which the cortex was supposed to play in movement" were made until 1870; and then, as Young remarks, "it is appropriate that Fritsch and Hitzig addressed their remarks directly to Flourens."[330]

In the course of this book we have repeatedly stressed the role that the intellectual milieu of early nineteenth-century Europe had in shaping the emergence and development of major innovations in the neurosciences. For the most part, we have argued that this influence was positive: it helped to direct thought and investigation into channels that led to fruitful new theories of the structure and function of the nervous system. In this section, however, we have described a contrasting case. The debates over brain localization in France between 1800 and 1850 were also structured by the wider intellectual context in which they occurred; but the effect of the philosophical issues that impinged upon them was, from a modern point of view, retrograde. Because of the complex of prejudices it offended, Gall's notion of cerebral localization was attacked and by the 1840s destroyed as a credible scientific hypothesis; and the ruin of Gall's system, by extension, discredited any other attempt to localize functions to discrete areas of the cerebral hemispheres.

Flourens, who was in terms of the sophistication of his experimental techniques and the precision and clarity of his reports an innovator, was in his concepts profoundly conservative. His eventual decision to conform and defer to the dominant metaphysics of his day was to have a decisive effect on theories of cerebral function for nearly forty years. The concept of cerebral localization could only regain scientific respectability in the 1860s, when the dominance of Flourens's work began to wane.

6.6. PIERRE FLOURENS: CEREBELLUM

6.6.1. Introduction

Unlike his research on the cerebrum, Flourens's investigations of the cerbellum did not involve him with the philosophical and cultural background of his times. They concerned somatic functions of the body and did not lead him into contentious areas as had been the case with his experiments on the cerebral hemispheres. But his renown as a brilliant experimental physiologist rests more on this part of his study of the brain, reported along with his experiments on the cerebrum in 1822, because it represents the most outstanding contribution to the subject in the first half of the nineteenth century. As we have seen, his opinions on the cerebrum had an immense negative influence on neurophysiology, for they retarded by several decades the evolution of the concept of a compound system of brain localization, even though many of his contentions were later disproved. In the case of the cerebellum, however, his observations and the interpretations he placed upon them have turned out to be mainly correct. In keeping with his *action propre* notion of brain localization, Flourens considered the whole organ to be devoted to one function, the coordination of movements.

Compared with the cerebral hemispheres, the cerebellum is a simpler structure for it is anatomically distinct from the rest of the brain, it consists of two halves and a midline portion, the vermis, and it is attached on each side to the brain stem by three stalks or peduncles. Paradoxically, its function is far from simple, and to no other part of the nervous system have so many concepts of action been applied, which fact is a measure of the complexity of the problem the organ presents to physiology. In 1842 Longet admitted that: "to ascertain precisely the functions of the cerebellum is one of the most perplexing problems in physiology."[331] At the end of the nineteenth century even after the remarkable advances that had been made in cerebellar physiology, the situation was much the same, as was testified to by Luigi Luciani (who had contributed importantly to this topic) when he confessed that "the experimental determination of the functions of the cerebellum is one of the most difficult problems in the physiology of the central nervous system."[332] The outcome of such investigations prior to 1921 was revealed by the renowned British neurologist Francis Martin Rous Walshe (1885–1973), when he declared that "perhaps no part of the nervous system has been more intensively studied than the cerebellum, and yet the final analysis of its symptom-complex and the determination of its functions have so far eluded us."[333] Although studies continue today, and a full elucidation of cerebellar function is still in the distant future, we can accept for our purposes that the cerebellum is an organ fundamentally concerned with correlating movement with proprioceptive impulses, in the interests of bodily stability. It regulates and controls balance and posture, and is in charge of the dynamic coordination of the numerous muscle groups necessary to produce normal and harmonious patterns of muscular movement.

In the following pages we shall trace the study of cerebellar function from the late eighteenth century to 1830. During this period the most outstanding advances were made by Rolando in 1809 and Flourens in 1822, although, as noted above, Rolando's work was virtually unknown in Europe until 1822. We can, therefore, discuss events in three phases: (1) before Flourens and Rolando; (2) their research; and (3) their reception. On the whole, secondary literature on this topic is sparse.[334]

6.6.2. The Cerebellum Before Flourens and Rolando

Among the scientific writers of antiquity whose works are available to us, Aristotle was the first to differentiate the cerebellum from the rest of the brain.[335] As mentioned above, Galen thought that the motor nerves ended in the cerebellum, which was, therefore, motor in function,[336] an idea transmitted through the Middle Ages by those who localized motion in it, rather than memory, which was the more usual faculty allocated to this organ or to the fourth ventricle by proponents of the cell doctrine of faculty psychology. At the end of the sixteenth century Constanzo Varolio (1543–1575), whose name is associated eponymously with the pons, claimed that the cerebellum was the origin of hearing, taste, and touch,[337] perhaps because the nerves responsible for these modalities lie close to it and were therefore thought to take their origin from it. However, the first experimental approach to the problem was made by Thomas Willis, who in 1664 applied to the cerebellum an *action propre* type of brain action, declaring that it governed the vital and involuntary activities of the body:

> The function of the *Cerebellum seems to be that of supplying the animal spirits to certain nerves, by which are carried out involuntary movements* (such as *the beating of the heart, respiration, the digestion of food, the secretion of chyle* and many others), *all of which occur continually without our knowledge or will.*[338]

Although his experimental results were due presumably to brain stem as well as cerebellar damage, there is no doubt that the modern history of the cerebellum begins with Willis. He also thought that it was the seat of musical ability, perhaps having been influenced by Varolio.[339] But, along with his concept of *action propre* in the other major anatomical subdivisions of the brain, the Hallerian doctrine of *action commune,* which endowed the whole brain with functional equivalence and its parts, such as the cerebellum, with no individual properties, completely suppressed Willis's opinions.[340]

In retrospect, however, there were during the eighteenth century at least two perceptive observations that were ignored at the time because of Haller's authority, but which foreshadowed nineteenth-century explanations of cerebellar function. The experiments on the medulla oblongata carried out by the French surgeon, Lorry, have already been discussed but, in addition, he thrust a needle through a cerebellar hemisphere of a pigeon and observed that the ipsilateral side of the body no longer functioned normally.[341] Thus, he not only refuted Willis's idea of the cerebellum being a center for the preservation of life but, as Neuburger has suggested, he was probably the first to report cerebellar incoordination.[342]

In 1773 this was also described by the French military surgeon, Jean Mehée de la Touche (fl. 1773–1800), together with other cerebellar signs such as forced rolling and circus movements, skew deviation of the eyes with nystagmus, and characteristic positioning of the head in animals after damage to the cerebellum had been inflicted.[343] Most of the clinical picture resulting from trauma to the cerebellum and its peduncles had, therefore, been described before the nineteenth century, but needless to say, despite this clear evidence of specific cerebellar functions, the Hallerian doctrine prevailed unscathed.

Also in the eighteenth century, there were important contributions to the anatomy of the cerebellum. The most noteworthy was that of Michele Vincenzo Giacinto Malacarne (1744–1816), who in 1776 provided the first detailed account, and introduced terms such as "tonsil," "pyramid," "lingula," and "uvula" that are still in use today.[344] His findings, however, had little impact at the time, and in Britain his book was completely unknown until reviewed in 1824.[345] Malacarne's proposals concerning cerebellar function were much less successful, and among them he argued that in humans the degree of intelligence was directly proportional to the number of the organ's folia,[346] a notion that Erasistratus had advanced a millennium and a half earlier in the case of the cerebral gyri.[347] Moreover, whereas Erasistratus assigned the soul to the fourth ventricle, Malacarne favored the cerebellum.

The famous German anatomist, J. C. Reil, extended Malacarne's morphological studies by providing remarkably detailed accounts of the cerebellum between 1807 and 1812.[348] He succeeded in carrying out accurate dissections because of his new hardening and preserving technique whereby the specimen was soaked in alcohol containing potassium or sodium carbonate or ammonia.[349] Reil explained that: "The chief merit of my work lies in the preparation of the brain for dissecting and the method of dissecting."[350] There is no doubt that this was the most detailed and precise description of any part of the brain, so far reported, and surprisingly little has been added since. It later received justifiable praise from anatomists, such as Bendikt Stilling, who recognized its merits from his own experience with the cerebellum. He commented that "By means of Reil's work the gross morphology of the cerebellum, that had been established by Malacarne, was placed for all time upon a firm and certain foundation."[351] Conversely, a comment from Britain is a measure of anatomical research in that country, rather than of Reil. His account of the cerebellum was depicted by an anonymous critic as "a description which we must characterize as tiresomely and uselessly minute, fitted to confuse the understanding of a student, and incapable of affording useful knowledge to a more mature enquirer."[352] Reil did, however, have some support in Britain. There was John Gordon (1786–1820) of Edinburgh, who alone taught his research there and described in a book of 1817,[353] but whose primary object was to denounce Gall's and Spurzheim's anatomical research by establishing Reil's priority and superiority. In fact, his book, which we have referred to already, was a biased and unbridled polemic. Herbert Mayo, however, was a more balanced advocate, and he published English versions of Reil's seven papers.[354] Reil also gave consideration to comparative aspects of the cerebellum, and his account of the increasing complexity of the vermis in the ascending scale of animals was in itself a notable advance, as was his pioneer and precise description of the cerebellar peduncles.[355]

Like Malacarne, Reil's opinions on the possible functions of the cerebellum were greatly inferior to his morphological data, and they did not survive for long. We have already discussed his notion of the organ as an electrometer, which may seem to us improbable, but was not the case at the time; this was also so with Rolando's similar suggestion (chap. 5.3.2). Moreover, Reil at least based his assumptions on anatomy, whereas his contemporaries used only speculation and analogy when they designated the cerebellum as the seat of the will, of animal instincts, or of irritability.[356] This was certainly true of some of Reil's fellow-*Naturphilosophen,* such as Carus, Jakob Fidelis Ackermann (1765–1815), Döllinger, and Eschenmayer.[357] Another was Treviranus, who, reasoning by analogy, declared that the vermis of the cerebellum must be concerned with respiratory movements because it was similar in size to the inferior cerebellar peduncle, which arose from near the origins of the vagus nerve.[358] The proximity of the cerebellum to the cranial nerves suggested other functions, and Carus believed that the flocculi were associated with the development of the organ of hearing, in view of their position close to the auditory nerve.[359] Schönlein had a similar view, but he envisaged the cerebellum as an enlarged auditory ganglion.[360] Both these opinions were reminiscent of Varolio and Willis.

We have already seen how Burdach, also a *Naturphilosoph,* was proposing a compound type of brain localization when he assigned specific functions to a variety of structures in the cerebral hemispheres. He treated the cerebellum in the same way, and in the 1820s suggested a number of functions for it, each ascribed to a precise, anatomical part. Thus, the vermis contained the center that allowed one to feel alive (coenesthesia); the flocculi, as suggested by Carus, were concerned with hearing; and the superior cerebellar peduncles brought into consciousness stimuli from autonomic activities, which he believed originated in the cerebellum.[361] The organ was also an intermediate link between spinal cord and cerebral hemispheres, and it represented the seat of visceral sensation and irritability, having a special relationship with sexual functions and the heartbeat.[362] In the case of cardiac action, Burdach was returning to Willis's views of 1664, and concerning procreative activity, he was in agreement with Gall.

The ancient Greeks had postulated a direct connection between the sexual organs and the brain by means of the spinal cord and "veins."[363] This idea was elaborated on by the Swedish mystic, Emmanuel Swedenborg (1688–1772) in the eighteenth century, for he contended that nerve fibers ran from the cerebellar white matter to the testes.[364] Gall arrived at a somewhat similar conclusion, presumably independently, that the cerebellum was the center of sexual feelings, and in his system of organology it was known in English as "the organ of amativeness." He based this idea on a wide range of evidence from his own and from others' observations, the majority being clinical.[365] Much of it we can judge to be unreliable, unconvincing, or both, and some of it bizarre.[366] However, part of it came from reputable clinicians, such as Serres, who reported priapism accompanying cerebellar apoplexy,[367] a well-recognized clinical event, also seen with cervical cord injury, such as that incurred, for example, by judicial hanging. On the basis of clinicopathological material Serres concluded that "there is a constant physiological relationship between the median lobe of the cerebellum and the genital organs,"[368] the former being the excitor of the latter.[369] In his view, the cerebellum was essentially the center for sensual pleasure.[370] A similar relationship was claimed by Pierre Salamon Ségalas d'Etchepare (1792–1875), when he discovered that needling the cerebellum of a capybara produced penile erection.[371] In this and other investigations, it seems likely that damage to the brain stem or to its cerebellar connections was responsible for such findings.

Gall, however, was able to assemble more apparent proof for this "organ" than for any of the others that constituted his system of organology, and the testimony of Georget in 1821 bears this out:

> M. Gall places the seat of physical love in the cerebellum. It is perhaps the part of the doctrine of plurality of brain organs and their particular functions, in support of which M. Gall has assembled the most evidence.[372]

It survives today along with the rest of the phrenologists' creed,[373] even though numerous medical scientists in the nineteenth century brought forward a variety of evidence to refute Gall's selection of the cerebellum as the "organ of amativeness."[374] Perhaps the most striking and most widely publicized case was that of (?) Combette (fl. 1831), reported in 1831. A girl of eleven was found at autopsy to have congenital absence of the cerebellum, but she had normal generative organs and "a precocious tendency to the passions of her sex, and was given to masturbation."[375] Flourens subjected the problem to experimental investigation, and in 1842 he described how he had removed about half of the cerebellum in a cock. He observed that not only was its desire to tread hens unabated but at postmortem eight months postoperatively the testes were enormous in size.[376] On the basis of this and other evidence, Gall's proposal was mostly rejected, and some, like W. B. Carpenter were highly critical of his reasoning with regard to cerebellar function: "If the evidence at present [1846] adduced in support of the Phrenological position be held sufficient to establish it, in defiance of so many opposing considerations, we must bid adieu to all safe reasoning in Physiology."[377] Nevertheless, there remained lingering doubts among nineteenth-century physicians, and William W. Hammond (1828–1900) in 1869 found it necessary to discuss Gall's notion in some detail before rejecting it.[378] Three years later Austin Flint argued that in addition to its somatic activity, the cerebellum "is in some way connected with the generative function."[379] Even in 1886 David Ferrier did not dismiss the idea out of hand, although he described it as "the most widely known but least well founded of all the hypotheses as to the functions of the cerebellum.[380]

6.6.3. Flourens and Rolando

Concerning the cerebellum, it will now be obvious that before the 1820s all was not darkness and confusion, as some writers would have us believe. But the next step was to apply new techniques in order to correct and extend the experimental evidence collected by Thomas Willis in the seventeenth century, and by all those since.[381] The main precautions necessary at operation were the avoidance of fatal damage to the brain stem, to which the cerebellum is attached, and of complications, such as uncontrollable bleeding with hematoma formation. Flourens's full-exposure method of operating, with visual control of ablation and the extent of the damage inflicted, was therefore particularly advantageous. The approach to the cerebellum was relatively easy, especially in birds, and it was probably this factor that determined his frequent use of them. A skillful operator like Flourens could therefore remove large amounts of the organ without incurring brain stem or cerebral damage or postoperative hemorrhage.

In 1822, Flourens reported one of the basic properties of the cerebellum: to coordinate voluntary muscle movements. He was using the same technique and reasoning he had employed with other subdivisions of the nervous system. If disturbing a piece of nervous tissue disturbed a function, the latter must reside in that piece of nervous tissue. Thus, he could state dogmatically: "The slightest disturbance of the cerebellum alters the harmony of coordinated movements (jumping, flying, standing, gripping, etc.); complete removal of it abolishes them completely. *The coordination of these movements,* therefore, derives exclusively from the cerebellum."[382] We can now discuss his ingenious research, which is no less remarkable and noteworthy than that on the cerebrum, already described. As Rolando's similar investigations, described in 1809, were not widely known until 1822–1823, we shall deal first with Flourens's, the announcement of which first drew attention to the Italian's book.

His research was first reported in his communication of 1822 to the Académie des Sciences;[383] it consisted of cerebellar ablation or damage, carried out on a variety of animals, but chiefly pigeons. Like his other experiments on the nervous system, they were characterized by precision, both in their execution and description, and they have received resounding praise ever since they were first scrutinized by Cuvier and his colleagues of the Académie in 1822,[384] and published again in 1823[385] and 1824.[386] John C. Dalton in 1861 commented: "There are few, if any, experiments which have been performed upon the nervous system, in which the phenomena produced are, at the same time, so striking and so invariable as in these."[387] One of the most singular features of Flourens's research was the way in which it revealed the obvious differences between the functional disturbances produced by removing the cerebrum and ablating the cerebellum, thus providing irrefutable proof that Haller's doctrine of functional equivalence throughout the brain could not be correct. The reporter of the Académie's proceedings for 1822 expressed it succinctly: "On depriving [the animal] of its cerebrum it was put into a state of sleep; on depriving it of its cerebellum it is put into a state of drunkeness."[388] As in the case of the cerebrum, Flourens carried out serial slicing of the cerebellum, and noted that the animal's ability to jump, fly, walk, and maintain the erect posture was successively impaired, although sensory faculties and volition were preserved. Combined movements could be performed, but coordination of them had been lost.[389] His conclusion was that "the cerebellum coordinates"[390] by means of a regulatory influence, but it was not responsible for the initiation of motor activity, a faculty demanded by Rolando as we shall see. Integrating this with the knowledge of motor function that he already possessed, Flourens described his motor system with admirable clarity:

> I have shown that all movements persist after ablation of the cerebellum; they lack only being regular and coordinated. From this I have been induced to conclude that the *production* and the *coordination* of movements constitute two classes of essentially distinct phenomena, and that they reside in two classes of organs also essentially distinct; to wit: *coordination* in the *cerebellum* and *production* in the *spinal cord* and *medulla oblongata*.[391]

We need only add that the will to call movements into action came from the cerebral hemispheres, as we have learned above. It has been claimed that Flourens's major mistake was to accord contralateral limb involvement to a cerebellar hemisphere lesion, but although this may have been unintentional and due to a faulty description of cerebellar signs in the pigeon, it was accepted in clinical medicine for some years.

Throughout his research, Flourens attempted to relate his findings to general principles or cognate phenomena, a technique that his contemporary, Magendie, never employed. Thus, he was the first to notice a similarity between the action of alcohol and the effects of cerebellar injury, and he declared that in each case there could be a drunken swim or flight, as well as a drunken gait.[392] As with the cerebrum, he recognized functional compensation, but he also found that deep lesions produced severe sequelae that usually persisted. In all Flourens's studies his operative techniques were revolutionary and based on new anatomical knowledge, his observations were penetrating, and his reports were elegant. However, his conclusions on cerebellar function, unlike those on some other nervous system subdivisions, the cerebrum in particular, have been proved to be mostly correct. In essence, he was promoting Gall's fundamental concept that morphological variation must be reflected in physiological differentiation. His assigning coordination of voluntary motor activity to the cerebellum provided a basis for modern views on synergia, defined as the cooperation between the various muscles that are concerned with movement and the maintenance of posture. Looking back at the end of the nineteenth century, Sherrington, who was himself an important contributor to cerebellar physiology, judged Flourens thus:

> Flourens translated the disturbances ensuing on destruction of the cerebellum to mean loss of a part possessing ability to co-ordinate the innervations which guide and execute complex movements. By his doing so, the idea of nervous co-ordination was, it seems to me, formally introduced into physiology.[393]

It is surprising that another pioneer of cerebellar physiology at the end of the century, Luigi Luciani, made the opposite assessment and described Flourens's theory as "obscure, garbled, and hardly intelligible."[394] On the other hand, his countryman, Luigi Rolando, had conceived a notion "lucid, well-defined, and complete in its fundamental elements."[395] We must now evaluate the significance of Rolando's investigations on the form and function of the cerebellum, which, like those of Flourens, were a part of a larger program of research on the nervous system.[396] In a variety of animals, including fishes, turtles, birds, guinea pigs, rabbits, and goats, he damaged the cerebellum or removed parts of it. Complete destruction of it led to paralysis of movement, whereas less severe trauma resulted in "staggering" (*incertezza,* uncertainty), a feature to which he paid little attention. But unlike cerebral damage, sensory, vital, and intellectual activities were unaffected nor was consciousness impaired. We have already considered Rolando's belief that the cerebellum was an electromotor similar to the electric organ of certain fishes, and that it secreted the motor fluid necessary for locomotion and other muscle action.[397] This, together with his other observations, provided the basis for his contention that the cerebellum initiated voluntary movements; this was, therefore, its *action propre.* It was, he said, "the organ upon which locomotion depends"[398] and "it must serve locomotion,"[399] for it was "the organ of movement,"[400] owing to the fact that "after injury, destruction, or removal of the cerebellum the locomotive power in all vertebrates ceases."[401] It thus worked with the cerebrum (6.4.3) to organize motor activity. Limb involvement was ipsilateral to a cerebellar hemisphere lesion, a correct observation, whereas Flourens's was incorrect. But, like Flourens, he recognized that recovery could follow cerebellar damage or ablation, providing it was neither severe nor too deep. The cerebral hemispheres, however, were the seat of sensory, vital, and intellectual faculties, but volition was in the cerebellum.

Rolando's belief that the cerebellum was a motor mechanism was in keeping with Galen's, who, as noted above, thought the motor nerves arose from it. Be this as it may, Rolando's erroneous basic concept of the organ being primarily responsible for motor functions, and his observations on the motor disability accompanying damage to it, were quite different from Flourens's. There were other fundamental differences between them, because whereas Rolando relegated volition to the cerebellum, Flourens placed it in the cerebral hemispheres, along with sensation and intellect, locations Rolando accepted. It followed that the charge of plagiarism made by Coster could not be substantiated. We should, of course, remember that Rolando in 1809 lacked the improved anatomical knowledge from which Flourens benefited, and his technique of carrying out ablations and traumatizing the brain by way of cranial holes was vastly inferior to Flourens's wide-exposure method. Also, most of his observations were made in animals during the acute postoperative phase, and therefore open to the various objections discussed above (chap. 1.2.2); he carried out no chronic experiments.

Despite these criticisms, however, Rolando's research cannot be dismissed lightly and some have even claimed them as "a foundation stone of cerebellar physiology";[402] and we have noted above Luciani's laudatory comment. He was working in virtual isolation from the scientific world of Europe, so that his endeavors were highly original, and with them he was contesting the dominance of the Hallerian school singlehandedly. Thus, although he may have made many errors in this work, he did reveal that cerebral and cerebellar functions were not the same, as Haller's doctrine of brain equipotentiality demanded. In the context of his time, Rolando occupied a unique position, and Flourens's criticisms, such as the following, were inaccurate as well as unwarranted. Because of his primitive techniques, Flourens declared:

> Rolando, therefore, confused all the phenomena, as he also confused all the organs from which these phenomena derived; and this happened because his method isolated nothing. With a *method of isolating,* he would have recognized the drowsiness deriving from cerebral lesions, the excitation of muscular contractions from the bigeminal or quadrigeminal bodies, the drunken state or disorder of movement from a cerebellar lesion.[403]

Like his contemporaries, such as Galvani, Gall, Reil, and Burdach, Rolando was a man of eighteenth-century origins, education, science, and culture, working in a period of revolution and change during the first decade of the nineteenth century, whereas Flourens belonged entirely to the new order and to the remarkable advances of the nineteenth century that had already been achieved.

A possible criticism of Rolando is to point out that he made no attempt to reassess and to modify if necessary his concepts of brain action. Thus in a further book of 1828,[404] he made no concessions to Flourens and his supporters, so that his original views like Flourens's changed little throughout his life. The cerebellum remained the motor organ of the brain and elaborated the motor nerve-fluid, although later he believed that it activated involuntary as well as voluntary musculature. Rolando had, therefore, incorporated Willis's theory of 1664 into his concept of cerebellar physiology. But his conceptual rigidity was no less than Flourens's, whose incorrect ideas of cerebral function remained unaltered until his death in 1867. As mentioned already, the ultimate irony is that, although there can be little doubt that Flourens was the better scientist and concerning the cerebellum made a memorable contribution to its physiology, his name is not widely known among the medical profession today, whereas Rolando's is universally associated with the cerebral "fissure of Rolando," described in the year of his death.[405]

It was unfortunate that Rolando's extremely interesting findings were at first unknown outside Italy, or perhaps even outside Sardinia, and that when they were given wider publicity they were immediately overshadowed and denied by Flourens's admittedly superior studies. The contrast between the two, while enhancing Flourens's position, showed Rolando's experiments and interpretations as seemingly crude and erroneous, whereas on the whole they do not deserve the severe censure that has been accorded them. Rolando's conclusions concerning cerebellar function were mostly wrong, but on the other hand Flourens's opinions on cerebral action were also mainly incorrect.

6.6.4. Reception of Flourens

Flourens's concept of cerebellar function was not accepted unanimously by any means, even though he had received the blessing of Cuvier and the Académie Commissioners. Thus, there were several investigators in the 1820s and 1830s who had interests vested in rival theories. Gall was bound to protest, just as he had concerning Flourens's views on cerebral action, and he made valiant efforts to amass supporting experimental data. We know that he was not enthusiastically in favor of animal experiments and lacked Flourens's technical skills. In Gall's hands, complete cerebellar ablation was invariably fatal, but the evidence he collected seemed to deny the existence of Flourens's incoordination, which he considered to be due to disturbances of motor function in dying animals, or to confusion with convulsions (see chap. 1.2.2). He also gleaned observations from comparative anatomy and the clinic, and he found it difficult to understand why two organs, the cerebrum and the cerebellum, should be needed for voluntary movements, one to direct and one to coordinate.[406] His conclusion was a scathing attack on vivisection as well as on Flourens's experiments, and he pointed out "that consequently these lesions provide nothing certain and useful, either for physiology or for human pathology; and that finally all these cruel mutilations have no other merit than that of vain curiosity."[407] Gall was clearly on the defensive, but not very successfully, as he strove to vindicate a very different concept of cerebellar function. A British contemporary described the situation sarcastically:

> M. Gall, incensed to find his organs of love, philoprogenitiveness, and many other propensities and noble faculties, all snatched from his hands to make up one poor, paltry machine for regulating the baser bodily motions . . . has vehemently resisted such an appropriation, and endeavoured to obstruct his adversary's progress.[408]

He considered that Gall's attack had, in fact, proved the validity of Flourens's proposals in view of the fact that "so acute and so captious a controversialist, on a point so injurious to his system, has made so weak an assault, and has been reduced to such sorry subterfuges."[409] However, one of Gall's followers, Broussais, leapt to his defense with an ingenious compromise, incorporating both theories of cerebellar function. The cerebellum, he avowed, controlled combined muscular actions and, therefore, the "muscles that contract with energy during the act of copulation."[410] He concluded by stating that "I attribute, therefore, the directions of the movements, the acts and the aptitudes that are related to generation to the influence of the cerebellum."[411] The attractiveness and suitability of Gall's notion had won it very wide acceptance, and a measure of its appeal is afforded by the opinion of the renowned physiologist, Longet, who although following Flourens faithfully, offered another compromise:

> However, we are a long way from wishing to affirm that the cerebellum has the exclusive role of *coordinating* voluntary limb movements, without venturing to believe, with Gall, that it might be the seat of the organ of the generative instinct.[412]

Opposition to Flourens's cerebellar physiology also came from two young postgraduate students at the Salpêtrière hospital in Paris, Foville and Pinel-Grandchamp, whose views on cerebral action also clashed with those of Flourens. In their monograph of 1823,[413] they rejected, "with the precious conviction of youth,"[414] Flourens's concept of cerebellar physiology in favor of a notion that had been discussed by Pourfour du Petit in 1710, whereby the cerebellum was claimed to be the seat of sensibility.[415] He had tested the notion that "it is the cerebellum that provides the spirits that produce sensation,"[416] and on the basis of animal experiments he reported: "It appears from these experiments that the cerebellum does not produce the spirits for sensation."[417] But what kind it did produce could not be determined with certainty. As we have noted, Foville distrusted animal experimentation, and preferred clinical and anatomical observations. In this instance he and his colleague reasoned, in keeping with the recent discovery of Magendie regarding the function of the spinal roots and the spinal cord pathways, that the posterior sensory columns and roots alone were connected to the cerebellum. This also accorded with Charles Bell's revised opinion on cerebellar and spinal root properties. As we have noted above (6.4.1), he had concluded in 1811 that the cerebellum controlled autonomic activities, but after Magendie's experiments of 1822 his views changed, and as part of his fraudulent priority claim he now thought it likely that the cerebellum was the seat of sensation. In the 1829 edition of his popular textbook produced jointly with John Bell (1763–1820), he conjectured that "If we were to indulge in opinions which we could not bring to the test of experiment, we should say that the cerebrum had power over the motions of the body, and the cerebellum over its sensibility."[418]

Foville expanded on this theme in 1831,[419] and considered "the cerebellum as the central focus of sensibility,"[420] whereas the cerebrum was in charge of voluntary motion with localized areas of specific action. He did, however, admit that sensation helped to coordinate voluntary motion: "the true regulator of movements is sensibility."[421] He thus associated himself with those, like R. B. Todd, who held that the cerebellum was the center of muscle sense. Todd had accepted the thalamus as the chief sensory center, and because of direct connections with it, the cerebellum seemed to be associated with "muscular sense," which was obviously involved with the coordination of movements.[422] But as he maintained that the cerebellum was linked with motor as well as sensory parts of the cerebrum and spinal cord, it was Todd's belief that it was a regulator of infinitely complex movements,[423] a notion akin to Broussais's. This idea represented another compromise that brought together motor and sensory functions, thus integrating two concepts of cerebellar action. It was to survive throughout the nineteenth century to the present day.[424]

Foville found another supporter in Britain, J. C. Prichard, who declared that the Frenchman's opinion on cerebellar function was "most probable."[425] However, he also assigned memory and imagination to the organ,[426] and was thereby returning to the faculty psychology of the Middle Ages, which located memory in the cerebellum or fourth ventricle. Another proposal based on an earlier speculation was that of Dugès[427] who, having observed the close juxtaposition of the cerebellum with the trigeminal, auditory, and glassopharyngeal cranial nerves, associated the organ with taste and hearing, a line of reasoning that had been adopted by Carus in 1814. He also agreed with Thomas Willis that, in addition, it presided over respiration and digestion.

Opponents of Foville's opinion were quick to point out that if the cerebellum were indeed a sensory center, it was strange that no sensory nerves seemed to be directly associated with it, and some already refuted its connection with the posterior spinal cord columns. It was also curious that pathological processes confined to it never gave rise to sensory disorders. And as Bouillaud reasoned:

> In fact, if the cerebellum was the unique center of sensibility what was the explanation for the paralysis of sensation that accompanies such a large number of diseases of the cerebrum?[428]

But the most damning evidence came from experimental physiology, the very source that Foville distrusted. Flourens could show that the cerebellum was seemingly unresponsive to noxious stimuli: "I exposed the cerebellum in another pigeon; I pierced it bit by bit in all directions with a needle; I cut serial slices: the animal did not budge."[429] Longet confirmed this,[430] and Magendie, although agreeing that superficial irritation produced no evidence of pain, found deeper structures, like the cerebellar peduncles to be sensitive.[431]

Flourens's conclusions regarding cerebellar function were also refuted on clinical grounds, because it was said that disturbances of coordination were rarely observed in diseases of the cerebellum. We can now assume, however, that this was due to the inadequate diagnostic methods then employed. One of the most puzzling features of cerebellar disease, as with cerebral, was the occasional absence of clinical manifestations in the presence of an extensive lesion. Charles Bell, when remarking on this, was correct when he attributed certain so-called cerebellar signs to brain stem involvement, an error of which Willis had not been aware.[432] By now, however, Bell changed his mind once more and had renounced his previous support for the sensory properties of the cerebellum, and he also denied that it was concerned with motor activity. "On the whole," he stated, "it does not appear to stand in direct relation to the motions of the frame, or to the common sensibility."[433] This part of the brain remained a clinical paradox, echoed in the words of Carl Wilhelm Hermann Nothnagel (1841–1905) later in the century: "There is no part of the brain other than the cerebellum where the significance of the symptoms, even at the earliest age, can be so contradictory."[434] What seemed to be the most influential clinical evidence against Flourens, however, appeared in a book by the renowned clinician and pathologist, G. Andral, early in the 1830s,[435] but when his material was later examined carefully, it turned out that most of the cases were unsuitable for the analysis to which they had been subjected.[436]

Outright denial of both Flourens's experimental observations and the conclusions he drew from them was uncommon. The way in which he had described his procedures allowed others to repeat them, and most found themselves in agreement, whereas some encountered features that he had overlooked. The first to confirm and extend Flourens's research on the cerebellum was Michel Foderà at Paris, who reported his results to the Académie des Sciences on 31 December 1822.[437] In retrospect, it is clear that he had seen and described the paleocerebellar syndrome consequent upon cerebellectomy, and due to the release of postural reflexes, such as those known as antigravity:[438]

> The animal bends its head backwards, with the hind legs held apart and the front ones straight and stiff. The position of the animal is as though it was about to move or fall backwards.[439]

He was not, however, the first to have encountered this for in 1773 Méhée de la Touche, as we have seen, had noticed the extension and rigid positioning of the head in animals after cerebellar injury,[440] and Saucerotte had made a similar observation in 1778.[441] Another significant, but little appreciated, observation reported by Foderà was that lesions of different parts of the cerebellum did not necessarily produce the same clinical picture.[442] But, in keeping with Flourens's principle of *action propre,* the organ was considered to be a single functional unit, like the other subdivisions of the nervous system. Foderà concluded: "It is probable that the cerebellum is an organ that presides over emotional and moral phenomena in particular."[443] Unfortunately, his excellent observations also induced him to adopt the extreme opinion that whatever motor or sensory effects might result from cerebellar lesions arose from disturbances of the medulla oblongata, the cerebellum being closely connected, but merely an appendage of it. His stance was, therefore, the precise opposite to that of Willis, who had attributed the sequelae of his experiments on the cerebellum to dysfunction of the latter, whereas most arose from interference with the brain stem. Nevertheless, Foderà correctly identified the signs of cerebellar hemisphere damage as ipsilateral, and thus agreed with Rolando and not with Flourens.

Magendie, Foderà's supervisor, was also interested in the cerebellum, especially the compulsive rotatory movements described by Saucerotte and others in the eighteenth century, and discussed by Foderà in his second paper, published in 1826. He was the first to describe them in detail and to produce them by sectioning the cerebellar peduncles. In an article of 1824, in which he reported these findings, Magendie presented the first certain evidence of the cerebellum's role in the maintenance of the body's equilibrium, now known to be a topic of immense complexity.[444] It was his opinion that the two halves of the cerebellum controlled the equilibrium of the body in the erect posture and in walking. They each exerted a force by way of the cerebellar peduncles, and one counterbalanced the other in the healthy animal. Thus, "it was through the equilibrium of these two forces that the state of standing and even the possibility of rest and of the various regular and voluntary movements of the animal resulted."[445] It followed that "the integrity of the organ [cerebellum] alone permits an equilibrium that is constant."[446] Magendie's view was to be widely accepted, in part owing to the great prestige he had acquired through his other research, but it seems likely that, unknown to him, some of his experimental results were due to damaging the vestibular nuclei in the brain stem and central vestibular pathways or, as now seems more likely, due to damage of that part of the cerebellum that inhibits muscle tone. In contradistinction to Flourens, he did not induce defects of movement performance in rabbits after cerebellar ablation, and he thought that coordination was a less important feature of cerebellar function than had been claimed. Disequilibrium seemed to him to be a much more potent factor in the disruption of voluntary movement.

But there were others who found themselves in complete unison with Flourens. Heinrich Hertwig (1807–?) agreed with his results and accepted his opinions, including the occurrence of contralateral cerebellar signs and the phenomenon of compensation.[447] Some tried, however, to reconcile Flourens's incoordination with Magendie's disequilibrium, the most noteworthy being Bouillaud. He accepted Flourens's experimental findings and concurred that the faculty of coordination was in the cerebellum, for he had carried out ablation as well as irritation by means of cautery, in dogs, rabbits, pigeons, and fowl.[448] Even so he disputed the notion that this involved all voluntary motion of the body. He regarded the cerebellum as "the legislator, so to speak, of the body's equilibrium, walking, running, jumping, and of various [similar] activities."[449] But it only presided over the coordination of muscles concerned with equilibration, posture, and progression, and had no power over the other voluntary bodily movements. Those concerned with speech, for example, were under the control of the cerebrum. The ocular manifestations of cerebellar damage were, he claimed, due to involvement of the neighboring quadrigeminal bodies, and the opisthotonus seen by Foderà did not escape his notice, although he drew no conclusions from it. It was Bouillaud's belief, in keeping with Magendie, that the cerebellum's only office was to maintain the equilibrium between the two sides of the body that was necessary for locomotion. He had thus harmonized and integrated two popular theories, but his main objective in doing so was to disprove Gall's theory of cerebellar action. To his experimental data he added cogent clinical arguments.[450]

A few, like Legallois, accepted the need for a mechanism that would regulate muscular movement, but instead of allocating it to the cerebellum he placed it in the medulla oblongata, thus perpetuating the confusion between brain stem and cerebellar activity that had begun with Willis in 1664. It was his belief that "it is somewhere in this part that resides the faculty by means of which animals regulate their movements."[451] But no matter how contrary other opinions on cerebellar functions were, their authors invariably praised Flourens's experimental prowess. John Bostock falls into this group, because his suggestion was that "the cerebellum is the centre of sympathetic or associated actions of the nerves that are concerned in voluntary motion."[452] He could not accept the existence of a specific nervous function that alone could coordinate. Coordination, he declared, existed, but it was due to several sympathetic and associated activities in the nervous system. Despite this and other differences from Flourens, Bostock was outspoken in his praise for such brilliant experimental investigations: "The experiments that were performed upon the cerebellum are very interesting, and are perhaps some of the most decisive in their results of any which are contained in the volume [P. Flourens, *Recherches* (1824)]."[453]

6.6.5. Summary

Following Flourens's main studies on the cerebellum carried out in the 1820s, together with the simultaneous resurrection of Rolando's earlier research, there were no further major advances in cerebellar physiology until the last decade of the nineteenth century. As in the case of Flourens's notion of the cerebral hemisphere's *action propre,* the one he enunciated for the cerebellum which made it the coordinator of voluntary movements was widely accepted, although challenged mainly by Magendie's concept of equilibration. The two provided guidelines to the future. Few rejected these opinions outright, and those who could not accept them in their entirety constructed various compromises to eliminate difficulties. Even so by 1862 the American physiologist, J. C. Dalton, could report that "of all the physiological theories with regard to the peculiar [specific] function of the cerebellum, the only one which has been received with any continued favour, is that first advocated by Flourens."[454]

The next outstanding contribution was made by Luigi Luciani in 1891.[455] As we have observed, he maligned Flourens's studies and favored Rolando's, and from the latter's idea of a diffuse cerebellar influence on all motor activities grew his own views, based on chronic cerebellar ablation experiments. His doctrine, like that of Flourens, included an *action propre* of the cerebellum, representing a facilitating effect upon central structures responsible for voluntary muscular motion. But although it pointed the way to several modern interpretations, by insisting on a unitary action, it in fact hindered progress for about fifty years, as the Hallerian and Flourentian teachings on the cerebrum had done earlier. One of the fundamental principles of cerebellar action is today known to be a compound type of functional localization, just as in other parts of the brain[456] and the unitarian or *action propre* concept of Galen, Willis, Haller, Rolando, Flourens, Luciani, and others in its various forms has eventually been shown to be erroneous.

6.7. SEQUEL

Despite the overwhelming support for Flourens's cerebral *action propre,* in opposition to Gall's compound localization, there were a few clinicians who although not necessarily accepting organology nevertheless had argued in favor of a punctate functional localization in the cerebral hemispheres. These men were to create a link between the early decades of the nineteenth century and the 1860s, when cerebral cortical localization became a scientific reality. We have examined in some detail Gall's assignment of the faculties of verbal memory and language to the frontal lobes of the cerebral hemispheres, and it was on this clinical phenomenon that the connection was established between the conjectures of the organologists and phrenologists and the scientific investigations culminating in the experimental verification of cortical localization in 1870.

The central figure was Bouillaud, already encountered, who argued in favor of cerebral motor areas, because limited palsies occurred in patients. On 21 February 1825 he presented a paper to the Académie Royale de Médecine in Paris,[457] and in the same year published a book on inflammatory disorders of the brain.[458] In them, he demonstrated not only his clinical acumen, but also his ability to pursue a logical line of reasoning. He advanced arguments opposing Flourens's opinion that the cerebrum had no direct influence on muscle contractions and could affect them only by means of its volition acting through lower centers. He continued:

> But it is not enough to know only in a general way that the cerebrum is indispensable for the production of many muscle movements; the question remains to find out if each of the various parts of which the cerebrum is composed controls particular movements; and finally to investigate if several cerebral nervous centers exist, which are related to muscle movements. Now the plurality of cerebral organs when considered from this latter point of view becomes an infinitely probable fact.[459]

But if limb muscles were controlled by the cerebral hemispheres, surely those concerned with speech should be similarly influenced. He then made the observation that was to lead in the 1860s to the downfall of Flourens's doctrine. Bouillaud's extensive clinical and pathological evidence deriving from his own and others' experience led him to state that patients who had lost their powers of articulate speech, but with preservation of intellect so that they understood everything and could express themselves by gesture or writing (or, as we would say, suffered from a motor aphasia) invariably had a lesion in their frontal lobes. He was not the first to make this association,[460] but his brilliant deductions from it were unique, and they represented one of the most noteworthy outcomes of the French school of clinicopathological correlation founded in the first few years of the nineteenth century. It seemed to him that there must be a nervous force that regulated and coordinated the organs of speech:

> Now from my personal observations and from those I have collected from other authors, I believe that the nervous principle in question, which may be termed the coordinating organ of speech (*organe législateur*), resides in the anterior lobes of the brain.[461]

One of the objects of Bouillaud's paper of 1825 was to announce his confirmation of Gall's organ of the faculty of speech, but in view of the way in which the latter had been conceived, we would judge the similarity to have been fortuitous. Although he seemed pleased to substantiate one aspect of organology, he did not subscribe to Gall's system and in the long run his evidence was to be used against it. In the meantime, he received more criticism than credit, because it seemed that he was supporting Gall's doctrine, which was already discredited as a scientific topic, and therefore tainted by the philosophical associations that had become attached to it. As well as being concerned with a particular problem, Bouillaud was also concerned with the basic principles of the medical sciences, and he voiced the feelings of his many colleagues, who, as we have noted above, had cited clinicopathological evidence to combat Flourens's doctrine of *action propre*. He stated:

> But if, on the one hand, physiology is the true torch of pathology, it is equally certain that pathology is for physiology an inexhaustible source of insights. It leads us in the most direct manner to a knowledge of the functions of organs; and, to observe that it is precisely the means which allows physiologists to discover the yet-unknown function of a given organ.[462]

In other words, experimental physiology was a kind of artificial pathology, for a lesion represented a "natural experiment,"[463] the importance of which to neurophysiology we have already discussed in chapter 1.2.5.

Bouillaud's general contribution to compound cerebral localization must also be emphasized, as well as his oft-repeated statement on the frontal lobes:

> It follows from all the facts that I have just set forth that disturbance of the speech following a local cerebral affection, is a sign that the disease occupies the anterior lobes of the brain.[464]

His most perceptive assertion concerned disorders of motor functions occurring with cerebral hemisphere disease:

> If I have committed several errors in determining the relations between the seat of the paralyses and that of the cerebral lesions, it will always remain demonstrated that there exist in the cerebrum many centers for movement, just as there exist many organs of intellect.[465]

There can, therefore, be no doubt of Bouillaud's commitment to a compound localization akin to Gall's, but composed of somatic and intellectual functions and not mental and moral propensities only. Unfortunately, this notion, later shown to be correct, received little support. In the first place, this punctate type of localization of cerebral action seemed too closely allied to Gall's organology, and some felt that Bouillaud's purpose was to support all aspects of it, which was not the case. Second, Flourens's experimental evidence was much more acceptable for many reasons, and one of them was their apparent reliability, owing to his stature as a scientist, and the precise and dogmatic way he had reported them. This could not be said of clinical material, renowned for its ambiguous, variable, capricious, and paradoxical behavior, which continued to be a problem throughout the nineteenth century, in particular exemplified by the false localizing signs of the intracranial space-occupying lesion.

These factors weighed against others who associated speech defects with frontal lobe lesions. Desmoulins, whose deviation from Flourens has already been mentioned, had this to say in 1825, that is, simultaneously with Bouillaud. In patients who seemed to have exhibited a motor dysphasia, he reported: "Now in all these cases the anterior part of the cerebral hemisphere was affected. . . . On the basis of this example, it is very likely that the different [mental] faculties each has a special site."[466] Thus, like Bouillaud, he was partly in favor of Gall's system, whereas Parchappe de Vinay in 1838 appears to have had no allegiance to it, when he equated the cortical decay characteristic of general paralysis of the insane with mental changes. Concerning speech, however, he wrote:

> In this regard the sole fact that seems to me worthy, of note is that the greatest embarassment of speech has generally appeared to coincide with the most extensive and deepest lesions of the anterior lobes.[467]

Naturally the criticisms leveled at Bouillaud were also leveled at Desmoulins and Parchappe. In addition, Bouillaud was attacked by both physiologist and pathologist. Longet, having sided with Flourens, predictably opposed Bouillaud, and concluded that there was no certain evidence approving a special location for the nervous principle that coordinated speech mechanisms.[468] He was joined by the influential clinicopathologists, Lallemand, Andral, and Cruveilhier.[469] Although Lallemand gave accounts of several cases that satisfied Bouillaud's criteria, he did not share the latter's convictions because the association of speech defect and frontal lobe lesion was not invariably clear.[470] Andral based his dissension on the grounds that one could be present without the other. Thus, patients with frontal lobe disease could have normal speech and some with speech disturbance had lesions in the parts of the cerebrum other than the anterior regions. "Loss of speech," he concluded, "is therefore not necessarily the result of a lesion of the anterior lobes, and, further, it can take place in cases where anatomy reveals no change whatever in these lobes."[471] Unknown, however, to these pioneers of the Parisian school of morbid anatomy as applied to clinical neurology, such evidence was of little value, because neuropathology was still at the macroscopical level, and the understanding of dysphasia, together with the clinical evaluation of it, was very limited.

Bouillaud, nonetheless, persisted in his opinion, and in 1848 produced further evidence supporting it. This conviction was so strong that he offered a sum of five hundred francs to anyone who could demonstrate a case of a deep frontal lobe lesion without an accompanying disturbance of the faculty of speech.[472] The fact that there was no response indicated either a lack of interest in the subject or, more likely, that Flourens's doctrine of cerebral *action propre* still ruled supreme. Moreover, under these circumstances to admit the existence of punctate, compound brain localization would not only have been interpreted as a heretical act, but it would also have revealed an acceptance of the despised organology of Gall and the phrenology of Spurzheim.

This attitude, however, was abruptly changed in 1861, six years before Flourens's death. During that year, a celebrated debate took place in Paris, involving Bouillaud's son-in-law Aubertin, Gratiolet, Broca, and others.[473] It had two outcomes. First, Bouillaud's clinicopathological deduction of a frontal lobe speech center was vindicated, and the left hemisphere was shown to be the one usually affected. Second, the scene was now set for the establishment of compound brain action, in the form of punctate localization of function in the cerebral cortex of humans and animals. This was made possible by two diametrically opposite approaches to the problem: John Hughlings Jackons's application of the philosophy of Herbert Spencer (1820–1903) to his own remarkable clinical observations and the inferences derived from them in the late 1860s; and the classical experiments carried out by Fritsch and Hitzig in 1870 and by David Ferrier in 1873.[474] Each in their own way detected circumscribed areas of cerebral cortex that represented contralateral motor functions of the body. It seems fitting that the clinical and experimental methods, which earlier in the century had opposed cortical localization, now combined to verify its existence. With these discoveries the topography of brain action was established, and regional delineations of function followed naturally.

In summary, we can point out that it had taken the first three-quarters of the nineteenth century to break free from first the universal influence of Haller's teaching of equipotentiality of brain function, and second from Flourens's equally ecumenical doctrine of *action propre*. Of all the many participants in this drawn-out conflict, perhaps the most interesting, yet enigmatic, was Franz Joseph Gall, who despite alleged personality defects deserves both praise and compassion. Although he formulated a basic principle of neurophysiology, compound cortical localization of function, he did so with data that were later shown to be worthless and his doctrine of organology was demolished by the experimental evidence of Pierre Flourens, which in turn proved to be erroneous. Gall was therefore rejected and reviled by most of his scientific contemporaries and in addition because his ideas contravened philosophical and theological tenets of early nineteenth-century France, he earned further repudiation. However, despite these judgments we should recognize his several momentous contributions to research on the form and function of the nervous system discussed in this book. They establish him as a prominent forerunner of today's neuroscientific concepts.

7

The Vegetative Nervous System

7.1. INTRODUCTION

The autonomic nervous system consists of elements in the central and the peripheral nervous systems, and it regulates the activities of structures not normally under voluntary control. It is the visceral component of the nervous system. However, for historical reasons to be discussed shortly, we have preferred to designate it "vegetative," a term that today is synonymous with "autonomic."

Before 1800, apart from its gross anatomy, little was known of this complex system, although numerous speculations concerning its functions had been made.[1] Much of our knowledge of it was accumulated in the nineteenth century, and we shall discuss below the period that extends from the beginning to about the middle of the century. This period was dominated by the theory of Bichat, which attested to the independence of the vegetative system from the brain and spinal cord, and its own nervous power. It is our purpose to discover the origins of his "ganglionic system" and the reception it received during the first half of the century. In fact, it survived until the 1880s, but thereafter it was rapidly destroyed by the work of two Cambridge scientists, Walter Holbrook Gaskell (1847–1914)[2] and John Newport Langley (1852–1925)[3] to be replaced by our present day concept of the autonomic nervous system. The complexity of the latter and the confusion and misunderstandings that have existed among investigators demand the following brief discussions of its structure, function, and terminology.

7.2. STRUCTURE AND FUNCTION

The terms autonomic or vegetative nervous system are applied to that aggregation of ganglia, nerves, and plexuses by means of which the abdominal viscera, heart, glands, blood vessels, and all nonstriated muscles elsewhere are innervated and connected to higher controlling centers in the spinal cord, brain stem, hypothalamus, and cerebral cortex. It is concerned chiefly, though not entirely, with the internal environment of the body, in contrast to the cerebrospinal system that deals mainly, but not exclusively, with the external world. It has relative independence but operates intimately, both centrally and peripherally, with the rest of the nervous system so that together they represent different aspects of a single integrated neural mechanism.

The peripheral part of the vegetative system is made up of ganglia, plexuses, and nerves, and is created by two outflows from the brain stem and spinal cord (see figure).

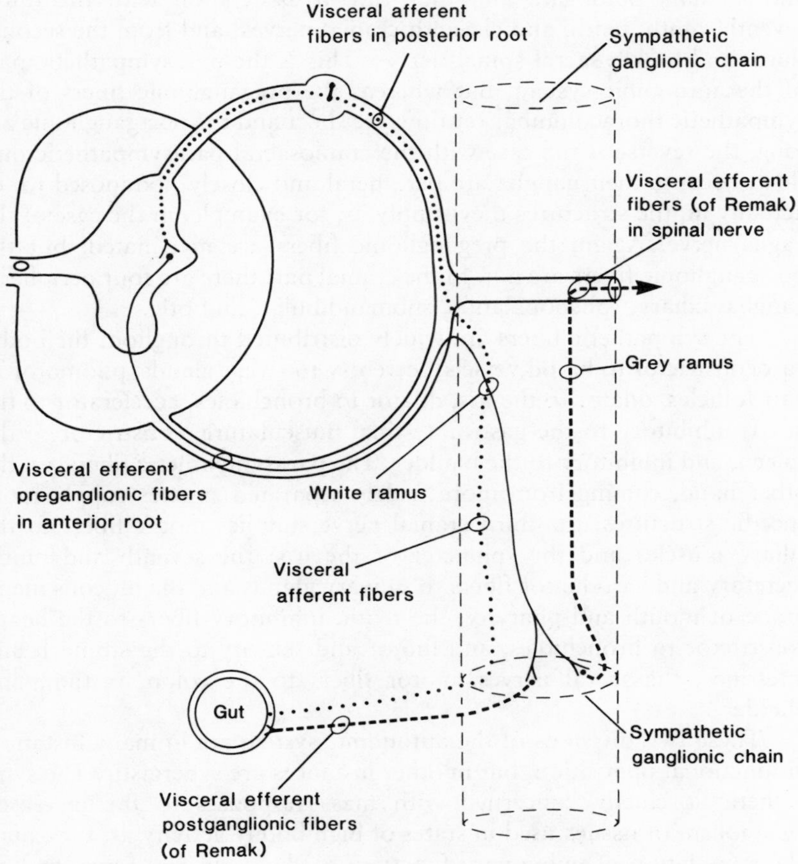

A diagram of the Vegetative Nervous System according to present-day concepts

1. *The thoracolumbar outflow* comes from all the thoracic and the upper two or three lumbar segments of the cord to form the sympathetic portion of the autonomic system. Its fibers arise from nerve cell bodies in the lateral horns of the cord's gray matter and leave by way of the anterior spinal root to travel through the fourteen or fifteen white rami communicantes to the ganglionic trunk as fine myelinated preganglionic visceral efferent fibers. They synapse with cell bodies in the ganglia to form mostly nonmyelinated postganglionic fibers that are much thicker than the preganglionic fibers, and they either pass through the gray rami to the somatic spinal nerves, in which they are distributed to the structures they innervate, or they course directly to them.

2. *The craniosacral outflow* follows much the same basic pattern. Its fibers arise from two areas: from cranial nerve nuclei in the midbrain and medulla oblongata and they run in association with the third, seventh, ninth, tenth, and eleventh cranial nerves; and from the second, third, and fourth sacral spinal nerves. This is the parasympathetic part of the autonomic system. But whereas the preganglionic fibers of the sympathetic thoracolumbar outflow are short and the postganglionic are long, the reverse is the case with the craniosacral parasympathetic outflow, because their ganglia are peripheral and closely juxtaposed to, or actually in, the structures they supply as, for example, in the case of the vagus nerve. Again, the preganglionic fibers are myelinated, but the postganglionic fibers are not. In the cranial part there are four peripheral ganglia: ciliary, sphenopalatine, submandibular, and otic.

The sympathetic fibers are widely distributed throughout the body: vasoconstrictor to blood vessels, secretory to sweat glands, pilomotor to hair follicles, dilator to the iris, dilator to bronchioles, accelerator to the heart, inhibitory to the gastrointestinal musculature, constrictor to the spleen, and inhibitory to the bladder. The parasympathetic fibers, on the other hand, coming from more widely separated sources supply more specific structures: the third cranial nerve supplies motor fibers to the ciliary muscles and the sphincter of the iris; the seventh and ninth, secretory and vasodilator fibers to salivary glands and the mucous membrane of mouth and pharynx; the tenth, inhibitory fibers to the heart, constrictor to bronchioles, and motor and sensory to the stomach and intestines; the sacral nerves, motor fibers to the colon, rectum, and bladder.

These two divisions of the autonomic system are in many instances in functional opposition, but in other instances are synergistic. The sympathetic is chiefly concerned with mass responses to the increased metabolism of tissues used in states of high bodily activity as, for example, stimulation of pulmonary function, cardiac rate and force, and all the sweat glands during exercise. The parasympathetic system, on the other hand, has to do mainly with localized responses involved in more sedentary activities, such as digestion and the emptying of bladder or bowels. The pupils, heart, and intestines receive fibers from both systems and take on their opposing actions. Blood vessels, however, receive mostly sympathetic influences, manifested by vasoconstriction. The most important role of the two systems is to preserve the body's ability to maintain internal stability or equilibrium, that is, its homeostasis, and they achieve this and other objectives by working together to balance their opposing actions under the control of the hypothalamus.

So far only the visceral efferent fibers have been described, but visceral afferents also exist, particularly for autonomic reflex activity. They are found in the ninth and tenth cranial nerves, and in many of the spinal nerves, especially thoracic, upper lumbar, and second, third and fourth sacral. They resemble their cerebrospinal, that is, somatic counterparts, because their cell bodies are in the ganglia of the cranial nerves or spinal roots and they are distributed peripherally; they proceed thence through autonomic ganglia, plexuses, and somatic nerves without synapsing, thus connecting the structures they innervate, like viscera and glands, directly with the spinal cord or brain stem, and thereby with higher centers. Along these fibers, which may be of the large or small myelinated or of the nonmyelinated variety, messages travel centripetally to initiate visceral reflexes that do not usually reach consciousness. However, these reflexes can also be evoked by somatic afferents, which illustrates the close association between the autonomic and the cerebrospinal nervous systems. The following definition summarizes their integrative activity: "the autonomic nervous system organizes the visceral support of somatic behaviour. The CNS integrates the activities of the body through these two complexes."[4]

7.3. TERMINOLOGY AND EARLY HISTORY

The history of the vegetative nervous system is in part also the history of the many attempts to find an appropriate name for it. We shall, therefore, survey them together here in order to understand the several terms used in the first few decades of the nineteenth century and to relate them to their modern equivalents.

The records of antiquity that have survived to the present day reveal that the chain of ganglia we call the sympathetic thoracolumbar outflow was first described by Galen in the second century A.D.[5] He claimed that it originated from the brain, because it arose from his third and fourth cranial nerves (our sensory and motor roots of the trigeminal nerve, respectively) and from his sixth nerve (our glossopharyngeal, vagus, and accessory).[6] It should be noted, however, that Galen did not dissect the human body, and that this erroneous description was based on animal anatomy only. Nevertheless, he identified the rami communicantes, an achievement made possible by skillful dissection and acute perception.[7] Differentiation between the sympathetic trunk and nearby cranial nerves, especially the vagus, was not made until the sixteenth century,[8] but the trunk's supposed cerebral origin was substantiated by eminent anatomists, such as Bartolomeo Eustachi (Eustachius, c. 1520–1574) in 1714,[9] and also by Thomas Willis,[10] who thought it arose from the trigeminal and abducens cranial nerves (of our classification). Despite the experiments of the remarkably able French investigator of the nervous system, Pourfour du Petit, reported in 1729, and which demonstrated the absence of a connection between the brain and the sympathetic trunk,[11] the error of Galen and Willis persisted, and it was still prevalent at the beginning of the nineteenth century.

We have already mentioned briefly the ancient concept of sympathy or consensus when discussing the history of reflex theory (chap. 4.2), but it was of equal significance in the history of the vegetative nervous system. Fundamentally, sympathy occurred when a change in the condition of one part of the body induced an alteration in the condition of another, or when a condition arising in one part had an effect that was felt elsewhere. The organs in particular reacted sympathetically to one another, even though there might be no anatomical connections between them. These numerous and frequent sympathetic associations, or "sympathy of the parts," were present in the healthy body, but more often in the diseased. At a time when the etiology of very few pathological processes were known and correct explanations for their multifarious manifestations usually impossible, sympathy was thought to account for some of the otherwise inexplicable combinations of clinical features, such as pain at a distance from the seat of disease; the malar flush with pulmonary tuberculosis; grinding of the teeth with intestinal worms; vomiting with renal calculi and with injury or disease of the brain; nasal symptoms with uterine disease; associations between uterus and breasts; and so forth. Today we explain such phenomena in the normal and abnormal body, previously attributed to sympathy, on a basis of reflex activity, hormonal or biochemical influences, allergy, bacterial toxins, referred pain, and many other physiological or pathological mechanisms.[12]

The involuntary interrelationships established between organs and regions that seemed to be satisfactorily explained by sympathy were accounted for by suggesting either nervous or vascular transmission between them, and Galen subscribed to both these methods.[13] Although his notions survived into the early nineteenth century, they were clouded by Renaissance physicians who postulated occult and often cosmic forces as the responsible agents. It was Thomas Willis who advocated a return to Galenic principles, and he popularized a mechanical explanation for sympathy that was still in vogue in the first few decades of the nineteenth century. He was an ingenious dissector and he had noted in greater detail than his predecessors the networks of autonomic and somatic nerves that were characteristic of all parts of the body. Moreover, in keeping with Galen, Willis held the erroneous opinion that the sympathetic trunk had its origins, like the cranial nerves, in the brain, and together with the vagus nerve it provided a wide distribution of nerves to the viscera and elsewhere, thereby establishing communications between the vital organs, such as the brain, heart, lungs, and intestines. These morphological arrangements, he claimed, permitted the "sympathy of the parts," and he thus revealed the anatomical pathways that appeared to him to allow both sympathy and reflexion to take place without involving the brain and, therefore, consciousness. It was characteristic of Willis to attempt a materialistic elucidation of physiological and pathological actions, based on contemporary neurological knowledge, much of which had derived from his own research. Furthermore, in doing so he helped in no small measure to fathom the nature of the peripheral parts of the vegetative and somatic nervous systems, as he also did for their central organs: he gave the first detailed description of their nerves, plexuses, and ganglia and at the same time suggested important functions for them in addition to innervating peripheral structures.

We have dealt with sympathy in some detail, because not only did Willis's theory of sympathetic neural transmission still find support in the early nineteenth century, but the basic idea of sympathy played a significant role in clinical medicine until the 1850s. This is vividly illustrated by the comment in 1821 that "a knowledge of sympathies is the foundation of medicine,"[14] made in a reputable and influential French medical encyclopedia. Even at midcentury, C. E. Brown-Séquard thought it appropriate to discuss the sympathies in relation to secretional, nutritional, and disease mechanisms, but equating them mainly, although not exclusively, with reflex phenomena.[15] It was also called upon to elucidate the pharmacological effects of therapeutic agents, for example, quinine, which in 1822 was thought "to excite a high degree of sympathy in the stomach."[16]

But despite the ancient origins of the notion that the vegetative nervous system provided a means of sympathetic communication throughout the body, the term "sympathetic" was not applied to the system until the eighteenth century.[17] Previously the commonest names for the sympathetic nerve or trunk were *nervus intercostalis* or *nervus intercostalis magnus,* usually said to have been introduced by Willis in 1664, along with the English equivalent, the "great intercostal nerve."[18] It had, however, been used earlier in the seventeenth century, for we find that Helkiah Crooke (1576–1653) referred to the *Intercostalis* nerve in 1616.[19] According to him it was a branch of the vagus nerve called by him the "gadding or wandering coniugation."[20] Willis, however, gave a better description of it, and like Galen he mentioned the rami communicantes:

> This [nerve] is commonly called the *Intercostalis,* because passing near the roots of the ribs it receives in every [intercostal] space a branch from the spinal cord.[21]

"Intercostal nerve," which was still being used in the nineteenth century, illustrates the problem of discovering what individuals meant by the terms they employed. It certainly embraced our sympathetic thoracolumbar outflow, but it also usually included part if not all the parasympathetic sacral outflow and some of the cranial, although excluding the vagus nerve even though it was recognized to be physiologically similar. In fact, there is a similar problem with all the terms used before the end of the nineteenth century, when a clearer distinction between the various components of the system was first made, although confusion did not end at once for it lasted well into the present century. Willis also introduced our term "solar plexus," for he compared the celiac plexus to the sun, and its nerves to the beams radiating from it.[22]

Although it was eventually employed almost universally, "intercostalis" was considered to be an inaccurate descriptive epithet in view of the fact its course extended far beyond the thoracic cage. Eventually a more appropriate one was introduced by Jacques-Bénique Winslow (1669–1760), a distinguished anatomist of Danish origin living in Paris. It is the one with which we are still familiar: the "sympathetic" nerve or trunk, his "grande sympathique," which for us designates the sympathetic thoraco-lumbar outflow of the autonomic nervous system.[23] Winslow, however, included in it the other outflow, but not the vagus nerve. His choice of the name was based on the fact that as Galen and especially Willis had already observed, it seemed to anastomose with the majority of the body's nerves, and thus as we have noted, furnished an anatomical explanation for the common phenomenon of sympathy, first advocated by Willis. Winslow also recognized a "petit sympathique" nerve, our facial nerve, and a "moyen sympathique" or "errand," our vagus, but these terms never became popular. "Sympathetic" nerve and system, on the contrary, soon received widespread approval, but, again, it is not always clear what individual authors included in the term. It was joined in the 1760s by "ganglionic" nerves and system of obvious derivation, which originated in the writings of James Johnstone (1730–1802), an English physician.[24] In the nineteenth century it was to become very popular, mainly because Bichat, in his attempts to establish the vegetative system as an independent source of nervous power, also employed "ganglionic," with "organic" as an alternative.

Other terms such as *"nerf trisplanchnique"* (F. Chaussier, 1807),[25] *Rumpfnervensystem* (K. F. Burdach, 1819),[26] "cycloganglionic system" (S. Solly, 1836),[27] "plexu-ganglionic system" (de Chaumont, 1854),[28] "secretory and excito-secretory system" (Henry Fraser Campbell [1824–1891], 1857),[29] never received acceptance, and the same fate has befallen more recent suggestions, such as *Lebensnerven* and *Lebenstrieb* (L. R. Müller, 1924, 1931),[30] and *système nerveux organo-vegetatif* (A. C. Guillaume, 1925).[31] *Halosympathique,* coined by Maxime Paul Marie Laignel-Lavastine (1875–1953) in 1923, meaning the "whole" autonomic system has also disappeared.[32] Mercifully, his *orthosympathomimetique* (our sympathetic) and *parasympathomimetique* have not survived, although "orthosympathetic" (sympathetic outflow), as opposed to "parasympathetic," is still occasionally used and should have been adopted because throughout the nineteenth and well into the present century "sympathetic" nervous system was often used synonymously with "autonomic" nervous system, with obvious confusion resulting. Another extinct term that gained only local popularity was *Grenzstrang* ("boundary cord"), used for a while in the school of pharmacology at Vienna to describe the (ortho-) sympathetic nervous system and to stress its intermediate position between the cranial and sacral (parasympathetic) outflow.[33]

In 1807, J. C. Reil proposed a new term, *vegetative Nervensystem,* because it seemed that the system was chiefly concerned with the organs and functions of nutrition, known since the seventeenth century as vegetative.[34] "Vegetative nervous system" has survived to the present day, mainly in Continental countries and in the United States, but is rarely used in Britain.[35] Because it was introduced early in the nineteenth century and has remained in currency ever since, we shall use it below, together with "ganglionic nervous system," to signify the combined outflows of the autonomic nervous system, usually excluding the vagus, with the understanding that it is not always clear what parts the early nineteenth-century individuals included in it. There are similar problems with Winslow's *grand sympathique* preferred almost universally in nineteenth-century France, and *Intercostalis* and *Sympathiens* in the German literature. Although they usually excluded the vagus nerve, the cranial and sacral outflows were often included, but at the same time some tried to restrict it to our sympathetic component. Thus, certainty concerning meaning is at times impossible to achieve, although the context in which the term appears sometimes helps. *Systema nervorum sympathicum* was adopted for the *Basle Nomina Anatomica* (B.N.A.) in 1895 to signify the sympathetic part as distinct from the vagus, thus leading to even more confusion.[36]

The prolonged search for a universally acceptable terminology to suit the nonsomatic nervous system has been in part due to its own complexity and to the obscurity that has consequently surrounded it. But more particularly it has been caused by the difficulty of discovering terms that would satisfy the different specialists involved in its elucidation. Thus, the anatomist demanded a morphological nomenclature, whereas the physiologist naturally insisted on a functional one. Then, as more data concerning the system's embryology and pharmacology became available, previously accepted terms were found to be no longer appropriate, and the problem of replacing them with entirely suitable and acceptable ones became increasingly urgent.[37]

Along with "vegetative," there is today another survivor from the nineteenth century, "visceral." It had been applied by Johnstone in 1795 to ganglionic nerves, which he called "visceral" nerves,[38] but it did not become widely popular until Gaskell used it late in the nineteenth century. Thus, "visceral nervous system" came to mean the two outflows and to this Langley objected, pointing out that "visceral" could not possibly be used in the case of nerves to the skin. It was chiefly to replace it that in 1898 he suggested "autonomic":

> I propose to substitute the word "autonomic." The word implies a certain degree of independent action, but exercised under control of a higher power. The "autonomic" nervous system means the nervous system of the glands and of the involuntary muscles; it governs the "organic" functions of the body.[39]

It was derived from the Greek (*autos,* self; *nomos,* law) and was applied to the two outflows, including the vagus nerve and is now synonymous with vegetative and visceral. Since the turn of the nineteenth century it has remained the most popular term, in the English-speaking countries at least, and is now almost universal.[40] However, it is ironic that today the word that vies with it for popularity is "visceral," the very one it was introduced to replace. Although "visceral" is less often used to describe the whole system, it is commonly applied to its nerve fibers as, for example, "visceral efferents" instead of "autonomic efferents," which, however, has been recommended, and to "visceral" reflexes.[41] "Autonomic" was also introduced to counter another name used by Gaskell, "involuntary nervous system," but although used by Gaskell during the remainder of his life,[42] understandably it has not survived.

One of the obvious objections to "autonomic" was the implication it made of autonomy. *The New English Dictionary* defines it as "Of, pertaining to, or possessing, autonomy; self-governing, independent." An 1854 usage is cited: "Reason is thus ever autonomic; carrying its own law within itself."[43] It might, therefore, be assumed that the autonomic system had a high degree of independent action, and yet, as critics could point out, the research of Gaskell and Langley had been aimed specifically at proving the opposite, by showing that Bichat's theory of an independent ganglionic system was untenable and that there were close links between autonomic and somatic nervous elements. Langley accepted this objection to his term, which some years later he justified as follows:

> The word "autonomic" does suggest a much greater degree of independence of the central nervous system than in fact exists, except perhaps in that part which is in the walls of the alimentary canal. But it is, I think, more important that new words should be used for new ideas than that words should be accurately descriptive. In any case, the old terms have no advantage as descriptive terms.[44]

Having grouped the thoracolumbar and the craniosacral outflows together, Langley retained the old term "sympathetic" for the first of these, but he was in need of a new epithet for the second. In 1905 he proposed "parasympathetic," which was accepted with little dissent: "I use the word para-sympathetic for the cranial and sacral autonomic systems."[45] The controversy over nomenclature did not, however, subside entirely and investigators continued to criticize Langley's terms, but without proposing attractive replacements.[46] "Autonomic" has therefore survived, and despite the objections to it, should be retained even if only to honor the man from whose work so much of our present knowledge of this part of the nervous system has stemmed.[47] As an authoritative modern textbook states:

> The term "autonomic" is convenient rather than appropriate. The "autonomy" of this part of the nervous system is illusory. It is intimately responsive to changes in the somatic activities of the body, and while its connections with somatic elements are not always clear in anatomical terms, the physiological evidence of visceral reflex activities stimulated by somatic events is abundant.[48]

But in the discussions below it would be anachronistic to make use of "autonomic," because it was not invented until the end of the nineteenth century and has a specific meaning unknown to workers earlier in the century. Hence, our choice of "vegetative" and "ganglionic." "Sympathetic" will only be employed to designate the conglomeration of ganglia, plexuses, and nerves in the thoracic and abdominal cavities, that is, the sympathetic trunk or nerve that forms our thoracolumbar outflow.

7.4. BICHAT'S DOCTRINE

By the end of the eighteenth century a considerable amount of knowledge concerning the gross anatomy of the vegetative nervous system was available, as revealed by the impressive and detailed anatomical illustrations published at that time. There is, for example, an accurate depiction of the human sympathetic trunk and vagus nerve published by Johann Ernst Neubauer (1742–1777) in 1772,[49] and there are excellent copper plates of 1794 based upon the pen drawings of the cardiac nerves executed by the celebrated anatomist Antonio Scarpa.[50] Nevertheless, the majority of medical authors were tied to the distant past and still under the influence of Galen. Thus, Simon August André David Tissot (1728–1797), whose popular books had a wide circulation, in 1800 gave an account of the form and function of the rami communicantes that differed little from that of Galen, recorded almost exactly sixteen centuries earlier.[51] However, the improvements made in anatomy by Neubauer, Scarpa, and their contemporaries were not accompanied by a similar increase in knowledge of the functions of the vegetative system. This topic was shrouded in confusion, contradiction, and obscurity, owing to factors that also inhibited research on other parts of the nervous system. Ancient concepts were well entrenched and rarely contested, experimental techniques were imperfect, and there was a willingness, stemming from credulity and a paucity of critical powers, to accept conclusions based on only a small number of observations, whether experimental or clinical.

Opinion at the close of the eighteenth century held that the normal movements of the thoracic and abdominal organs were provoked by stimuli acting locally on their nerves, and that they could also be produced by reflected action through the vegetative ganglia. The role of the brain in these activities for which the system had responsibility was undecided, although it was clear that emotions presumably emanating from it influenced the functions of the viscera, and that stimulation of the medulla oblongata and occasionally of the cardiac nerves, also had an effect on them. Even this evidence had been denied. Little or nothing was known of the mechanism of blood flow or the production of secretions, but the brain seemed able to increase them. Healthy viscera gave rise to little or no sensation, whereas disease processes were able to produce acute pain, which could be referred to other parts of the body, thus providing an example of sympathy that was made possible (as Galen and Willis had suggested), by the "sympathetic" nerve, still known by some as the *intercostalis*. Most observers held that the latter arose not only from the spinal roots by way of the rami but also from cranial nerves and thus from the brain, according to the erroneous conclusion of Galen and Willis that was still widely accepted at the end of the eighteenth century, even though Pourfour du Petit in 1729 had demonstrated by experiment that it was fallacious.[52]

The *intercostalis* was known to supply viscera, glands, and blood vessels, but the viscera also received branches from the vagus nerve and apparently from the sacral somatic nerves that we now know belong, like the vagus, to the parasympathetic craniosacral outflow. Most accepted that nerves ran through the ganglia to other destinations or formed a kind of plexus in them, whereas others claimed that they were reorganized therein. They received additional nerve energy from the ganglia and from the latter new fibers arose. The idea that the central mechanism of the reflex lay in the ganglia, introduced in the eighteenth century, still held sway. As noted above, at the beginning of the nineteenth century the vagus nerve, although seeming to perform functions similar to those of the vegetative system, was not usually included in expressions like "vegetative," "organic," "ganglionic," or "sympathetic" nervous system, terms that, however, commonly included the two outflows.

In the absence of microscopical data, investigators could rely only on the gross features of the vegetative nervous system, and the most striking and intriguing were its ganglia. They had presented an enigma since Galen first described them and hazarded the opinion that they provided the nerves with a form of strengthening.[53] Before 1800 there were several further attempts to elucidate their function,[54] but we need discuss only the three that survived into the nineteenth century. The first was the oldest, having been conceived by Willis in 1664.[55] He believed that the ganglia and their nerves were merely an appendage of the cerebrospinal axis, stating that the vegetative system "grows like a bush upon another bush or tree."[56] He compared the ganglia to the knots in a tree trunk and ascribed to them the function of receiving the nerve "spirits," then thought to account for nerve conduction, and guiding their flow in various directions. This, he declared, was the mechanism that kept each part of the body in sympathy with all the others.

In 1749 the idea was adopted and extended by J. F. Meckel, the Elder, who speculated that ganglia were structures in which entering nerves could divide, thus allowing a wider distribution of them throughout the body as also happened in a plexus.[57] In addition they could change direction or unite with one another. Meckel had only gross anatomical evidence to sustain his opinion, but he claimed that the nerves leaving a ganglion were more than those entering it and thus that ganglia could generate fibers and the claim was substantiated by his son, J. F. Meckel, the Younger.[58] This was accepted by a sequence of distinguished anatomists, including Zinn, Haller, Johann Gottlob Haase (1739–1801), Scarpa, Johann Pfeffinger (1728–1782), Alexander Monro *secundus,* Blumenbach, and E. H. Weber.[59] In modern parlance the ganglion, therefore, resembled a railway marshaling yard. When the ganglion was investigated microscopically in the nineteenth century and the fibers better identified, it could be shown that Meckel's elaboration of Willis's assumption contained considerable truth. Willis, and those who followed him, thought that the nerves and ganglia of the vegetative system were of secondary importance to the brain and spinal cord. This downgrading was in sharp contrast to the theory Bichat advanced in 1800.

The second theory of ganglionic function was suggested by Winslow in 1732, when he introduced the term *sympathetic* nerve. He too believed that the system explained the phenomenon of sympathy, but in addition he asserted that the ganglia were small brains serving as sources of nervous power and thereby having some degree of independence from the cerebrospinal system.[60] It, too, still received attention at the beginning of the nineteenth century, usually combined with the first theory.

The third attempt to explain the function of the ganglia was the most influential of the three in the early nineteenth century. It was proposed by Johnstone in 1771[61] and will be discussed in detail later. Briefly, he accepted Winslow's concept of the ganglion as a small brain, but in his view it also functioned as a selective filter, as we might interpret it. It prevented the passage of motor signals that reached it from the brain, and thus accounted for the lack of voluntary control over visceral and other vegetative functions. In health it also blocked sensory messages from the viscera so that they could not reach the brain and therefore consciousness. In the presence of disease, however, pain could achieve this journey because of a change in the ganglion's discriminatory powers. Johnstone also subscribed to Meckel's idea of the ganglia serving as places for the realignment of nerves or fibers.

Each of the three theories found its advocates in the first few decades of the nineteenth century. Moreover, certain elements from them were incorporated into a new doctrine that was to dominate research into the vegetative system for decades. This was the scheme put forward by Bichat at the turn of the century, proclaiming the complete independence of this system from the cerebrospinal and its ability to produce and dispense its own nervous power. Thus the turn of the nineteenth century saw the opening of a new chapter in the history of the vegetative nervous system, due entirely to Bichat, whose opinions are to be found in three treatises published in 1800,[62] 1801,[63] and 1801–1803;[64] he died in 1802 before the last of these had been completed. By means of them, together with further editions and translations, Bichat's works had immense influence, for among other contributions, they established his ganglionic nervous system which was not entirely rejected until the 1880s.[65]

First, Bichat created a basic physiological system founded on three tenets: (1) fundamentally, life could be characterized as resistance to death, that is, opposition to decomposition; (2) life was made up of two components, animal (somatic) and organic (vegetative); (3) tissues had two vital properties, sensibility and contractility (the Hallerian doctrine). It is the second that concerns us here: Bichat's *vie animale,* or *vie de la relation,* and his *vie organique* or *vie de la nutrition.*[66] The notion of the body having two kinds of life, animal and organic, which survives in modern ideas of cerebrospinal and autonomic functions, was by no means new for its roots lie in Greek antiquity. Living beings were seen to have two main groups of functions: those related to the maintenance and preservation of their individual existence and to the reproduction of their species; and those that brought them into relation with the external world, so that natural phenomena, together with the laws governing them, could be recognized, understood and, if necessary for protection, could be avoided. Aristotle was well aware of this distinction between vital and animal functions, and Galen derived from it the vital and animal "spirits" that were the regulating powers in his general concept of bodily activity.[67] In the eighteenth century this ancient doctrine was still widely accepted, and we need only mention two expressions of it, by Frenchmen who are known to have influenced Bichat and in whose writings lie the germs of the system he created. Théophile de Bordeu (1722–1776) in his book of 1751 on glandular secretion, spoke of intermediate forms of life between plants and animals. These he termed *végétaux animalisés,*[68] and he asked:

> Must it not be admitted that in the more perfect animals there are certain parts that approach the vegetable kingdom more closely than others? Should it not be found that there may be intermediaries between the two kingdoms? Thus an animal is composed of different parts, each of which belongs to a different kingdom of nature.[69]

Bichat's idea of animal and vegetative life within the same organism is here clearly foreshadowed. More immediately, Bichat had been influenced by Jean Charles Marguerite Guillaume de Grimaud (1750–1789) of Montpellier, who in 1787 had also proposed that the body possessed two types of function:

> I shall divide the functions into two classes; I shall consider them to be internal and external.
>
> The internal functions are accomplished in the interior of the living being, and they relate to the body in an exclusive manner. By means of the

> exterior functions the animal can extend outside of itself; it expands and enlarges its existence, and it entertains interest in, and sorts out, the objects that surround it; it studies these objects, it judges their qualities according to ideas [established] prior to all tuition, in spite of what most Philosophers of this century say, and by its *locomotive* faculty, it approaches some and withdraws from others.[70]

Bichat accepted the existence of two distinct and separate lives in the organism, and then enlarged the theme more than anyone before him. He was a master at deriving general principles from a mass of anatomical, physiological, and clinical data collected by means of dissections, animal experiments, and hospital practice, and then organizing them into systems. He depended primarily upon "the living books, the sick and the dead," rather than entirely upon the many volumes available to him in the libraries of Paris.[71] His aim was to carry out an orderly analysis of the body's vital functions. The "animal" or "animalic" life (*vie animale* or *vie de la relation*) resided in the parts of the body that permitted the individual to react and relate to its external environment and thus to the world at large. It was intermittent because it ceased with sleep; it was affected by experience, practice, and habit. The brain was its central organ. Its basic activities were concerned with sensory perception and motor responses, but it also had to do with understanding and will. "Organic" or "vegetative" life (*vie organique* or *vie de la nutrition*), however, was contained within the individual's internal world. It was concerned with metabolic and catabolic processes; in other words, with "assimilative" activities, involving digestion, absorption, and so forth; and with "dissimilative" activities, comprising the opposites, such as decomposition, distribution, and excretion. It was continuous, it was not influenced by habit, but it responded to the emotions. The heart was its central organ. The various opposing properties of these two inherent lives of the body are shown in table 1. Next, taking further inspiration from Isaac Newton's ability to delineate the basic properties of the physical world, Bichat related tissue propensities to the two kinds of life, and thereby created a doctrine of properties that was basic to his system of physiology.

Of equal importance were the associations Bichat made between the animal and organic lives and the nervous system. Whereas the ancients, in particular Galen, had allocated the power that regulated and presided over the two lives to "spirits," Bichat claimed that it was dependent upon the nervous system. This led him to equate the two classes of life with the two apparently separate nervous systems: animal life in the cerebrospinal system and organic life in the vegetative. He was, therefore, the

TABLE 1
BICHAT'S SYSTEM

Principal features	*Organic life and ganglionic system*	*Animal life and cerebrospinal system*
Purpose	Inner life: heart, lungs, intestines, etc.	Externally directed body activities
Associated with	Circulation, respiration, digestion, secretion: i.e., anabolism and catabolism	Volition and sensations from external world
Action	Continuous	Intermittent
Structure of parts innervated	Asymmetrical, disharmonious, centrally placed	Symmetrical, harmonious, peripherally placed
Principal center(s)	Multiple. Ganglia, especially in epigastrium	Single. Brain
Habit and education	Independent of them	Formed by them
Will or intellect	Independent of them	Controlled by them
Passions	Influenced by them	Not influenced by them
Consciousness	Absent	Present
Existence	Terminates with death of heart	Terminates with death of brain and dies before many organs

first to establish the association of vegetative nerves with the metabolic functions of the body. The most important feature of his scheme was the strict independence of the two, so that the brain, spinal cord, and somatic nerves on the one hand, and the ganglia with their vegetative nerves and ganglia on the other, functioned autonomously, each with its own source of nervous power.[72] The two systems are contrasted in table 1.

Concerning its anatomical features, the ganglionic nervous system was composed of structurally distinct units, the ganglia. Those on the cranial nerves (ciliary, sphenopalatine, submandibular, and otic) were homologues of the ones of the thoraco-abdominal cavity. From the ganglia arose nerve fibers, the analogues of the cerebrospinal nerves. Here Bichat was merely accepting the opinions of many of his predecessors,[73] but in view of the fact that more fibers left than entered a ganglia, it followed that it could generate them, just like the brain and spinal cord, a property that obviously further established the autonomy of the ganglionic system.[74] The sympathetic trunk was equivalent to the spinal cord, and the celiac ganglion to the brain, which had already been called by some the *cerebrum abdominale*.[75] Bichat described his system thus:

> Now the nerves of the ganglia cannot transmit the activity of the brain, for we have seen that the nervous system derived from these bodies must be considered as entirely independent of the cerebral nervous system; that the great sympathetic [nerve] does not at all take its origin from the brain, the spinal cord or from the nerves of animal [somatic] life; that its origin is in the ganglia exclusively; that this nerve indeed does not exist at all, properly speaking, and that it is only an aggregate of as many little nervous systems as there are ganglia, which are the special centers of organic life, analogous to the great brain and unique center of animal life, which is the brain.[76]

His assertion that the ganglia of the sympathetic nerve represented small nervous systems echoes Winslow's view that the ganglia were small brains but, in addition, the sentence in which he made this comment is reminiscent of that of Johnstone, when the latter claimed that the sympathetic nerves, "truly derived from the spinal marrow have in their numerous Ganglions proper to them, so [as] many receptacles of nervous energy, so [as there are] many subordinate Brains."[77] This aspect of Bichat's scheme will be discussed later, but it should be noted here that the concept of ganglia acting as independent sources of nervous energy, and thus equivalent to the brain, was central to his theory.

Nevertheless, the two systems of life were thought not to be completely separate and distinct, and this was also an essential part of his theory, created presumably to account for the effects of emotions on the viscera and for involuntary movements of voluntary muscles and vice versa. Concerning the two systems, he stated:

> Each is not at all confined strictly to the organs belonging to one or other of the lifes. Thus the nerves of the brain send several prolongations into the glands, into the [involuntary] muscles, etc.; likewise, the ganglionic nervous system has several branches to the voluntary muscles.[78]

This feature of his doctrine is usually overlooked, but it is difficult to justify it in view of the fact that Bichat elsewhere claimed total independence for his system. Presumably it did not (in his own eyes) necessarily undermine his main thesis of an autonomous system. Whatever the explanation for it, concerning the muscles Bichat was merely repeating what S. T. Soemmerring had declared in 1798:

> not only the muscles of spontaneous [involuntary] movements, but also the muscles that are purely voluntary such, for example, as those of the arms and feet, receive nerve fibers from the ganglia.[79]

In other respects, Soemmerring, like most anatomists of the time, accepted and reiterated the opinions of Johnstone.

But if the ganglionic nervous system was relatively morphologically distinct from and physiologically independent of the brain and spinal cord, what about the rami communicantes that ran between the spinal roots and the vegetative ganglia and seemed to link them, as Willis had remarked long ago? They surely indicated that it had a spinal cord and, therefore, presumably a cerebral origin.

As we have seen, they had been described by Galen as well as by Willis and their division into white and gray was reported in 1749 by Meckel, the Elder,[80] who had noted that some were white whereas others were redder and softer, and these were later termed gray. In 1743 Winslow had given the following somewhat erroneous account: "The ganglia connect posteriorly with the ganglia of the spinal cord by means of quite short collateral threads."[81] However, their functional significance had never been established, and in fact they remained an enigma to some extent until Gaskell's work during the 1880s. In the absence of histological data, Bichat was at liberty to deny that they represented true functional pathways. According to him they were only anastomoses, or a series of nervous links that merely joined the two systems together structurally, but not necessarily functionally. The same argument was mounted to account for the decussation of the pyramids in the medulla oblongata, when Gall, among others, described it.[82] Certainly the two sides of the cord were connected for this could not be denied, but to claim that nervous energy could therefore cross over in the links did not follow. In the same way, Bichat maintained that the rami did not convey nervous power from the cerebrospinal system to the ganglia, as some before him had contended.[83] Again, it is to be noted that no microscopical evidence was available for the defense or refutal of either of these hypotheses. On the whole, however, Bichat's elucidation of the rami remained the weakest part of his scheme, and one of his German followers, J. C. Reil, had to elaborate further their function, as we shall see later.

A link between the sympathetic trunk and the cerebrospinal system cephalad to the rami, that is, with the brain by way of cranial nerve connections, was still accepted by some, but it offered no difficulty to Bichat. He could cite Pourfour du Petit who in 1729 had correctly disproved its existence (n. 52 above).[84] Bichat's denial of an association between the ganglionic and cerebrospinal nervous centers by means of rami or cranial nerves allowed him to make the claim (nn. 76, 92) that the sympathetic nerve was not a nerve as such and in fact did not exist. Thus, the ganglionic system was functionally, as well as morphologically, autonomous. Taking into account the data that was available to him, Bichat's brilliant concept would seem to be both attractive and acceptable. He was able to muster additional proof, as he thought, that the sympathetic trunk was a series of independent ganglia linked together and not a nerve at all in the usual sense of the term.[85] He pointed out that although gaps in the rami were occasionally encountered, for example, at the lower thoracic and upper lumbar levels, the organs usually supplied by those missing appeared to suffer no inconvenience. He could therefore argue that connections between the ganglionic and cerebrospinal systems were not essential as functional pathways. Anatomists, however, were able to deny this claim, and those who did so included E. H. Weber,[86] Baron Antoine Portal,[87] and also J.G.C.F.M. Lobstein,[88] who, as we shall see, made an important contribution to our theme in his treatise of 1823 which received considerable acclaim. They declared never to have seen such gaps, although they admitted that on superficial examination an interruption might occasionally appear to exist.

Further evidence favoring Bichat's contention of an isolated ganglionic system came from the observation that the ciliary and sphenopalatine ganglia were always found in an isolated state, with communicating branches going to the cranial nerves only. Also, in birds the superior cervical ganglion was always isolated and it never communicated with the inferior. As Bichat admitted, this latter evidence came from Cuvier, who had declared: "No trace of the great sympathetic nerve can be found in the necks of birds."[89] This statement, however, was subsequently refuted by a number of anatomists.[90] Another comment made by Cuvier must also have been helpful to Bichat as he accumulated evidence in support of his assertions that the so-called sympathetic nerve was not a nerve. In the first place the rami were not its roots of origin, and second it did not arise from the brain like a cranial nerve. Cuvier announced that "this [sympathetic] nerve can in no way be considered to issue from the brain,"[91] and that it only "communicated" with cranial and spinal nerves, thus putting the stamp of authority on Pourfour du Petit's perceptive observation of 1729 and further consolidating Bichat's position.

Concerning the sympathetic chain and his system Bichat could now summarize his opinions:

> These diverse considerations make very probable the opinion I have held for some time, that the great sympathetic nerve does not really exist at all, that the cord it presents is only a series of communications between small nervous systems [ganglia], arranged one above the other, and that these communica-

> tions are only accessory and perhaps need not exist . . . I began to consider each ganglion as the specific center of a small nervous system, quite different from the brain and quite distinct from the small nervous systems of other ganglia. On considering the functions of the nerves issuing from these centers, I am more and more convinced that in no way do they belong to the cerebral system.[92]

The nerves of the ganglionic system mediated organic functions, but the precise nature of the latter and how they were brought about remained a mystery. Bichat's final view on this point was fully justified in the light of the limited knowledge available in 1801. It is to his credit that he admitted ignorance and did not spin webs of hypotheses, as many did at that time in a futile attempt to answer questions that for the moment were unanswerable. The following statement represents an accurate assessment of the situation in the year before his death: "But whilst recognizing the functions they do not perform, we are ignorant of those for which they are actually destined."[93] Three decades later Charles Bell described the same state of affairs, and it is of some interest that his pronouncement was curiously similar to the one made by Bichat. Writing of the sympathetic trunk, he stated: "In short, we only know what the sympathetic is not; and by that means we are left to conjecture what really are its functions."[94] Thus, there was, he stated, no evidence to suggest that it was a nerve of the emotions or that it had control over voluntary motions. There was likewise nothing to indicate that it possessed sensibility, because as we shall see this possibility had been ruled out by experiments. It is revealing to observe that in 1829 one of Britain's most outstanding scientists knew of no irrefutable evidence that could elucidate the precise functions of the vegetative nervous system.

7.5. THE ORIGINS OF BICHAT'S DOCTRINE. JOHNSTONE'S SYSTEM

Bichat's role, like that of any genius, was to amass evidence to establish a completely new concept, in this case his revolutionary view of the two nervous systems. Much of the evidence came, as we have seen, from his own observations and reasoning, but an equal amount derived from the ideas of others, and some of these have been mentioned above. His doctrine, therefore, in part reflected the views of earlier investigators, and we can now consider in more detail the apparent influence on him of three of them: Winslow, Johnstone, and Cuvier.

Winslow. In 1732, Winslow stated that the ganglia characterizing the nerve to which he had given the name of great sympathetic represented "so many little brains."[95] As this nerve did not descend from the cranial cavity and as it appeared to be essentially a product of its ganglia, Winslow argued that it was an independent structure, even though he had entertained the possibility of it having a spinal cord origin by way of the rami communicantes.[96] Here then were the basic requirements for an autonomous, self-powered ganglionic nervous system.

Johnstone. Johnstone's influence on Bichat, however, seems to have been greater than that of Winslow. Johnstone had much the same opinion regarding the ganglia as Winslow, for he declared that they were analogous to the brain itself: they were "subordinate springs and reservoirs of nervous power,"[97] comments reminiscent of Bichat's. But, unlike the latter, he believed that the ganglia were in contact with the spinal cord and thus with the brain.[98] Johnstone also subscribed to Willis's view that the multifarious phenomena of sympathy were made possible by means of contacts made in the ganglia. Johnstone was supported in this notion of the ganglia being subsidiary centers of nervous energy by Alexander Monro *secundus,* who in 1783 offered an explanation of how they acquired and dispensed it. Meckel the Elder had noted that the nerves issuing from a ganglion were bulkier than those that entered,[99] and Monro suggested that this was due to the addition of nervous matter to the nerve as it passed through the ganglion:

> We shall more readily receive the opinion that the ganglia are additional sources of nervous energy, if we are persuaded, from what has been before observed, that every nerve, is in its course [through a ganglion], covered with cineritious [gray] matter, from which energy is added to it.[100]

In addition they "seem to receive new energy from the vascular matter of the ganglion."[101] The significance of this hypothesis relates not only to Bichat's ganglionic system, but also to Gall's proposal that cerebrospinal nerves received additional nerve energy by traversing gray matter (chap. 2.4). The occurrence of gray matter in the ganglia had been agreed by Winslow in 1732, and was still accepted by Charles Bell a century later,[102] but on macroscopical grounds only. We have already discussed the way in which this macroscopical concept was transposed to the microscopical level by Purkyně (chap. 3.4).

Johnstone also included the spinal root ganglia in his ganglionic system, and their function was to control involuntary movements of the voluntary musculature, such as tremor, spasms, and the like, just as the nerves of the vegetative ganglia were thought by him to control involuntary movements of the vital organs. We have already observed that Soemmerring and Bichat also sought to explain these movements. Johnstone's was a particularly ingenious proposal, and, in the light of contemporary knowledge, quite acceptable. According to him, although the ganglionic system was linked to the cerebrospinal, it retained a degree of independence so that its organs could still function when their connections with it were severed.[103] The ganglia had the task of converting voluntary motor messages into involuntary messages, and brief mention has already been made of this selective filtering mechanism. It proved to be one of the most adroit features of his scheme and one that survived well into the nineteenth century. Voluntary motor messages from the brain to the viscera were rendered involuntary, uniform, and unconscious by the nervous matter generated by the ganglion, and they were filtered off, thus preventing the will from reaching and affecting the vital organs, in particular the heart and the intestines.[104] This is how Johnstone in 1771 described the benefits deriving from such a resourceful arrangement:

> In a word, *Ganglions* limit the exercise of the soul's authority in the animal economy; and put it out of our power by a single *volition* to stop the motions of our heart, and in one capricious instant irrevocably to end our lives.[105]

In 1795 he gave his final account of how the ganglia functioned. He knew that in the cerebrospinal system the somatic nerves from different parts of the body were brought together in plexuses for the purpose of voluntary movements. However:

> The ganglions, on the contrary, are organized for the purpose of separating from the power of volition, all the organs, moved by stimuli, acting on irritable parts. –The heart, –the intestines, –the abdominal viscera and glands in general,—the *Fallopian* tubes, and uterus—the iris.[106]

He made no provision for sympathetic associations.

Subsequently there were many references to Johnstone's highly original contribution to ganglionic function, but often no allusion was made to the man who had devised it, as he himself complained: "My opinion has been silently attacked, and as silently adopted, without any explicit acknowledgement of the author, or, any direct quotation from his work."[107] This was the case with one of Bichat's contemporaries, the celebrated French physiologist Anthelme Balthasar Richerand (1779–1851), who failed to cite Johnstone by name in an authoritative and popular textbook of physiology,[108] by means of which his opinions were widely disseminated.[109] In the third edition of 1804 he approved of Bichat's system,[110] but claimed priority for some of his ideas, which he said he had published in 1799.[111] But similarly he made no reference to Bichat by name, and in any case his claim is untenable. Richerand believed that the ganglionic system connected together all the organs concerned with the assimilation of food, by withdrawing these vital activities: "from the influence of volition, which is such a fickle and variable faculty of the mind that life at each instant would be exposed to great dangers if it was in our power to stop or interrupt the exercise of functions to which existence is absolutely linked."[112] This seems to have been taken directly from Johnstone's writings, (see e.g., n. 105 above), but no reference was made to him. It appeared in succeeding editions and was transmitted by other authors.

As in the case of much of Bichat's system, Johnstone's speculation was a simple and easily comprehended explanation of a mysterious process that made possible the separation of voluntary from involuntary motion. But some of its popularity may have been due to its additional theological appeal, for as Johnstone himself pointed out, the remarkable arrangement that he had proposed was clear proof of God's mercy and unerring wisdom in providing man with an inbuilt mechanism necessary for his preservation. Johnstone's idea of a method whereby the body's essential and vital activities could be safeguarded was also referred to in later nineteenth-century physiological literature. Thus, Claude Bernard in his celebrated book on experimental science cited "a philosophical physiologist," who had pointed out that in the case of circulation, secretion, digestion, and so forth "nature had prudently wished to screen these important phenomena from the caprices of an ignorant will."[113] Again, Johnstone received no credit, except that he was designated a "philosophical physiologist," and modern writers who have quoted from Bernard, likewise do not identify him.[114]

This interpretation, however, dealt only with the motor messages from the brain. What about the sensory impressions that arrived at the ganglia from the organs? Here Johnstone provided an equally subtle elucidation. It was a matter of common observation that in the healthy state sensations from the viscera were few, vaguely localizable, and never of a prominent intensity. The reason for this, Johnstone maintained, was because the ganglia were again acting as filters, as we may phrase it, by preventing entering sensations from reaching the *sensorium commune*, or as we would express it, consciousness. In the presence of disease of the organs, however, the ganglionic filters allowed sensory messages to pass and so reach the brain, there to be registered as pain.

The presumption that the ganglia were able to produce new nerves was a vitally important factor for the assumed independence of the ganglionic system, and J. F. Meckel the Elder, as already noted, and others had argued that this must take place, in view of the fact that often more nerves left a ganglion than entered it.[115] Johnstone agreed with his predecessors, such as Giovanni Battista Morgagni (1682–1771), that the ganglia consisted of "a mixture of cortical and medullary substance nourished by small blood vessels,"[116] an opinion that he had deduced from gross anatomical examination, analogy with the brain and spinal cord, and from speculation. By means of these constituents the ganglia were able to produce new fibers and so to create their own nerves and plexuses, an ability that confirmed their autonomous separation from the brain and spinal cord. But it seems that Johnstone assented only partly to this latter proposal, because he maintained that nerves from the brain and cord supplied the heart and intestines, which could survive for a while after these nerves were cut.[117] We shall see that the ability of the ganglia to "generate" new fibers was confirmed by Remak and by others on the basis of microscopical observations, so that the early gross anatomists were proved correct (see 7.7.5).

There is no doubt that Johnstone had a wide following, and his scheme received frequent mention in the literature of the late eighteenth and early nineteenth century, even if at times anonymously. In particular, Alexander Monro *secundus,* while expressing doubt concerning part of Johnstone's scheme, agreed with him that the ganglia acted as subsidiary sources of nervous energy. The widely influential Tissot also accepted Johnstone's thesis, although he did accuse him of laying little emphasis on facts that conflicted with it.[118] But the man who at the time was said to have afforded him the strongest support was Jean Frédéric Lobstein (1736–1784), the Elder, whose evidence had come from meticulous dissections reported in 1760.[119]

Cuvier. The third person who exercised a significant influence on Bichat was his illustrious contemporary Cuvier, to whom reference has already been made. In the first lecture of his celebrated course on comparative anatomy given in 1795,[120] he discussed the animal and vital functions of the organism, finding the brain responsible for its ability to avoid deleterious influences. He continued:

> These actions of the nervous system are dependent upon the numerous communications that special nerves called *sympathetics* establish between the various ramifications of the body (*tronc générale*) and by means of which impressions are transmitted more rapidly than by the brain. These nodes, that have the name of *ganglions* when they are of considerable size are a kind of secondary brain, and it can be observed that they are larger and more numerous in the same proportion as the main brain is smaller in size.[121]

As in the case cited above, there can be no doubt that Bichat was well aware of Cuvier's opinions, which, unlike those of many of his predecessors, were founded on a vast number of animal dissections, just as Bichat had derived his from an extensive series of human dissections, autopsies, and physiological experiments. It is clear, however, that Cuvier was mostly supporting existing notions, and it cannot be said that he expoused the theory of an independent ganglionic system as has been suggested.[122] Nevertheless, his comments, made before Bichat published his system, must have had an effect.

Of these three sources of influence, the most significant seems to have been that of Johnstone. His views were based on anatomical, clinical, and experimental observations, and their importance warrants the prominence we have given them. Not only were they of consequence in the discussion of Bichat's writings, in which incidentally no reference seems to have been made to Johnstone, but also in their own right. Thus they were accepted until almost the middle of the nineteenth century, mainly on account of their simplicity, coherence, and basis of common sense. Some in Britain, however, judged that Bichat had appropriated Johnstone's opinion without acknowledgment.[123] As we have seen, there were indeed similarities, but a charge of plagiarism would be as unwarranted as one arising from Johnstone's own use of earlier notions. Each of these two authors added something significantly new to the body of ideas that he inherited from his predecessors.

7.6. THE RECEPTION OF BICHAT'S SYSTEM

Bichat was in no doubt about the important role played by his ganglionic nervous system in the physiology of the organism. Nor did he overlook how limited contemporary knowledge of it was:

> Let us remark in concluding this system that there is nothing more deserving of the attention of physiologists. All the others present a series of phenomena already well-known. In this one we have hardly perceived anything.[124]

Like any substantial theory, it presented medical science with a new field of research, but unfortunately Bichat died in 1802, soon after announcing it. It was left to his successors to establish it more securely and to extend it.

On the whole it won immediate and wide approval. One of its main attractions must have been the use it made of a simple and tidy division of the numerous and complex bodily phenomena into two kinds of life belonging to two distinct and independent nervous systems. It seemed to alleviate much of the current confusion due to conflicting theories and contradictory observations, and it promised a degree of order instead of the chaos arising from the rapidly accumulating mass of data concerning the nervous system. Moreover, Bichat advanced his doctrine with compelling logic and a masterly presentation. But, the premature demise of a remarkable young genius destined for an outstandingly brilliant career and assured of a prominent place in the ranks of French medical savants may have been an additional attraction for the pious, who were mindful of the regrettable loss suffered by science.

Among the many prominent medical scientists who accepted Bichat's views was Reil, who became one of his most influential supporters and in 1807 published an important paper purporting to improve the system, and in which he introduced the term "vegetative nervous system."[125] In particular, Reil tackled the vital problem of the anatomical links between the cerebrospinal and ganglionic systems provided by the rami. Bichat had recognized the problem they posed to his attempts to establish the ganglionic system as an autonomous unit, but he had not probed them deeply. His only argument was to admit that they existed as structural links, but to deny the possibility of them being functional connections. Johnstone had faced the same enigma long before. Reil now took up the task, and he asserted that each ramus acted like a semi- or part-conductor appliance (*Apparat der Halbleitung*),[126] thus resembling in modern terms an electrical "make-and-break" key between the circuits of the ganglionic and the cerebrospinal system:[127]

> I call the semi-conductor a nervous appliance, which under certain circumstances and in normal conditions is an isolator, but under different circumstances can be a conductor.[128]

Normally it prevented transmission of messages, but in an abnormal state it became a transmitter. For example, in health sensory impressions from the intestines were prevented from reaching consciousness, but disease allowed this transfer by increasing the conductivity of the rami, thus permitting sensations to reach the brain and to enter the realm of consciousness.[129] Thus, basically the *Apparat der Halbleitung*, situated as it was between the cerebrospinal and vegetative systems, was "a functional isolator, which, under abnormal circumstances, is a conductor and can connect the vegetative with the animal sphere."[130] In reality, this was merely a more technical and therefore more modern version of Johnstone's original idea for ganglionic action now applied to the rami. Extending his electrical analogy, Reil stated that the ganglia were not the origins of the nerves, but simply semiconductors, and able selectively to enforce obstruction to traffic through them. This was also the role of the spinal root ganglia:

> Moreover, the ganglia that isolate a certain part [of the body] are numerous, and, in addition, this part is cut off from the brain's influence. A cut nerve regenerates with the restoration of movement, but not the consciousness of sensation, because it possesses a ganglion, which acts as a semiconductor.[131]

Reil was again following Johnstone, who also attributed this intervention to the spinal ganglia, claiming them to be "the first checks to the usual powers of Volition."[132]

Reil's general concepts were as follows. The vegetative nervous system was completely different from the cerebrospinal, for it belonged only to the organs and functions of nutrition. It presided over this activity alone, and by its influence the materials dissipated or consumed by the processes of life were reproduced.[133] It could, therefore, be considered as a truly "vegetative" function. From this belief arose the name that he gave to the system:[134]

> By means of the vegetative apparatus (*Apparat der Vegetation*), the ganglionic system gives the parts their vitality, and at the same time it is the means by which the dispersed and isolated organs are brought together into a dynamic whole.[135]

Reil was also referring here to the Willisian notion of sympathy, expressed here more in the form of what was to be known as integration later in the century.

Reil agreed with Bichat that in the lower orders of animals only the vegetative system existed.[136] In higher species it was intimately connected with the cerebrospinal system, but, nevertheless, was independent of it. There was no way by which it could develop embryologically from the brain and spinal cord, nor could it originate from it by means of nerve fibers. The two systems had several differences, one of the most significant being that in the case of the cerebrospinal, the nerves coursed toward the brain in which they terminated and it was therefore the system's central organ. In contrast, the ganglia formed no similar single focus of action, for they were widely dispersed.

Basically, the sympathetic trunk first ensured that the power of volition over the internal organs could be diminished, as Johnstone had originally proposed. Second, it restrained within their proper sphere the sensory impressions that were constantly produced by vital processes in the healthy organs, so that they could not be transmitted to the brain, again in keeping with Johnstone. Had the cardiac nerves been allowed to proceed directly from the cranial or spinal nerves to the heart, and there were no cervical or thoracic ganglia intervening, the heart would be under the power of the will, just like the voluntary muscles of the body. Again, if nature had placed no ganglia between the abdominal plexus of vegetative nerves and the cord, the irritation that food might excite in the intestinal tract would be carried to the brain. In the case of the cerebrospinal nervous system, determinations of the will were usually transmitted to the *sensorium*. In the ganglionic system, on the other hand, the nervous energy was developed slowly by an obscure process and only in disease were sensory impressions from the viscera transmitted to the brain, with the rami taking part in this process.[137] Reil also dealt with the role of the ganglionic system in sleep and in certain diseases.[138] In summary, from a survey of his proposals, it seems that Reil was elaborating, and making more scientific, the concepts of Johnstone, rather than those of Bichat!

These opinions of Reil, which defended Bichat's system by grafting onto it an electrical analogue of Johnstone's concept of the ganglionic filter in order to strengthen its weakest part, received approbation from Karl Wilhelm Wutzer (1789–1863), along with some censures.[139] He agreed with Winslow that the ganglia were independent nervous centers, and he endeavored to support with new arguments and experiments this idea that was central to Bichat's concept of an autonomous ganglionic center. Like Johnstone, Wutzer believed that the ganglia diminished and impaired the action of the brain and spinal cord on the ganglionic system, and under certain conditions destroyed it altogether. In the same way they interrupted the transmission of sensation from the vegetative to the animal sphere. But, as we can now judge, none of Wutzer's contentions was new; he was merely attempting to substantiate speculations that had been absorbed into Bichat's system, but he was not extending it by original contributions. He did not accept that the ganglia were structurally distinct units from which new fibers could originate independently of the cerebrospinal system.[140] His *Habilitationsschrift* of 1817 is nevertheless a valuable source of evidence supporting Bichat, although its greatest value to us lies in the historical introduction.

A more critical appraisal of Bichat's system was made by Gall. His opinion on whether it was independent of the brain and spinal cord appeared in his report to the Académie des Sciences in Paris, submitted on 14 March 1808 (see chaps. 2.1 and 6.3.7). In it he stated:

> Although we consider all the nerves, not only those of organic life along with Bichat, but also those of animal life, as so many independent systems, there are however many communications between them. The systems of organic life sometimes actually appear to be in absolute isolation; however, in keeping with the customary laws, they turn out to be intimately connected together by means of anastomoses. Similarly, all organic life is in reciprocal connection with animal life by means of communicating branches: of the spinal cord [rami]; of the vagi, and glossopharyngeal nerves; [and] of the fifth and sixth pairs [trigeminal and abducens cranial nerves], which run to the intercostal [sympathetic] nerve.[141]

In 1810 the first volume of the monumental treatise on Gall's theory of organology and its anatomical basis appeared, and it is noteworthy that its opening chapter dealt with the ganglionic nervous system.[142] It was entitled "On the intercostal nerve or the great sympathetic nerve," indicating that the former term was still in current use; it probably included both autonomic outflows, but not the vagus. The reason they gave for beginning with this topic is also of interest, for they stated that they wished to proceed "from the simple to the complicated."[143] Gall was evoking here an important principle, the so-called "genetic" approach of Henle (see chap. 1.2.3). This was the method of proceeding from the simple or lower neural system to the more complex or higher. Gall considered the vegetative ganglia as the "preparatory apparatus" for the spinal cord, and their morphology was "simple" or "primitive" because they represented an earlier stage in the evolution of the more complicated or "higher" cord (see chap. 2.4). Gall's procedure of going from the simple to the more complex nervous system morphology has been discussed in chapter 2.1,3,4.

Gall did not, however, agree with the widely accepted belief that the ganglionic system could diminish the influence of the brain by obstructing the operation of the will, or that the size of the ganglia necessarily indicated their independence. His conclusion was as follows:

> These observations suffice also to prove that the division of the nervous system into a system of the brain and one of the ganglia made by Bichat and Reil, to which Bichat adds the ganglia of the spinal cord and the head, not only does not establish a precise difference [between the two], but [proves] that still less is it founded on physiological considerations.[144]

On the whole Gall found himself more in agreement with Bichat than opposed to him, but had no additions or modifications of note to propose.

The British physiologist, Wilson Philip, was also skeptical of the ganglionic system as enunciated by Bichat, Reil, Wutzer, and others. Basically, he contested the concept of its autonomy, and instead believed that it was, in fact, secondary to the cerebrospinal axis. He was, therefore, in a direct line of descent from Willis, who had judged the ganglia and their nerves to be appendages of the brain and spinal cord, a notion that had received considerable support when associated with his idea that sympathy operated through them. The ganglionic system could not, Wilson Philip declared, be independent and of equal ranking with the cerebrospinal, as Bichat had maintained. In this view, he had been preceded in the nineteenth century by François Chaussier (1746–1828) and Legallois.

In 1807 Chaussier had accepted Willis's concept of the intercostal nerve and ganglia, his "nerf trisplanchnique."[145] Legallois in 1812 thought similarly and had carried out extensive experimental research on the physiology of the spinal cord, especially its effect on the circulation of the blood. He did not investigate the ganglionic system primarily, but he concluded that:

> It is from the great sympathetic [nerve] that the heart receives its principal nerve fibers, and it is solely by this nerve that it can derive its powers from all parts of the spinal cord. The great sympathetic must therefore have its roots in this cord.[146]

Presumably he was referring to the sympathetic trunk only, excluding the vagus. Legallois also emphasized the new and powerful role for physiology in solving the questions concerning the origin of the trunk when he stated that: "all the questions, I say, insoluble until now by means of anatomy are completely resolved by the experimental approach, and it is demonstrated at the same time that the ganglia can no longer be compared with little brains."[147] The last statement was of considerable significance, because here in 1812 was experimental evidence refuting Winslow's concept of 1732. According to Legallois, the spinal cord belonged to both animal and vegetative life, but the truth of this view was not revealed until much later in the century. He was directly opposing Bichat's scheme of an independent ganglionic system, but his defiance seems to have had a negligible effect, and subsequent writers made little reference to his findings. Another of his conclusions, which opposed the venerated view of Haller that the heartbeat was dependent solely on its muscular irritability, was that the state of the spinal cord also played a role, and later this revolutionary idea became part of the neurogenic theory of cardiac action.

Wilson Philip's basic thesis was similar:

> Thus the sympathetic nerves, conveying the influence of the spinal marrow, and the *par vagum* [vagus nerve], that of the brain, unite in forming the ganglions, which with their plexuses, constitute a secondary centre of nervous influence, a channel through which the influence of every part of the brain and spinal marrow flows, to be bestowed on the thoracic and abdominal viscera, on the [blood] vessels and all secreting surfaces; the most important of which parts we have by direct experiment found subjected to every part of the brain and spinal marrow.[148]

Antonio Scarpa, who had also accepted Willis's downgrading of the ganglionic system, had made a comparable statement in 1779,[149] and Wilson Philip was now agreeing with him and providing experimental proof. But J.G.C.F.M. Lobstein proffered the cogent criticism that if the ganglia were connected with the brain and spinal cord and acted as their nervous centers, how was it that the nerves issuing from them did not have the same function as the nerves of the cerebrospinal system? Moreover, if they acted only as nerve centers or rendezvous, why should they have a different structure and different properties from somatic nerve ganglia and plexuses?[150]

According to Wilson Philip, the powers of the various organs were independent of the cerebrospinal system, yet, at the same time, they were subject to influences communicated to them by way of the ganglia. However, basing his opinion on experimental evidence, he claimed that the ganglia could not intercept stimuli traveling through them from the brain or cord, and that likewise the effects of sedatives applied to the nervous system could not be blocked by them.[151] This proved to be the death knell for Johnstone's brilliant concept of the ganglionic selective filter, which had already been of service for about fifty years.

Only about a decade after Gall had inferred that the ganglionic system presented a relatively "simple" or lowly arrangement, Wilson Philip admitted that superficially it seemed easy enough to comprehend but, nevertheless, it was a difficult and obscure area of research, concerning which no definitive statements could be ventured. Unlike many of his predecessors, the opinions he offered were derived from animal experimentation only which, of course, introduced the hazard of species variations. Nevertheless, his conclusions provided significant advances away from Bichat's doctrine. Thus, his view that the ganglionic system was not able to produce its own nervous power and was therefore dependent upon the brain and spinal cord, provided, in later elaborated forms, the mainstay of those who refuted the system's autonomy. Others expressed a similar view, for example, John Mason Good (1764–1827), whose book on the study of medicine was widely influential, stated in 1822 that concerning the ganglionic system: "It is connected both with the brain and spinal marrow, and may be said to arise from either."[152] This statement, and his account of the "system and ganglions of the intercostal nerve" were the same in the fourth edition of his book, published in 1840.[153]

We have noted that Willis's concept of a system that provided a morphological basis for sympathy was still present early in the nineteenth century. It was further publicized by the distinguished French physician, Paul Joseph Barthez (1734–1806),[154] who in his book of 1806 on the science of man, stated with assurance, that the sympathetic nerves with their ganglia and plexuses accounted for sympathy. However, he also subscribed partially to Bichat's scheme, because like Winslow and Johnstone he declared that "the ganglia can be regarded as small brains, or sites of growth (*glèbes*) of the nerves."[155] In other words, they possessed nervous power and could give birth to new fibers. He was one of the few who combined Willis's theory of sympathy with Bichat's ganglionic system.

Béclard also supported Willis, and thus was not in full agreement with Bichat. First, it is interesting to observe his comments on the theory of Willis, made in 1823, that "Willis had an idea concerning the ganglia and the sympathetic nerve that is very similar to that which is generally held today."[156] Béclard declared that the sympathetic trunk had its roots in the spinal, but not in the cranial nerves and thus could not enjoy full autonomy. Its function was to direct nutrition and secretion, to distribute the nervous agent to the heart, digestive tract, and genito-urinary organs, and "to establish a sympathetic liaison between all of the principal organs."[157] He summarized his opinion thus:

> This [sympathetic] nerve thus forms a specific system in the general [nervous] system; it has its own sphere of action contained within a general sphere [of nervous activity]. This [ganglionic] nervous system and the other one [cerebrospinal] have intimate connections; their influence is reciprocal, especially in the state of disease.[158]

This reveals that Béclard was close to the Willisian doctrine, and at the same time his definition of the vegetative nervous system was not very far from that enunciated by Langley at the end of the nineteenth century, who declared that the autonomic system had "a certain degree of independent action, but exercised under the control of a higher power."[159] The notion of a truly "sympathetic" nervous system derived considerable support from the authority and eminence of those individuals who had subscribed to it in the past, and those who continued to do so. Its basic principles of linking the somatic with the vegetative system and a general downgrading of the latter, placed it in direct opposition to Bichat's doctrine. Like the opinions of Wilson Philip, it acted as a useful antithesis, but on the whole it competed feebly for attention, and it gradually fell into decay as the notion of sympathy itself declined in popularity.

A partial opponent of the ganglionic system hypothesis as proclaimed by Bichat was J.G.C.F.M. Lobstein, whose treatise of 1823 on the vegetative system has already been referred to. First of all, he strenuously denied Bichat's central contention that his system was made up of independent centers of nervous power, isolated from brain and spinal cord, and he was able to marshal effective evidence to refute it.[160] Some of the arguments he employed were as follows:

> Indeed, if each of these bodies [ganglia] constitutes a specific center of action, I believe there will result a certain confusion that will disturb the functional harmony; and if these same ganglia came to be considered as laboratories of the nervous principle, and as a center of activity, one cannot see why

> there should be a relatively large ganglion just for the sake of one or two insignificant [nerve] fibers that issue from it.[161]

In Lobstein's view, the vegetative system worked side by side with the cerebrospinal, the two systems having a reciprocal influence the one upon the other. There were, he claimed, sixty connections between the spinal cord and the sympathetic trunks and the vagus nerve permitted a consensus between the encephalic and abdominal centers:

> It is therefore quite true that man and perfected animals possess two separate and distinct nervous systems, but having numerous connections between them, having mutual dependence, and exercising actions that counterbalance each other.[162]

Their independence was, therefore, functional only, and Lobstein insisted that both systems would be better understood if they were studied from the comparative viewpoint, and the parallelism between them thus traced carefully. His three conclusions were as follows:

> 1. That the trisplanchnic [sympathetic] nerve, although forming a system separate from the cerebral nervous system, has the greatest analogy with the latter, and it possesses the same vital characteristics.
> 2. That although each system presides over diverse functions, they both operate on the organs subjected to their authority by the same mode of action.
> 3. That finally, the nervous system of nutritive [vegetative] life, and that of the life of communication [somatic], exercise on each other a constant influence, but which manifests itself especially in the state of disease.[163]

We have spent some time discussing the opposition that was mounted against Bichat in the first few decades of the nineteenth century, because it contained the germs of discontent that eventually swept his system away. Although the majority of opinion agreed with him, we have seen that little new was added by such supporters as Reil and Wutzer to his original scheme. Frequently, unsubstantiated hypotheses were introduced to elucidate its obscurities, but they did little to advance its basic precepts, thus leaving it vulnerable to the inroads of contrary evidence that was based more securely on scientific principles.

Such was the case with Broussais, who offered additional backing from theoretical sources. He was concerned in particular with the relationship of sensation to the ganglionic nervous system of Bichat. In a long and rambling paper he postulated the existence of a special kind of sensibility, by which he meant irritability, in the system.[164] All the organs destined for nutrition, secretion, circulation, and other vegetative activities were endowed with it. He was, however, in favor of connections between the ganglionic and cerebrospinal complexes, so that functional contact could be made between them, and he gave several examples of this two way-process in health and in disease.[165] Broussais was, therefore, like Béclard, Lobstein, and others, a patron of the midway school, which rejected the extreme view of Bichat and preferred the notion that allowed the two systems to exist in a state of symbiosis. Emendations concerning sensation as proposed by Broussais led to no great advance in elucidation, but they did not detract from the popularity of a scheme that was to survive, admittedly modified, until the 1880s. But, as the century advanced, the midway position came to be the more commonly accepted method of relating organic and animal functions.

Broussais, however, like Legallois and Lobstein, placed the issue in its wider context, and made an important observation on its contribution to medical science in general. It had, he asserted, opened up new horizons for both physiology and pathology and had provided a certainty and simplicity that previously had been lacking:

> the knowledge of the functions of the great sympathetic [nerve] is a unique means we have of providing physiology and pathology with a degree of certainty and simplicity that the immense progress in all the sciences today demands, for it is truly shameful to see medicine still drifting amid vagueness and uncertainty.[166]

We can note here that John Fletcher, in keeping with Broussais, thought that the ganglionic nervous system was the source of irritability. He was also one of the most fervent proponents of the independence of the system, but his carefully selected arguments sanctioning this thesis need not concern us here.[167]

Having dealt with the more important proponents and opponents of Bichat's scheme, who, early in the nineteenth century, applied both speculation and experimentation to justify, sustain, extend, or refute the idea of an independent ganglionic nervous system, we will now examine the way in which the findings of particular disciplines were brought to bear on the problem. Embryology, comparative anatomy, pathology, and clinical medicine, together with further experimentation on the ganglionic system, and the new insights derived in the 1830s from the progress of microscopical anatomy all played significant roles.

7.7. FURTHER EVALUATION OF BICHAT'S SYSTEM

7.7.1. Embryology and Teratolology

The results of Bichat's efforts to recruit proof for his system from developmental anatomy were not impressive. This is not in any way a criticism of a man whose brief years of professional life were crammed with hectic activity, as manifested by the remarkable series of dissections and autopsies carried out, the number of patients observed and treated, and the classic works written. Had he lived, no doubt he would have evaluated and expanded some of the findings discussed below. The few pieces of evidence that he did cite concerned the differences between the development of the ganglionic and cerebrospinal systems, but they were based on scanty as well as precarious data.[168] The general background to this approach to the vegetative nervous system has been discussed in chapter 2.2. Here we noted that certain tenets of romantic biology vitiated Bichat's doctrine of a complete separation of the vegetative from the cerebrospinal system. Thus, as Gall maintained, growth was thought to take place in each by means of accumulations of gray matter, that is, ganglia. Only the arrangement of the latter distinguished the two systems, which implied similarity rather than contrariness.

However, in general, it seemed that confirmation of ganglionic independence could be gained from embryological observations. Thus J. F. Ackermann reported in 1813 that the sympathetic trunk of the human embryo appeared at an early state of development in parallel with the abdominal organs that it supplied. The precocious appearance of other organs innervated by the ganglionic system, especially the heart, seemed, he thought, to confirm his opinion, and he confidently asserted that the development of the ganglionic system preceded that of the cerebrospinal. The heart was, of course, the source of vital energy, and thus the center of organic life. In fact, he contended that the bodily systems all developed from the cardiac ganglion.[169] He concluded that the two nervous systems were independent from each other, both morphologically and functionally; but his opinion won little support, and most anatomists dismissed it on the grounds that it lacked sufficient proof.[170]

The embryological studies carried out by Lobstein ten years later were more accurate and received more approval. In 1823, he described the sympathetic nerve in three human embryos of fourteen weeks, five months, and eight months, together with a fetus at term.[171] It first became visible at three months, and Lobstein concluded that the relatively poor development of the celiac ganglion could be explained by the torpidity of intrauterine life. On the whole, the ganglionic system was more highly developed before birth than the cerebrospinal, which agreed with the predominance of organic life in the fetus. These observations favored its partial functional independence, which we have seen was Lobstein's opinion. However, he deviated from Bichat's notion of complete autonomy, because each system although functionally distinct worked in parallel and could influence the other. Broussais, who endorsed this concept of function in tandem, also believed that the sympathetic nerve alone demonstrated vigor and activity in the fetus, for it directed the secretory and nutritive organs and sustained the energy of the heart.[172] The predominance of the ganglionic system in the early stages of life was thus evident.

These early and primitive observations on the embryology of the ganglionic system are worthy of special attention, not because of their scientific merit but for two opposing reasons. First, they seemed to provide support for Bichat, although the crude evidence assembled by no means warranted the opinions derived from them. Second, later in the century, when histogenesis based on microscopical techniques had been established as a new and reliable science, embryological research gave results diametrically opposed to those just cited. It was this more trustworthy evidence that contributed to the downfall in the 1880s of the very doctrine that developmental anatomy at first seemed to support.

In the early decades of the nineteenth century teratology as well as embryology was appealed to in the hope of yielding support for ganglionic independence. On many occasions since the seventeenth century, monstrosities with deficiencies affecting the nervous system in various ways had been made use of to contest or to confirm theories concerning its function. For example, at a time when it was commonly considered that motion was brought about by a "spirit" or fluid produced in the brain, the absence of the brain in anencephalics that could move presented crucial evidence against the notion (see chap. 1.2.5). Similarly, those who sought proof for an independent ganglionic system of predominant importance to the body, enlisted observations made on human fetuses with defective nervous systems. They pointed out that no instance was on record of a monster in which the ganglionic system had been totally absent. Obviously, it could be deduced from this that a part never found wanting must be more fundamental to the organism than one often missing or defective as in the case of the cerebrospinal axis, and that it must therefore serve some specific and vital purpose in the economy of the body.[173] Lobstein in particular advanced what seemed to be impressive data, for in six malformed fetuses he found that whereas the brain and other organs could be deficient, the ganglionic system was usually, if not always, quite perfect, as long as the monster did not vary considerably from the human form.[174] Breschet also drew evidence from his experience with normal and monstrous fetuses, similar to that of other investigators. His conclusion was:

> The [vegetative] nerve ganglia appear and develope independently of the nerves of animal life; for the proportions of these ganglia were much greater than those of the nerves of the brain; and these ganglia were also very prominent in monstrous fetuses, particularly in monsters in which the brain and spinal cord did not exist.[175]

Other observers added material of a similar nature, including Marshall Hall, who in 1842 described a human fetus of six months with brain and spinal cord entirely absent. Nevertheless all parts of the ganglionic system were perfect.[176] These teratological observations, like the embryological, were macroscopical only, but they each seemed to prove the greater significance of the ganglionic nervous system over the cerebrospinal, and even its autonomy. Later in the century, however, they were shown to be erroneous.

7.7.2. Comparative Anatomy

Comparative anatomy also played a role, and we have already discussed its contemporary general principles above (see chap. 2.1, 2). Bichat had placed great stress on it, and S. Langston Parker (fl. 1831) of Birmingham between 1830 and 1831 explored its possibilities.[177] He pointed out that lower classes of animals appeared to possess only one nervous system, analogous to the ganglionic system of vertebrates, the brain and spinal cord being entirely wanting. This notion was consonant with efforts made by many investigators of this period to discover a single "type" from which all forms of the nervous system found in the animal kingdom could be seen to derive. Its ramifications in early nineteenth- century biological thought were explored in chapter 2.2. As Gall asserted, in this view the vegetative nervous system constituted a more primitive (hence its priority of appearance in the embryo and its dominance in the simplest animals) and therefore more typical form of organization than the cerebrospinal. Although this seemed an attractive hypothesis, the greater weight of evidence was against it. Lobstein's opinion, however, was that if it could be proven it would constitute a very favorable argument for Bichat's supporters.[178]

7.7.3. Pathology and Clinical Medicine

The pathology of the nervous system in children and adults was also thought to contribute to the elucidation of the problem, by giving further evidence of the indispensability of the ganglionic system to the vital functions, and thus verifying its predominance in the overall activity of the body. Its autonomy could also be revealed, it was thought, by autopsy findings in idiots in whom the cerebrospinal system was diseased and atrophied, but the ganglia with their nerves and plexuses were said to be perfectly healthy.[179]

There was also the role of the ganglionic system in the practice of medicine. Richerand in 1799 had discussed the outcome of pathological influences on the solar plexus with the production of a variety of symptoms, some of them psychological:

> In all cases the internal sensation of a shock more or less acute is experienced. From the solar plexus of the great sympathetic [trunk], which, according to quite widely received opinion, is regarded as the seat of this sensation, its effects are transmitted to the abdominal and thoracic plexuses.[180]

The application of a new concept such as the ganglionic nervous system to the problems of clinical medicine was a natural development in the search for the etiology of diseases and the provision of specific therapy. Both Bichat and Reil had pointed out the benefits that might accrue from this approach, and with their followers they hastened to apply the system's principles to medical practice. If it were completely separate from the brain and spinal cord, one could expect that specific disease processes would occur in it. One of the earliest suggestions complying with this possibility was made by Bichat, who, following Richerand and others (see chaps. 6.3.1, 6.5), located mental disease in the abdominal ganglia and plexuses:

> Some doctors have believed, and I also suspect, that hysterical fits that begin with an oppression of the epigastrium, in which the patient feels thereafter a ball rising to the gullet, can be due to certain lesions of the semilunar [celiac] ganglion, the solar plexuses, and of the connections which run from ganglion to ganglion into the neck.[181]

This was an ingenious physical elucidation of a psychiatric disorder, *globus hystericus,* but autopsies in two such patients not surprisingly revealed no pathological changes. However, just as experience had shown that cerebral disease could leave no (macroscopic) traces in the brain so it could be argued that the same might be the case with diseased ganglia and epigastric plexuses. Bichat suggested that "This point merits special examination,"[182] and Philippe Pinel followed his lead. According to him the onset of mania was defined as follows:

> An acute malady, or to speak more generally, a stimulus of any kind acting vigourously on the epigastric center of forces [the *cerebrum abdominale*] and producing there a profound commotion, which is repeated in the abdominal plexuses, and giving rise to spasmodic contractions, and to an obstinate constipation and intense heat of the bowels.[183]

He was, however, merely elaborating Richerand's suggestion. Lobstein, too, subscribed to this etiology, and he considered that hypochondria, hysteria, melancholia, and mania were all due to disorders of the ganglionic nervous system.[184] As we have seen, it was Gall who countered this notion by insisting that the brain was the only seat of the mental processes and therefore of their disorders (chap. 6.3.4). Even so, a certain John Smith Waugh (d. ?1858) in 1838 gave further support for the brainlike qualities of the abdominal ganglia. It is not only surprising that he located the soul's habitat in the *cerebrum abdominale,* but also that at this late date he was seeking its anatomical site:

> There are many anatomical, physiological, and pathological considerations in support of the semilunar [celiac] ganglion being the organ of the soul in man, or where this is impressed by the perceptive influence, which I have not space to dwell upon.[185]

It was Lobstein who made the first attempt to list diseases other than psychiatric that arose from disturbances of the ganglionic nervous system.[186] It seemed to him that a wide variety of common ailments could be included, such as arthritis, intermittent fever, angina pectoris, malaria, migraine, insomnia, toothache, lead colic, and many more. This bewildering collection rivaled that proposed by the supporters of Willis's concept of sympathy operating through the intercostal nerve. In the 1870s, fifty years after Lobstein, the conglomeration of diseases thought to be produced by malfunction of the ganglia, nerves, and plexuses was much the same, despite the fact that the role of these structures as an independent system was by then under widespread attack. Thus, in 1873, two German physicians named at least eighteen diseases of the vegetative system, ranging from migraine to diabetes mellitus.[187] Even at the end of the nineteenth century the list was still impressively long and varied. By then the morbid influence of the vegetative system on diseased states was thought to be extensive and due to very frequent reflex irritation.[188] These attempts to give the ganglionic nervous system a special place in pathology were as fruitless as the efforts to establish the system itself as an autonomous unit, and Ackerknecht has concluded that "our knowledge of the vegetative nervous system . . . has not been a useful foundation of a patho-physiological system."[189]

7.7.4. Experimental Physiology

A few early physiologists, like Legallois and Wilson Philip, had carried out animal experiments on the ganglionic system, although mostly indirectly. They had, however, been almost alone in this, and procedures involving the system directly were equally uncommon, because of the hazards likely to be encountered. Bichat had explained that as the ganglia were deeply situated, physiological experiments on animals were difficult to perform. He forecast correctly when he declared that "[I]t is this that will undoubtedly perpetuate for a long time the obscurity that prevails concerning the functions of these organs."[190]

One of the problems confronting Bichat and his followers was the role of sensation in the ganglionic system, and efforts were made to tackle it experimentally. If the system were an independent unit, it would be expected that stimulation of it could not evoke sensation as in the case of the cerebrospinal axis. Moreover, Johnstone's and Reil's selective filter mechanisms in a normal animal would prevent pain passing centrally. To test these propositions Bichat had examined the response of a dog to vigorous mechanical and chemical irritation of the celiac ganglion and its nerves and had observed that it expressed not the slightest evidence of distress or agitation. On the other hand, the same animal struggled violently when a spinal or cranial nerve was similarly stimulated. He concluded: "In general it appears that the sensibility of the ganglia is infinitely less marked than that of many other organs."[191] Reil also experimented on this problem and he agreed with Bichat's findings,[192] as did Gall who wrote:

> Let us admit with Bichat, Reil, and other authors that living animals when opened up do not cry out if the abdominal nerves are pricked, but give signs of suffering as soon as the nerves of animal life are traumatized.[193]

One of the first to contradict Bichat's opinion on the inaccessibility of the ganglia was J[?]. M[?]. Dupuy (1771–c. 1830), who in 1806 and 1815 excised the superior cervical sympathetic ganglion in living horses and described the operation as an easy one.[194] However, removal excited no pain, but produced the usual sequelae due to the interruption of vasomotor nerves. In dogs, Wutzer observed the same lack of response to irritation of the lumbar ganglia by various methods, except in the case of galvanic excitation which induced contractions of abdominal and thigh muscles, due no doubt to the spread of abnormally strong currents.[195] The investigations of Lobstein were more ambitious, but the results were the same; animals did not react to irritation of ganglia,[196] and in a full-term human fetus almost dead from birth trauma, electrical stimulation of the sympathetic nerve (not unexpectedly) similarly produced no reaction.[197]

It seems very likely that these and other early experimental results were incorrect owing to several factors. There were the operative difficulties predicted as an impediment by Bichat, the defective techniques of stimulation, species variations, inadequate anatomical knowledge and powers of observation, the shock accompanying extensive surgical procedures on conscious animals, and the formulation of opinions based on too few experiments. Without taking these into account, it is otherwise difficult to explain why later investigators consistently reached opposite conclusions. But it is also possible that individuals approached the problem with a preconceived acceptance of the insensibility of the ganglionic system and found what they were seeking. This seems to have been the case with Brachet, who had accepted Bichat's doctrines. He reported in 1830[198] that after exposing the abdominal and thoracic ganglia in calves, dogs, and in other animals he found them to be at first insensitive, but after a few minutes, pricking with a pin produced clear manifestations of pain. Nevertheless, these seemingly contrary findings did not necessarily refute Bichat's thesis. Brachet argued that the response to pain occurred because of "inflammation" of the ganglia and viscera, brought about by "exposure to the air." This is an interesting notion common in the first half of the nineteenth century and earlier, based presumably on a pre-germ theory explanation for the peritoneal infection that must have followed most experimental laparotomies. In accordance with the concepts of Johnstone and Reil, disease (in this instance, "inflammation") allowed stimuli to reach the brain and be perceived as pain. Brachet's opinion was in keeping with this:

> Thus we shall conclude that in the normal state the ganglionic nerves are unable to transmit to the brain the sensations they receive, or, in other words, they do not at all possess the animal sensibility of Bichat, cerebral sensation.[199]

In fact, his results varied for some animals reacted as described above while others did not,[200] so that his experimental evidence apparently favoring Bichat must be regarded as untrustworthy. Additionally, we might even judge his interpretations as contrived. We should recall here that Brachet had also been responsible for an erroneous theory linking the ganglionic system with reflex activity (see chap. 4.3).

With the advent of physiologists of the caliber of Johannes Müller, E. H. Weber, Flourens, and Longet, this experimental support for Bichat rapidly evaporated. Müller in 1835 reported that in the rabbit mechanical or chemical irritation of the celiac ganglion could produce pain. The section in his textbook of physiology dealing with this was headed, "The sympathetic nerve has sensation."[201] It was now evident that Johnstone's original hypothesis of the ganglion blocking the progress of sensory impulses to the brain in health but not in disease, could no longer be sustained. Thus, Müller asserted that the pain caused by disease processes in parts supplied by the ganglionic system gave eloquent testimony to their endowment with sensation, and Weber also preferred to take account of events in the pathological, rather than in the physiological, state:

"For my part, the everyday observation of pain in those parts, that [according to Bichat's theory] ought be insensitive, I hold to be more worthy of notice than these experiments."[202] Flourens, like Müller, encountered adequate evidence that in the rabbit pinching the celiac ganglion was painful, and he also found the cervical and first thoracic ganglia feebly sensitive.[203] He did not accept the complete independence of the ganglionic system, but thought instead that it acted as an intermediary between the cerebrospinal nervous system and the heart and gut, which is one of our current ways of defining the autonomic nervous system. He stated:

> the movements of the heart and intestines still [depend upon] the [cerebrospinal] nervous system, but only in a mediate and consecutive manner; and on the union of these viscera to this system [by way of] the great sympathetic.[204]

This is much the same position arrived at earlier by Legallois, Lobstein, and others.

Overwhelming confirmation of the existence of sensation in the ganglionic system also came from the careful studies of Longet, whose experiments reported in 1850 were judged to be the most carefully executed and reliable so far.[205] They revealed beyond any doubt that the cervical and lumbar, as well as the celiac, ganglia were sensitive. He could claim that: "The great splanchnic nerves seem to me always to possess a most appreciable sensibility, at least in dogs."[206] His qualification of the type of experimental animal was a seemingly small, yet important, advance in research methods which would eventually help to account for the conflicting results that plagued this field of investigation. Longet also pointed out correctly, and for the first time, that the sensibility of the ganglionic system was low compared with that of the cerebrospinal nerves, which agreed with the known fact that visceral sensations were vague and poorly localized. This attempt to grade sensation according to intensity was another notable contribution to research methodology. However, the dissimilarity he had detected gave some support to those who were still seeking fundamental differences between the two nervous systems in order to confirm their functional autonomy. Nevertheless, the knowledge that sensations (e.g., from colon and bladder) could be perceived in health might have called into question the independence of the ganglionic nerves from the brain. The possibility, however, exists that the sacral outflow that provides these organs with part of their vegetative supply was mistaken for somatic nerves.

The problem of whether the ganglionic system possessed consciousness had also been discussed earlier, along with sensation. If the latter emanating from the healthy system was not appreciated, it could be argued that the ganglionic system lacked consciousness. This seemingly significant difference between the two systems, which one would have expected to become a controversial aspect of Bichat's theory, in fact, received little attention. One of the few to comment on it was Friedrich Arnold, who in 1831 declared that the ganglionic system lacked consciousness, indicating yet another fundamental contrast to the cerebrospinal system.[207]

The varieties of evidence we have just surveyed seemed mostly to confirm Bichat's doctrine of an independent system. Rather than from speculation, most derived from observations made by astute and accurate investigators. However, the interpretations they arrived at could not always be justified by the data they had accumulated. There was a willingness to erect unrealistic hypotheses often based on a small number of observations, whether from laboratory or clinic, and the influence of preconceptions that allowed the individual to arrive at the conclusion he had already accepted, consciously or unconsciously, must have played a part. The end result was that Bichat's system continued to be bolstered by an unsubstantial framework of apparent proof that provided it, however, with only a limited survival.

7.7.5. Histology

7.7.5.1. *Introduction.* By the 1830s most had accepted Bichat's scheme, although some had reservations concerning certain aspects of it. Research methods, however, were still primitive and had not advanced much since Bichat's day. The few available had provided as much as could be expected at this stage of their evolution. Gross anatomy, embryology, teratology, and pathology seemed to have supported him, but what was the evidence beyond that appreciated by the naked eye? As discussed elsewhere (chap. 3.1), in the early 1830s there were very few reliable microscopes, no histological techniques, and no cell theory. Tissue from vegetative and spinal root ganglia and from nerves was examined more frequently than samples from the brain and spinal cord, merely because it was more readily obtainable, and in the absence of adequate fixation and sectioning methods it was easier to handle than the pulpy brain or cord substance. Also, we should recall that throughout the period we are studying (i.e., up to the 1850s), there were no staining techniques, and pieces of tissue were usually mounted in water only, with the inevitable creation of confusing artifacts due to the passage of water by osmosis into the nervous elements, usually the nerve fiber. But despite these technical and conceptual hazards, a great deal of information regarding the microscopical structure of the ganglionic system was amassed from 1833 onwards. In view of the complexity of the system and the fact that proper elucidation of it could not begin until the 1880s when other methods than histological were essential for elucidation, it is not surprising that on the whole more confusion than enlightenment was generated by the pioneers we shall now discuss. From a faltering start, however, this method of neuroscientific research was to lead at the end of the century to the destruction of Bichat's doctrine.

7.7.5.2. *The early microscopists.* We have dealt elsewhere with the early years of the nerve cell concept and we have seen how Remak in particular was concerned to derive physiological significance from the histological aspects of the vegetative nervous system (see chap. 3.5.2). Nevertheless some of that discussion will be considered again here, with special reference to the ganglionic system. One of the first to exploit the new achromatic microscope in the study of nervous tissue was C. G. Ehrenberg, and his general theoretical scheme, in the light of which his neurohistological findings must be assessed, has already been described (chap. 3.1). In 1833 he reported that in a vegetative ganglion he had seen "irregular bodies which produce the actual swelling of the ganglion and give it more the appearance of a glandular substance."[208] Some have claimed that Ehrenberg was describing nerve cell bodies and this was no doubt so, but he could not have recognized them as such, because, as we have explained, the cell theory of animal life had not yet been enunciated (see chap. 3.1). He may also have encountered the myelinated and nonmyelinated nerve fiber, although he was unaware of their significance, and his accounts are not easy to follow. Nevertheless, Ehrenberg's further comments on the ganglia are of great interest:

> An understanding of their structure favors the idea that the ganglia are comparable to small brains. However, the universally accepted theory that they are comparable to the cortical substance of the cerebrum must be corrected since, although their color is similar, the cortical substance consists of a mixture of vessels and very delicate articulating (varicose) fibers that can scarcely be differentiated.[209]

He thus supported with histological evidence the time-honored belief that the ganglia resembled small brains as originally proposed by Winslow in 1732, but he correctly denied the "universally accepted theory" that they consisted of cortical gray matter. This notion had also been advanced early in the eighteenth century[210] and was part of Johnstone's concept of the ganglionic system, for he had stated that ganglia were "a mixture of cortical and medullary substance."[211] Even though it might be true that the vegetative ganglia acted like independent cerebral organs, and the claim for autonomy of the ganglionic system was thus greatly enhanced, Bichat nevertheless had rejected this part of Johnstone's theory, although he did insist that the ganglia had independent nervous power. Bichat's opinion thus seemed to be vindicated by Ehrenberg's microscopical findings.

Ehrenberg was followed three years later by another talented observer, G. G. Valentin, who gave a detailed account of the nerve fiber and the nerve cell body in a classic paper[212] that has been discussed in detail elsewhere, along with an account of the general characteristics and background philosophy of his neurohistological and other microscopical research (chap. 3.2, 3). He called the nerve cell body "globule," and there is no doubt that in his case these were true cells. Those he found in the ganglia he termed "ganglionic globules," and together with "ganglionic corpuscles," this became a generic term for the nerve cell body. Valentin's most valuable contribution to neurohistology at this time was to suggest that nervous tissue in both cerebrospinal and vegetative nervous systems was made up exclusively of these cell bodies and nerve fibers, his *Grundtypus*, but he did not believe that they were connected to one another.[213] He refuted this possibility in the case of ganglionic elements. One might think that the tail-like appendix of some cells was prolonged into a ganglionic fiber, but this was not so. He explained that:

> Apart merely from the great differences between the contents of the primary fibers and the parenchyma of the globules, the fact alone that one occasionally finds such a tailed globule completely enclosed by its sheath of cellular tissue must bring this assumption to naught.[214]

Valentin also examined the rami communicantes and concluded correctly that fibers in the white variety came only from the spinal roots and traveled to the ganglionic system. They must therefore be efferent in direction and function (? our preganglionic visceral efferents). In addition some of these fibers entered a ganglion and terminated there, whereas others passed through it without interruption (? visceral efferents on their way to the splanchnic nerves or to other ganglia of the sympathetic trunk, and perhaps visceral afferents). Valentin's further studies reported in 1839 will be discussed below, but first we must consider the work of his most prominent rival in the field of neurohistology, Robert Remak.

Without doubt Remak was the most outstanding contributor to the earliest phase of achromatic microscopy applied to the nervous system (see chap. 3.5.2). In his inaugural dissertation of 1838, the main aim of which was to accumulate histological data that would provide elucidation of the functions of the vegetative nervous system, he gave the first adequate description of the nonmyelinated or gray fiber, known today as the "fiber of Remak":[215] "They are not tubular, that is, surrounded by a [myelin] sheath, but naked, being transparent as if gelatinous, and much finer than most of the primitive tubes [myelinated fibers]."[216] He maintained that whereas the larger (myelinated) fibers were found only in the cerebrospinal nervous system and had motor or sensory functions, the finer ones (nonmyelinated) occurred exclusively in the ganglionic system and had quite different properties. Thus, the ganglia from whence the fine fibers mainly arose must be centers for the regulation of the organs that were supplied by these fibers. Remak was, therefore, supplying microscopical proof for the old concepts of the ganglia being small brains. In keeping with Bichat's nomenclature, Remak called these fine fibers "organic," and occasionally they were termed "gelatinous." Today they include the postganglionic visceral efferents and the nonmyelinated type of visceral afferents. However, Remak's finding provoked more opposition than acceptance, and his organic fibers were not fully approved until about 1860. The cell bodies and nerve fibers in nervous tissue had been judged by Valentin to be its fundamental elements, but that they were components of the same structure, the "nerve cell," later known as the "neuron," was first proposed by Remak, as related in chapter 3.5.1. From his suggestion the neuron doctrine eventually developed. This immensely important discovery was made while examining "the sympathetic and spinal ganglia, the centers of the organic [vegetative] nervous system."[217] In 1838 he stated:

> *The organic fibers originate from the very substance of the nucleated globules.* This observation, although very difficult to make and requiring great skill in preparation as well as in observation, is nevertheless so clear that it cannot be doubted.[218]

This finding represents one of the most noteworthy advances in nineteenth century neuroscience, although at the time it was hotly contested. But Remak went further and identified the function of the ganglion's cells and fibers:

> Now since the same organic fibers constitute the larger part of the sympathetic nerves and originate from the nucleated globules, which together make up the ganglia, the *sympathetic ganglia must be considered the true centers of the nervous system.*[219]

His strict division of nerve fibers into primitive tubules (myelinated fibers) of the cerebrospinal system and organic (nonmyelinated) fibers of the vegetative system, although later shown to be too rigorous, was of the utmost significance because it provided strong support for Bichat's erroneous notion of two autonomous systems, each with its own morphological and physiological characteristics. It, therefore, offset to some degree Remak's positive benefactions to neurohistology. Another perceptive proposal made by Remak, but not properly understood until much later in the century, was that the posterior spinal root ganglia belonged partly to the ganglionic system, in view of their similar structure, and the presence in them of organic fibers:

> the *spinal ganglia seem to relate to the organic nervous system*. . . . I suspect that the spinal ganglia were specially constructed to receive the necessary organic fibers from the sympathetic ganglia by way of the posterior and mainly sensory spinal nerve roots.[220]

It may be that Remak had identified the nonmyelinated type of visceral afferent neurone, with its cell body in the spinal root ganglion and its axone an organic fiber passing to it from a viscus or other structure, and found only in the thoracic, upper lumbar, and some of the sacral spinal cord segments. It should be recalled that Johnstone in 1771 had advanced the same claim concerning the spinal ganglion, but on the basis of very different and, to us, unacceptable evidence. Reil had done likewise.

In keeping with Valentin, Remak concluded correctly that the white rami were efferent pathways leading to the vegetative ganglia, and in 1838 A. W. Volkmann also accepted that in the frog the sympathetic nerve was connected with the anterior spinal roots, because fibers from the spinal cord (our preganglionic visceral efferents) traveled through these roots on their way to the white rami and thence to the ganglia.[221] This is now known to be the case. Having noted that the fibers in the white rami were thickest nearest their spinal root origin, Volkmann agreed with Valentin and Remak that they must contain efferent fibers proceeding from the cerebrospinal to the vegetative system. In agreement with Valentin and in opposition to Remak, Volkmann denied that there was any connection between the ganglion's cell bodies and fibers.

Remak's ideas on the rami communicantes confirmed the views of his teacher and main advocate, Johannes Müller. In 1832 Müller had agreed with Wutzer's speculation[222] that the sympathetic trunk received fibers from both roots of the spinal cord, and that in consequence it must contain both motor and sensory elements.[223] Although Scarpa had denied this,[224] Wutzer and Müller gained support from two equally outstanding anatomists, Anders Adolf Retzius (1796–1860)[225] and August Franz Joseph Carl Mayer (1787–1865).[226] In general, we would accept this differentiation of rami fibers, because the preganglionic visceral efferents emerge from the anterior spinal roots and myelinated visceral afferents pass into the posterior, as we have just mentioned. Müller also concluded that because the white rami seemed to contain mainly tubular (i.e., myelinated) fibers (more delicate, however, than those in somatic nerves, and which gave the rami their white color) they must originate in the cerebrospinal system.[227] As Valentin, Remak, and Volkmann also asserted, these rami must be efferent. On the other hand Müller stated that the gray rami carried organic fibers arising from cells of the vegetative ganglia (? our postganglionic visceral efferents). Remak agreed with this arrangement:

> the communicating branch, according to the distinguished *Müller*'s and my own observations, often displays a distinctly gray color, which I have learned with the help of the microscope, is produced by the great number of organic gray fibers in it.[228]

Müller's observations on the organic fibers had first appeared in 1833.[229] In general, the white and gray rami maintained a reciprocal relationship between the two nervous systems. Cerebrospinal nerves could contain motor and sensory fibers, together with organic fibers that arose in the vegetative ganglia and ran through the gray rami to the cerebrospinal nerves, in which they were distributed to the structures they innervated. This was his opinion in 1840:

> From all the foregoing facts I arrived at the conclusion that in the cerebrospinal nerves three kinds of fibers must be distinguished; the sensitive and motor, which are both white [myelinated], and come from the roots of the cerebro-spinal nerves,–and gray [nonmyelinated] organic fibers, which have their origin in the ganglia of the ganglionic or sympathetic nerve itself.[230]

The efferent fibers of the vegetative system (pre- and postganglionic) carried messages for involuntary movements, nutrition, secretion, and chemical processes in general, and the motor and sensory somatic fibers traveled to and from cerebrospinal centers. Müller's findings did not necessarily weaken the argument that the ganglionic system was functionally independent, and in fact, along with Remak, he helped to sustain Bichat's doctrine with this new and persuasive evidence. Henle also favored Remak's microscopical findings. Although at first he suggested that the organic fibers were perhaps nonnervous structures such as blood vessels or epithelial tissue,[231] he was eventually able to help in substantiating their existence, for in 1840 he declared that:

> the organic nerves are the motor nerves of the involuntary muscles, and perhaps of the cellular [i.e., connective] tissue and the blood vessels, and as such they merely constitute a subdivision of the class of motor nerves.[232]

Remak was concerned not only with the microscopical structure of the ganglionic system but being a physiologist as well as a histologist, he was interested, like Müller and Henle in its function, and we have looked at some of his opinions in this field (chap. 3.5.2). In 1840 he advanced a physiological theory that contained a number of perceptive notions, and it is in these that his importance also lies.[233] There was, he said, an obvious functional difference between myelinated fibers from the brain and spinal cord and the nonmyelinated, organic fibers from the ganglionic system. The properties of the former were relatively well understood, but the latter, he asserted, influenced the action of involuntary muscle and secretory organs throughout the body, thus being concerned with the activities of the thoracic and abdominal viscera, the blood vessels, the mucous and serous membranes, and possibly the skin.[234] Organic nerves were not, however, in full command of organs, because it was common knowledge that the latter continued to function when their nerve supply was interrupted, as Johnstone and others had pointed out. Nevertheless, Remak insisted that the ganglia represented central points of the vegetative nervous system. Remak also proposed organic (visceral) reflexes, and held that reflex activity initiated secretion,[235] which Kisch has surmised was an anticipation of Pavlov's conditioned reflex.[236] As we have just noted, Müller had arrived at similar conclusions regarding ganglionic function, and in 1833 had described the organic fiber as "corresponding with its distribution to parts which serve principally for the production of chemical changes in the fluids of the body."[237] It should, however, be recalled that Johnstone in 1771 had preceded Müller and Remak, when he claimed that "Ganglions probably have some use in Secretion, by securing a more uniform motion of the liquors in secreting organs."[238] Also, that:

> the nervous twigs on which they [ganglia] have been observed, being chiefly distributed to the salivary and mucous Glands, about the jaws, tongue, palate, throat, and nostrils; may they not be supposed to have some use in glandular secretion?[239]

However, Remak went further than his predecessors when he suggested that nervous control by organic fibers influenced both the quality and quantity of secretions, and that they produced these effects indirectly by acting on the gland's blood vessels, the truth of which was eventually to be revealed (see chap. 3.5.2). He also elaborated a postulate of Bichat that voluntary muscles received vegetative as well as somatic fibers, and he contended that they were mainly responsible for muscle tone.[240] In 1844 this was denied by Volkmann,[241] and it now seems likely that the organic fibers Remak had traced to these muscles were vasomotor in function. However, Volkmann upheld Remak's further suggestion that motor activity of involuntary muscles was invariably controlled by their vegetative nerve supply.[242]

Remak had several opponents, but the most virulent was Valentin, whose opposing views were ventilated in a monograph of 1839.[243] In its first section he extended the account of the cerebrospinal nerves that he had published three years earlier,[244] in the second he discussed the physiology of the vegetative system,[245] in the third the laws governing the peripheral nerves, and in the fourth gave his opinions on the influence in general of nerves on organic and animal functions.[246] This work was of high merit, and the following is one of the compliments accorded it:

> we would again express our conviction of the great importance of this work, and of the high rank which we think it ought to take amongst physiological treatises. We have never met with a work on any subject in which so much original matter of sterling value is so judiciously mixed up with the knowledge previously obtained from other sources.[247]

Such was the unstinted praise of a British writer, but it is a measure of the interest in scientific medicine manifested in Britain at the time that whereas works of greatly inferior quality on clinical subjects were translated into English, this declared classic was not. In it Valentin joined Johnstone, Müller, and Remak when he asserted that the ganglionic system directed and controlled the functions of nutrition, secretion, circulation, and so forth. But, unlike them his considered view was comparable to Willis's, that the sympathetic trunk was an offshoot or dependency of the brain and cord from which all its fibers originated. He based this on his correct conclusion that the greak bulk of the sympathetic trunk consisted of fibers deriving from the cerebrospinal system by way of the white rami, and on his incorrect belief that the organic fibers described by Remak and Müller did not in fact exist.[248] Ganglionic fibers were neither peculiar in their structure nor in their relations. They were, he contended, extensions of the cell body's capsule, and he agreed with other German microscopists, such as Henle (who later recanted), Volkmann, and Wagner, who declared them to be artifacts or a kind of connective or epithelial tissue and not a neural structure.[249] This denial was unfortunate for it helped others less gifted than he to reach similar mistaken conclusions.

Later, Valentin argued cogently, as others had before him, that if, as appeared likely, certain fibers from the cerebrospinal system passed through the ganglia unhindered the ganglionic system could no longer be said to possess independence.[250] We now know that preganglionic efferents to the splanchnic nerves along with the visceral afferents do just this. However, he was cautious to admit that such a hypothesis could not be verified until the complete course of each entering fiber could be traced microscopically. His rejection of connections between a ganglion's incoming fibers and its cells caused him no problem, because as mentioned, according to Henle, fibers in the ganglia could influence one another without making direct contact. In other words, crossover transmission took place (see chap. 4.6). As Henle asserted, "The nerves may also communicate their excitability to one another in the ganglia, and the ganglia may thus be considered in some degree as central [nervous] organs, and as the mediators of the sympathies."[251] He was therefore not only agreeing with Bichat's ganglionic autonomy but was also providing those like Valentin who did not accept Remak's notion of cell body-fiber union, with a nonanatomical means of communication between nerve fibers.

The histological data so far available to Valentin induced him, contrary to the opinion of most other physiologists, to reject Bichat's concept of a system complete in itself.[252] The ganglionic system was, he declared, entirely derived from the cerebrospinal. The account he gave of the properties of the vegetative ganglia, although ingenious, was, however, unconvincing. He concluded that they must be associated with those of the cerebrospinal system, because in his opinion vegetative ganglion cells had no specific activities of their own, although they added strength to the operations of nervous fibers passing through the ganglia.[253] Valentin's contradictory and incorrect views were only a part of his denial of Remak's microscopical discoveries, which we now know were not only mostly true but also represented exceedingly significant advances in the histology of nervous tissue. Remak's techniques were superior to those of Valentin, as were his powers of observation and interpretation, but another factor may have been a conflict of personalities. Whatever the cause, the outcome of their disagreements led to an acrimonious debate that hindered rather than promoted research in this area of microscopical anatomy. It was not until 1842 that Valentin admitted that he had been wrong to deny the existence of Remak's organic fibers.[254]

It is a difficult task to interpret and to compare and contrast minutely the findings of these outstanding early microscopists. Their work, which admittedly produced remarkable results, was bedeviled by at least two consequential variables: their crude and unreliable microscopes and histological techniques; and the lack of attention they paid to species differences. Each induced confusion, but to discover exactly how the varying results and explications came about would be a formidable exercise, involving the careful repetition of their experiments. Unfortunately, detailed information sufficient to permit this is rarely available, so that in most cases attempts to achieve a practical analysis of a microscopist's observations and to compare them with contemporary as well as modern data may never be possible. Nevertheless, important advances had been made. The pathways of certain fibers in spinal roots, spinal root ganglia, white and gray rami, vegetative ganglia, and somatic nerves had been vaguely discerned, but the main stumbling block, as we now appreciate was the unwillingness of some microscopists to accept the cell body-fiber connection and the existence of organic fibers in the ganglionic system. On the whole, however, those who interpreted their findings in favor of Bichat's doctrine were in the ascendancy. The discovery that fibers seemed to connect the spinal cord with the ganglia by way of the white rami, which to us would seem to be conclusive proof against an autonomous vegetative system, did not, however, have the same significance in the 1830s and 1840s. It could still be argued then that these need not be functional links, except as pathways for the influences from the mind that acted on the viscera. In any case the ganglia could produce their own fibers and in addition were invested with independent nervous power. Valentin was almost alone in his rejection of Bichat's doctrine, but his opinion was based on two grave errors: the rejection of Remak's proposed cell body-fiber union and of Remak's organic fibers. Like Gall, Valentin was right, but for the wrong reasons.

7.7.5.3. *Bidder and Volkmann.* In 1844 it was reported that "It is not yet decided by anatomists and physiologists whether the sympathetic [vegetative] be an independent system of nerves, or dependent on the cerebro-spinal system."[255] Although considerable histological evidence now existed both accepting and denying Bichat's ganglionic system, the problem remained. However, about two years earlier two German scientists had for the first time instituted anatomical studies with the express purpose of solving it. They were F. H. Bidder and A. W. Volkmann, and their report appeared in 1842.[256] The merits of their labors were extolled by an anonymous British critic as follows:

> We feel inclined to place much confidence in the observation detailed in this essay. Professors Bidder and Volkmann seem to have taken great pains, not so much to show themselves learned and deep-thinking, [but] as truth-loving and industrious inquirers.[257]

They began by examining in great detail the microscopical constituents of the ganglionic and cerebrospinal systems.[258] In line with Valentin and others, they denied the existence of the organic fibers that Remak claimed were characteristic of the ganglionic system, but at the same time contested Valentin's other conclusions that rejected ganglionic autonomy. In the place of organic fibers, Bidder and Volkmann recognized two kinds of fibers in the vegetative system: small ones that predominated in number and characterized the system; and large ones that seemed to come from the cerebrospinal system and were equally characteristic of it. It is difficult to identify these fibers in the light of modern knowledge and it is perhaps foolhardy to attempt to do so. However, it seems that they were both myelinated, and no doubt the crude techniques available to Bidder and Volkmann induced deception, for their small fibers must have been the nonmyelinated organic fibers of Remak. No other interpretation is possible. Likewise the large fibers must have been myelinated autonomic and somatic components.

Attempting to differentiate more precisely between these basic elements of the vegetative system, Bidder and Volkmann made use of a new microscopical procedure, already employed by the latter.[259] Thus, together they introduced mathematical precision by inventing ways of measuring the caliber of nerve fibers, and popularized the numerical method in biological microscopy. Before the photomicrograph was available, a microscopist had to rely on his powers of observation and description, as well as on his own or his draftsman's artistic skills and accuracy in order to convey the precise nature of his findings. A micrometric approach, therefore, added a new dimension to histological research, because not only was precision increased but in addition it was now possible for an investigator to test another's accuracy. The technique was to prove most valuable to later anatomists, like Gaskell, who in the 1880s began to sort out the vegetative fibers, and incidentally in so doing overturned Bidder and Volkmann's conclusions.[260] But, meantime, armed with this new technique they could now quantify the differences between the two varieties of fibers, the small and the large. They confirmed that despite considerable differences among species of animals and humans, the large fibers were cerebrospinal in origin and the small fibers were invariably vegetative.

The second part of their treatise considered the connections between the vegetative and spinal nerves. First they studied the frog's rami communicantes carefully, attempting like Reil to account for their existence and to prove that they were not functional links between the two nervous systems. Subjecting them to numerical analysis, they discovered that more than two-thirds of the fibers in the white rami were large and took a centrifugal course toward the periphery of the body. These were cerebrospinal fibers. The remainder, however, were small and proceeded centripetally to the spinal root ganglia. These were ganglionic fibers. Bidder and Volkmann had thus proved quantitatively the opinion formulated earlier by Volkmann, Remak, and others that the white rami were chiefly efferent. They could now argue that in the frog the majority of rami fibers were not vegetative, but cerebrospinal, and that less than a third came from the spinal root ganglia and could be regarded as part of the ganglionic system. Next they subjected various somatic nerves of the body to a similar analysis with the object of finding out the relationships between the small and the large fibers:

> The nerves supplying the voluntary muscles contain very few of the small fibers; about ten percent on average. We have encountered no exception to this rule in the four classes of vertebrates.[261]

If the large fibers predominated in a somatic nerve, the reverse should be the case in a ganglionic nerve:

> In the healthy state, the nerves of the mucous membranes convey little or no sensibility and are composed almost exclusively of small fibers; we can therefore conclude that the nerves distributed to the oesophagus, stomach, gut, and bladder are composed almost entirely of them.[262]

They could illustrate this with several examples, and so were able to conclude that the degree of vegetative activity in an organ was directly proportional to the number of small-caliber fibers in the nerve supplying it. They could also demonstrate that these small fibers could not have come from the brain or spinal cord, by contrasting the fiber content of a ramus with that of a peripheral twig of a ganglionic nerve. The former could contain 2 percent, whereas the latter had 100 percent of small fibers. It followed that if the small fibers did not originate in the cerebrospinal system they must arise in the vegetative, and the obvious and widely accepted site was its ganglia. Again using their measuring procedures, Bidder and Volkmann estimated the number of fibers entering a frog's ganglion and the number leaving it. With numerical precision they confirmed an opinion that had been based upon cruder research methods.[263] In the cat, efferent fibers were four times more numerous than afferent, and similar results were obtained in other species. There was no doubt in Bidder's and Volkmann's minds that the vegetative nervous system had anatomical autonomy and, therefore, could function as a unit independent of the brain and spinal cord and not as an appendage of them. This conclusion was stated in the title of their report of 1842: *The Independence of the Sympathetic Nervous System proved by means of anatomical Investigations*.[264] But, as we can now judge, Bidder and Volkmann were basing it on erroneous evidence, and they were introducing additional confusion into an already contradictory debate. However, in common with all early microscopists, they were facing insurmountable barriers, the most formidable being the absence of adequate methods of preparing and staining the tissues they were studying. In their case there was, in addition, a deterrent of equal dimension and this was the immense complexity of the fiber system under investigation. In fact, later in the century the histological approach used on its own was shown to be incapable of elucidating fully the various components of the vegetative system and their alignments. Pharmacological techniques had to be employed in order to supplement microscopy. Nevertheless Remak, working under similar restrictions and with the same methods and materials, approximated so much more closely to the truth as we with hindsight can judge.

The eminent Swiss microscopist, R. A. von Koelliker also contributed to the discord of the early 1840s when he opposed some of Bidder's and Volkmann's theories. In 1844 he published a monograph with a title very similar to that used by the two Germans, but in addition to "independence" of the vegetative system he included "dependence": *The Independence and Dependence of the Sympathetic Nervous System proved by means of anatomical Observations.*[265] He dealt in turn with the four elements said to make up the vegetative ganglia of the vertebrate: connective tissue, the so-called organic fibers of Remak, other nerve fibers, and ganglionic corpuscles.[266] Concerning the organic fibers he joined those who refused to acknowledge their existence, stating that they were not nervous elements, but instead were imperfectly developed fibro-cellular bundles deriving from the nerve's coverings.[267]

In opposition to Bidder and Volkmann, but in agreement with Valentin, Koelliker considered that the small fibers of the ganglionic system did not constitute a special class.[268] Moreover, he did not accept the significance they had placed on the morphological differences between these small ganglionic fibers and the large somatic type. He dismissed it thus:

> Indeed a difference exists between the thick and the fine fibers of the sympathetic nerve and other nerves. Nevertheless this in itself does not mean that there are two special kinds of nerve fibers, sympathetic and cerebrospinal.[269]

More important were the differences in their individual origins and the courses they ran. Whereas Bidder and Volkmann thought that in the frog most of the fibers of the rami were somatic and were carried to the periphery of the body in the spinal nerves and that the rest arose from the spinal root ganglia to form the sympathetic trunk, together with fibers from the vegetative ganglia, Koelliker, working with rabbit and human material, thought the reverse to be true. The contents of the rami, he declared, ran principally in a central not a peripheral direction, thus indicating a dependence on the cerebrospinal system. He did agree with them that small myelinated fibers arose from the vegetative and spinal and cranial nerve ganglia, and that these represented the independent elements of the ganglionic system. He did not, however, believe that they were confined to the latter, because they were connected with the cerebrospinal nervous system, that is, to the ganglia just mentioned and so to brain and spinal cord cells. Furthermore, somatic fibers passing through the rami and vegetative ganglia, likewise meant that the system was partly dependent on the brain and cord. But like Bichat, Koelliker considered that each of its ganglia was a repository of a special nervous power, all constituting in unison a functional whole, and thereby allowing the ganglionic system a degree of autonomy. One of his more significant findings for the current debate was that when teasing out the fourth sympathetic ganglion of the cat, he thought he could trace the nonmyelinated process of a nerve cell body into a myelinated fiber, indicating that the same nerve fiber could have a nonmyelinated and myelinated part, which we now accept. But of much greater moment, Koelliker was agreeing that the process of a ganglion nerve cell was, in fact, the beginning of a nerve fiber (see chap. 3 n. 143), and he proposed this as a general law.

The variations between the observations and interpretations of experienced microscopists such as Bidder, Volkmann, and Koelliker, and those between Remak and Valentin, illustrate well the difficulties facing investigators in the 1840s. In particular there was the hazard of ignoring species differences, and even these men of genius did not seem always to be immune from it. As noted above, the title of Koelliker's publication on the vegetative system, as in the case of Bidder's and Volkmann's revealed his conclusion regarding its basic features. Whereas they proclaimed it independent of the cerebrospinal system, he contended that it was partly independent and partly dependent, thus strengthening with morphological data the case put forward by Lobstein, Béclard, Broussais, and others, who had adopted a midway or compromise position. He argued that some independence of the system could be assumed, not because it contained unique elements absent from other parts of the nervous system as Remak and Bidder and Volkmann had claimed but because of its many ganglia and the numberless fibers that arose from their cells, together with the general complexity of its composition.

The ganglionic system's dependence upon other parts of the nervous system was due, however, to the fact that it received fine fibers from the spinal and cerebral nerve ganglia, and both fine and large fibers from the brain and spinal cord. In this respect it was probably more dependent in higher than in lower vertebrates, a view with which we would agree. Koelliker's ideas concerning the possible functions of the vegetative system[270] were not entirely in keeping with contemporary assessments, for he stated: "In the first place, I propose the thesis that the sympathetic nerve has nothing to do directly with nutrition."[271] Its effect was exerted indirectly by means of vasomotor influences. But otherwise he accepted its properties as designated by Müller, Remak, Valentin, and others.

The outcome of Bidder's and Volkmann's research was further support for Bichat's doctrine of an autonomous ganglionic complex, although it would seem that their opinions were based on faulty microscopical observations. Nevertheless, as we have mentioned (chap. 3 n. 191), Bidder later added more evidence for this by agreeing with Remak's concept of the ganglia as "central organs," and that their cells were responsible for their physiological activity. Koelliker, however, offered only partial confirmation of Bichat's theory and could agree wholeheartedly with neither Valentin's opposition to Bichat nor with Bidder's and Volkmann's approval. As time went on, however, the observations of Bidder and Volkmann on the "small" myelinated fiber of the ganglionic system became increasingly difficult to defend, for they were often incompatible with the results of other investigators, probably due to the use of different animal material and to microscopical techniques. Less and less attention was paid to them, and some ignored the problem whereas others were content to accept Remak's organic, nonmyelinated fibers. After midcentury, discussions on the differentiation by means of morphological criteria between fibers entering a ganglion, those arising from it, and those passing through it to pursue a direct course to an organ or tissue, gradually subsided. By 1870, although Remak's fibers had been accepted for about a decade, this problem was not thought to be of sufficient importance even to warrant notice by Maximilian Johann Sigismund Schultze (1825–1874) in his authoritative account of nerve fibers, written in 1871 for the widely approved treatise on histology edited by Salomon Stricker (1834–1898).[272]

But meantime important evidence contesting Bidder's and Volkmann's conclusions had been advanced by Thomas Snow Beck (1814–1877). The problem that still proved most difficult, and yet so vital, concerned the role of the rami. Several suggestions have already been discussed, but a unique observation made by Beck in 1846 on their arrangement, although receiving little attention at the time, pointed to modern concepts. In humans he found that the cervical and sacral regions possessed only gray rami.[273] Thus, he alone cast doubt on the universal view that ganglionic fibers derived from all the spinal nerves by way of the white rami. As we now know, each spinal nerve has a gray ramus, but the white are limited to the thoracic and upper lumbar levels, although variations in different animals exist.

This was the first foreshadowing of the autonomic outflows that Gaskell and Langley eventually differentiated. Thus Gaskell was to show that only those spinal nerves with white rami sent fibers to the sympathetic or thoracolumbar outflow. However, Beck's main intention was to disentangle the microscopical complexities of the ganglionic system, and in the first place he accepted Remak's organic fibers, thereby refuting the opinion of Bidder and Volkmann, and of all those who had disputed the existence of these elements of the vegetative system. He assembled anatomical evidence from humans to show that they were true nervous structures, and neither connective nor any other kind of nonneural tissue. As Remak had claimed, they made up the ganglionic system and they originated in its ganglia, being quite distinct in both form and function from cerebrospinal fibers. Thus, despite the contrary opinions that we have discussed, Beck insisted that there were important distinguishing morphological features of the two nervous systems. In particular the latter were separate at their origins and at their terminations, but connected together by the rami:

> We have thus distinct and separate systems of nerves; one composed of gelatinous [organic] nervous fibres which have their origins at the different ganglia; and the other composed of tubular [somatic] nervous fibres which arise at the brain and spinal cord.[274]

Like many before him, Beck differentiated between the two kinds of rami by the direction of their constituent fibers as well as by their appearance. In keeping with Müller and others he believed that the white contained animal fibers from both spinal roots in equal proportions and thus carried both motor and sensory messages (our preganglionic visceral efferents and visceral afferents). They, therefore, could be thought of as branches of the spinal nerves, sending fibers outward to the viscera (visceral efferents). The gray rami also linked spinal and vegetative nerves, and like other ganglionic nerves contained mainly organic fibers along with some animal fibers. The splanchnic nerves were essentially branches of the intercostal nerves reaching their destination directly without anastomosing in the ganglia and coming from the spinal cord. In a second paper Beck discussed the physiological implications of his anatomical findings.[275] The two nervous systems, he maintained, although independent units, had considerable reciprocal influences as Müller, Remak, and others had insisted. Whether appealing to microscopical, physiological, or to clinical evidence the answer was always the same. He concluded:

> that the different viscera receive their nervous supply from a system of nerves, which, with the various ganglia from which they take their origin, form a system distinct from, and independent of, the cerebro-spinal system; and that the modifications of function which are observed in the different viscera, are clearly to be traced to the varying proportions of tubular [animal] fibres which they receive, associated with the gelatinous [organic] fibres.[276]

Beck was probably referring here to Bidder's and Volkmann's view that the nerve to an organ provided it with both organic and somatic influences. Beck was agreeing with them that the degree of influence that the former had on a viscus was directly proportional to the percentage of organic fibers the nerve contained.

The contradictory results arising from the various investigations of the rami, ganglia, and splanchnic nerves were due, Beck explained, to an ignorance of the compound nature of these structures. They were by no means as simple as many had thought for they contained variable numbers of organic and animal fibers, each of which possessed different functions and varying degrees of excitability. On the whole, he had provided a much more lucid account of the vegetative nervous system than the majority of his contemporaries. But, he was primarily concerned with presenting evidence for a modified form of Bichat's scheme, not destroying it, and his discovery concerning the disposition of the rami, so important in retrospect, passed mainly unnoticed. In 1854, Remak reported further research especially on ganglion cells and the constituents of the white and gray rami.[277] His account of the rami was the best that could be hoped for in the period before Gaskell's studies utilizing new techniques, and Langley's pharmacological differentiation of ganglionic fibers. It also provided a summary of his own and others' findings. The white rami contained myelinated fibers from each anterior and posterior spinal root and therefore from the cord (? preganglionic efferents and myelinated afferents). The gray were made up of nonmyelinated fibers arising from cells in the ganglia, and distributed to the periphery in the cerebrospinal nerves (? postganglionic efferents or fibers of Remak). Remak, therefore, maintained that the gray rami were peripheral (i.e., centrifugal) nerves, but he seems to have been ignorant of Beck's discovery regarding the distribution of the rami.

7.7.5.4. *Conclusion.* Following the appearance in the 1830s of the first reports on the microscopical aspects of the fibers and cells contained in the vegetative system controversy persisted intermittently until the 1880s when Gaskell and Langley began to sort out the constituents of the system, employing new research methods. Thus at the middle of the nineteenth century there existed several opinions on the arrangement of its fibers. Some believed that the rami communicantes carried only fibers arising in the spinal cord and traveling to the ganglia, others that fibers in the rami passed in both directions, and another suggestion was that the fibers all originated in the ganglia and that their course could be either in a central direction by way of the rami and spinal roots, or peripherally in the somatic nerves of the cerebrospinal nervous system. Despite the confusion generated by multiple opinions, it seemed that microscopy had provided more evidence in support of Bichat's doctrine than against it. But in the absence of any firm knowledge of the origins of the myelinated white ramus fibers and of the organic fibers of the gray, it is not surprising that chaos continued and interest in the problem gradually declined. For the time being Bichat's doctrine was widely accepted, having been bolstered by the quantitative, yet incorrect, results of Bidder and Volkmann, along with the partial support of Koelliker and Beck. In fact, by midcentury it seemed to be more intact than ever for histological research seemed mostly to confirm it. Even in 1865 Polaillon was using histological findings to support Bichat, as well as Remak (see chap. 3.5.2).

7.8. CONCLUSION AND SEQUEL

For a review of midcentury concepts of the vegetative nervous system, Todd's *The Cyclopaedia* is a valuable source. His comments serve not only to illustrate the confusion and contradictions but in addition they indicate the survival of the speculation first advanced by Alexander Monro, *secundus,* in 1783,[278] adopted by Bichat, and subscribed to by men such as Koelliker, that the ganglionic, like the cerebrospinal, system had its own inherent nervous force located in the ganglia:

> [ganglia] are the seat of a special development of nervous power, whether spontaneously arising in the nutrient changes of ganglia, or by the reflexion of a change propagated to them by afferent nerves implanted in them.[279]

The persistence of this notion is of considerable significance, because it was vital to Bichat's ganglionic system and acceptance of it helped to guarantee approval of his doctrine, which had now thrived for half a century. Although its morphology and physiology were shrouded in doubt and darkness, there was as yet little sign of its decline, let alone its demise. At the same time, some felt that it was not entirely satisfactory, for numerous inadequacies, contradictions, anomalies, and unanswered questions were apparent. In retrospect it is obvious that the methods of investigation then available were unable to provide adequate and reliable answers, and in 1847 Todd admitted that "these questions cannot be satisfactorily solved in the present state of our knowledge."[280]

A midcentury assessment would be that owing to the complexity of the vegetative and cerebrospinal nervous systems and the crudity of current research techniques, conflicting theories were rife. Nevertheless, it seemed that on the whole the evidence so far brought forward from the fields of embryology, teratology, comparative anatomy, pathology, clinical medicine, experimental physiology, and histology favored Bichat's concept. Further elucidation of the vegetative system was to depend largely upon revelations made possible by the microscope, but up to 1850 it had provided only a mass of data with an accompanying variety of opinions concerning its fibers that supplied vegetative structures in the trunk and limbs. The cranial part of the ganglionic system was no better understood, and although by this time, the coccygeal,[281] ciliary,[282] sphenopalatine,[283] otic,[284] and other ganglia had been added to the system,[285] their relationship with it— like those of the vagus nerve and the plexuses, submucous (of Meissner) and myenteric (of Auerbach), of the intestines—was obscure.

Whereas most research in the first half of the nineteenth century was interpreted as sanctioning an autonomous ganglionic system, in the second half, the reverse was the case. The period after 1850 was characterized by the gradual accumulation of observations, overwhelming in both quality and quantity, that cast increasing doubt on the existence of two independent parts of the nervous system—the cerebrospinal and the ganglionic—and on the notion that the latter was a separate source of nervous energy. This shift in opinion was due chiefly to the demonstration that specific parts of the spinal cord and brain had controlling influences over the structures included in the ganglionic system's territory of supply, thus demolishing the whole concept of its autonomy. Rather than being morphologically distinct and able to act on its own, it could be shown beyond doubt that it was subjugated to higher spinal cord and brain centers. First there was the *piqûre diabétique* of Claude Bernard, which in 1849 provided unassailable evidence of a connection between the medulla oblongata and carbohydrate metabolism, an activity of the ganglionic system.[286] Three years later Budge and Augustus Volney Waller (1816–1870) discovered the cilio-spinal center, thus indicating the central connections of the cervical sympathetic chain of ganglia.[287] One of the last strongholds of those who accepted Bichat's independent system was the notion that visceral (autonomic) reflexes were limited to the ganglia and their nerves, as Willis in the seventeenth century and Unzer, Procháska, and others in the eighteenth had suggested. As we have seen,

Müller in 1835[288] and Grainger in 1837[289] also upheld the existence of reflexes taking place only by way of the vegetative ganglia, and in chapter 3.5.2 we discussed Remak's important contribution to sensorimotor, and therefore, reflex physiology of the vegetative system. However, the idea of an independent vegetative reflex system was demolished when visceral reflexes were shown to operate by way of the central nervous system.[290]

The influence of the cerebral cortex on ganglionic activities could also be demonstrated, as soon as cortical function became a research field after 1870 (see chap. 6.7).[291] Yet another factor in the decline of Bichat's system was further evidence from the new science of microscopical developmental anatomy. We have already seen how earlier in the century gross embryological observations were thought to support the system's autonomy (7.7.1), but histiogenetic evidence now refuted it, and the reverse judgment was made.[292]

Thus by the 1880s there seemed to be sufficiently reliable facts to overturn Bichat's theory and the need now was for a synthesis of these facts, and the provision of an acceptable alternative system. These were the tasks undertaken by Gaskell and Langley in Cambridge.[293] Whereas Gaskell investigated mainly the anatomical aspects of the vegetative nervous system, Langley adopted a completely new line of research: the use of drugs to distinguish between different parts of what Gaskell called the "visceral" or "involuntary" nervous system, and Langley the "autonomic" made up of "sympathetic" and "parasympathetic" parts. By combining their morphological, physiological, and pharmacological data they were able to create a firm foundation upon which modern concepts of autonomic functions have been built. The picture is still very far from completion, and Johnstone's comment of 1795 is as appropriate today as it was then, at the opening of the era we have surveyed. Having discussed the reception of his doctrine of the ganglia, he speculated on the future:

> In the next age, consequences of these truths, will be unveiled, to an extent not now to be conceived, but of the greatest importance in the healing art: in the mean time, what is here proposed, will furnish some direction to a sagacious searcher into the seat and nature of internal diseases.[294]

Johnstone's comments can also be applied to the other neuroscientific concepts that we have discussed in this book. Moreover, they remind us that the underlying purpose of investigating the nervous system has been and always will be a vital step towards the understanding and the ultimate conquest and elimination of diseases that attack it. This objective was by no means unique to the eighteenth century, because as we noted in chapter 1, Thomas Willis in 1664 expressed similar sentiments when he pointed out that the nervous system not only explained many properties of the body and of mental processes, but also that by means of this system "no less than the hidden causes of diseases and symptoms, which are commonly ascribed to the incantations of witches, may be discovered and satisfactorily explained."[295]

Notes

1. INTRODUCTION

1. See D. von Engelhardt, "Einheitliche," (1972), pp. 169–171; T. Lenoir, *The Strategy* (1982), p. 1.

2. There is no definitive work on the romantic philosophy of nature in English, but the following are useful sources: C. Siegel, *Geschichte* (1913); F. H. Garrison, "The Romantic period" (1931); O. Temkin, "German concepts" (1950); G. Rosen, "Romantic medicine" (1951); M. H. Abrams, *The Mirror* (1953); A. Lovejoy, *The Reason* (1961); A. Gode-von Aesch, *Natural Science* (1966); D. M. Knight, "The physical sciences" (1970); B. Gower, "Speculation in physics" (1973); J. L. Esposito, *Schelling's Idealism* (1977); T. Lenoir, "Generational factors" (1978); idem, *The Strategy* (1982). For its influence on pre-Darwinian British biology, see P. F. Rehbock, *The Philosophical Naturalists* (1983); on clinical medicine, see N. Tsouyopoulos, "German philosophy" (1984).

3. The treatment of *Naturphilosophie* by historians is discussed in T. Lenoir, *The Strategy* (1982), p. 5.

4. D. von Engelhardt, "Grundzüge" (1972), p. 301.

5. T. Lenoir, *The Strategy* (1982), pp. 5–6.

6. E. S. Russell, *Form and Function* (1916), pp. 100–101.

7. On the dissemination of transcendental ideas in Britain, see P. F. Rehbock, *The Philosophical Naturalists* (1983).

8. T. Lenoir, *The Strategy* (1982), p. 68. We shall mention the "organic physicists" in chap. 5.5.

9. E. S. Russell, *Form and Function* (1916), p. 89.

10. The changing fortunes of *Naturphilosophie* are charted in D. von Engelhardt, "Naturphilosophie" (1975).

11. In C. G. Carus, *Traité Élémentaire* (1835), 1:XXXIV. For biography of Carus, see M. Neuburger (1981), pp. 308–309.

12. T. Willis, *Cerebri Anatome* (1664), chap. 19. "De systemate nervoso in genere . . . ," p. 124. The phrase "incantations of witches" has been taken from Samuel Pordage's trans., in T. Willis, *Dr Willis's Practice* (1684), see *Five Treatises . . . The Anatomy of the Brain* (1681), chap. 19, p. 125. The Latin translates as "tricks of conjurors," but we prefer the contemporary interpretation. For biography of Willis, see *DSB;* A. Meyer, "Karl Friedrich Burdach" (1966); K. Dewhurst, *Thomas Willis's Oxford Lectures* (1980); idem, *Willis's Oxford Casebook (1650–1652)* (1981); and M. Neuburger (1981), p. 372.

13. K. M. Figlio, "Theories of perception" (1975), pp. 177–178.

14. For biography of Gall, see J. A. L. Fossati, "GALL (François-Joseph)" (1858); B. Hollander, *The Unknown Life* (1909); O. Temkin, "Gall" (1947); E. H. Ackerknecht and H. V. Vallois, *Franz Joseph Gall* (1956); R. M. Young, *Mind, Brain and Adaptation* (1970); idem, *DSB;* E. Lesky, ed., *Franz Joseph Gall* (1979); and M. Neuburger (1981), p. 323. For biography of J. C. Spurzheim, see A. Carmichael, *A Memoir* (1833); *DSB;* and M. Neuburger (1981), p. 361.

15. For a modern justification of this, see W. S. McCulloch, "Why the mind is in the head" (1951). For a discussion of relationships between brain and mental state, see J. Fodor, *The Language of Thought* (1974).

16. F. Magendie, *Précis* (1816–17), 1 (1816), "De l'intelligence," 170. For biography of Magendie, see J. M. D. Olmsted, *François Magendie* (1944); O. Temkin, "The philosophical background" (1946); *DSB;* Clarke and O'Malley (1968), pp. 299–304, 682–683, 732–737, and elsewhere; and M. Neuburger (1981), pp. 273–276, 340. Lesch's analysis of Magendie's experimental physiology, experimental pharmacology, and "pathological physiology" as he called it (see chap. 1.2.5) is the best available: J. E. Lesch, *Science and Medicine in France* (1984), pp. 89–124,136–137, 140–196, and passim.

17. J. E. Lesch, *Science and Medicine in France* (1984), pp. 167–168.

18. For biography of Cuvier, see W. Coleman, *Georges Cuvier* (1964); R. Dujarric de la Rivière, *Cuvier* (1969); *DSB;* and M. Neuburger (1981), p. 314.

19. For biography of Bell, see G. Gordon-Taylor and E. W. Walls, *Sir Charles Bell* (1958); and M. Neuburger (1981), p. 301. See also Clarke and O'Malley (1968), pp. 269–299, 303–305, and elsewhere.

20. See J. E. Lesch, *Science and Medicine in France* (1984), pp. 100–108.

21. G. R. Treviranus, in G. R. Treviranus and L. C. Treviranus, *Vermischte Schriften* (1816–1821), 4 (1821):226. For biography of G. R. Treviranus, see *DSB;* A. Meyer, *Historical Aspects* (1971); and M. Neuburger (1981), p. 365.

22. For a classic discussion of priority in scientific discovery see R. K. Merton, "Singletons and multiples" (1961).

23. A whole book on this celebrated dispute is available, P. F. Cranefield, *The Way In* (1974).

24. For biography and work of Rolando, see E. Manni, "Luigi Rolando" (1973); *DSB;* Clarke and O'Malley (1968), pp. 480–484, 653–657, and elsewhere; and M. Neuburger (1981), pp. 263–265, 355, and elsewhere.

25. For biography and work of Flourens, see J. M. D. Olmsted, "Pierre Flourens" (1953); *DSB;* Clarke and O'Malley (1968), pp. 483–490, 656–662, and elsewhere; and M. Neuburger (1981), pp. 276–278, 321, and elsewhere.

26. For biography of Hall, see [C. Hall], *Memoirs* (1861); *DSB;* M. Neuburger (1981), p. 327; chap. 4 n. 56 below; and Clarke and O'Malley (1968), pp. 347–351.

27. For one aspect of this conflict, see T. Lenoir, "Teleology without regrets" (1981).

28. See, for example, the views of J. C. Reil: M. Neuburger, *Johann Christian Reil* (1913), p. 17. See also, A. Lewis, "J. C. Reil's concept of brain" (1958); idem, "J. C. Reil" (1965); *DSB;* and M. Neuburger (1981), pp. 353–354. See also chap. 2 n. 5.

29. His idea first appeared in 1715, in the inaugural dissertation of one of his pupils: A. Kock, *De Generatione* (1715), §. V (pp. 9–11).

30. E. Clarke, "The neural circulation" (1978).

31. G. Rath, "Albrecht Thaer" (1958).

32. W. Cullen, *Institutions of Medicine* (1772). This edition was not seen nor was the second of 1777. The 3d ed. was used: idem, *Institutions of Medicine, Part I* (1785). It is also in idem, *The Works* (1827), 1:1–224. See I. A. Bowman, *William Cullen* (1975).

33. The final form of this notion is in W. Cullen, *The Works* (1827), vol. 1, para. 30 (pp. 16–17). It was an extension of the usual seventeenth- and eighteenth-century physical theories of nerve conduction. See chap. 5; E. Clarke, "The doctrine" (1968); Clarke and O'Malley (1968), pp. 155–177; and G. S. Rousseau, "Nerves" (1976).

34. It was also termed a "vital principle," W. Cullen, *A Treatise* (1789), 1:59.

35. W. Cullen, *Institutions of Medicine* (1785), para. 125 (pp. 93–95). For quote on this, see chap. 5 n. 49 below.

36. Ibid. para. 27 (p. 23).

37. G. Rath, "Neural pathology" (1959).

38. For an account of the debate between Virchow and a proponent of neural pathology, Gustav Adolf Spiess (1802–1875), see G. Rath, "Neural pathology" (1959), pp. 533–541.

39. He did so when describing inflammation: F. G. J. Henle, *Handbuch* (1846–1853), 1:244. However, he was by no means fully committed to it. For biography of Henle, see *DSB*.

40. See E. R. Long, *A History of Pathology* (1965), pp. 76–88; E. H. Ackerknecht, *Medicine at the Paris Hospital* (1967); and J. E. Lesch, *Science and Medicine in France* (1984), pp. 5, 54, 166–196, and elsewhere, who also

provides a penetrating analysis of the medical and scientific background. For an excellent nineteenth-century survey of its genesis and practice, see F. J. V. Broussais, *Examen* (1829–1834), vol. 2 (1829), "Chapitre XXIV. Naissance de l'anatomie pathologique," pp. 217–314; and vol. 4 (1834), "Chapitre XXXVII. De l'anatomie pathologique moderne et de quelques nouvelles doctrines," pp. 82–141 and remaining chapters of book. See in particular chaps. 41–45 on the application of morbid anatomy to diseases of the nervous system (pp. 600–758).

41. See J. W. Wilson, "Virchow's contribution" (1947); and L. J. Rather, ed., *Disease, Life, and Man* (1958).

42. J.G.C.F.M. Lobstein, *Discours* (1821). He also proposed a new theory of disease based on anomalies of innervation (*Essai* [1835]). For biography, see A. Brunschwig, "Jean Fréderic Lobstein" (1933); and M. Neuburger (1981), p. 338. See chap. 7 nn. 88, 119.

43. J.G.C.F.M. Lobstein, *Discours* (1821), p. 20.

44. Ibid., p. 33.

45. Ibid., p. 40.

46. Ibid., p. 42.

47. Ibid., p. 43.

48. Anonymous, "[Recent discoveries]" (1824), p. 142.

49. These were papers or reports by Flourens, Cuvier, Rolando, Coster, Foderà, and Magendie. The first five will be discussed in chap. 6, and Magendie's in chap. 4.

50. J. C. Dalton, *Experimentation* (1875), p. 32.

51. J. C. Dalton, *The Experimental Method* (1882), p. 2.

52. A. Brigham, *An Inquiry* (1840), pp. 26–27. For a nineteenth-century survey of the aims and methods of physiological research in general, see M. Verworn, *General Physiology* (1899), chap. 1, pp. 1–54.

53. A. Brigham, *An Inquiry* (1840), p. 27.

54. See H. McIlwain, "Chemical contributions" (1958); and D. B. Towers, "Origins" (1958).

55. See J. E. Lesch, *Science and Medicine in France* (1984), pp. 100–108.

56. P. Flourens, "Note touchant les effets de l'inhalation etherée" (1847); and idem, "Note touchant l'action de l'ether" (1847).

57. C. Bell, "On the nerves" (1821), p. 399.

58. This was privately printed for friends and colleagues in 1811: *Idea* (1811). From it arose the priority dispute with Magendie mentioned above and discussed below in chap. 4.

59. F. J. Gall, *Revue Critique* (1825), p. 118.

60. F. J. Gall, *Influence du Cerveau* (1825), pp. 145–146.

61. Most biographers have referred to them (n. 14, above). See also chap. 2, n. 26. For an early review of Gall's anatomy of the brain, see T. C. Rosenmüller, "Account" (1806). Gall and Spurzheim's detailed description of the nervous system is in their *Anatomie et Physiologie* (1810–1819), vol. 1 (1810).

62. M. Neuburger (1981), p. 334. Flourens's neurophysiology is discussed mainly in chap. 6.4, 6.

63. H. Mayo, *Outlines* (1827), p. 225. His use of the word "theoretical" is curious, because we know that Gall was a "practical" anatomist and mainly a "theoretical" physiologist. For biography of Mayo, see *DSB;* and M. Neuburger (1981), pp. 341–342.

64. S. Solly, *The Human Brain* (1836), p. xii. For biography of Solly, see *Plarr's Lives* (1930–1970).

65. J. J. C. Legallois, *Expériences* (1812), p. 151. (Also quoted in chap. 7 n. 147.) The celebrated writer, Hippolyte Adolphe [Henri] Taine (1828–1893), made a similarly sweeping claim that "vivisections have produced almost all the physiology of the nervous system" (cited by J. Schiller, "Claude Bernard and vivisection" [1967], p. 252, but not found in H. Taine, *On Intelligence* [1871]). Legallois's report on his research was presented to the Institut Impériale de France on 11 September 1811. See J. J. C. Legallois, "Rapport [1811]" (1812). For biography of Legallois, see E. Legallois, "Notice" (1830); *DSB;* G. Legée, "M.J.P. Flourens" (1975); and M. Neuburger (1981), p. 336.

66. F. Magendie, "Quelques idées" (1809). There is an analysis of this by W. R. Albury, "Physiological explanation" (1974). For an excellent account of Magendie's physiology, see W. R. Albury, "Experiment and explanation" (1977). J. Schiller ("Claude Bernard and vivisection" [1967]) gives a brief history of experimental physiology.

67. W. R. Albury, "Physiological explanation" (1974), p. 96.

68. For *idéologie,* see F. Picavet, *Les Idéologues* (1891); G. Boas, *French Philosophies* (1925); E. Cailliet, *La Tradition* (1943); P. Delaunay, "La médecine" (1920); G. Rosen, "The philosophy of ideology" (1946). More recent literature is cited in M. S. Staum, "Medical components" (1978), and in idem, *Cabanis* (1980). See also E. Haigh, "Medicine and ideology" (1984).

69. O. Temkin, "The philosophical background" (1946).

70. For a detailed discussion of their different approaches, see J. M. D. Olmsted, *François Magendie* (1944), chap. 7, pp. 93–122.

71. F. Magendie, *Leçons* (1841), 2:6.

72. C. Bernard, *Introduction* (1865). See also J. Schiller, "Claude Bernard and vivisection" (1967); and idem, "The genesis and structure" (1973). For biography, see J. M. D. Olmsted, *Claude Bernard* (1939); J. M. D. and E. H. Olmsted, *Claude Bernard* (1952); and *DSB*.

73. P. Flourens, *Recherches* (1842), p. 502.

74. This is the title of chap. 9 of his *Recherches* (1842), pp. 502–511. He also discussed the subject in his "Préface," pp. VII–X. For excellent surveys of Flourens's experimental method, see R. M. Young, *Mind, Brain and Adaptation* (1970), pp. 58–63; and M. Neuburger (1981), pp. 276–278.

75. P. Flourens, *Recherches* (1842), p. 511.

76. Ibid. It is important to note that Flourens and his contemporaries referred to the cerebral hemispheres as *le cerveau proprement dit* (p. 510).

77. R. M. Young, *Mind, Brain and Adaptation* (1970), p. 62.

78. M. Neuburger (1981), p. 276.

79. For a contemporary discussion of the problem, see J. H. Bennett, *Inaugural Dissertation* (1837), pp. 44–54. Little seems to have been written on the early history of experimental animal psychology, but see E. G. Boring, *A History* (1957); idem, "The beginning" (1961); and M. Neuburger (1981), pp. 265–270, 286. A. Meyer ("Karl Friedrich Burdach" [1970], p. 559) mentions comparative behavior studies. For an account of how the understanding of the minds of animals and of human behavior evolved 1870–1930, see R. Boakes, *From Darwin to Behaviorism* (1984). See also B. R. Singer, "History of the study" (1981) for a history of views on instinctive behavior, and of ethology.

80. S. Solly, *The Human Brain* (1836), p. 325.

81. F. B. Hawkins, *Elements* (1829). Despite their titles, the following articles are not helpful here, O. B. Sheynin, "On the history" (1980); E. Schultheisz, "The beginning" (1982).

82. P. Flourens, *Recherches* (1824), p. v. He stated: "This agent acts in too special a manner for it to be used indiscriminately with the others [methods of stimulation]" (p. v.). His comment in the 1842 edition (p. IX) was exactly the same, and a special work on galvanism was still promised. For the history of electrical excitation of nervous system structures, see A. E. Walker, "Stimulation and ablation" (1957); K. E. Rothschuh, "Zur Geschichte der physiologischen Reizmethodik" (1966); M. A. B. Brazier, *A History of Neurophysiology* (1984); and L. A. Geddes, *A Short History* (1984). D. Rapp (*Die Entwicklung* [1970]) and K. E. Rothschuh ("Die Bedeutung apparativer Hilfsmittel" [1971]) have followed the development of physiological methodology and apparatus (1784–1911), and their publications are most valuable. See Bibliographical Notes.

83. J. C. Dalton, *The Experimental Method* (1882), p. 22.

84. F. Magendie, *Leçons sur les Fonctions* (1841), vol. 1, "Onzième leçon. 23 janvier 1839," pp. 198–199. The episode was related by J. M. D. Olmsted, *François Magendie* (1944), pp. 135–136. While operating at the base of the brain, he damaged a large blood vessel and soon afterward the animal was thought to be dead. Removal of the cranial vault and cerebral hemispheres, however, resuscitated it immediately.

85. He discussed Flourens's work in F. J. Gall, *Influence du Cerveau* (1825), pp. 379–415. One of his conclusions was: "Thus everything goes to prove that the idea of the cerebellum being the balancing mechanism and the regulator of movements is a curious notion rather than a true discovery" (p. 405). See chap. 6.6

86. This was true in the few experiments he carried out on the healing of brain wounds, P. Flourens, *Recherches* (1842), chap. 9, pp. 155–168.

87. V. Horsley and E. A. Schäfer, "A record" (1888), p. 5.

88. P. Flourens, *Recherches* (1842), chap. 9, pp. 155–168, see also 6.7, below.

89. Luigi Luciani (1840–1919) achieved and reported this in 1891. See 6.7.

90. R. M. Young, *Mind, Brain and Adaptation* (1970), pp. 62–63.

91. F. J. Gall, *Influence du Cerveau* (1825), p. 156. For the defense of a contemporary against allegations of "cruel experiments," see A. P. Wilson Philip, *An Experimental Inquiry* (1818), pp. 363–384. For biography of Wilson Philip, see W. H. McMenemey, "Alexander Philips Wilson Philip" (1958); *DSB;* and M. Neuburger (1981), p. 349.

92. P. Flourens, *Recherches* (1842), p. VII. A young Italian contemporary, Michel Foderà (1793–1848), pointed out another advantage: in young animals, compensation to brain injury was greater and more rapidly achieved than in older ones (idem, "Recherches" [1823]). For biography of Foderà, see M. Neuburger (1981), p. 321.

93. W. B. Carpenter, *Principles of Human Physiology* (1846), para. 459, p. 344. For biography of Carpenter, see *DSB*.

94. [A. L.] Foville, "Researches" (1829), p. 279. For biography of Foville, see M. Neuburger (1981), p. 322.

95. R. S. Dow, "Thomas Willis" (1940). For biographies of Aristotle and Galen, see *DSB;* and M. Neuburger (1981), pp. 296–297 and 323, respectively.

96. W. Lawrence, *Lectures on Physiology* (1819), Lecture 3, p. 86. They were given in 1818.

97. S. Solly, *The Human Brain* (1836), p. xv.

98. Anonymous, ["Review of "*Report on Animal Physiology*"] (1836), p. 393.

99. F. G. J. Henle, *Handbuch* (1846–1853), 1 (1846):25. See T. Lenoir, "Generational factors" (1978).

100. F. G. J. Henle, *Handbuch* (1846–1853), 1 (1846):25.

101. On the doctrine of parallelism, see E. S. Russell, *Form and Function* (1916), pp. 81–83, 89–94; S. J. Gould, *Ontogeny* (1977), especially chap. 3; T. Lenoir, *The Strategy* (1982), pp. 42–44.

102. F. Tiedemann, *Anatomie* (1816), p. 4. See Clarke and O'Malley (1968), pp. 395–397; 827–829. For biography of Tiedemann, see *DSB;* and M. Neuburger (1981), p. 364.

103. F. Tiedemann, *Anatomie* (1816), p. 4.

104. Ibid., p. 2.

105. N. Steno, *Discours* (1669), p. 54. This lecture had been delivered at Paris in 1665.

106. T. Willis, *Cerebri Anatome* (1664), chap. 13, p. 83. See M. Neuburger (1981), p. 48; and A. Meyer and R. Hierons, "A note" (1964).

107. M. Neuburger (1981), p. 6. He discussed the natural experiment on a number of occasions (see his index). His chap. 11 deals with "The influence of surgery on the experiment" (pp. 169–182).

108. Ibid., p. 6.

109. S. Solly, *The Human Brain* (1836), p. 325.

110. C. F. Lallemand, *Recherches Anatomico-Pathologiques* (1820–1821). Cited by S. Solly, *The Human Brain* (1836), p. 326. For biography of Lallemand, see M. Neuburger (1981), p. 334. See also a contemporary account of his work, F. J. V. Broussais, *Examen* (1829–1834), 4 (1834):692–711. For biography of Broussais, see *DSB.*

111. The first systematic textbook of neurological diseases by Moritz Heinrich Romberg (1795–1873)—*Lehrbuch* (1840–1846)—reveals the state of clinical neurology toward midcentury. English trans., idem, *A Manual* (1853).

112. A. W. Otto, *Lehrbuch* (1830), vol. 1, pt. 2, sect. 20, §. 216 n. 3 (p. 375). There is an English trans.: idem, *A Compendium* (1831), see p. 365 n. (3).

113. See, for example, the case reported by E. Clarke and J. L. Laidlaw in "Silent hydrocephalus" (1958).

114. See H. M. Thomas, "Decussation" (1910); Clarke and O'Malley (1968), "Pyramidal tract," pp. 280–290; and M. Neuburger (1981), "Experiments on contralateral innervation," pp. 53–63.

115. J. H. Bennett, *Inaugural Dissertation* (1837), p. 37.

116. S. Solly, *The Human Brain* (1836), pp. 325–326.

117. Ibid., p. 327.

118. Ibid.

119. For details of this classic, see Bibliographical Notes. For an analysis of it and the authors cited in it, see P. Schmidt, *Zu den geistigen Wurzeln* (1973). For biography of Müller, see R. Virchow, *Eulogy of Johannes Müller* (1858); W. Haberling, *Johannes Müller* (1924); G. Koller, *Das Leben* (1958); *DSB;* and M. Neuburger (1981), p. 345.

120. J. Müller, *Handbuch* (1835–1840), vol. 1 (1835, 2d ed.), Book 3, sect. 5, chap. 3, "Vom Gehirn," "VI. Von den Hemisphären des grossen Gehirns," pp. 837–838. Quote on p. 837; English trans. by W. Baly (vol. 1, 1838), p. 839.

121. Two of the most commonly recognized today are the symptomless, slowly developing brain lesion and the false localizing signs of a space-occupying intracranial lesion.

122. J. E. Lesch, *Science and Medicine in France* (1984), pp. 178–191.

123. Ibid., p. 172.

124. P. Pinel, "Recherches" (1822), pp. 209–210. We are indebted to J. E. Lesch for this quotation.

125. J. B. Bouillaud, *Traité Clinique* (1825). Cited by S. Solly, *The Human Brain* (1836), pp. 467–468. For biography of Bouillaud, see J. D. Rolleston, "Jean-Baptiste Bouillaud" (1930–1931). See also a contemporary account of his work, F. J. V. Broussais, *Examen* (1829–1834), 4 (1834):711–734.

126. J. B. Bouillaud, *Traité Clinique* (1825), p. 295.

127. D. J. Larrey, *Clinique Chirurgicale* (1829–1836), 1 (1829):vi, 157–159. "I believe that I have been the first amongst French surgeons to verify

the principal tenets of Dr. Gall's doctrine: following physical lesions of various parts of the brain and according to the signs that characterize each of these lesions, the resultant effects correspond with the damaged functions." (p. vi).

128. C. F. Lallemand, *Observations Pathologiques* (1818), p. 53. This was his M.D. thesis.

2. THE CEREBROSPINAL AXIS

1. R. D. Grainger, *Elements of General Anatomy* (1829), p. 474. For biography of Grainger, see *Plarr's Lives* (1930–1970). For Galen's physiology and anatomy of the nervous system, see J. Wieberg, "The anatomy of the brain" (1914); Clarke and O'Malley (1968), pp. 14–19, 147–153, 260–265, 291–294, and passim; R. E. Siegel, *Galen on Psychology* (1973); idem, *Galen on the Affected Parts* (1976); and M. Neuburger (1981), pp. 6, 7, 11, and passim.

2. J. G. Spurzheim, *The Anatomy of the Brain* (1826), p. 10. For an example of this old view of the nervous system, see J. A. Unzer, *Erste Gründe* (1771), p. 14.

3. C. Bell, *The Nervous System* (1830), p. 3.

4. J. J. C. Legallois, *Expériences* (1812), p. 4. See chap. 1 n. 65.

5. W. B. Carpenter, *Principles of Human Physiology* (1846), p. 352.

6. See E. Lee, "The brain" (1849); E. G. T. Liddell, *The Discovery,* (1960), pp. 65–68; R. Leys Fried, *Alison versus Hall* (1976), pp. 126–127.

7. [W. B. Carpenter], ["Review of *The Brain and Its Physiology*"] (1846), pp. 511–512.

8. Ibid., p. 512. We shall discuss in chap. 7 this attempt to provide the vegetative (autonomic) nervous system with autonomy.

9. M. Krishaber, *Considérations,* (1864), p. 20.

10. [W. B. Carpenter], ["Review of *The Brain and Its Physiology*"] (1846), p. 512.

11. R. B. Todd and W. Bowman, *The Physiological Anatomy* (1845–1856), 1 (1845):246–247. For biography of Todd, see *DNB;* of Bowman, see *DSB.*

12. See, for example, W. B. Carpenter, *Manual of Physiology* (1846), p. 504.

13. P. A. Béclard, "Additions au système nerveux de la vie organique" (1821), pp. 402–403, 407–408. For biography of Béclard, see M. Neuburger (1981), p. 301.

14. See R. A. von Koelliker, *Die Selbständigkeit* (1844), pp. 29–30. For biography of Koelliker, see W. F. R. Weldon, "Albert von Koelliker" (1898); A. Koelliker, *Erinnerungen* (1899); G. R. Cameron, "Rudolf Albert Kölliker" (1955); and *DSB.* We have noted above the first use in the seventeenth

century of the comparative approach to the study of neuroanatomy, especially by Thomas Willis and Nicolaus Steno. See also n. 90 below. For Willis, see R. S. Dow, "Thomas Willis" (1940).

15. C. Bell, *The Nervous System* (1830), pp. 5–6.

16. W. Lawrence, *Lectures on Physiology* [1818] (1822), pp. 50–51.

17. M. Gross, "The lessened locus of feelings" (1979), especially pp. 259–260.

18. Anonymous, ["Review of *The Human Brain*"] (1837), p. 478. For similar statements see Anonymous, ["Review of *On the Physiological Inferences*"] (1839), p. 506; W. B. Carpenter, *Principles of Human Physiology* (1855), p. 441.

19. F. Tiedemann, "Beobachtung" (1824), p. 57.

20. F. J. Bérard, *Doctrine des Rapports* (1823), pp. 122–124. For biography, see *DSB*.

21. Ibid., pp. 102–103.

22. For summaries of Gall's neurology see O. Temkin, "Remarks" (1953); R. M. Young, "Franz Josef Gall" (1972).

23. Anonymous, ["Researches of Malacarne and Reil"] (1824), p. 107.

24. Ibid.

25. J. Elliotson (trans): J. F. Blumenbach, *Elements of Physiology* (1815), p. 203. See also Anonymous, "Dr. Gall's second dissection" (1823).

26. S. Solly praised Gall's and Spurzheim's dissection technique: "Every honest and erudite anatomist must acknowledge that we are indebted mainly to Gall and Spurzheim for the improvements which have been made in our mode of studying the brain." (*The Human Brain* [1836], pp. x–xi). J. C. Reil was also laudatory: "The worthy Reil, says professor Bischoff, who as a profound anatomist and judicious physiologist does not need my commendations, has declared when raising himself above the trivialities of egotism 'that he had discovered more in the dissections of the brain made by Gall than he had believed possible to be discovered in his whole lifetime.'" (Cited by F. J. Gall, *Revue Critique* [1825], pp. 490–491.) See also E. Lesky, ed., *Franz Joseph Gall* (1979), p. 39. As Blainville pointed out, however, Gall's claims were somewhat exaggerated (H. M. D. de Blainville, *Histoire des Sciences* [1845], 3:303–304. For biography of Blainville, see M. Neuburger [1981], p. 317). There was also the biased attack on Gall and Spurzheim by John Gordon (1786–1820) in *Observations* (1817), who declared that they were merely copying earlier anatomists such as Raymond de Vieussens (ca. 1635–1715), F. Vicq d'Azyr, and Reil. In it he adopted his usual abrasive and intemperate style: "I cannot believe that their pretensions while they carry with them a charge of neglect and ignorance against every preceding inquirer, in contempt of much well-earned reputation, are yet as unfounded as they have been confidently advanced; and are, both in their results and in their principles, calculated to retard the progress of real Knowledge" (pp. 2–3). Gordon's book is, however, a useful source of information on the history of

brain dissection. For Gall's method of dissecting the brain, see Clarke and O'Malley (1968), pp. 825–827.

27. F. J. Gall and J. C. Spurzheim, *Recherches* (1809), p. 19.

28. C. H. E. Bischoff and C. W. Hufeland, *Darstellung* (1805), p. 14.

29. This is Blainville's expression, *Histoire des Sciences* (1845), 3:318.

30. J. C. Spurzheim, *The Physiognomical System* (1815), pp. 14–16.

31. G. Cuvier et al., *Rapport* (1808), pp. 20–21, reported in Anonymous, "Report on a memoir" (1809); see also F. J. Gall and J. C. Spurzheim, *Anatomie et Physiologie,* (1810–1819), 1 (1810):39 and pl. II, fig. 3.

32. G. Cuvier et al., *Rapport* (1808), p. 21.

33. On this aspect of Gall's system, see E. Lesky, "Structure and function" (1970), pp. 308–309. Thomas Willis in 1664 (*Cerebri Anatome* [1664], chap. 26, "Nervorum paris, intercostalis . . . ") had also compared the ganglion to "a knot in the stem of a flourishing tree . . . and a diverting place for the many directions the [nerve] spirit can take" (p. 185).

34. G. Cuvier et al., *Rapport* (1808), p. 48.

35. F. J. Gall and J. C. Spurzheim, *Recherches* (1809), p. 92.

36. Ibid., p. 99.

37. J. Soury, *Le Système Nerveux Centrale* (1899), 1:501.

38. G. G. T. Keuffel, "Ueber das Rückenmark" (1811), pp. 148–149.

39. T. A. Appel, *The Cuvier-Geoffroy Debate* (1975), p. 290.

40. A. Dugès, *Mémoire* (1832), pp. vii–viii. For biography of Dugès, see [?]. Hoefer, ed., *Nouvelle Biographie* (1855–1866), vol. 15 (1858).

41. A. Dugès, "Mémoire" (1826), pp. 44–45.

42. A. Dugès, *Mémoire* (1832), p. vii.

43. Ibid., p. 65. Italics added.

44. E. Lesky, "Structure and function" (1970), p. 303.

45. K. E. Rothschuh, *History of Physiology* (1973), pp. 156–157.

46. H. B. Nisbet, *Goethe* (1972), pp. 6–7.

47. See B. Hoppe, "Le concept de biologie" (1971). He introduced the term "biology."

48. G. R. Treviranus, *Biologie* (1802–1822), 1 (1802):7–8.

49. Ibid., p. 119.

50. See P. Flourens, "Éloge" (1860), pp. xix–xx on Blainville; and [W. B. Carpenter], ["Review of *The Brain and Its Physiology*"] (1846), p. 544.

51. Quoted in W. H. Bruford, *Culture and Society* (1962), p. 146.

52. C. S. Sherrington, *Goethe* (1942), p. 21.

53. A. Gode-von Aesch, *Natural Science* (1966), p. 55.

54. G. G. Valentin, *Handbuch* (1835), p. 573. For biography of Valentin, see E. Hintzsche and W. Rytz, *Gustav Gabriel Valentin* (1953); B. Kisch, "Forgotten leaders" (1954), pp. 141–192; and *DSB*.

55. H. M. D. de Blainville, *Histoire des Sciences* (1845), 3:511. On the developmental aspect of romantic thought, see W. H. Bruford, *Culture and Society* (1962), p. 222; O. Temkin, "German concepts" (1950); K. E.

Rothschuh, *History of Physiology* (1973), pp. 161–162. For general discussions, see chap. 1 n. 2.

56. A. Gode-von Aesch, *Natural Science* (1966), p. 93.

57. Quoted in W. H. Bruford, *Culture and Society* (1962), p. 201.

58. J. J. Virey, *Philosophie* (1835), p. 387.

59. I. Döllinger, *Grundriss* (1805), p. 2.

60. C. A. Philites, "Von dem Alter" (1809), pp. 53–54, 56.

61. F. Tiedemann, *Zoologie* (1808–1810), 1 (1808):64–65.

62. See E. S. Russell, *Form and Function* (1916), pp. 69–70, 80–83, 91–93. S. J. Gould, *Ontogeny and Phylogeny* (1977), pp. 33–68.

63. I. Döllinger, *Von den Fortschritten* (1824), pp. 10–11.

64. P. Flourens, *Recueil* (1862), p. 288.

65. G. R. Treviranus, *Biologie* (1802–1822), 1 (1802):161. See also idem, *Die Erscheinungen und Gesetzte* (1831), p. 25.

66. J. Fletcher, *Rudiments of Physiology* (1835–1837), Pt I (1835), p. 36. For biography of Fletcher, see *DNB*.

67. J. J. Virey, *Philosophie* (1835), pp. 6–7.

68. Anonymous, ["Review of *Histoire Générale*"] (1839), p. 4.

69. See H. B. Nisbet, *Herder* (1970), pp. 30–31.

70. J. Fletcher, *Rudiments of Physiology* (1835–1837), Pt I (1835), pp. 36–37.

71. R. D. Grainger, "Illustrations" (1842–1843), p. 93.

72. F. Tiedemann, *Zoologie* (1808), 1:vii.

73. W. B. Carpenter, *Principles of General and Comparative Physiology* (1839), p. 162.

74. R. D. Grainger, "Illustrations" (1842–1843), p. 93. See also J. Anderson, *Sketch* (1837), p. 1.

75. On the vertebral theory of the skull, see E. S. Russell, *Form and Function* (1916), pp. 96–99.

76. H. M. D. de Blainville, *Histoire des Sciences* (1845), 3:511.

77. J. Müller, *Vergleichende Anatomie* (1835), p. 234.

78. G. R. Treviranus and L. C. Treviranus, *Vermischte Schriften* (1816–1821), 4 (1821):226. We have already referred to this statement (see chap. 1 n. 21).

79. J. Fletcher, *Rudiments of Physiology* (1835–1837), Pt I (1835), p. 59.

80. J. F. Blumenbach, *Handbuch* (1805), p. 291.

81. J. Müller, "Ueber die Metamorphosen" (1828), p. 16.

82. F. Tiedemann, *Anatomy of the Foetal Brain* (1826), pp. 121–122; F. von P. Gruithuisen, *Anthropologie,* (1810), pp. 239–240.

83. E. R. A. Serres, *Anatomie Comparée* (1824–1826), 1 (1824):lxiv.

84. F. J. Gall and J. C. Spurzheim (1809), pp. 94–95.

85. F. Tiedemann, *Anatomy of the Foetal Brain* (1826), p. xi.

86. F. J. Gall and J. C. Spurzheim, *Anatomie et Physiologie* (1810–1819), 1 (1810):21.

87. Ibid., p. xiii.

88. J. Anderson, *Sketch* (1837), p. 4.

89. J. Müller, "Ueber die Metamorphosen" (1828), p. 1.

90. See R. S. Dow, "Thomas Willis" (1940). See also Pieter Camper (1722–1789), "Deux discours" (1778). To some eighteenth-century anatomists, however, even such limited analogies between humans and the lower animals seemed strange and provoked resistance: see W. F. Bynum, "The anatomical method" (1973), p. 447.

91. See, for example, P. A. Béclard, "Additions" (1821), pp. 398–409, 407–408.

92. G. R. Treviranus and L. C. Treviranus, *Vermischte Schriften* (1816–1821), 3 (1820):56.

93. F. J. Gall and J. C. Spurzheim, *Anatomie et Physiologie* (1810–1819), 1, (1810):25.

94. See E. Lesky, "Structure and function" (1970), pp. 304–305.

95. J. C. Reil, "Das verlängerte Rückenmark . . . Funfte Fortsetzung" (1809), p. 485.

96. F. Tiedemann, *Zoologie* (1808–1810), 1 (1808):107.

97. F. Tiedemann, *Anatomie der Röhren-Holothurie* (1816), p. 90, pl. 9, fig. 2.

98. S. Solly, *The Human Brain* (1836), p. 14.

99. J. L. Schönlein, *Von der Hirnmetamorphose* (1816), pp. 4–6, 16–17. For biography of Schönlein, see E. H. Ackerknecht, "Johann Lucas Schoenlein" (1964); and M. Neuburger (1981), p. 359.

100. J. Anderson, *Sketch* (1837), p. 6.

101. Ibid., pp. 7–8.

102. C. A. Philites, "Von dem Alter" (1809), p. 56.

103. F. J. Gall and J. C. Spurzheim, *Anatomie et Physiologie* (1810–1819), 1 (1810):138.

104. Ibid., pp. 139, 149; E. Lesky, "Structure and function" (1970), pp. 308–309. A. L. Foville, *Traité* (1844), p. 357; J. Quain, *Elements of Anatomy* (1837), p. 108.

105. See K. F. Burdach, *Vom Baue und Leben* (1819–1826), 1 (1819):62 (for biography of Burdach, see A. Meyer, "Karl Friedrich Burdach" [1966]; idem "Karl Friedrich Burdach" [1970]; *DSB;* and M. Neuburger [1981], p. 308); J. F. Meckel, the Younger, *Beyträge* (1808–1811), 2 (1811):85; J. Fletcher, *Rudiments of Physiology* (1835–1837), Pt. I (1835), pp. 26–30. For biography of Meckel, see *DSB;* and M. Neuburger (1981), pp. 342–343.

106. F. Tiedemann, "Beobachtung" (1824), p. 58.

107. J. H. F. Autenrieth, "Bemerkungen" (1807), pp. 55–56.

108. F. J. Gall and J. C. Spurzheim, *Recherches* (1809), pp. 89–90. See also idem, *Anatomie et Physiologie* (1810–1819), 1 (1810):38–39; and J. C. Spurzheim, *The Physiognomical System* (1815), pp. 25–26.

109. L. A. Desmoulins, *Anatomie* (1825), 1:129–130.

110. J. Swan, *Illustrations* (1835), pp. 42–44.

111. Anonymous, ["Review of *Illustrations*"] (1840), pp. 230–231.

112. Anonymous, [Review of *Illustrations*] (1836), pp. 193–194.

113. G. R. Treviranus and L. C. Treviranus, *Vermischte Schriften* (1816–1821), 4 (1821):227.

114. K. F. Burdach, *Vom Baue und Leben* (1819–1826), 1 (1819):67.

115. J. Fletcher, *Rudiments of Physiology* (1835–1837), Pt. I (1835), p. 46.

116. J. Anderson, *Sketch* (1837), p. 13.

117. S. Solly, *The Human Brain* (1836), p. 36.

118. Ibid. (1847), p. 331.

119. H. Mayo, *The Nervous System* (1842), pp. 18–19; R. B. Todd and W. Bowman, *The Physiological Anatomy* (1845–1856), 1 (1845):319; A. Dugès, *Traité* (1838–1839), 1 (1838):81–83.

120. J. Goodsir, "On the morphological relations" (1856), p. 83.

121. H. M. D. de Blainville, *Histoire des Sciences* (1845), p. 327.

122. J. C. Spurzheim, *The Anatomy of the Brain* (1826), pp. 47–48. He was, however, only reflecting views of his predecessors, in particular, Legallois.

123. J. Copland, "Appendix" (1829), p. 672.

124. R. D. Grainger, *Observations* (1837), pp. 26, 44–45.

125. [W. B. Carpenter], ["Review of *The Brain and Its Physiology*"] (1846), p. 494.

126. J. H. F. Autenrieth, "Bemerkungen" (1807), p. 57.

127. F. Leuret and L. P. Gratiolet, *Anatomie Comparée* (1839–1857), 2 (1857):6 (by Gratiolet). Conrad Eckhard (1822–1905) in 1849 and Ludwig Türck (1810–1868) in 1856 were the first to make certain reference to what later became known as "dermatomes" and "myotomes." See Clarke and O'Malley (1968), pp. 310–316. For biography of Leuret and Gratiolet, see pp. 399 and 403, respectively. For Leuret, see *DSB* also.

128. F. Leuret and L. P. Gratiolet, *Anatomie Comparée* (1839–1857), 2 (1857):8–9 (by Gratiolet). An early example of the theory that the cord is made up of several partly autonomous locally functioning centers is found in Johann Peter Frank (1745–1821), "Untersuchungen" (1791), pp. 284–285.

129. Legallois was aware of Gall's anatomical ideas at the time of his experiments: J. J. C. Legallois, *Expériences* (1812), p. ix.

130. A. Dugès, *Mémoire* (1832), pp. 348–349.

131. A. Vulpian, *Leçons* (1866), p. 12. That the spinal cord had an intrinsic power was echoed by the neurologist Romberg in his *Lehrbuch* (1840–1846), the widespread influence of which was greatly increased by an English translation, *A Manual* (1853). Complete copies of the 1st, 2d, and 3d German editions could not be traced, and the following quotations are from the English version. The spinal cord "is a central organ of the nervous system, and as such possesses peculiar endowments" (2:42). And "[T]he

spinal cord viewed as a central organ, not only serves as an agent for the mutual transmission of stimuli, but also as a source of nervous power, of the principle of motor and sensory tension, by which the continuance and vigour of motion and sensation is secured, and a general stimulus for the entire organism provided" (2:395). The intrusion of this new concept into clinical neurology was of great consequence for the interpretation of spinal cord disorders.

132. F. J. Gall and J. C. Spurzheim, *Anatomie et Physiologie* (1810–1819), 1 (1810):25.

133. Ibid., p. 165.

134. Ibid., 2 (1812):258–259.

135. F. J. Gall and J. C. Spurzheim, *Recherches* (1809), pp. 150–151.

136. See especially F. Tiedemann, *Anatomy of the Foetal Brain* (1826), pp. 150–151.

137. R. D. Grainger, *Elements of General Anatomy* (1829), pp. 497–498.

138. For a summary of this literature, see M. Krishaber, *Considérations* (1864), pp. 26–28.

139. G. Cuvier et al., *Rapport* (1808), p. 48.

140. See K. F. Burdach, *Die Physiologie* (1826–1840), 2 (1828):418.

141. J. C. Reil, "Untersuchungen . . . Vierte Fortsetzung" (1809), p. 147.

142. Ibid., p. 151.

143. F. Arnold, *Handbuch* (1851), p. 682. See also E. Huschke, *Schaedel, Hirn und Seele* (1854), p. 146.

144. J. C. Reil, "Das verlängerte Rückenmark . . . Funfte Fortsetzung" (1898), p. 486.

145. See H. M. D. de Blainville, *Histoire des Sciences* (1845), 3:315–316.

146. H. M. D. de Blainville, "Considérations" (1821), p. 49.

147. W. B. Carpenter, *Principles of Human Physiology* (1846), p. 266.

148. J. H. F. Autenrieth, "Bemerkungen" (1807), p. 56.

149. F. von P. Gruithuisen, *Anthropologie* (1810), p. 240.

150. See F. Tiedemann, *Zoologie* (1808), vol. 1, pp. 106–107; J. Müller, "Ueber die Metamorphosen" (1828), p. 13; A. Dugès, *Mémoire* (1832), pp. 62–63; C. G. Carus, *Traité* (1835), 3:37.

151. J. L. Schönlein, *Von der Hirnmetamorphose* (1816), pp.17–18.

152. Ibid., pp. 18–19.

153. Ibid., pp. 19–20, 35.

154. [W. B. Carpenter,] ["Review of *The Brain and Its Physiology*"] (1846), pp. 500–501.

155. K. F. Burdach, *Die Physiologie* (1826–1840), 2 (1828):418–419, 422–427.

156. F. Tiedemann, *Anatomy of the Foetal Brain* (1826), pp. 6–7, 122.

157. J. Fletcher, *Rudiments of Physiology* (1835–1837), Pt. I (1835), p. 60.

158. E. R. A. Serres, *Anatomie Comparée* (1824–1826), 1 (1824):xi.

159. F. J. Bérard, *Doctrine des Rapports* (1823), p. 119. See also G. Büchner, "Probevorlesung" (1836).

160. W. Griesinger, *Pathologie und Therapie* (1845), pp. 10–11. For biography, see chap. 4 n. 150, below.

161. F. Leuret and L. P. Gratiolet, *Anatomie Comparée* (1839–1857), 2 (1857):82–83, 162 (by Gratiolet).

162. S. W. Ranson, *The Anatomy of the Nervous System* (1959), p. 2.

163. Ibid., p. 24.

164. Ibid., pp. 5–6.

165. Ibid., p. 7.

166. Ibid., pp. 8, 12.

167. Ibid., pp. 21–22. See also A. C. Guyton, *Textbook of Medical Physiology* (1976), pp. 610–611.

168. See W. Coleman, "Morphology" (1976).

3. THE NERVE CELL

1. M. F. X. Bichat, *Traité des Membranes* (1800), pp. 30–32. For biography of Bichat, see [?]. Hoefer, ed., *Nouvelle Biographie* (1858–1866), vol. 6 (1862); E. H. Ackerknecht, *Medicine at the Paris Hospital* (1957), pp. 51–58; *DSB;* and M. Neuburger (1981), p. 303. For a discussion of the epistemological and methodological differences between Bichat's physiology and that of Magendie, see J. V. Pickstone, "Bureaucracy, liberalism and the body" (1981). See also E. Haigh, *Xavier Bichat* (1984). There is no adequate history of histology, but A. Hughes, *A History of Cytology* (1959) is valuable. See also T. S. Hall, *Ideas of Life and Matter* (1969), 2:121–304, for an excellent account of plant and animal microanatomy, 1800–1860. For the role of the microscope in biological research, see S. Bradbury, *The Evolution of the Microscope* (1967). For the history of neurohistology, see (1) L. F. Barker, *The Nervous System* (1899). Chaps. 1 and 2 contain critical analyses of advances in the nineteenth century; (2) C. H. L. Stieda, "Geschichte" (1899). Deals with period 1790–1865. More detailed but less reliable than Barker's account and especially unfair to Robert Remak; (3) A. T. Rasmussen, *Some Trends in Neuroanatomy* (1947), see chap. 2, "The microscopic structures of nervous tissues and the development of the neuron concept," pp. 31–35. No references and not entirely reliable; (4) H. Spatz, "Neuronenlehre und Zellenlehre" (1952); (5) A. Andreoli, *Zur geschichtlichen Entwicklung* (1961). Balanced, but not entirely reliable account; (6) Clarke and O'Malley (1968), pp. 27–138, Leeuwenhoek to Ramón y Cajal (1933); (7) A. Meyer, *Historical Aspects* (1971), Part 3,"15. Some problems concerning the discovery of the neurone." Early history only of cell and fiber.

2. F. J. Gall and J. C. Spurzheim, *Anatomie et Physiologie* (1810–1819), vol. 1 (1810): A knowledge of the microscopical elements of nerve fibers, whether globules or other structures, "gives no hint as to how their functions can be ascertained" (p. xix).

3. P. A. Béclard, *Élémens d'Anatomie Générale* (1823), pp. 96–97.

4. A. van Leeuwenhoek, "An abstract of a letter" (1685), written at Delft and dated 25 July 1684. The complete letter is "De structura cerebri" (1722). See Clarke and O'Malley, pp. 418–420. For Leeuwenhoek, see C. Dobell, *Anton van Leeuwenhoek* (1932). Other prominent globulists were: G. M. della Torre, *Nuove Osservazioni Microscopiche* (1776); F. G. F. Fontana, *Traité sur le Vénin* (1781), 2:209–221 (see n. 10 below); J. Procháska, *De Structura Nervorum* (1779), sect. 2, chap. 5, "De nervorum medulla," pp. 66–73 (for biography, see *DSB;* and M. Neuburger [1981], p. 352); J. Wenzel and C. Wenzel, *De Penitiori Structura Cerebri* (1812), p. 24; G. R. Treviranus, in G. R. Treviranus and L. C. Treviranus, *Vermischte Schriften* (1816–1821), 1:128. The globule was an optical illusion, spherical in form, with a bright center and a dark outline, and due to the optical aberrations of crude lens systems. Nevertheless, descriptions of them have deceived those investigating early microscopy, as, for example, in the case of René Joachim Henri Dutrochet (1776–1847), who in his book, *Recherches Anatomiques* (1824) described globules, which were interpreted as cells by A. R. Rich, "The place of R.-J.-H. Dutrochet" (1926). Rich therefore claimed priority for Dutrochet and accused Schwann of plagiarism! F. K. Studnička, "Aus der Vorgeschichte" (1931–1932) fell into the same error, but J. W. Wilson in "Dutrochet" (1947) has set the record straight. However, Dutrochet played an important part in French physiology of the early nineteenth century. See J. V. Pickstone, "Globules and coagula" (1973); J. Schiller, *Physiology and Classification* (1980), pp. 63–66. Rudolf Virchow explained that Milne-Edwards's notion of globules, for example, was "in part attributable to optical illusions in microscopical observation. The inferior method that prevailed during the whole of the last [eighteenth] and part of the present [nineteenth] century of making observations in direct sunlight, caused a certain amount of dispersion of light in nearly all microscopical objects, and the impression communicated to the observer was that he saw nothing but globules (*Kügelchen*)." (*Die Cellularpathologie* [1858], p. 23.) Moreover, the tissue used was unstained. See also J. W. Wilson, "Virchow's contribution" (1947). J. R. Baker, in "The cell-theory" (1948–1955), has made a critical appraisal of the cell theory, including its prehistory. He explains that particles smaller than cells may have presented a globular appearance due to light haloes surrounding them and arising from spherical aberration. On the other hand, the globules may have been fat droplets or products of degeneration. They certainly were not cells. An alternative notion of the ultimate elements of nervous substance was that of Haller. As with other tissues it was made

up of the theoretical "fiber," equivalent to the physicist's theoretical atom, and a gluelike material (A. von Haller, *Elementa* [1757–1766], vol. 1 [1757], bk. 1, "Corporis humani elementa," "Sectio I. Fibra," pp. 2–8). For biography of Haller, see M. Neuburger (1981), p. 327.

5. The Meckel and Milne-Edwards versions of globulism are found in J. F. Meckel, the Younger, *Handbuch* (1815–1820), 1 (1815):4–8; and H. Milne-Edwards, *Mémoire sur la Structure Elémentaire* (1823); and idem, "Recherches microscopiques" (1826). On Home, see below. For a discussion of globulism, see J. Pickstone, "Globules and coagula" (1973).

6. E. Home, *The Croonian Lecture* (1799), p. 7.

7. E. Home, *Lectures on Comparative Anatomy* (1814–1828), 5 (1828): 193–194. For Bauer's life and work, see G. Meynell, "Francis Bauer" (1983).

8. E. Home, *Lectures on Comparative Anatomy* (1814–1828), 3 (1823):37.

9. Ibid., pp. 37–39.

10. The existence of threads or fibers in the peripheral nerves had been established macroscopically by Andreas Vesalius (1514–1564) in 1543: the nerve was "a thick cord, twisted from many threads." (*De Humani Corporis Fabrica* [1543], p. 633). The microscopical nerve fiber, however, was not recognized until 1781, by the Italian scientist Felice Gaspar Ferdinand Fontana (1730–1805) in his book on snake venom: "I finally succeeded in finding several very small, more or less transparent cylinders which seemed to possess a pellicle and to be partly filled with a transparent, gelatinous fluid and small globules or bodies of unequal size . . . which I shall call primitive nerve cylinders" (*Traité sur le Vénin,* [1781], 2:204). See M. A. B. Brazier, "Felice Fontana" (1963); Clarke and O'Malley (1968), pp. 35–38; and E. Clarke and J. G. Bearn, "The spiral nerve bands" (1972). For bibliography of Fontana, see P. K. Knoefel, *Felice Fontana* (1980). Fontana's descriptive terms reflected the concept of the hollow nerve functioning as a tube to carry messages (see chap. 5). Therefore, the term "nerve fiber" used before 1780 did not refer to the microscopical structure, see A. Berg, "Die Lehre von der Fraser" (1942); and L. J. Rather, "Some relations" (1969); and M. D. Grmek, "La notion de fibre" (1970). See F. G. F. Fontana, "Observations sur la structure des nerfs faits à Londres en 1779," in *Traité sur le Vénin* (1781), 2:187–208. It has been claimed that he described the myelinated nerve fiber (B. Zanobio, "Le osservazioni" [1959], p. 162). A similar claim for G. R. Treviranus is more substantial: see his *Vermischte Schriften* (1816–1821) compiled with L. C. Treviranus, vol. 1 (1816), "4. Ueber die organischen Elemente des thierischen Körpers," pp. 117–144, see p. 128. He produced the first illustration of it and used the terms "nerve medulla" (*Nervenmark*) and "nerve tube" (*Nervenröhr*).

11. E. Home, *Lectures on Comparative Anatomy* (1814–1828), 5 (1828):242.

12. Ibid., p. 194.

13. Ibid., 3 (1823):41, 43.

14. He invented an achromatic objective (G. B. Amici, *De' microscopii* [1818]); see also V. Chevalier and C. L. Chevalier, *Microscopes Catadioptriques* (1827); and V. Ronchi, "Giovanni Battista Amici's" (1969). This was improved by J. J. Lister, the wine merchant father of Joseph, Lord Lister (1827–1912), the surgeon.

15. J. J. Lister, "On some properties" (1830). For details of his life and work, see J. Lister, "Of the late Joseph Jackson Lister" (1870); and *DSB*.

16. G. F. Hildebrandt, *Handbuch* (1830–1832), 1 (1830):131–133.

17. R. D. Grainger, *Elements of General Anatomy* (1829), pp. 26–27. T. Hodgkin and J. J. Lister, "Notice" (1827); A. Hughes, *A History of Cytology* (1959) commented, "With this paper animal histology may be said properly to begin" (p. 8). Hodgkin and Lister reported that in brain tissue "one sees instead of globules a multitude of very small particles, which are most irregular in shape and size" (p. 137).

18. F. B. Churchill, "Rudolf Virchow" (1976); A. Baxter and J. Farley, "Mendel and meiosis" (1979); L. S. Jacyna, "John Goodsir" (1983).

19. L. J. Rather, *The Genesis of Cancer* (1978), p. 77.

20. A. Andreoli, *Zur geschichtlichen Entwicklung* (1961), p. 10. See also Clarke and O'Malley, (1968), pp. 39–43.

21. C. G. Ehrenberg, "Nothwendigkeit" (1833), pp. 449–450.

22. C. G. Ehrenberg, *Beobachtung* (1836), p. 10; English trans., 1837, pp. 267–268.

23. Ibid., p. 14; English trans., 1837, p. 274.

24. F. von P. Gruithuisen, *Anthropologie,* (1810), pp. 41, 106–108, 258–260.

25. F. von P. Gruithuisen, *Organozoonomie* (1811), p. 212.

26. C. G. Ehrenberg, "Nothwendigkeit" (1833), pp. 451–452.

27. See I. Jahn, "Ehrenberg" (1971), p. 290; W. G. Siesser, "Christian Gottfried Ehrenberg" (1981), pp. 171–172.

28. T. Hodgkin and J. J. Lister, "Notice" (1827), p. 137; H. M. D. de Blainville, *Cours* (1829), 1:387; G. R. Treviranus, *Neue Untersuchungen* (1835), p. 33.

29. G. F. Hildebrandt, *Handbuch* (1830–1832), 1 (1830):266.

30. See E. Hintzsche and W. Rytz, *Gustav Gabriel Valentin* (1953), p. 5; and V. Kruta, "Les relations" (1966).

31. R. Remak, "Ueber die physiologische Bedeutung" (1840), p. 236. For biography and work of Remak, see B. Kisch, "Forgotten leaders" (1954), pp. 227–296; Clarke and O'Malley (1968), pp. 46–52; A. Meyer, *Historical Aspects* (1971), pp. 162–169; and *DSB*.

32. R. Toellner, "Naturphilosophische Elemente" (1971), p. 35. See also H. J. John, *Jan Evangelista Purkyně* (1959), pp. 5, 9; E. Witte, "Beitrag" (1942); V. Kruta, *The Poet and the Scientist* (1968).

33. M. Teich, "The world outlook" (1962), pp. 130–131.

34. V. Kruta, "J.E. Purkyně's conception of physiology" (1971), p. 29; idem, "G. Prochaska's and J.E. Purkyně's contributions" (1964), p. 140.

35. J. E. Purkyně, ["Review of K. F. Burdach"] (1833), pp. 118, 121–122.

36. J. E. Purkyně, "Ueber den Begriff" (1852), p. 66. Purkyně's views corresponded with those of the organic physicists, such as E. du Bois-Reymond (see chap. 5.5), on this issue. But it is unlikely that either was directly influenced by the other; rather, both should be seen as responding to the powerful drive to unification of the sciences in contemporary German philosophy. On the organic physicists, see C. A. Culotta, "German biophysics" (1974); P. F. Cranefield, "The organic physics" (1957); idem, "The philosophical and cultural interests" (1966).

37. J. E. Purkyně, ["Review of K.F. Burdach"] (1833), p. 121.

38. V. Kruta, "J.E. Purkyně" (1962), p. 79.

39. See F. K. Studnička, "Joh. Ev. Purkinje" (1927), esp. pp. 117, 121; Z. Frankenberger, "J.E. Purkyně" (1959). A summary of these earlier researches is found in J. E. Purkyně, "Ueber die Analogieen" (1839).

40. G. Sarton, "The discovery of the mammalian egg" (1931).

41. V. Kruta, "K.E. von Baer" (1971–1972), p. 97.

42. J. E. Purkyně, "Ei" (1834), pp. 160–161. Purkyně omitted some words from Harvey's original text. The full sentence reads: "Natura enim divina, et perfecta, in iisdem rebus semper sibi consona est." W. Harvey, *Exercitationes* (1651), p. xiii.

43. J. E. Purkyně, "Ueber den Typus" (1843), p. 104; see also idem, "Ueber die Struktur" (1842), p. 95.

44. J. E. Purkyně, ["Review of Carl Friedr. Burdach"] (1828), pp. 62–63, 66.

45. B. Kisch, "Forgotten leaders" (1954), pp. 146–147.

46. E. Hintzsche and W. Rytz, *Gustav Gabriel Valentin* (1953), p. 22. For biography of Wagner, see *DSB*.

47. See E. Hintzsche, *Zellen und Gewebe* (1963).

48. G. G. Valentin, "Feinere Anatomie" (1836), pp. 303–304; see also idem, "Die Entwickelung der Pflanzengewebe" (1837), p. 161.

49. G. G. Valentin, *Lehrbuch* (1844), 1:1.

50. The influence of *Naturphilosophie* on the microscopy of this period is discussed in B. Hoppe, "Discussions" (1968).

51. See K. E. Rothschuh, "Von der Histomorphologie" (1971), pp. 204–206; and M. Teich, "Purkyně and Valentin" (1970).

52. F. K. Studnička, "J.K. Purkinje's 'Physiology'" (1936), p. 476. A summary of previous researches on ciliary motion is found in J. E. Purkyně and G. Valentin, *De Phaenomeno* (1835), pp. 287–314.

53. E. Hintzsche and W. Rytz, *Gustav Gabriel Valentin* (1953), p. 12.

54. J. E. Purkyně and G. G. Valentin, *De Phaenomeno* (1835), p. 286.

55. J. E. Purkyně and G. G. Valentin, *De Motu Vibratorio* (1835), p. 15.

56. B. Kisch, "Forgotten leaders" (1954), p. 158.

57. J. E. Purkyně and G. G. Valentin, *De Phaenomeno* (1835), p. 360. See also G. G. Valentin, "Fortgesetzte Untersuchungen" (1836), p. 148.

58. G. G. Valentin, "Flimmerbewegung" (1842), p. 484.
59. J. E. Purkyně, "Einbildungskraft" (1834), p. 194.
60. Ibid., pp. 198–199.
61. J. E. Purkyně ["Review of Carl Friedr. Burdach"] (1828), p. 62.
62. J. E. Purkyně ["Review of K.F. Burdach"] (1833), p. 119.
63. J. E. Purkyně, "Mikroskop" (1844), p. 122.
64. E. Hintzsche and W. Rytz, *Gustav Gabriel Valentin* (1953), p. 43; H. Van der Loos, "The history of the neuron" (1967), p. 26.
65. E. Hintzsche, *Zellen und Gewebe* (1963), pp. 33–34.
66. F. Leuret and L. P. Gratiolet, *Anatomie Comparée* (1839–1857), 1 (1839):81–82 by (Leuret). For biography of Leuret, see chap. 2 n. 127.
67. G. G. Valentin, *Handbuch* (1835), p. 586.
68. Ibid., pp. 586–587.
69. Ibid., p. 588.
70. Ibid., pp. 26–27.
71. F. K. Studnička, "Joh. Ev. Purkinje" (1927), esp. pp. 121–122; idem, "John. Ev. Purkinjes histologische Arbeiten" (1936), esp. p. 53; E. Hintzsche and W. Rytz, *Gustav Gabriel Valentin* (1953), pp. 18–20; E. Hintzsche, ed., *Zellen und Gewebe* (1963).
72. G. G. Valentin, "Über die Entwickelung" (1842), p. 138.
73. G. G. Valentin, "Ueber die Scheiden" (1839), p. 157.
74. G. G. Valentin, "Ueber den Verlauf" (1836), pp. 127–128.
75. Ibid., pp. 157–158.
76. Ibid., pp. 184, 188.
77. Ibid., pp. 195–196.
78. Ibid., p. 201.
79. Ibid., p. 202.
80. Ibid., p. 204.
81. Ibid., p. 208.
82. Ibid., pp. 214–215, 218.
83. Ibid., pp. 218–219.
84. In S. T. Soemmerring, *Hirn und Nervenlehre* (1841), pp. 45, 124–125.
85. T. Schwann, *Mikroskopische Untersuchungen* (1839), pp. 181–182. For Valentin's reactions to cell theory, see G. G. Valentin, "Die Fortschritte der Physiologie (1839), pp. 6–7. Lenoir has pointed out that Schwann was also indebted to von Baer's work on the mammalian ovum in formulating his model of the animal cell (T. Lenoir, *The Strategy* [1982], p. 116).
86. In S. T. Soemmerring, *Hirn und Nervenlehre* (1841), pp. 14–17.
87. See F. K. Studnička, "J. E. Purkyně's 'Physiology'" (1936), 475; idem, "Joh. Ev. Purkinjes histologische Arbeiten" (1936), p. 49; A. Andreoli, *Zur geschichtlichen Entwicklung* (1961), p. 11; V. Kruta, "J. E. Purkyně" (1962), p. 89; H. Van der Loos, "The history of the neuron" (1967), pp. 29–30; Clarke and O'Malley (1968), pp. 53–56; and V. Kruta, "J. E. Purkyně's contribution" (1971), p. 114.

88. J. E. Purkyně, "Neueste Beobachtungen" (1837), p. 88.

89. J. E. Purkyně, "Neueste Untersuchungen" (1837), p. 47. For the description of his cerebellar cell, see H. R. Viets and F. H. Garrison, "Purkinje's original description" (1940); Clarke and O'Malley (1968), pp. 55–56; and V. Kruta, "A note" (1971).

90. J. E. Purkyně, "Neueste Untersuchungen" (1837), pp. 48–49.

91. Ibid., p. 47.

92. O. Matoušek, "Purkinje's contributions" (1970), pp. 32, 37–38.

93. H. Boerhaave, *Academical Lectures* (1742–1746), 2 (1743):129.

94. F. von P. Gruithuisen, *Anthropologie* (1810), p. 398.

95. F. Tiedemann, *The Anatomy* (1826), pp. 147–148.

96. H. M. D. de Blainville, *Cours de Physiologie* (1829), 2:372–373.

97. A. Dugès, *Traité* (1838–1839), 1:349.

98. A. W. Volkmann, "Gehirn" (1842), pp. 570–571; see also G. G. Valentin, "Gewebe" (1842), p. 704.

99. J. E. Purkyně, "Neueste Untersuchungen" (1837), pp. 48–49.

100. S. Ochs, "Waller's concept" (1975), p. 256; and see chap. 5 n. 47.

101. F. von P. Gruithuisen, *Organozoonomie* (1811), pp. 113–114.

102. A. H. Hassall, *The Microscopic Anatomy* (1849), 2:356–357, 373.

103. C. G. Ehrenberg, "Nothwendigkeit" (1833), p. 458.

104. E. Hintzsche, ed., *Zellen und Gewebe* (1963), pp. 41, 54.

105. J. E. Purkyně, "Über den Bau" (1837).

106. Ibid., p. 45.

107. F. von P. Gruithuisen, *Organozoonomie* (1811), pp. 131–132, 208, 212–214. See also F. W. J. Schelling, *Von der Weltseele* (1798), pp. 297–298; C. Siegel, *Geschichte* (1913), pp. 194–195.

108. J. E. Purkyně, "Papierstreifen" (1850), p. 254.

109. Ibid., pp. 254–255.

110. Ibid., p. 258.

111. F. W. J. Schelling, *Von der Weltseele* (1798), p. 213.

112. S. C. Wagener, *Das Leben des Erdballs* (1828), pp. 15–17. See also K. F. Burdach, *Die Physiologie* (1826–1840), 1 (1826):421.

113. J. E. Purkyně, ["Review of Carl Friedr. Burdach"] (1828), pp. 61–62.

114. K. F. Burdach, *Vom Baue und Leben* (1819–1826), 1 (1819):23–24.

115. G. G. Valentin, "Über den Verlauf" (1836), pp. 175–176.

116. C. [?] von W.[erner], *Critische Darstellung* (1802), p. 33.

117. F. W. J. Schelling, *Einleitung* (1799), pp. 1–2. See also K. F. Burdach, *Die Physiologie* (1826–1840), 6 (1840):523.

118. J. E. Purkyně, "Sinne im allgemeinen" (1846), p. 155.

119. In S. T. Soemmerring, *Hirn und Nervenlehre* (1841), p. 15.

120. G. G. Valentin, "Über den Verlauf" (1836), p. 195.

121. J. E. Purkyně, "Papierstreifen" (1850), pp. 256–257.

122. Ibid., p. 257.

123. Ibid.

124. A. Gode-von Aesch, *Natural Science* (1966), pp. 252–256.

125. B. G. Ernst, *Neues Planetenbuch* (1847), p. 25.

126. Ibid., pp. 28, 48.

127. J. E. Purkyně, "Papierstreifen" (1850), pp. 258–259.

128. Ibid., pp. 257–258.

129. B. Stilling, "Fragmente" (1842), p. 92. For biography and work of Stilling, see Clarke and O'Malley (1968), pp. 270–275, 833–837 and elsewhere; and F. Schiller, "Stilling's nuclei" (1969). See also Anonymous ["Volkmann"] (1844).

130. F. H. Bidder, *Zur Lehre* (1847), pp. 3–4. For biography of Bidder, see T. Achard, *Die Physiologe F. Bidder* (1969).

131. B. Kisch, "Forgotten leaders" (1954), pp. 245–250.

132. B. Stilling, *Anatomische und mikroskopische Untersuchungen* (1856), p. 101.

133. R. Remak, *Observationes* (1838), p. 9. For review, see Anonymous ["Remak on the structure"], (1839).

134. B. Stilling, *Anatomische und mikroskopische Untersuchungen* (1856), p. 101.

135. R. Remak, *Observationes* (1838), pp. 15–16.

136. R. Remak, "Anatomische Beobachtungen" (1841), p. 510; idem, "Über den Inhalt" (1843), p. 200.

137. A. Hannover, "Die Chromsäure" (1840), pp. 555–556. See Clarke and O'Malley (1968), pp. 59–61, 833.

138. H. L. F. Helmholtz, *De Fabrica* (1842), pp. 22–33. Cited by Clarke and O'Malley (1968), p. 59. See Clarke and O'Malley (1968), p. 207 for biography.

139. J. G. F. Will, "Vorläufige Mittheilung" (1844).

140. E. Harless, "Briefliche Mittheilung" (1846), pp. 286, 290–291; R. Wagner, *Neue Untersuchungen* (1847), p. 7.

141. F. H. Bidder, *Zur Lehre* (1847), pp. 4–5.

142. R. Wagner, *Neue Untersuchungen* (1847), p. 7.

143. R. A. von Koelliker, *Die Selbständigkeit* (1844), p. 17. For biography of Koelliker, see chap. 2 n. 14 above.

144. Ibid., p. 19.

145. R. A. von Koelliker, "Neurologische Bemerkungen" (1848), pp. 135–136.

146. A. W. Volkmann, "Nervenphysiologie" (1844), p. 481.

147. Ibid., pp. 565, 613n.

148. J. F. B. Polaillon, *Étude* (1865), pp. 24, 28.

149. R. Remak, "Ueber multipolare Ganglienzellen" (1854), p. 26; B. Stilling, *Über den Bau* (1846), p. 29 (see F. Schiller, "Stilling's nuclei" [1969]); L. P. Gratiolet, "Structure de la moelle épinière" (1852), p. 272.

150. J. Paget, "Report" (1846), p. 273; William Sharpey (1802–1880) in J. Quain, *Elements of Anatomy* (1848), 1:cci–ccii.

151. B. Stilling, *Anatomische und mikroskopische Untersuchungen* (1856), pp. 131–135.

152. J. F. B. Polaillon, *Étude* (1865), p. 28.

153. See L. G. Stevenson, "Anatomical reasoning" (1959); G. L. Geison, "Social and institutional factors" (1972).

154. G. L. Geison, *Michael Foster* (1978), pp. 47–48; L. S. Jacyna, "Principles of general physiology" (1984).

155. B. Stilling and J. Wallach, *Untersuchungen* (1842), p. 13; B. Stilling, *Untersuchungen über die Functionen des Rückenmarks* (1842), p. 8. For Stilling's research on the spinal cord, see G. Aumueller, "Benedict Stillings (1810–1879)" (1984).

156. B. Stilling and J. Wallach, *Untersuchungen* (1842), pp. 14–16, 27–28.

157. R. A. Koelliker, "Neurologische Bemerkungen" (1848), p. 148.

158. R. A. Koelliker, "Nervenzellen" (1892), p. 33.

159. R. A. Koelliker, *Die Selbständigkeit* (1844), pp. 34–35.

160. R. Remak, "Weitere mikroscopische Beobachtungen" (1837), col. 36.

161. R. Remak, "Vorläufige Mittheilung" (1836), p. 146. For the "Bell-Magendie" theory of spinal root function, see chap. 4.3.

162. R. Remak, "Ueber die Verrichtungen" (1838), col. 67.

163. R. Remak, "Ueber die physiologische Bedeutung" (1840), pp. 245–246.

164. R. Remak, "Nervensystem (physiologisch)" (1841), pp. 179–180.

165. B. Stilling and J. Wallach, *Untersuchungen* (1842), pp. 31–32.

166. J. F. B. Polaillon, *Étude* (1865), p. 22.

167. R. Remak, "Ueber die physiologische Bedeutung" (1840), p. 225.

168. Ibid., p. 231.

169. Ibid., pp. 236–237.

170. R. A. von Koelliker, *Die Selbständigkeit* (1844), p. 38.

171. R. Remak, "Nervensystem (histologisch)" (1841), p. 150.

172. R. Remak, "Ueber die physiologische Bedeutung" (1840), p. 253.

173. R. Remak, "Ueber die Verrichtungen" (1838), p. 69.

174. A. W. Volkmann, "Nervenphysiologie" (1844), p. 481.

175. F. H. Bidder, *Zur Lehre* (1847), p. 32.

176. G. G. Valentin, "Ueber den Verlauf" (1836), p. 61.

177. G. G. Valentin, "Ueber die Scheiden" (1839), pp. 156–157.

178. B. Stilling, "Fragmente zur Lehre" (1842), p. 92.

179. R. Remak, "Nervensystem (physiologisch)" (1841), p. 152.

180. R. Remak, "Ueber die Verrichtungen" (1838), pp. 66–67.

181. R. Remak, "Ueber die physiologische Bedeutung" (1840), p. 258. See also idem, "Nervensystem (physiologisch)" (1841), pp. 153–154.

182. R. Remak, "Ueber die physiologische Bedeutung" (1840), pp. 260–265.

183. Ibid., pp. 256, 264, 253.

184. R. Remak, "Nervensystem (physiologisch)" (1841), pp. 172, 179, 183, 186.

185. W. B. Carpenter, *Prize Thesis*. (1839), pp. 184–185; see also p. 147.

186. W. B. Carpenter, *A Manual of Physiology* (1846), pp. 221–222, 491.

187. R. B. Todd, *The Descriptive and Physiological Anatomy* (1845), p. xii. See also W. Sharpey in J. Quain, *Elements of Anatomy* (1848), 1:ccxxxiv–ccxxxv.

188. R. A. von Koelliker, *Die Selbständigkeit* (1844), pp. 34–35.

189. R. Remak, "Ueber die physiologische Bedeutung" (1840), p. 237.

190. R. Remak, "Nervensystem (histologisch)" (1841), pp. 143–144.

191. F. H. Bidder, *Zur Lehre* (1847), p. 36.

192. R. A. von Koelliker, "Neurologische Bemerkungen" (1848), p. 150.

193. B. Stilling, "Fragmente zur Lehre" (1842), p. 136.

194. B. Stilling, *Ueber die Medulla Oblongata* (1843), p. 54.

195. F. Schiller, "Stilling's nuclei" (1969), p. 80. B. Stilling, *Neue Untersuchungen* (1856–1859), pp. 268–269.

196. R. Remak, "Ueber multipolare Ganglienzellen" (1854), pp. 27–28.

197. R. Wagner, "Sympathischen Nerv" (1846), pp. 398–400.

198. F. Leuret and L. P. Gratiolet, *Anatomie Comparée* (1839–1857), 2 (1857):3–4 (by Gratiolet).

199. L. Hermann, *Grundriss der Physiologie* (1863), pp. 330–331.

200. Ibid., pp. 332, 335–336.

201. See, for example, R. Wagner, "Sympathischen Nerv" (1846), p. 398.

202. T. H. Huxley, "On the present state" (1854–1858), p. 436.

203. R. A. von Koelliker, "Neurologische Bemerkungen" (1849), p. 146.

204. He was working under the supervision of Rudolph Wagner, who described his findings in R. Wagner, "Neurologische Untersuchungen" (1850), pp. 41–56.

205. Ibid., pp. 185–196.

206. R. Wagner, "Ueber die Elementar—Organisation des Gehirns" (1854), pp. 25–44, see pp. 35–36.

207. Ibid., p. 36.

208. The term *nerve cell* caused confusion because until the end of the nineteenth century it was often used to signify the cell body without its processes. The modern term *nerve cell*, synonymous with "neuron" did not come into universal use until the late 1890s, after the invention of "neuron" by Wilhelm Waldeyer in 1891 (see n. 222 below). See E. A. Schäfer, "The nerve cell" (1893).

209. For the history of tissue coloring methods, see H. J. Conn, ed., *The History of Staining* (1933); E. Hintzsche, "Die Entwicklung" (1943); J. R. Baker, "The discovery" (1945); H. J. Conn, "Development" (1946); Clarke and O'Malley (1968), pp. 839–851. For fixation and sectioning, see B. Bracegirdle, *A History of Microtechnique* (1978). See also C. B. Farrar,

"The growth" (1905); A. Hughes, *A History of Cytology* (1959).

210. J. C. Reil, "Untersuchungen . . . Vierte Fortsetzung" (1809), pp. 137–142. See Clarke and O'Malley (1968), pp. 830–832.

211. A. Hannover, "Die Chromsäure" (1840), pp. 549–550, 555. See Clarke and O'Malley (1968), p. 833.

212. See, for example, the work of Otto Friedrich Karl Deiters (1834–1863), *Untersuchungen* (1865). See also Clarke and O'Malley (1968), pp. 66–70, fig. 16; and F. Schiller, "The intriguing nucleus" (1974).

213. J. von Gerlach, *Mikroscopische Studien* (1865), pp. 1–3. See Clarke and O'Malley (1968), pp. 840–841. It should be noted, however, that Marquese Alfonso Corti (1822–1888) used it in "Recherches" (1851), and is, therefore, the real discoverer of histological dyeing.

214. J. von Gerlach, "Über die Structur" (1872). See Clarke and O'Malley (1968), pp. 88–90, fig. 24.

215. The best account is in C. Golgi, "Sulla fina struttura" (1875). See idem, "Professor Golgi's method" (1886); and Clarke and O'Malley (1968), pp. 842–845.

216. C. Golgi, "Recherches" (1883–1884). See also Clarke and O'Malley (1968), pp. 91–96.

217. "Neuron" is today defined as "A complete nerve cell, consisting of a cell body containing the nucleus and its processes, axonal and dendritic. The term implies that the nerve cell is structurally independent of other cells and not part of a syncytium." McD. Critchley, ed., *Butterworths Medical Dictionary* (1978).

218. W. His, "Zur Geschichte" (1887). See Clarke and O'Malley (1968), pp. 99–104.

219. A. H. Forel, "Einige hirnanatomische Betrachtungen" (1887). See Clarke and O'Malley (1968), pp. 104–109. For the research of His and Forel, see H. Buess, "Vom Beitrag der schweizer Ärzte" (1964).

220. S. Ramón y Cajal, "Estruttura" (1888). See also Clarke and O'Malley (1968), pp. 109–113; and S. Grisolía et al., eds. *Ramón y Cajal's Contribution* (1983), pp. 3–31, 249–258.

221. P. Ehrlich, "Über die Methylenblaureaction" (1886). See Clarke and O'Malley (1968), pp. 97–99.

222. W. Waldeyer, "Über einige neuere Forschungen" (1891). See Clarke and O'Malley (1968), pp. 113–117. For the history of the neuron doctrine, see publications cited in n. 1 above. For end-of-century surveys of the neuron, see L. F. Barker, "On the validity" (1898); idem, *The Nervous System* (1899); and G. H. Parker, "The neurone theory" (1900).

223. W. Waldeyer, "Über einige neuere Forschungen" (1891), p. 1352.

224. S. Ramón y Cajal; "¿Neuronismo o reticularismo?" (1933). It contains an excellent review of the evidence favoring the existence of the neuron. English trans. in idem, *Neuron Theory* (1954).

4. THE REFLEX

1. There are the following general accounts: C. Eckhard, "Beiträge zur Geschichte" (1881). Accurate, fully documented and used by most subsequent writers. Deals chiefly with experimental aspects; C. F. Hodge, "A sketch" (1890); R. H. Gault, "A sketch" (1904); F. Fearing, *Reflex Action* (1930) is the most comprehensive survey, with frequent quotations, but opinions not always reliable, and the author's dependence on secondary sources has led to some distortions; H. E. Hoff and P. Kellaway, "The early history" (1952), with long translated quotations; G. Canguilhem, *La Formation* (1955), the most scholarly and thoughtful survey; M. A. B. Brazier, "Historical development" (1959), part of an excellent account of the history of neurophysiology; E. G. T. Lidell, *The Discovery* (1960) is not always accurate, and references scanty, Sherrington being dealt with at disproportionate length, but with excellent results; G. Canguilhem, "Le concept" (1964); Clarke and O'Malley (1968), pp. 323–382; J. P. Swazey, *Reflexes* (1969); M. Neuburger (1981), pp. 237–246 and *passim*.

2. (1) Aristotle, *De Motu Animalium,* 11 (703 b:2–21), in idem, *De Motu Animalium . . .* (1912). See Clarke and O'Malley (1968), p. 325. (2) Galen, *Du Mouvement des Muscles,* bk. 2, chaps. 5–6, in C. Daremberg, *Oeuvres Anatomiques* (1854–1856), 2 (1856):362–367. See Clarke and O'Malley (1968), pp. 326–328.

3. For Descartes and reflex action, see F. Fearing, "René Descartes" (1929); idem, *Reflex Action* (1930), pp. 18–28; H. E. Hoff and P. Kellaway, "The early history" (1952); G. Canguilhem, *La Formation* (1955), pp. 26–56; Clarke and O'Malley (1968), pp. 329–333.

4. G. Canguilhem, *La Formation* (1955), pp. 138–159.

5. For Willis and reflex action, see F. Fearing, *Reflex Action* (1930), pp. 54–59; H. E. Hoff and P. Kellaway, "The early history" (1952); G. Canguilhem, *La Formation* (1955), pp. 57–78; A. Meyer and R. Hierons, "On Thomas Willis's concepts" (1965); Clarke and O'Malley (1968), pp. 333–335; K. Dewhurst, *Thomas Willis's Oxford Lectures* (1980), p. 74. For Willis's highly original contribution to the concept of sympathy, and its evolution before his time, see R. Y. Meier, "'Sympathy'" (1982), which is derived from idem, "Sympathy as a Concept" (1979).

6. The reference made by John Locke (1632–1704) to reflex action, for example, was brief and direct: "If, for example, something is tickling one's skin, a corresponding motion is communicated to the spirits in the brain, and being thus aroused, they affect those nerves concerned with moving the hand to rub that part. This often happens even when we are not thinking about it or sleeping." From K. Dewhurst, *Thomas Willis's Oxford Lectures* (1980), p. 79.

7. A von Haller, "De partibus" (1753). See idem, *A Dissertation* [1755]

(1936); Clarke and O'Malley (1968), pp. 170–174; M. Neuburger (1981), pp. 114–116, 145–146, and passim.

8. For Whytt and reflex action, see L. Carmichael, "R. Whytt" (1927); F. Fearing, *Reflex Action* (1930), pp. 74–83; H. E. Hoff and P. Kellaway, "The early history" (1952); G. Canguilhem, *La Formation* (1955), pp. 101–107; Clarke and O'Malley (1968), pp. 336–342; R. K. French, *Robert Whytt* (1969).

9. Whytt's ideas are to be found chiefly in his *An Essay* (1751) and *Observations* (1765).

10. Whytt cited Hales in "Physiological essays. II" (1755), p. 290.

11. C. Eckhard, "Beiträge zur Geschichte" (1881), p. 43.

12. R. Whytt, *An Essay* (1751), p. 384.

13. J. A. Unzer, *Erste Gründe* (1771), pp. 396, 410–412, 493. See Clarke and O'Malley (1968), pp. 342–345.

14. J. Procháska, *Adnotationum* (1784), "Sectio primus. De functionibus systematis nervosi commentatio," pp. 1–164. English trans. in idem, *. . . and a Dissertation* (1851). See V. Kruta "The physiologist" (1962) in which the author's claims for Procháska are at times excessive; M. Neuburger, "Streiflichter" (1909); Clarke and O'Malley (1968), pp. 345–346; M. Neuburger (1981), pp. 166–168, 240–244, and passim.

15. J. Procháska, *Adnotationum* (1784), p. 114. We should note at this point an assessment of Procháska's work by the greatest contributor to reflex physiology, C. S. Sherrington. In 1900 he stated: "The part that Prochaska took in the development of the study [of the reflex] appears over-estimated; his experimental contributions are negligible" (C. S. Sherrington, "The spinal cord" [1900], p. 786). Admittedly Procháska's experiments were relatively few, but judging by contemporary literature, he had a wide and significant influence which continued well into the nineteenth century, as we shall see.

16. J. Procháska, *Adnotationum* (1784), p. 117.

17. F. H. A. von Humboldt, *Versuche* (1797), 1:231. For biography of Humboldt, see C. Kellner, *Alexander von Humboldt* (1963); *DSB;* and M. Neuburger (1981), pp. 331–332.

18. J. Procháska, *Physiologie* (1820), pp. 85–86.

19. See, for example, J. Procháska, *Versuch* (1815).

20. F. Vicq d'Azyr "Recherches" (1784), pt. 3, "XX. La moelle épinière," pp. 597–603.

21. J. J. C. Legallois, *Expériences* (1812), p. 140.

22. Ibid., pp. 140–141.

23. E. Darwin, *Zoonomia* (1794–1796), 1 (1794):135–139. They were acquired *"by the repeated efforts of our muscles under the conduct of sensations and desires"* (p. 137).

24. J. Cruveilhier, *Anatomie Pathologique* (1829–1842), 1 (1829), "Livraison III. Maladies de la moelle épinière," p. 5.

25. L. A. Desmoulins, *Anatomie* (1825), 2:552–559.

26. C. P. Ollivier, "*Traité*" (1827), 1:103–105. He made more extensive reference to Legallois in this edition than in the first of 1824.

27. L. F. Calmeil, "Sur la structure" (1828), pp. 87–96.

28. A. P. Wilson Philip, *An Experimental Inquiry* (1817), pp. 97, 103–104. See chap. 1 n. 91.

29. Ibid., p. 210.

30. A. Flint, *The Physiology* (1872), p. 299.

31. H. Mayo, *Outlines* (1829), p. 282.

32. H. Mayo, "On the cerebral nerves" (1823), p. 6. French extract in idem, "Sur les nerfs" (1823).

33. H. Mayo, "Remarks" (1823), p. 136.

34. Ibid., p. 135.

35. H. Mayo, *Outlines* (1829), p. 282.

36. The role of Mayo's discovery in the history of the reflex demands further elucidation.

37. J. L. Brachet, *Recherches Expérimentales* (1830), chap. 8, "Influence du système nerveux ganglionaire sur les sympathies," pp. 285–367.

38. Hall refuted the idea in "On the reflex function" (1833), pp. 660–661.

39. C. Bell, *Idea* (1811), p. 23. We shall discuss further the outcome of Bell's proposal as it concerned functional brain localization in 6.4 and 6.6.4.

40. F. Magendie, "Expériences" (1822).

41. For this literature, see Clarke and O'Malley (1968), pp. 296–303; and, more importantly, P. F. Cranefield, *The Way In* (1974); also, M. Neuburger (1981), pp. 247–258.

42. Cranefield has shown that even historians of Max Neuburger's stature were deceived by Bell's deceitful textual emendations. Like other German readers, Neuburger based his paeons of praise for Bell, rather than for Magendie, not on the 1811 *Idea,* but on a translation into German of Bell's texts published after Magendie's article of 1822, by which time they had been suitably but fraudulently "improved" (as Cranefield ingeniously styles it) and the original opinions of 1811 carefully suppressed. (See P. F. Cranefield, *The Way In* [1974], pp. 33–34.) Thus, in M. H. Romberg's *Karl Bell's* (1832), which is a translation of Bell's *Nervous System* (1830), could be found Bell's conclusions on root function based on the experiments of Magendie rather than on his own. These conclusions were quite different from the ones in Bell's 1811 tract which had a very limited circulation and probably never reached Germany. See also J. M. C. Olmsted's "The Aftermath" (1943).

43. J. Müller, "Bestätigung" (1831). See Clarke and O'Malley (1968), pp. 304–305.

44. C. Bell, "On the nervous circle" (1826), p. 170.

45. S. Solly, *The Human Brain* (1836), p. 141.

46. F. Magendie, *Mémoire* (1823), p. 17: "le sanctuaire le plus caché."

47. B. Stilling and J. Wallach, *Untersuchungen über den Bau . . . Erstes Heft* (1842), p. 14. See Clarke and O'Malley (1968), pp. 270–275.

48. Anonymous, "Versuch" (1842), p. 296. The author used the term *Lex Belliana,* and, as this was introduced by Valentin, it is possible that he wrote this article.

49. R. Leys Fried, "Alison versus Hall" (1976); and idem [Ruth Leys], "Background" (1980).

50. W. P. Alison, "Observations" (1826). The "peculiar doctrines" mentioned in the title of this article refer to Bell's theory of the respiratory nerves, a doctrine Alison rejected (pp. 189–228). See also idem, *Outline* (1831), pp. 345–354, where he supported Whytt and Alexander Monro *secundus* and attacked Bell's materialistic idea of sympathy, for example, between the respiratory muscles (see below). It is curious that historians have not before introduced Alison so prominently into the reflex debate. This may be due to their negligence or, as seems more likely, Dr. Fried has overemphasized the role of a previously little recognized participant in the controversy. Nevertheless, she has provided a valuable survey of many aspects of research in reflex physiology, taking Alison as a nineteenth-century representative of the vitalistic interpretation.

51. R. Leys Fried, "Background" (1980), pp. 24–34, gave a full account of the system and of Alison's critique of it, which is in W. P. Alison, "Observations" (1826), pp. 189–228.

52. A. Comparetti, *Occursus* (1780), "§. IV. Effectuum propagatio, & varietas," see paragraphs 87–94 (pp. 173–182).

53. F. Tiedemann, "Über den Antheil" (1825).

54. According to Volkmann, J. Müller had refused to accept fiber anastomoses and G. R. Treviranus had not seen them. Remak, in many observations made on spinal cord fibers, noted anastomoses on only four occasions. E. H. Weber claimed to have seen them, but in only three instances was the ramification beyond doubt. In very many claimed cases, it turned out that the appearances were due to the crossing of fibers, without any evidence of communication between them (A. W. Volkmann, "On reflex motions" [1838], p. 215n). See 3.5.1 for detailed discussion of nerve-fiber connection.

55. [?] Kronenberg, "Versuche" (1839); and I. van Deen, *Traités* (1841). For van Deen, see Anonymous ["Volkmann"] (1844).

56. For biography and work of Hall, see [C. Hall], *Memoirs* (1861); *DNB*—based on a curiously biased article by [T. H. Wakley], "Biographical sketch" (1850); F. Fearing, *Reflex Action* (1930), pp. 122–145; G. Jefferson, "Marshall Hall" (1953); *DSB*. See also chap. 1 n. 26. D. E. Manuel has given a good account of Hall's various activities ("Marshall Hall" [1980]), but it is overly sympathetic in tone and she makes no reference to the foibles that account for his unfortunate personality and thus for his behavior and for the reactions of his peers to it.

It has been claimed that Hall's son was an "eminent barrister" (E. Clarke, in W. Haymaker and F. Schiller, eds., *The Founders* [1970], p. 223), but this is incorrect. As John D. Spillane has explained (in *The Doctrine of the Nerves* [1981], p. 245), a Dr. Alfred Hall of Brighton attended Marshall Hall in his last illness and was permitted to christen his son Edward Marshall Hall, who eventually entered the legal profession. (See E. Marjoribanks, *The Life of Sir Edward Marshall Hall* [1929], p. 16.)

57. In a copy of J. F. Clarke, *Autobiographical Recollections* (1874), there is a penciled comment in a contemporary hand concerning Hall: "The most conceited man I ever knew."

58. Ibid., p. 327.

59. In an unsigned article, T. H. Wakley remarked that Hall's discoveries "will henceforth rank him with Harvey in the field of science and experiment" ([T. H. Wakley] "Biographical sketch" [1850], p. 124).

60. M. Hall, *Synopsis* (1850), p. 2. He estimated that he had spent at least 25,000 hours on experimental and clinical investigations.

61. [C. Hall], *Memoirs* (1861).

62. Ibid., p. 104.

63. See, for example, his review of M. Hall's *New Memoir* (1843), in T. H. Wakley, [Review] (1846). In it he awarded Hall, "SECOND place in physiology" after Harvey (p. 154). See also idem, "Biographical sketch" (1850). In fact Hall's *New Memoir* (1843), despite its title, was mainly a presentation of previously published material, with little new added.

64. [C. Hall], *Memoirs* (1861), pp. 107–110.

65. M. Hall, *On the Diseases* (1841), p. 38. More than a third of this book deals with his opinions on the reflex.

66. M. Hall, " . . . a brief account" (1832).

67. Ibid., p. 191.

68. M. Hall, "On the reflex function" (1833). Its title in the abstracts of papers presented, was "On the reflex function of the medulla oblongata and spinalis, or the principle of tone in the muscular system."

69. Ibid., p. 635.

70. M. Hall, *On the Diseases* (1841), pp. vii–viii.

71. M. Hall, "On the reflex function" (1833), p. 658.

72. J. A. H. Murray et al., eds., *A New English Dictionary* (1888–1928) accepted this priority.

73. M. Hall, "On the reflex function" (1833), p. 663.

74. R. B. Todd was one of Hall's most virulent critics and, in his *The Cyclopaedia* (1835–1859), vol. 3, (1839–1847), he gave a lengthy review (pp. 721U–722A) of Hall's opinions published 1835–1846, the originality of which he denied. In the case of Hall's 1833 paper he noted in particular a similarity with statements made by Procháska in 1784. Todd believed that Hall had merely revived Procháska's views without acknowledgment, had amassed additional experimental support for them, and had applied them to diseases of the nervous system. See n. 85 below.

75. Cited in W. Stirling, *Some Apostles* (1902), p. 86.

76. M. Hall, *Lectures* (1836). They had been delivered during 1835. For the anatomy and physiology of his system as applied to diseases of the nervous system, see pp. 11–31.

77. M. Hall, "On the function" (1837). An abstract of the three presentations he made was recorded in the report for 2 March 1837.

78. However, the article "On the function" (1837) appeared in two Continental periodicals. See Bibliography.

79. M. Hall, *A Letter* (1848).

80. P. F. Cranefield in the 1975 reprint of H. Mayo, *Anatomical* (1822–1823), p. v, footnote, claimed that Hall's paper was rejected on the advice of Herbert Mayo. If he was in fact referring to the 1837 paper, this does not accord with Hall's accusations directed at Peter Mark Roget (1779–1869), whom he suspected as the responsible person. See M. Hall, *A Letter* (1848), pp. 6–8.

81. Ibid., p. 6.

82. [W. P. Alison], "Travers, Mayo, Ley, Hall" (1837).

83. R. Leys Fried, "Background" (1980), p. 4. We should mention here an American, Martyn Paine (1794–1877), whose book of 1847 (*The Institutes*) was permeated with vitalism similar to Alison's. His ideas also followed Whytt's and included a sentient principle. He believed "that the power by which motion is carried on is implanted in all parts, and that the nervous power is simply a stimulus in developing motion, and, therefore, on common ground with other stimuli" (p. 806). He described the brain as "associating in harmonious action the immaterial with the material parts" (p. 284), and sympathy was modified sensibility (p. 101). Quotes are from 4th ed. (1858), but much the same statements are in all editions from 1847 to 1867. Paine's influence in Europe was probably small.

84. M. Hall, *Memoirs* (1837). The rejected paper is "Memoir II. On the true spinal marrow, and the excito-motory system of nerves" (pp. 41–113).

85. The main attack was by J. D. George, a president of the Medical Society of University College, London, in "Contribution" (1837–1838). This provoked a long series of leaders and letters in this and other British medical periodicals. See n. 74 above.

86. One of the beneficial effects of this dispute was a translation of parts of Procháska's 1784 book into English, idem, . . . *and a Dissertation* (1851).

87. The respected physician, R. B. Todd (see n. 74 above), probably did not qualify for these epithets. Nevertheless he made a detailed comparison between the books of Procháska and Hall, and his considered opinion was "to refuse assent to his [Hall's] claims to original discovery as well as to his hypothesis, and even to the accuracy of his experiments." (R. B. Todd, ed., *The Cyclopaedia* [1835–1859], 3 [1839–1847]:722A).

88. The need for an organizing body for Britain independent of the Royal Colleges was now being voiced, and Hall was actively involved in the estab-

lishment of what eventually became the British Medical Association. This aspect of Hall's career has yet to be fully investigated.

89. M. Hall, *Synopsis* [1850], p. vii. It seems a curious use of "diastaltic," previously used only in reference to music: "music able to expand and exalt the mind" (J. A. H. Murray et al., eds., *A New English Dictionary* [1888–1928]). Hall used it to mean "acting through or along" and it replaced the earlier term "kinetic" he had proposed.

90. M. Hall, "On the anatomy" (1846).

91. M. Hall, *The Gulstonian Lectures* (1842), p. 32.

92. M. Hall, "On the anatomy" (1846).

93. J. Müller, *Zur vergleichenden Physiologie* (1826). See also W. Riese and C. E. Arrington, "The history" (1963); and Clarke and O'Malley (1968), pp. 203–206.

94. M. Hall, *New Memoir* (1843), p. 45.

95. Hall was a compulsive classifier, as can be seen best in his *Principles* (1837), where his cataloguing of diseases is reminiscent of the eighteenth-century nosologists.

96. For Hall's practical application of the diastaltic system to the interpretation of neurological disorders, see idem, *On the Diseases* (1841).

97. This was especially true of the work of Gilbert Blane (1749–1834), who in 1788 had reported experiments on decollated animals, concluding that "instinctive movements may be exerted, without the intervention of the *sensorium commune,* and therefore without sensation or consciousness" (G. Blane, *A Lecture* [1788], p. 37). Observations on an anencephalic monster in 1822 confirmed for him this opinion (idem, *Select Dissertations* [1822], "Dissertation" VIII, pp. 229–283, see pp. 262–263). His contribution was, in fact, quite modest, but as it agreed with Hall's doctrine, he was given more praise than he deserved, and some historians have been deceived by Hall's biased judgment.

98. P. Flourens, *Recherches Expérimentales* (1824), p. 35: "The cerebral hemispheres are, therefore, the specific organ of sensation."

99. Ibid., p. 15: "the spinal cord then is the organ or instrument of the general sympathies [reflexes]."

100. In a letter to Hall dated 3 February 1839, and cited in M. Hall, *New Memoir* (1843), p. 40. Hall added, "I consider this testimony as the best reward of my labours" (ibid.). He dedicated his *New Memoir* (1843) to Flourens in glowing terms.

101. R. D. Grainger in a letter to Hall dated 3 April 1837 and cited by [C. Hall], *Memoirs* (1861), p. 108. I. van Deen wrote with similar effusive phraseology, in a letter dated 14 October 1839 (ibid., p. 105).

102. M. Hall, *New Memoir* (1843), p. 10.

103. M. Hall, *Synopsis* (1850), p. 31.

104. M. Hall, "Theory of the inverse ratio" (1832).

105. D. Ferrier, "An address" (1883), p. 805. Admittedly he had just received the Marshall Hall Prize for 1883.

106. J. Müller, *Handbuch* (1834–1840), (vol. 1, 1834). This book was published in parts (see Bibliographical Notes), and Müller's account of his work on the reflex was in the first part of vol. 1, which appeared in Spring 1833, pp. 333–335. It has not been seen, but he referred to it in the 2d ed. of 1 (1835):689–690. See also ibid., pp. 696–698.

107. J. Müller, *Handbuch* (1841–1844 to ?), 1 (1841–1844, 4th ed.): 610 n.

108. J. Müller, *Handbuch* (1835–1840), 1 (1835, 2d ed.):697. This did not appear in Baly's English version (1838–1842).

109. M. Hall, "On the reflex function" (1837).

110. J. Müller, *Handbuch* (1835–1840), 1 (1835, 2d ed.):690.

111. Ibid., p. 798.

112. J. Müller, *Handbuch* (1841–1844 to ?), 1 (1841–1844, 4th ed.):622.

113. A. W. Volkmann, "Ueber Reflexbewegungen" (1838).

114. A. W. Volkmann, "Nervenphysiologie" (1844), p. 546.

115. For the debate on the "spinal-cord soul," mainly between Lotze and Pflüger, see F. Fearing, *Reflex Action* (1930), pp. 161–186.

116. A. W. Volkmann, "Nervenphysiologie" (1844), p. 546.

117. J. W. Arnold, *Die Lehre* (1842), p. 86.

118. A. W. Volkmann, "Ueber Reflexbewegungen" (1838), p. 23.

119. J. Müller, *Handbuch* (1835–1840), 1 (1835, 2d ed.):699.

120. J. W. Arnold, *Die Lehre* (1842), p. 86.

121. For C. S. Sherrington's contributions to reflex physiology, see E. G. T. Lidell, *The Discovery* (1960); R. Granit, *Charles Scott Sherrington* (1966); Clarke and O'Malley (1968), pp. 370–382; J. P. Swazey, *Reflexes* (1969); J. C. Eccles and W. C. Gibson, *Sherrington* (1979). For a concise account of Sherringtonian reflex physiology, see R. S. Creed et al., *Reflex Activity* (1932).

122. W. Griesinger, "Ueber psychische Reflexactionen" (1843), pp. 81–82.

123. Ibid., p. 82.

124. R. Leys Fried, "Alison versus Hall" (1976), p. 2.

125. M. Hall, *New Memoir* (1843), pp. 36–37.

126. M. Hall, *Memoirs* (1837), pp. 70–71.

127. R. Leys Fried, "Alison versus Hall" (1976), pp. 17–18.

129. R. B. Todd and W. Bowman, *The Physiological Anatomy* (1845–1856), 1 (1845):201, 204.

130. Ibid., pp. 26–27.

131. Ibid., p. 262.

132. [C. Hall], *Memoirs* (1861), pp. 58, 61; G. Wilkins, *Body and Soul* (1822), pp. 103–104.

133. A. Gode-von Aesch, *Natural Science* (1966), p. 57; J. C. A. Grohmann, "Physiologie" (1820), p. 285.

134. A. Gode-von Aesch, *Natural Science* (1966), p. 57.
135. Ibid.
136. Ibid., pp. 66–67.
137. A. W. Volkmann, "Ueber Reflexbewegungen" (1838), pp. 37–38.
138. J. Müller, *Handbuch* (1835–1840), 1 (1835, 2d ed.):816–818. A. W. Volkmann, *Die Lehre* (1837), p. 159.
139. J. Müller, *Handbuch* (1835–1840), 1 (1835, 2d ed.):820.
140. A. W. Volkmann, *Die Lehre* (1837), pp. iii–iv.
141. Ibid., p. 159.
142. Ibid., p. 161–162.
143. See n. 115 above.
144. It should be noted, however, that at least one British physiologist, John Hughes Bennett, arrived in 1837 at a notion of brain reflexes. Bennett rested his claim on what he saw as the "strong analogy" between the arrangement of the sensible and volitional nerves of the brain and the motor and sensory fibers of the spinal cord; in fact, he pointed out that the anterior and posterior columns of the cord originated in the corpora striata and the thalami, respectively. On these grounds he held that Müller's claim that the brain also possessed a reflex function was entirely plausible and Hall's idea of the concept of the reflex too restricted. In short, the latter's excito-motory acts "differ in *degree,* not in *kind* from involuntary movements generally." (J. H. Bennett, *Inaugural Dissertation* [1837], p. 67, where he was citing from a review of the work of Hall and others, said to be written by W. P. Alison: see [W. P. Alison], "Travers, Mayo, Ley, Hall" [1837], p. 37.) Bennett did not, however, extend the reflex to the cerebral cortex (J. H. Bennett, *Inaugural Dissertation* [1837], pp. 60–61, 66–67). Nevertheless, in an 1860 letter to Hall's widow, Bennett did pretend that his work of 1837 "was the first attempt to explain the true connexion between the spinal and cerebral functions, on the principles originated by Dr. Hall." (J. H. Bennett, "Letter" [1860].) Bennett, however, had been anticipated in his view that the spinal cord columns were continued into the cranium by C. Bell, A. L. Foville, and others (C. Bell, *Idea* [1811], p. 21; A. L. Foville, "Researches" [1829] and "Encéphale" [1831]).
145. J. Müller, *Handbuch* (1835–1840), 1 (1835, 2d. ed.): 690, 717–720. For Remak, see 3.5.2.
146. M. Hall, *Memoirs* (1837), p. vii. See also idem, "The true spinal marrow" (1856) where Hall denied that reflex action, as he defined it, took place in the cerebral or the vegetative ganglia.
147. A. W. Volkmann, "Nervenphysiologie" (1844), p. 543.
148. A. W. Volkmann, *Die Lehre* (1837), p. 119.
149. A. W. Volkmann, "Ueber Reflexbewegungen" (1838), p. 39.
150. O. M. Marx, "Nineteenth-century medical psychology" (1970), p. 358. For biography of Griesinger, see A. Mette, "Wilhelm Griesinger" (1963); K. Fichtel, "Wilhelm Griesinger" (1965).

151. E. H. Ackerknecht, *A Short History* (1959), p. 63.

152. W. Griesinger, *Die Pathologie* (1845), pp. 1–2. There is an English translation, *Mental Pathology* (1867).

153. W. Griesinger, "Ueber psychische Reflexactionen" (1843), pp. 76, 113.

154. See K. Fichtel, "Wilhelm Griesinger" (1965), p. 1034.

155. W. Griesinger, "Ueber psychische Reflexactionen" (1843), p. 82.

156. W. Griesinger, *Die Pathologie* (1845), pp. 10–11.

157. W. Griesinger, "Neue Beiträge" (1844), p. 10.

158. Ibid., p. 10.

159. Ibid., p. 11.

160. W. Griesinger, "Ueber psychische Reflexactionen" (1843), pp. 71–78.

161. Ibid., pp. 86–87.

162. Ibid., p. 87. See also n. 115 above.

163. Ibid., pp. 87–88.

164. Ibid., pp. 90, 96.

165. Ibid., p. 96.

166. Ibid., p. 98.

167. Ibid., pp. 100, 107. See E. H. Ackerknecht, *A Short History* (1959), pp. 57–58; and O. M. Marx, "Nineteenth-century medical psychology" (1970), pp. 357–358.

168. W. Griesinger, "Ueber psychische Reflexactionen (1843), pp. 111–112.

169. Ibid., p. 112.

170. See L. S. Jacyna, "Principles of general physiology" (1984).

171. R. D. Grainger, *Observations* (1837), p. 106.

172. Ibid., p. iv (italics added).

173. Ibid., p. 108.

174. L. S. Jacyna, "Principles of general physiology" (1984), pp. 68–74.

175. R. Owen, *Lectures* (1843), p. 363; see also p. 207.

176. W. B. Carpenter, "On the voluntary and instinctive actions" (1837), pp. 24–25.

177. Ibid., pp. 26–27, 30–31.

178. [W. B. Carpenter], ["Review of *The Brain and its Physiology*"] (1846), p. 513.

179. W. B. Carpener, *Manual* (1846), p. 439.

180. Ibid., p. 536.

181. See T. Laycock, "On the reflex function" (1845).

182. W. B. Carpenter, *Principles of Human Physiology* (1853), p. 672.

183. T. Laycock, "A Journal, 1833–1857," pp. 26–27. For biography, see K. Macleod, *Laycock* (1908); and M. P. Amacher, "Thomas Laycock" (1964).

184. T. Laycock, "Phrenology" (1859), p. 556. Phrenology will be discussed in chap. 6. It was based on the supposed localization of psychological and moral attributes to specific areas or "organs" on the surface of the brain.

185. Ibid., p. 560. The term "organology" was used by Gall, but he never employed "phrenology."See 6.3.

186. T. Laycock, *Mind and Brain* (1860), 1:67.

187. T. Laycock, "Analytical essay" (1839), pp. 49–50.

188. T. Laycock, "Reflex, automatic, and unconscious cerebration" (1876), pp. 484–485.

189. T. Laycock, "Analytical essay" (1839), pp. 50–52.

190. T. Laycock, *A Treatise* (1840), p. 107.

191. Ibid., p. 108.

192. T. Laycock, "Letter to George Combe, 3 June 1845," ff. 12–13.

193. T. Laycock, "On the reflex function" (1845), p. 298.

194. T. Laycock, "Letter to George Combe, 27 February 1845," f. 3.

195. T. Laycock, "On the reflex function" (1845), p. 303.

196. Ibid., p. 309.

197. Ibid., p. 311.

198. Ibid.

199. A. Mette, "Wilhelm Griesinger" (1963), p. 59. See also K. Fichtel, "Wilhelm Griesinger" (1965), p. 1032; and M. P. Amacher, "Thomas Laycock" (1964), pp. 168–169.

200. I. M. Sechenov, "Physiologische Studien" (1863). For biography, see M. N. Shaternikov. "The life" (1935); N. Ischlondskey, "The life and activity" (1958); I. M. Sechenov, *Autobiographical Notes* (1965). See also Clarke and O'Malley (1968), pp. 361–365. For his writings, see I. M. Sechenov, *Selected Works* (1935); idem, *Selected Physiological and Psychological Works* (1962); and A. M. Costa, *Psychologie Soviétique* (1977), chap. 2. See also M. P. Amacher, "Thomas Laycock" (1964).

201. T. Laycock, "Further researches" (1855), p. 155. We shall encounter this attitude again in 6.3.1.

202. R. M. Young, *Mind, Brain and Adaptation* (1970), p. 74.

203. T. Laycock, "Further researches" (1855), p. 156.

204. Ibid., pp. 156–157. See K. Macleod, *Laycock* (1908), pp. 10–11.

205. K. Dewhurst, *Hughlings Jackson* (1982), pp. 7–9.

206. J. H. Jackson, "On the scientific and empirical investigation" (1876), p. 167.

207. H. T. Engelhardt, "John Hughlings Jackson" (1975), pp. 143, 148.

208. M. Hall, *New Memoir* (1843), p. 37.

209. M. Hall, *Synopsis* (1850), p. 13.

210. M. Hall, *New Memoir* (1843), pp. 37–38.

211. R. D. Grainger, *Observations* (1837), p. v.

212. Ibid., p. 57.

213. Ibid. The complex fiber system of the vegetative nervous system will be discussed in chap. 7.5.

214. R. D. Grainger, *Observations* (1837), p. 34.

215. W. B. Carpenter, *Prize Thesis* (1839), para. 76 (pp. 57–58), "The divisions of the nervous apparatus in Myriapoda." G. Newport, "On the structure" (1843), pp. 243–272; this is the best account of his meticulous studies on the nervous system of the *Articulata.* For further discussion of these investigations, see R. Leys Fried, "Alison versus Hall" (1976).

216. W. B. Carpenter, *Prize Thesis* (1839), pp. v–vi.

217. Ibid., pp. 76–77. See also idem, *Principles of General and Comparative Physiology* (1841), para. 733 (pp. 553–554).

218. Ibid., p. 550n.

219. Ibid., para. 725 (pp. 549–550).

220. R. B. Todd, *The Cyclopaedia,* ed. R. B. Todd (1835–1859), 3 (1839–1847):722C. For a detailed discussion of his objections, see R. B. Todd and W. Bowman, *The Physiological Anatomy* (1845–1856), 1 (1845):321–341.

221. M. Hall, *Synopsis* (1850), p. 33.

222. R. B. Todd, *The Cyclopaedia,* ed. R. B. Todd (1835–1859), 3 (1839–1847):722D.

223. For example, B. Schulz, *Die Physiologie* (1842). For review, see Anonymous ["Volkmann"] (1844), p. 403. The anonymous reviewer stated that "our author, like most of his countrymen, takes the opportunity of doubting the anatomical existence of Dr. Hall's excito-motory nerves" (p. 403).

224. A. W. Volkmann, "Ueber Reflexbewegungen" (1838), pp. 39–40.

225. Ibid., p. 40.

226. F. G. J. Henle, "Ueber Nervensympathie" (1840).

227. Ibid., p. 83.

228. Ibid., "Krankhefte Sympathien" (1840).

229. A. Dupré, "Expériences" (1843).

230. A. W. Volkmann, "Nervenphysiologie" (1844), p. 528.

231. Ibid., pp. 547–548.

232. G. Kirschner, *M. Hall. Abhandlungen* (1840). "Appendix," p. 216. This is a translation of Hall's *Memoirs* (1837), thus bringing his articles of 1833 and 1837 to a wider German audience.

233. R. Wagner, "Sympathischen Nerv" (1846), pp. 398–400.

234. Ibid., p. 398.

235. G. A. Spiess, *Physiologie* (1844), pp. 159–177.

236. R. A. von Koelliker, *Mikroskopische Anatomie* (1850–1854), 2, pt. 1 (1850):443.

237. J. L. C. Schroeder van der Kolk, *Bau und Functionen* (1859), chap. 4, para. 5 (pp. 63–64). The English translation (1859) was added to by the author, so that it can be regarded as the 2d ed. The original Dutch edition of 1854 was not seen.

238. J. L. C. Schroeder van der Kolk, in "Professor Schroeder" (1859), p. 73. In this English version, the sentence has been amplified when contrasted with the German version (p. 69).

239. R. Wagner, "Ueber die Elementar-Organisation" (1854).

240. R. Wagner, "Ueber den Bau" (1854).

241. G. H. Lewes, *The Physical Basis* (1877), p. 425.

242. C. E. Brown-Séquard, *Course of Lectures* (1860), p. 156. Marshall Hall, who had died three years earlier, would have been justifiably outraged by the omission of his name from this roll of honor, and by the use of the term "sympathy" instead of "reflex." It is possible that these were deliberate distortions arising from personal antipathy. For Martyn Paine, see n. 83 above. The contributions of Tissot and Barthez were of no consequence whatever, and F. Fearing in his exhaustive survey of reflex physiology (*Reflex Action* [1930]) made no reference to them.

243. See literature cited in n. 121 above.

244. For Pavlov's work, see I. P. Pavlov, *Lectures* (1928–1941); E. A. Asratyan, *I. P. Pavlov* (1953); *DSB*.

245. R. Granit, "Interactions" (1982).

5. NERVE FUNCTION

1. There exists no comprehensive account of the history of nerve function, but the following sources can be recommended: K. E. Rothschuh, "Vom spiritus animalis" (1958); M. A. B. Brazier, "The historical development" (1959); Clarke and O'Malley (1968), pp. 139–259. There is also J. F. Fulton, "The history of the physiology of muscle" (1926), but it is not entirely reliable. M. A. B. Brazier's recent *A History of Neurophysiology* (1984) gives an excellent account of nerve function in the seventeenth and eighteenth centuries, with a large part devoted to electrophysiology; it can be strongly recommended.

2. L. Galvani, *De Viribus Electricitatis* (1791). See n. 50 below for details.

3. For modern accounts of nerve function, see R. D. Keynes, "Ion channels" (1979); and R. D. Keynes and D. J. Aidley, *Nerve and Muscle* (1981).

4. E. Clarke, "The doctrine" (1968).

5. *Galen on the Natural Functions* (1916), bk. II, chap. VI, p. 153. In C. G. Kühn, *[Galen] Medicorum Graecorum Opera* (1821–1833), 2 (1821):97. See also Clarke and O'Malley (1968), pp. 144–146.

6. The following deal with animal electricity before Galvani: J. Priestley, *History and Present State* (1767); H. E. Hoff, "Galvani" (1936); W. C. Walker, "Animal electricity" (1937); I. B. Cohen, "Introduction" (1953); M. A. B. Brazier, "The evolution of concepts" (1958); P. C. Ritterbush, "Electricity" (1964), whose criticisms of eighteenth-century workers identifying electrical with nervous fluid have been challenged by R. W. Home,

"Electricity" (1970); E. Snorrason, *C.G. Kratzenstein* (1974); B. I. Williams, *The Conceptual and Empirical Basis* (1975); M. Neuburger (1981), pp. 141–143, 191–199; M. A. B. Brazier, *A History of Neurophysiology* (1984), pp. 107–217. There is also E. G. Gartrell, *Electricity, Magnetism* (1975), a checklist of primary sources, 1600–1850. For a history of physical electricity in the seventeenth and eighteenth centuries, see J. L. Heilbron, *Electricity* (1979).

7. S. W. Jackson, "Force" (1970); not entirely reliable and most of the material is from sources in English. For eighteenth-century accounts of nerve fluid, see D. Bayne (alias Kinneir), *A New Essay* (1739); and M. Flemyng, *The Nature* (1751). For a more complex eighteenth-century view of nerve action, see S. Musgrave, *Speculations* (1776).

8. A. von Haller, *Elementa* (1757–1766), vol. 4 (1762), bk. 9, sect. 2, "Motus musculorum phaenomena," § 15. "Vis nervosa" (pp. 467–468). This motor force was termed *vis motoria* by J. Müller and *excitabilité* by P. Flourens, and Marshall Hall was still using *vis nervosa* in 1840, arguing that it was responsible for sensory, as well as motor, nerve messages. (See M. Hall, "Briefe" [1840]; and "Memoirs . . . Memoir III" [1840]).

9. R. W. Home, in "Electricity" (1970), dealt mainly with Haller's rejection of this identity, and how his objections were met by Galvani. It is interesting to note that the term "electrical fluid" survived into the present century. See also n. 6 above.

10. S. Hales, *Statical Essays* (1733), pp. 58–59. German writers have usually attributed the first mention of this possibility to Christian August Hausen (1693–1743) in his *Novi Profectus* (1743). They include A. von Haller, *Elementa* (1757–1766), vol. 4 (1762), bk. 10, sect. 8, § 15. "Num aether," see pp. 378–379; E. du Bois-Reymond, *Untersuchungen* (1848–1884), 2, pt. 1 (1849):210–211, but he was citing Haller; L. Hermann, *Lehrbuch* (1892), p. 388. M. Neuburger (1981) also placed Hausen's name first and omitted that of Hales (p. 95 n. 38). See also J. Fisher, "The history of electricity" (1956), p. 50.

11. S. Hales, *Statical Essays* (1733), p. 59.

12. M. Adanson, *A Voyage* (1759), pp. 244–245. The electric eel's effect "did not appear to differ sensibly from the electrical motion of the Leyden experiment." It was not until 1777 that the electrical nature of the shocks of *Torpedo* and *Gymnotus* was established and generally accepted (W. C. Walker, "Animal electricity" [1937], p. 87).

13. For the early history of electric fish, see P. Kellaway, "The part played" (1946); and W. C. Walker, "Animal electricity" (1937), pp. 87–101; and M. Neuburger (1981), pp. 193–196. For a survey of early nineteenth-century knowledge of the electric fish, see J. Coldstream, "Electricity, animal" (1837).

14. Plato referred to the numbing and paralyzing effect of the sting of the flat sea-fish, *narke;* see his *Menon,* 80a, in *Platonis Opera Omnia* (1873),

p. 206. Avicenna (980–1037) also cited its therapeutic use; see J. O. Leibowitz, "Electroshock therapy" (1957). See also P. Kellaway, "The part played" (1946), pp. 129–133, "Electrotherapy introduced."

15. J. Walsh, "Of the electric property" (1774); J. Hunter, "Anatomical observations" (1774); idem, "An account" (1775); H. Cavendish, "An account" (1776); F. H. A. von Humboldt, *Versuche* (1806); idem, *Aspects of Nature* (1849), 1:21–23, 186–187; H. Davy, "An account" (1829); J. Davy, "An account" (1832); idem, "Observations" (1834). For discussion of work of Walsh, Hunter, and Cavendish, see W. C. Walker, "Animal electricity" (1937), pp. 90–100.

16. These included A. Michelitz (1747–1818) in "Scrutinium" (1782); and F. A. Reuss (1761–1830) in *Ergo Spirituum Animalium* (1783). See also E. Clarke, "The doctrine" (1968).

17. M. Neuburger (1981) in his n. 38 (p. 195) claimed that these were: C. A. Hausen, François Boissier de Sauvages de la Croix (1706–1767), Jean Étienne Deshais (fl. 1749), J. Priestley, Anton de Haën (1704–1776), E. Darwin, C. Bonnet, Jan Ingen-Housz (1730–1799), F. H. A. von Humboldt, Ritter, Procháska, Aldini, Cabanis, "Herschel" [?], Thomas Young (1773–1829), Wilson Philip, and K. A. Weinhold.

18. R. Whytt, *An Essay* (1751), p. 239.

19. See R. K. French, *Robert Whytt* (1969), pp. 63–76.

20. A. von Haller, *Primae Lineae* (1747), chap. 12, "De cerebro," § 391 (p. 201). For a detailed discussion of Haller's opinions on the nature of the nerve fluid, and of the reasons why he rejected the possibility of it being the same as the electrical fluid, see R. W. Home, "Electricity" (1970).

21. See the 2d edition of A. von Haller, *Primae Lineae* (1751), para. 391 (pp. 240–241); and the 3d edition idem, *Primae Lineae* (1767), para. 379 (pp. 196–197). Also in idem, *Dr. Albert Haller's Physiology* (1754), vol. 1, § 391 (p. 315).

22. A. von Haller, *Elementa* (1757–1766), vol. 4 (1762), bk. 2, sect. 8, "Conjecturae," § 16. "Quaenam ergo spirituum materies sit" (p. 381). For full details, see also § 15. "Num aether" (pp. 378–380). His objections to electricity are also in L. M. A. Caldani, "Lettre" (1762), and "Sur l'insensibilité" (1762); and in F. G. F. Fontana, "Dissertation epistolaire" (1762).

23. A. Monro, *secundus, Observations* (1783), p. 75.

24. Ibid., p. 76.

25. J. A. Unzer, *Erste Gründe* (1771), pt. 2, chap. 1, "Von den Nervenkräften und Nervenwirkungen überhaupt," (pp. 344–406). English trans., idem, *The Principles of Physiology* (1851), pp. 189–221.

26. J. Procháska, *Adnotationum Academicarum* (1784), pt. 1, chap. 3, "Functiones nervorum," § 1, p. 77. English trans. idem, . . . *and a Dissertation* (1851), p. 407. For Procháska's neurophysiology, see V. Kruta, "The physiologist" (1962); and *DSB*.

27. This later statement appeared in a footnote on p. 390 of the English

translation but is absent from the original Latin text (p. 47). See, however, J. Procháska, *Physiologie* (1820) in which he expounded his theory that life in general derived from the principles of the electrical process, "Dritter Abschnitt," pp. 26–72. However, as noted in chap. 4, he had by now descended into mystical obscurity.

28. W. D. Hackmann, "The researches" (1972).

29. L. Galvani, *De Viribus Electricitatis* (1791). See n. 50 below.

30. For the invention of the Leyden jar, see J. Priestley, *History and Present State* (1767), p. 282; C. Dorsman and C. A. Crommelin, "The invention" (1957); J. L. Heilbron, "À propos de l'invention" (1966); and idem, "G.M. Bose" (1966). See also H. E. Hoff, "Galvani" (1936); and other references cited in n. 6 above.

31. O. von Guericke, *Experimenta Nova* (1672), bk. 4. "De virtutibus mundanis," chap. 15. "De experimento . . . " (pp. 147–150); and "Iconismus XVIII," p. 148. See H. Schimank, "Geschichte" (1935); W. D. Hackmann, *John and Jonathan Cuthbertson* (1973); B. S. Finn, "Output" (1971); and W. D. Hackmann, "Electricity from glass" (1978).

32. L. M. A. Caldani, "Lettre" (1762), dated 30 October 1756; and "Sur l'insensibilité" (1762), dated 30 December 1757.

33. G. Beccaria, *Dell'Elettricismo* (1753), bk. 1, chap. 7, § 430, p. 129. Described in greater detail in idem, *A Treatise* (1776), chap. 3, sect. 1, §§ 632–637 (pp. 270–272). See also M. Neuburger (1981), p. 192; and M. Gliozzi, "Giambattista Beccaria" (1935).

34. A. Schierbeek, *Jan Swammerdam* (1967), pp. 72, 77–79. However, his account was not published until 1738, in *Bybel der Natuure* (1737–1738), 2 (1738):839. In English, idem, *The Book of Nature* (1758), pt. 2, p. 123. See also G. A. Lindeboom, "Jan Swammerdam" (1982); and M. A. B. Brazier, "The problem" (1982).

35. E. du Bois-Reymond, *Untersuchungen* (1848–1884), 1 (1848):37.

36. B. I. Williams, *The Conceptual and Empirical Basis* (1975).

37. Ibid., p. 1.

38. The more noteworthy works dealing with galvanism (animal electricity) or its history mostly contain an account of Galvani's studies: P. Sue ainé, *Histoire du Galvanisme* (1802–1805); C. H. Wilkinson, *Elements* (1804); J. Bostock, *An Account* (1818); E. du Bois-Reymond, *Untersuchungen* (1848–1884), 1 (1848):31–93; H. E. Hoff, "Galvani" (1936); I. B. Cohen, "Introduction" (1953); M. A. B. Brazier, "The evolution of concepts" (1958); idem, "The historical development" (1959); K. E. Rothschuh, "Aus der Frühzeit" (1959); idem, "Von der Idee" (1960); G. C. Pupilli and E. Fadiga, "The origins" (1963); Clarke and O'Malley (1968), pp. 177–237; *DSB;* B. I. Williams's *The Conceptual and Empirical Basis* (1975) is the best and most detailed discussion in English on the origins and contents of Galvani's ideas, but she was concerned primarily with muscular motion rather than with nerve function; M. Neuburger (1981), pp. 141–143, 191–199; and

M. A. B. Brazier, *A History of Neurophysiology* (1984), pp. 205–217. See also n. 6 above. For individuals, see B. Dibner, *Ten Founding Fathers* (1954). P. F. Mottelay's *Bibliographical History* (1922) is valuable for reference.

39. L. Galvani, *De Viribus Electricitatis* (1791). See n. 50 below.

40. This succinct summary was made by a contemporary, C. H. Pfaff (1773–1852) of Kiel, who was in agreement with Galvani: *Über thierische Elektricität* (1795), pp. 329–330.

41. T. Schwann, *Mikroscopische Untersuchungen* (1839), see pp. 174–175. See also Clarke and O'Malley (1968), pp. 56–58.

42. L. Galvani, *De Viribus Electricitatis* (1791), p. 39. Taken from L. Galvani, *Luigi Galvani . . .*, trans. M. G. Foley (1953), p. 76.

43. L. Galvani, *De Viribus Electricitatis* (1791), p. 42.

44. It should be noted that "animal electricity" referred to electricity in animals, whereas "animal spirits" meant psychic or mental spirits, "animal" here being derived from *animus,* the mind, soul, etc.

45. C. Bernard, *Leçons sur la Physiologie* (1858), 1:4.

46. The notion that the brain secreted a substance, "animal spirits" (see n. 44 above), fundamental to nerve function, began with the Hippocratic Writers. See F. Solmsen, "Greek philosophy" (1961).

47. M. Malpighi, "De cerebri cortice," in *De Viscerum* (1666), pp. 50–72; and T. Wharton, *Adenographia* (1656), chap. 3, "Num cerebrum ad glandula num numerum vel viscerum accedat . . . ?" pp. 8–13. See L. Belloni, "Neuroanatomie" (1968); E. Clarke and J. G. Bearn, "The brain 'glands'" (1968); and M. Neuburger (1981), pp. 10n, 25–26, 81.

48. Sir J. Elliot, *Elements* (1786), chap. 9, "Of the glands," p. 246: "THE BRAIN seems to secrete a substance which, being conveyed by the nerves, assists in nutrition. By means either of the same, or some other matter or fluid, sensation and motion are probably performed."

49. W. Cullen, *The Works* (1827), 1:118.

50. The periodical publication was "De viribus electricitatis" (1791), and the book *De Viribus Electricitatis* (1791). All references to this report will be to the book. There is an English translation of it by R. M. Green: L. Galvani, *A Translation* (1953). A more reliable version, however, is by M. G. Foley: L. Galvani, *Luigi Galvani* (1953), in a book that also contains an excellent introduction by I. B. Cohen ("Introduction" [1953]), together with a facsimile reprint of Galvani's book, and a bibliography of his writings (pp. 157–176), which is a revised version of the inaccurate bibliography of J. F. Fulton and H. Cushing, "A bibliographical study" (1936). For further biographies of Galvani, see M. Neuburger (1981), p. 324.

51. E. du Bois-Reymond, *Untersuchungen* (1848–1884), 1 (1848):50–51.

52. I. B. Cohen, "The two hundredth anniversary" (1952).

53. See P. C. Ritterbush. "Electricity and vital energy," in idem, "Electricity" (1964), pp. 28–35; and T. S. Hall, *Ideas* (1969), 2:223–228.

54. J. Abernethy, *Physiological Lectures* (1822), p. 26. They had been

delivered in 1814. For the full development of this theme, with the inclusion of all known physical forces, and its extension into the bizarre and occult, see Baron C. von Reichenbach (1808–1869), *Physico-physiological Researches* (1851). Also of interest is the work of A. Smee (1818–1877) in electrical physiology. The titles of his books indicate the central role he accorded electricity in biological processes: *Elements of Electro-biology* (1849); *Instinct and Reason* (1850). The ability of electricity to produce epidemics was an equally curious aspect of bioelectricity: W. Craig, *On the Influence of Variations* (1859). There must be many similar examples. For a modern interpretation of these possibilities, see H. S. Burr and F. S. C. Northrop, "The electrodynamic theory of life" (1935).

55. J. Abernethy, *Physiological Lectures* (1822), p. 33.

56. T. S. Surr, *A Winter in London* (1806), 2:179.

57. W. Lawrence, *Lectures* (1819), p. 76: "the contrast between the animal functions and electric operations is so obvious and forcible, that the attempts to assimilate them do not demand further notice."

58. J. C. Prichard, *A Review* (1829), pp. 32–33.

59. J. Fletcher, *Rudiments* (1835–1837), pt. Ia (1836), p. 120n.

60. F. A. Mesmer, *Mémoire* (1779), pp. 6–7. He referred here to his medical dissertation at Vienna: idem, *Dissertatio* (1766). In it he drew upon *De Imperio* (1704) of R. Mead (1673–1734); English version, idem, *Of the Power* (1712). For an English trans. of Mesmer's memoir, see F. A. Mesmer, *Mesmerism* (1948); see also F. A. Pattie, "Mesmer's medical dissertation" (1956).

61. Anonymous, *Rapport* (1841), pp. 26–91; for other reports, see pp. 92–236. The *Rapport* was first published in 1784, but the comments (in C. Burdin and E. F. Dubois d'Amiens, *Histoire Académique,* (1841), pp. 26–91) on this 1841 reproduction are of interest. One of the commissioners was Benjamin Franklin (1706–1790), and an English version of the *Rapport* is B. Franklin et al., *Report of Dr. Benjamin Franklin* (1785). See E. J. Dingwall, "The French Commissions" (1967); G. Zorab, "Electrical and galvanic theories" (1967); R. Darnton, *Mesmerism* (1968), pp. 10–12, 14–16, 28–29, 60; and G. Sutton, "Electric medicine" (1981).

62. The best review of this is in B. Dibner, *Galvani-Volta* (1952). For biographies of Volta, see R. Appleyard, *Pioneers* (1930), pp. 55–83; and *DSB*.

63. The controversy began with a paper read by Volta at the University of Pavia on 5 March 1792, which was published with additional observations as "Memoria prima" (1792). It was followed by "Memoria seconda" (1792). These papers were reprinted in idem, *Collezione* (1816), vol. 2, pt. 1, pp. 13–52 and 55–118, respectively. In 1791 Volta was elected a foreign Fellow of the Royal Society (London), and in 1792 sent two papers to the Society, dated 13 September and 25 October 1792. They were read on 31 January 1793 and published in French: A. Volta, "Account" (1793). Also in idem,

Collezione (1816), 1:121–160. They were addressed to Tiberius Cavallo (1749–1809), an Italian electrician residing in London. There followed a stream of publications from Volta, and in 1792 alone at least 12 were published; see B. Dibner, *Galvani-Volta* (1952), pp. 24–32.

64. A. Volta, "Account" (1793), p. 36.

65. A. Mauro, "The role of the Voltaic pile" (1969), p. 144.

66. [L. Galvani], *Dell'Uso e dell'Attività* [1794]. Not seen, but see idem, *Luigi Galvani* (1953), the M. G. Foley translation, pp. 28–29, 160–162, and 174–175. English translation of crucial experiment report is in B. Dibner, *Galvani-Volta* (1952), pp. 50–51.

67. H. B. Jones, ed., *On Animal Electricity* (1852), p. 13. This is a translation of an account of E. du Bois-Reymond's research results by the Freiburg-im-Breisgau physicist Johannes Müller (1809–1875): *Bericht* (1849), pp. 768–844. Not seen, but cited by Estelle du Bois-Reymond and P. Diepgen, eds., *Zwei grosse Naturforscher* (1927), p. 207 n. 181; English trans., *Two Great Scientists* (1982), p. 149 n. 181. It has, therefore, been impossible for us to differentiate between Müller's original text and Jones's many additions.

68. B. I. Williams, *The Conceptual and Empirical Basis* (1975), pp. 412–413.

69. G. Aldini, *De Animali Electricitate* (1794). Two papers read at Bologna, the first in 1793, the third in 1792. English trans. in idem, *An Account* (1803), pp. 133–185. Expanded French version in idem, *Essai Théoretique* (1804). See Clarke and O'Malley (1968), pp. 183–185. The bibliography of Aldini's writings by J. F. Fulton and H. Cushing, "A bibliographical study" (1936) is unreliable.

70. E. du Bois-Reymond, *Untersuchungen* (1848–1884), 1 (1848):95.

71. F. H. A. von Humboldt, *Versuche* (1797), "Zehnter Abschnitt," 1:367–381. See K. E. Rothschuh, "Friedrich Alexander von Humboldt" (1959); idem, "Alexander von Humboldt" (1959); and idem, "Alexander von Humboldt et l'histoire" (1960).

72. F. H. A. von Humboldt, *Versuche* (1797), 1:379–380.

73. Ibid., p. 367.

74. G. V. M. Fabbroni, "Sur l'action chimique" (1799), p. 357. Also cited by P. Sue ainé, *Histoire du Galvanisme* (1802–1805), vol. 1 (1802), § 3. "Extrait de l'ouvrage de Fabroni [*sic*] sur l'irritation métallique," pp. 229–234. "Fabbroni" is the correct spelling. For biography, see *DSB*.

75. J. Bostock, *An Account* (1818), pp. 21–22. For a brief discussion of the Voltaic pile and electrochemical theory in 1800, see W. M. Sudduth, "The Voltaic pile" (1980).

76. F. H. A. von Humboldt, *Versuche* (1797), 1:1.

77. Ibid., p. 398.

78. A. Volta. "On the electricity excited [text in French]" (1800). English version in "On the electricity excited" (1800), and facsimile reprints of this

in B. Dibner, *Galvani-Volta* (1952); and in G. Sarton, "The discovery" (1931), pp. [129–157]. For the genesis of this invention and an explanation for the lengthy period of time that Volta took to devise it, see S. Gill, "A Voltaic enigma" (1976). Gill criticized some of the arguments advanced by A. Mauro, "The role of the Voltaic pile" (1969).

79. For a history of the Voltaic pile, see G. Sarton, "The discovery" (1931). See also B. Dibner, *Alessandro Volta* (1964), and for the background to the development of the pile, see G. Sutton, "The politics of science" (1981).

80. W. C. Walker, "The detection and estimation" (1936), p. 100.

81. B. Dibner, *Heralds of Science* (1969), p. 31.

82. For a discussion of them, see S. Gill, "A Voltaic enigma" (1976). See also W. C. Walker, "The detection and estimation" (1936), who described events leading up to Volta's discovery of the electric current.

83. For a review of French contributions, see T. M. Brown, "The electric current" (1969).

84. For Galvani's application of galvanism to clinical medicine, see E. Benassi, "Ipotesi elettropathogenetiche" (1963). In 1803 a Société de Galvanisme was founded in Paris for the examination of the effects, especially medical, of galvanism. Its *Journal du Galvanisme, de Vaccine* . . . (vols. 1–2, 1803) described the therapeutic value of galvanic shock, which was but a repetition of the eighteenth-century procedures that employed electrostatic machines and the Leyden jar as sources of electricity. For a detailed account of the medical application of Voltaic electricity at this time, see J. A. Sigaud la Fond (1740–1810), *De l'Électricité Médicale* (1802). See also P. Laurentius, *Geschichte* (1936); E. Charbonnel-Duteil, *Les Debuts* (1943); F. Schiller, "Neurology" (1982); and, in particular, M. Rowbottom and C. Susskind, *Electricity and Medicine* (1984). For a study of eighteenth-century electrotherapy as practiced by John Wesley (1703–1791) and Jean Paul Marat (1743–1793), see F. Schiller, "Reverend Wesley" (1981). See also L. A. Geddes, *A Short History* (1984).

85. G. Aldini, *An Account* (1803). He discussed this on pp. 14–18. See especially "Experiment I" (pp. 14–15) and pl. 1, fig. 3. Also in idem, *Essai Théoretique* (1804), pp. 11–16. See also Clarke and O'Malley (1968), pp. 183–185.

86. G. Aldini, *An Account* (1803), p. 14.

87. For biography, see *DSB;* and M. Neuburger (1981), p. 355. Bibliography in *DSB,* and in J. C. Poggendorff, *Biographisch-literarisches Handwörterbuch* (1863–1926), vol. 2 (1863).

88. For Ritter's philosophical associations, see A. Gode-von Aesch, *Natural Science* (1966); and B. Gower, "Speculation in physics" (1973), pp. 327–328.

89. J. W. Ritter, *Beweis* (1798). Not seen, but cited by J. C. Poggendorff, *Biographisch-literarisches Handwörterbuch* (1863–1926), vol. 2 (1863); and *DSB.*

90. J. W. Ritter, ed., *Beyträge* (1800–1805). A collection of lengthy articles on galvanic electricity, mostly by Ritter. It contains the earliest account of the decomposition of electric current (J. W. Ritter, "Beweis," [1800]); and a description of his invention of a storage battery (idem, "Von der Galvanischen Batterie," [1802]). He reported a few of his experiments in "New Galvanic discoveries" (1806).

91. E. G. T. Liddell, *The Discovery* (1960), p. 42.

92. J. W. Ritter, "Versuche und Bemerkungen" (1801), p. 437.

93. Little reference to Ritter was made in the British literature, and there are very few copies of his writings in British libraries that were collecting actively at the beginning of the nineteenth century. As far as his electrophysiological research is concerned, however, the stagnancy of physiology in early nineteenth-century Britain makes this country a special case, and Ritter was by no means the only Continental scientist whose work was ignored. See G. L. Geison, "Social and institutional factors" (1972).

94. See *DSB* biography of Ritter.

95. Anonymous, ["Review of *Darstellungen*"] (1807), pp. 240–241. See J. W. Ritter, "Darstellungen des Gegensatzes" (1805).

96. Anonymous, ["Review of *Darstellungen*"] (1807), p. 228.

97. D. Hüffmeier-von Hagen, "J. W. Ritter" (1964).

98. E. du Bois-Reymond, *Untersuchungen* (1848–1884), 1 (1848):263; and ibid., "Ritter's Arbeiten über das Gesetz der Zuchungen," pp. 313–333; and ibid., passim. See also D. Hüffmeier, "Johann Wilhelm Ritter" (1961), who agreed with du Bois-Reymond's assessment of Ritter.

99. J. Teichmann, in "Beziehungen" (1974), argued that the addition of Ritter's opinions to the work of Volta was fruitful for the development of science.

100. B. Gower mentioned examples of this in "Speculation in physics" (1973), pp. 301–302. See also C. A. Culotta, "German biophysics" (1974).

101. For example, J. H. D. Petetin (1744–1808), *Électricité Animale* (1808). See also E. Stainbrook, "The use of electricity" (1948).

102. J. J. Berzelius, *A View* (1818), p. 9. This was first written in 1810.

103. J. C. Reil, "Fragmente," (1807–1808), pp. 26–29.

104. J. J. Berzelius, *A View* (1818), p. 11.

105. J. C. Reil, "Fragmente" (1807–1808), p. 27.

106. Ibid., p. 29.

107. L. Rolando, *Saggio* (1809), pp. 62–63.

108. Ibid., pp. 31–32.

109. Ibid., pp. 60–62.

110. Ibid., p. 62.

111. J. Müller, *Handbuch* (1835–1840), 1 (1835, 2d ed.):830.

112. K. A. Weinhold, *Versuche* (1817), § 32. "Versuch mit einem künstlichen Hirn und Rückenmark," pp. 35–37.

113. M. Neuburger (1981), p. 199.

114. See Clarke and O'Malley (1968), pp. 425–428.

115. J. G. F. Baillarger, "Recherches sur la structure" (1840), "Art. X.—Applications physiologiques," see pp. 174–178; and also pp. 180–181.

116. Ibid., p. 181.

117. R. B. Todd and W. Bowman, *The Physiological Anatomy* (1845–1856), 1 (1845):237–244.

118. Ibid., p. 239.

119. Ibid., p. 241. Charles Bell had made a similar comment in 1823 when discussing nerve function, although he was referring only to gross anatomy: J. Bell and C. Bell, *The Anatomy and Physiology* (1823), 2:363.

120. J. F. W. Herschel, *A Preliminary Discourse* (1831), p. 343n. For an analysis of this book, see J. Agassi, "Sir John Herschel's philosophy" (1969).

121. J. F. W. Herschel, *A Preliminary Discourse* (1831), pp. 342–343.

122. P. T. Meissner, *System* (1832), § 70 (pp. 63–64), §§ 73–87 (pp. 66–86), § 126 (pp. 142–144).

123. Ibid., § 45, p. 45.

124. E. Huschke, *Schaedel, Hirn und Seele* (1854), p. 173.

125. Ibid., pt. 3, "Die Seele," chap. 2, "Das Hirn, ein elektrischer Apparat," pp. 168–174.

126. Ibid., p. 168.

127. Ibid. In the present century there were still relics of this belief; for example, in R. L. Watkins, "The brain" (1906).

128. For a modern account of these creatures, see R. D. Keynes, "The generation of electricity" (1956).

129. See n. 12. Conclusive proof was provided by J. Walsh, "Of the electric property" (1774). See W. C. Walker, "Animal electricity" (1937), pp. 90–92 for a discussion of his experiments.

130. F. H. A. von Humboldt, *Versuche* (1806).

131. C. G. Carus, *Lehrbuch* (1834), 1:314n.

132. The results were described in A. C. Becquerel, *Traité Expérimental* (1834–1840), vol. 4 (1836), para. 946 (pp. 264–265). His chap. 3 dealt entirely with "Des poissons électriques," pp. 255–278. Quote on p. 265.

133. W. H. Wollaston, "On the agency" (1809).

134. G. R. Treviranus, *Biologie* (1802–1822), vol. 5 (1818), bk. 7, sect. 3, "Thierische Elektricität," p. 179. He gave an excellent survey of eighteenth- and early nineteenth-century studies together with his own views on the electric fish, pp.144–180.

135. A. P. Wilson Philip, *An Experimental Inquiry* (1817), p. 139. His article, "On the effects of galvanism" (1817) dealt only with its alleged beneficial effect on asthma.

136. Idem, *An Experimental Inquiry* (1817), experiments 46–47 (pp. 127–133). Perhaps the editor of *The Anatomy* (1820) by A. Monro, *secundus,* was referring to Wilson Philip among others when he stated that: "The

identity of the nervous fluid with the electric or galvanic power, has been lately revived by the chemical philosophers of the present day" (p. 343n).

137. C. G. Carus, *Lehrbuch* (1834), vol. 1, § 376, p. 315.

138. Attempts to do so in the eighteenth century were discussed by W. C. Walker, "The detection and estimation" (1936). See also A. W. Humphreys, "The development" (1937).

139. B. Dibner in *Oersted* (1961) gives an excellent survey of the 1800–1820 period (p. 12n). Sixty-eight books, pamphlets, and notices from nine countries on constant-flow electricity were published during it: see W. D. Weaver, ed., *Catalogue* (1909), 1:253–282. Further biography on Oersted: R. Appleyard, *Pioneers* (1930), pp. 142–176; and *DSB*.

140. G. D. Romagnosi, "Articulo sul Galvanismo" (1802). Not seen, but English trans. are J. J. Fahie, *A History of Electric Telegraphy* (1884), p. 259; and B. Dibner, *Oersted* (1961), p. 31.

141. H. C. Oersted, *Experimenta* (1820). Facsimile reprints of this 4-page tract are in G. Sarton, "The foundation" (1928), and B. Dibner, *Oersted* (1961), pp. 23–27. English version in H. C. Oersted, "Experiments" (1820), which is reproduced by G. Sarton "The foundation" (1928), and B. Dibner, *Oersted* (1961), pp. 22, 27.

142. G. Sarton, "The foundation" (1928), p. 435.

143. R. C. Stauffer, "Speculation and experiment" (1957); and B. Gower, "Speculation in physics" (1973), pp. 339–349. See also D. M. Knight, "The physical sciences" (1970).

144. R. C. Stauffer, "Persistent errors" (1953), p. 310. He has corrected errors in dates, thus eliminating the possibility of chance.

145. J. S. C. Schweigger, "Electromagnetischer Multiplicator" (1821).

146. For an excellent account of the earlier part of this history, see H. E. Hoff and L. A. Geddes, "The rheotome" (1957), pp. 213–217. See also E. Gerland and F. Traumüller, *Geschichte* (1899); and L. A. Geddes and H. E. Hoff, "The capillary electrometer" (1961).

147. H. A. M. Snelders, "J. S. C. Schweigger" (1971).

148. J. C. Poggendorff, "Physikalisch-chemische Untersuchungen" (1821). See E. Gerland and F. Traumüller, *Geschichte* (1899), pp. 375–376.

149. L. Nobili, *Descrizione* (1825). For biography of Nobili, see *DSB*.

150. A. M. Ampère, "Mémoire" (1820). Read at the Académie Royale des Sciences, 2 October 1820. He enunciated fundamental principles of electrodynamics which determined the exact relationships between the flow of electrical current and magnetism. For a concise account of his researches, see A. M. Ampére and J. Babinet, *Exposé* (1822); and *DSB*.

151. L. Nobili, "Comparaison" (1828).

152. L. Nobili, "Analyse" (1830).

153. T. M. Brown, "The electric current" (1969).

154. F. A. Longet, *Anatomie et Physiologie* (1842), vol. 1, chap. 6. "De

la force nerveuse," pp. 120–146. In his "Bibliographie" (pp. 145–146), Longet cited fourteen authors for the period 1820–1840: eight were French, four Italian, one Swiss, and one German (J. Müller). For biography of Longet, see H. Larrey, [Obituary of F. A. Longet] (1871); and M. Neuburger (1981), p. 338.

155. O. Temkin, "Materialism" (1946), p. 326.

156. G. Cuvier, *Le Règne Animal* (1817), vol. 1, "Des forces qui agissent dans le corps animal," see p. 31.

157. P. A. Béclard, *Élémens* (1823), § 632 (pp. 632–633).

158. Ibid., § 786 (pp. 668–669).

159. J. L. Prévost and J. B. A. Dumas, "Sur les phénomènes" (1823).

160. G. Cuvier, *Le Régne Animal* (1817), 1:32.

161. J. J. Berzelius, *Läërbook* (1817–1830), 1 (1817):126. This was not seen but was cited by D. Nachmansohn in "Electricity" (1940), who pointed out the modern finding of high concentrations of choline esterase and acetylcholine in the electric organ. Nachmansohn has proposed a connection between Berzelius's contention and this finding but such retrospective judgment is unhistorical to say the least.

162. J. J. Berzelius, *A View* (1818), pp. 5–6.

163. I. S. David, *Identité du Fluide Nerveux* (1830). Not seen, but cited by F. A. Longet, *Anatomie et Physiologie* (1842), 1:121, 135–136.

164. J. Müller, *Handbuch* (1835–1840), vol. 1 (1835, 2d ed.), bk. 3, sect. 1, chap. 3, "Von dem wirksamen Princip der Nerven," p. 620.

165. C. C. Person, "Sur l'hypothèse" (1830).

166. A. Donné, "Recherches" (1834).

167. F. A. Longet, *Anatomie et Physiologie* (1842), 1:138–139.

168. Ibid., p. 143.

169. Ibid., pp. 120–121.

170. Estelle du Bois-Reymond and P. Diepgen, eds., *Zwei grosse Naturforscher* (1927), pp. 88–89, in a letter from Paris dated 9 April 1850; in English trans., *Two Great Scientists* (1982), p. 58. The reference here to F. A. Longet's new work was to his *Traité de Physiologie* (1850–1861), "Sens de la vue," 2 (1850):17–128. The reference to Carl Ludwig's textbook was to his *Lehrbuch der Physiologie* (1852–1856). See also Estelle du Bois-Reymond and P. Diepgen, eds., *Two Great Scientists* (1982), pp. 57–61; and W. Haberling, "du Bois-Reymond in Paris 1850" (1926).

171. R. B. Todd and W. Bowman, *The Physiological Anatomy* (1845–1856), "Nervous and electrical forces compared," 1 (1845):237–244.

172. Ibid., pp. 240–241.

173. G. L. Geison, "Social and institutional factors" (1972).

174. See L. P. Williams, *Michael Faraday* (1965), chap. 4, "The discovery of electromagnetic induction" (pp. 137–190). He had discovered that electricity could be generated in a wire by means of the electromagnetic effect of a current in another wire. This revelation, made in the autumn of 1831,

forms the basis of modern electrical technology for Faraday had invented the first electrical transformer and the first electrical generator.

175. M. Faraday, "Experimental researches in electricity.—Fifteenth series" (1839).

176. Ibid., p. 1.

177. Ibid., p. 12.

178. The most important contribution to medical electricity in Britain is said to have been made by Thomas Addison (1793–1860), published in "The influence of electricity" (1837). It was, however, only a clinical report on its effects in patients, who, unknown to Addison, could well have been suffering from psychological ailments! See also n. 84 above.

179. In a letter to Carl Ludwig dated 2d August 1852, published in Estelle du Bois-Reymond and P. Diepgen, eds., *Zwei grosse Naturforscher* (1927), p. 111; in English trans., *Two Great Scientists* (1982), p. 73. Thirty years earlier, W. Lawrence had commented thus on Haller's *Elementa* (1757–1766): "It is no slight proof of its merits, that although published in the middle of the last century, it remains the book of authority; and particularly in this country, which is still destitute of original standard works in anatomy and physiology." (W. Lawrence, *Lectures,* 1822, p. 54.)

180. J. S. Burdon Sanderson, ed., *Translations* (1887), p. xii.

181. The best accounts of Matteucci's work are by G. Moruzzi: "The electrophysiological work" (1963); "L'opera" (1964), with partial bibliography; *L'opera* (1973); and *DSB*. Complete bibliography in N. Bianchi, *Carlo Matteucci* (1874). See also Clarke and O'Malley (1968), pp. 185–192.

182. C. Matteucci, "Sur le courant électrique" (1838), p. 95.

183. C. Matteucci, "Expériences" (1836). Two further papers were idem, "Nouvelle expériences" (1837); and idem, "Recherches physiques" (1837).

184. C. Matteucci, *Essai* (1840), p. 62.

185. C. Matteucci, "Ueber die electrischen Erscheinungen" (1839), column 133.

186. C. Matteucci, "Sur le courant électrique" (1838), "Première section. – Des diverses parties du corps de la grenouille qui développent le courant électrique, et des propriétés de ce courant," pp. 95–101.

187. C. Matteucci, "Deuxième mémoire" (1842). The first memoir was idem, "Sur le courant électrique" (1838), despite the fact that "second mémoire" was in its title. See Clarke and O'Malley (1968), pp. 186–188.

188. G. Moruzzi, "The electrophysiological work" (1963), p. 142.

189. C. Matteucci, "Deuxième mémoire" (1842), p. 331. See Clarke and O'Malley (1968), p. 188.

190. He described it in detail in C. Matteucci, *Traité* (1844), pp. 28–30.

191. Ibid., p. 52. Concerning muscles, he came to the same conclusion that an electrical current was present in them during life and even after death. In these experiments he collaborated with F. H. A. von Humboldt: C. Matteucci and F. H. A. von Humboldt, "Sur le courant" (1843).

192. C. Matteucci, *Traité* (1844), p. 29.

193. Ibid., pp. 55–57. See Clarke and O'Malley (1968), pp. 189–190. Modifications and refinements were possible; see C. Matteucci, *Lectures* (1847), "Lecture IX. Electric currents of muscles," pp. 192–194.

194. C. Matteucci, *Traité* (1844), p. 56.

195. C. Matteucci, "[Report on muscle contraction current]" (1842). This was his original, sealed report of 1841—"Expériences rapportées dans un paquet cacheté deposé par M. [J.B.A.] Dumas au nom de M. Matteucci, et dont l'auteur, présent à la séance, désire aujourd'hui l'ouverture."

196. C. Matteucci, "Sur un phénomène physiologique" (1842). Matteucci's experiments are all reported in idem, *Traité* (1844), pp. 130–141.

197. C. Matteucci, "[Report on muscle contraction current]" (1842), p. 797.

198. Ibid.

199. Ibid.

200. S. T. Soemmerring, *Über den Saft* (1811), § 5 (pp. 17–18).

201. Becquerel reported his findings in a note sent to Matteucci. See C. Matteucci, *Traité* (1844), pp. 133–134. See also Becquerel's later report, "Note relative" (1849).

202. A. H. Bequerel, in C. Matteucci, *Traité* (1844), p. 134.

203. C. Matteucci, "Expériences" (1845), p. 70.

204. C. Matteucci, "Electro-physiological researches.—Third memoir" (1845), p. 317.

205. C. Matteucci, *Lectures* (1847), p. 319. These lectures were given in 1844, but this translation from the Italian was corrected and expanded by the author, so that the opinions expressed here can be dated 1847.

206. C. Matteucci, "Electro-physiological researches—Ninth series" (1850), pp. 648–649.

207. Ibid., p. 649.

208. C. Matteucci, "Electro-physiological researches.—Eighth series" (1850), p. 296.

209. C. Matteucci, "Electro-physiological researches.—Ninth series" (1850), p. 649.

210. E. du Bois-Reymond, *Untersuchungen* (1848–1884), 2, pt. 1 (1849):29.

211. C. Matteucci, "Sur le courant électrique" (1838), "Seconde section.—Des causes qui modifient le courant de la grenouille," pp. 101–104.

212. Ibid., pp. 102–103.

213. C. Matteucci, "Deuxième mémoire" (1842), p. 325.

214. Ibid., p. 327.

215. E. du Bois-Reymond, "Vorläufiger Abriss" (1843), para. 32, pp. 12–13; and para. 49, p. 19.

216. C. Matteucci, "Expériences sur les phénomènes" (1845).

217. E. du Bois-Reymond, *Untersuchungen* (1848–1884), 2, pt. 1 (1849):425–430. See also idem, "On Signor Carlo Matteucci's letter" (1853), § 9. "On the negative variation of the muscular current during contraction," pp. 27–30.

218. C. Matteucci, *Essai* (1840), p. 81.

219. C. Matteucci, "Deuxième mémoire" (1842), p. 339.

220. C. Matteucci, "Electrophysiological researches.—First memoir" (1845), p. 294.

221. F. A. Longet, *Anatomie et Physiologie* (1842), 1:126–129.

222. C. Matteucci and F. A. Longet, "Note sur l'hypothèse" (1844), p. 580.

223. E. du Bois-Reymond, "Vorläufiger Abriss" (1843).

224. F. A. Longet, *Anatomie et Physiologie* (1842), 1:123.

225. E. du Bois-Reymond, *Untersuchungen* (1848–1884), 1 (1848): XIV–XV.

226. J. Müller, *Handbuch* (1835–1840), vol. 1 (1835, 2d ed.), "Prolegomena," pt. 4, "Physicalische Erscheinungen," sect. 1, "Entwickelung von Electricität," p. 72.

227. Ibid., book 3, "Physik der Nerven," pt. 1, chap. 2, "Reizbarkeit der Nerven. Electrische Reize," p. 600.

228. Ibid., bk. 3, pt. 1, chap. 3, "Von dem wirksamen Princip der Nerven," pp. 616–625.

229. Ibid., p. 624.

230. C. Matteucci, "Electro-physiology" (1866), p. 302.

231. E. du Bois-Reymond, *Untersuchungen* (1848–1884), 1 (1848):XXI.

232. It was donated by Antoine Jean Baptiste Robert Auget, Baron de Montyon (1733–1820). See N. Egli, *Der "Prix Montyon"* (1970); and M. Crosland, "From prizes to grants" (1979).

233. C. Matteucci, "Electro-physiological researches.—First memoir" (1845), p. 294.

234. C. Matteucci, "Electro-physiological researches.—Second memoir" (1845), p. 301.

235. For biography of E. du Bois-Reymond, see H. Boruttau, *Emil du Bois-Reymond* (1922); and *DSB,* where the entry by K. E. Rothschuh is the best account in English, although it has suffered in translation. A list of biographies and obituaries is in Estelle du Bois-Reymond and P. Diepgen, eds., *Zwei grosse Naturforscher* (1927), p. 221; in English trans., *Two Great Scientists* (1982), p. 165. For discussions of his work, see K. E. Rothschuh, "Emil du Bois-Reymond" (1964); Clarke and O'Malley (1968), pp. 192–203. For bibliography, see K. E. Rothschuh and E. Tutte (1975) where there is a list of ninety-five secondary sources.

236. O. Temkin, "Materialism" (1946); P. F. Cranefield, "The organic physics" (1957); idem, "The philosophical and cultural interests" (1966);

D. H. Galaty, "The philosophical basis" (1974); C. A. Culotta, "German biophysics" (1974); F. Gregory, *Scientific Materialism* (1977).

237. E. du Bois-Reymond, *Untersuchungen* (1848–1884), 1 (1848):XV.

238. H. L. F. Helmholtz, "Vorläufiger Bericht" (1850). See H. E. Hoff and L. A. Geddes, "Ballistics" (1960); and Clarke and O'Malley (1968), pp. 206–209.

239. A. Flint, *The Physiology of the Nervous System* (1872), "Nerve-force," pp. 97–98; and ibid., "Non-identity of nerve-force with electricity (pp. 98–99).

240. For Hermann's work, see Clarke and O'Malley (1968), pp. 209–213. G. Moruzzi in *L'Opera* (1973), pp. 44–53 has discussed Matteucci's influence on Hermann's theory of nerve impulse conduction.

241. For twentieth-century advances, see H. H. Dale, "Acetylcholine as a chemical transmitter" (1938); Clarke and O'Malley (1968), pp. 213–259; Z. M. Bacq, *Chemical Transmission* (1975); and A. L. Hodgkin et al., *The Pursuit of Nature* (1977).

242. L. Galvani, *De Viribus Electricitatis* (1791), p. 42.

6. BRAIN FUNCTIONS

1. This topic has generated a large amount of secondary literature, and the best bibliography of its general aspects is in E. Clarke and K. Dewhurst, *An Illustrated History* (1972), pp. 144–148, where each entry has a brief critical annotation. See also Clarke and O'Malley (1968), pp. 458–575. The best account of the period from the seventeenth to the early nineteenth century is in M. Neuburger (1981), chaps. 2, 3, 11, 18, and passim. For an excellent survey of the nineteenth century, see A. E. Walker, "The development" (1957). See also J. Hunt, "On the localisation" (1868–1869).

2. H. Head, *Aphasia* (1926), 1:1.

3. For Lashley's holistic theory, see his "Integrative action" (1933); and "Functional determinants" (1937). See also Clarke and O'Malley (1968), pp. 570–575. In 1937, he declared that "nearly a century of psychologizing concerning the cerebral cortex has added practically nothing to knowledge of its fundamental activities" (idem, "Functional determinants" [1937], p. 386). For an appraisal of Lashley's views, see J. Orbach, ed., *Neuropsychology* (1982).

4. J. P. Swazey in "Action propre" (1970) has discussed the pendulum swings between the two types of actions, and was following E. G. Boring, *A History* (1957) and B. Tizard, "Theories of brain" (1959). She has, however, confused the meaning of the two types of *action* as defined by Flourens.

5. G. T. Fritsch and E. Hitzig, "Über die elektrische Erregbarkeit" (1870). English trans. in G. von Bonin, *Some Papers* (1960), pp. 73–96; and in R. H.

Wilkins. "Neurosurgical classics XII" (1963), and in idem, *Neurosurgical Classics* (1965), pp. 15–27. See Clarke and O'Malley (1968), pp. 507–511.

6. Galen, *De Usu Partium,* bk. 8, chap. 11, in C. G. Kühn, ed., *[Galen] Medicorum Graecorum Opera* (1821–1833), 3 (1822):667. See M. T. May, *Galen* (1968), 1:415.

7. Galen, *De Usu Partium,* bk. 8, chap. 6, in C. G. Kühn, ed., *[Galen] Medicorum Graecorum Opera* (1821–1833), 3 (1822):636–637. See M. T. May, *Galen* (1968), 1:398; and Clarke and O'Malley (1968), pp. 148–149, 460–463.

8. The so-called cell doctrine of brain function has received considerable attention. See E. Clarke and K. Dewhurst, *An Illustrated History* (1972), pp. 10–48. A more recent work, E. R. Harvey, *The Inward Wits* (1975), is not recommended. For Nemesius, see Clarke and O'Malley (1968), pp. 463–465.

9. T. Willis, *Cerebri Anatome* (1664). For details of his scheme and a discussion of his work, see M. Neuburger (1981), pp. 17–45.

10. F. Pourfour du Petit, *Lettres* (1710), pp. 5–6, 7–8. See M. Neuburger (1981), pp. 59–60. For biography of Pourfour du Petit, see L. Kruger, "Francois Pourfour du Petit" (1963); E. Zehnder, *François Pourfour du Petit* (1968); *DSB;* and M. Neuburger (1981), p. 351.

In about 1745, Emanuel Swedenborg made some remarkable statements concerning the cerebral cortex and its sensory and motor functions. Concerning the latter, he described their location as in our present day motor homunculus:

> The muscles and actions which are in the ultimates of the body or in the soles of the feet depend more immediately upon the highest parts [of the cortex]; upon the middle lobe the muscles which belong to the abdomen and thorax, and upon the third lobe those which belong to the face and head; for they seem to correspond to one another in an inverse ratio" (E. Swedenborg, *The Brain* [1882–1887], 1 [1882]:58–59).

The precise origins of some of his opinions are unknown, but is likely that Pourfour du Petit was responsible for the above. Another possible source is Raymond de Vieussens, writing in 1684 (see O. M. Ramström, "Swedenborg" [1911], p. 68). There is also the unreliable paper of K. Akert and M. P. Hammond, "Emanuel Swedenborg" (1962). For papers on neurological aspects of Swedenborg's writings, see Swedenborg Congress, *Transactions* (1911).

11. The best account of Haller's research on the brain and the opinions he derived from it is in M. Neuburger (1981), pp. 118–152, and passim.

12. M. Neuburger (1981), p. 116.

13. Haller did encounter cortical excitability on one occasion, but being a single observation and as it was opposed to his precept, he ascribed it to the abnormal thinness of the gray matter in the particular animal employed,

an insupportable conjecture. (*Mémoires* [1762], 1:204, Experiment 148 on 22 March 1752.) See this report for his experiments on both gray and white matter.

14. A. von Haller, *Elementa* (1757–1766), vol. 4 (1762), bk. 10, sect. 7, "§ XXI. Adversariorum experimenta," p. 315.

15. Ibid., p. 352.

16. J. G. Zinn, "Experimenta" (1749). See M. Neuburger (1981), pp. 133–137.

17. One of the best surveys is L. D. Arnett, "The soul" (1904). See also B. Révész, *Geschichte des Seelenbegriffes* (1917).

18. J. Procháska. *Adnotationum* (1784), chap. 5, "Functiones animales," § 3. "[Whether or not there is a special site in the brain for each part of the intellect]," pp. 141–143. See Clarke and O'Malley (1968), pp. 474–475. See J. Procháska, . . . *and a Dissertation* (1851), pp. 446–447. For a discussion of the seat of the *sensorium commune,* see ibid., pp. 429–430.

19. C. Bell, *Idea* (1811), p. 4. Similar passages have already been quoted in chap. 2 (nn. 3, 15), where they serve as examples of the "Galenic" concept of nervous structure and function.

20. J. Baader, *Observationes Medicae* (1762). A series of case reports of patients seen in Vienna, 1746–1750. See "Observatio XXII," pp. 28–30.

21. Ibid., p. 30.

22. M. Neuburger (1981), p. 173. Pourfour du Petit's should be claimed as another.

23. L. S. Saucerotte, "Mémoire [1768]," (1778), p. 399. M. Neuburger (1981) deals with the fascinating research of these eighteenth-century surgeons (pp. 169–182).

24. This explanation has been made by A. E. Walker, "Stimulation and ablation" (1957), pp. 436–437.

25. J. Sabouraut, "Mémoire [1768]" (1778), p. 485. A comment by Galen is appropriate here: "A physician who knows from dissection the origin [in the nervous system] of the nerves supplying each part will more successfully treat the loss of sensibility or movement of each part," *On the Affected Parts,* bk. 3, chap. 14, in R. E. Siegel, *Galen on the Affected Parts* (1976), p. 102.

26. J. Gregory, *Lectures* (c. 1770), 2:149. We are indebted to Dr. Chris Lawrence for this reference.

27. Galen, *The Differentiation of Symptoms,* bk. 3. In C. G. Kühn, ed., *[Galen] Medicorum Graecorum Opera* (1821–1833), 7 (1824):55–62. See Clarke and O'Malley (1968), pp. 462–463.

28. See A. E. Walker, "Stimulation and ablation" (1957); and K. E. Rothschuh, "Zur Geschichte" (1966).

29. G. T. Fritsch and E. Hitzig, "Ueber die elektrische Erregbarkeit" (1870). See n. 5 above.

30. P. J. G. Cabanis, *Rapports* (1805), 1:174. The 1st ed. of 1802 was not seen, but this passage is doubtless in it, for it is alluded to by M. A. B.

Brazier ("Challenges" [1979], p. 15) although without a precise reference to it. Moreover, it appears in identical form in the 2d, 3d, and 4th eds. Cabanis's arguments in favor of compound brain localization are impressive and demand further study. His basic assertion was: "But it is not only for sensations, but also for movements that the spontaneous action of the nervous system is often restricted to certain specific areas [of the brain]" (P. J. G. Cabanis, *Rapports* [1805], 1:172).

The editor of the 4th ed. (1824) published 6 years after Cabanis's death (Étienne Pariset [1770–1847]) added a note (1:154); not present in the 2d and 3d editions. It is especially revealing and supported Cabanis's opinions. It reported a case of focal epilepsy: "In a case of epilepsy, the *aura* began in the little finger of the right hand, and the actual cause of the disorder had its seat in the parietal [lobe] of the left side [presumably of the brain]." The lesion was a musket ball, the removal of which dispelled the symptoms.

31. These studies were discussed by M. Neuburger (1981), pp. 141–143, but were concerned mainly with cardiac activity.

32. F. H. A. von Humboldt, *Versuche* (1797), 1:280n.

33. L. Rolando, *Saggio* (1809), p. 31. See Clarke and O'Malley (1968), p. 481.

34. Rolando, pp. 67–68.

35. See H. Hastings, *Man and Beast* (1936).

36. T. Willis, *De Anima* (1672), chap. 4, p. 43. See Clarke and O'Malley (1968), p. 473.

37. Anonymous, "Prof. Bischoff's account" (1806), p. 362. Epicurus, the Greek philosopher, lived about 341 to 270 B.C.

38. F. Jeffery, "Criticism" (1826), p. 257. A long reply in defense came from G. Combe, *Letter* (1826).

39. J. Bostock, *An Elementary System* (1828–1830), vol. 3 (1830), chap. 16, "Of the connexion of the physical and the intellectual faculties," p. 199.

40. F. J. Gall, *Philosophisch-medizinische Untersuchungen* (1791). O. Temkin has summarized the contents of the 2d ed. of 1800 in "Gall" (1947), pp. 313–314.

41. For references to Gall and Spurzheim biography, see chap. 1 n. 14, above.

42. This plan was also adopted by E. H. Ackerknecht and H. V. Vallois, *Franz Joseph Gall* (1956), p. 13 n. 3; and by E. Lesky, "Structure and function" (1970).

43. Some of the more recent literature is O. Temkin, "Gall" (1947), which remains the best short account in English; idem, "Remarks" (1953); J. D. Davies, *Phrenology* (1955); E. H. Ackerknecht and H. V. Vallois, *Franz Joseph Gall* (1956); Clarke and O'Malley (1968), pp. 476–480; G. Lanteri-Laura, *Histoire de la Phrénologie* (1970); R. M. Young, *Mind, Brain and Adaptation* (1970); J. P. Swazey, "Action propre" (1970); E. Clarke and K. Dewhurst, *An Illustrated History* (1972), pp. 91–98; D. de Guistino,

Conquest of Mind (1975); R. J. Cooter, "Phrenology and British alienists" (1976); idem, "Phrenology: The provocation of progress" (1976), with extensive bibliography; and idem, *The Cultural Meaning* (1985), which is the most recent and best survey of the ramifications of nineteenth-century phrenology; together with its exhaustive bibliography it can be strongly recommended. See also W. Riese, "F.-J. Gall" (1936); and idem, "Les discussions" (1936). A selection of Gall's writings, translated into German where necessary, is in E. Lesky, ed., *Franz Joseph Gall* (1979). See additional literature in n. 115 below.

44. Anonymous, *Craniologie* (1807). This seems to be one of the first detailed accounts of Gall's doctrine and is translated from the German. An earlier one, Anonymous, *Exposition* (1803), used the term "la doctrine physionomique de Gall," as in Anonymous, *Some Account* (1807). The authors could not be traced.

45. F. J. Gall, *Organologie* (1825).

46. J. C. Spurzheim, *The Physiognomical System* (1815).

47. T. I. M. Forster, "Sketch" (1815). "Phrenology" used thus by Forster: "The objection therefore falls to the ground, which accuses the new Phrenology of supporting the doctrine of Fatalism" (p. 222). In his book of the same year, *Sketch,* "phrenology" was replaced by "zoonomy" in its title; "phrenology" was used (on pp. 88 and 102, for example), but it was not defined.

48. P. S. Noel and E. T. Carlson, "Origins" (1970), p. 695. This was found in a manuscript, but it is also in B. Rush, *On the Utility* (1811), p. 271. Not seen, but cited by the above authors.

49. P. S. Noel and E. T. Carlson, "Origins" (1811), p. 695. This was also found in a manuscript, but is in B. Rush, *On the Opinions* (1811), p. 293. Not seen, but cited by above authors. See also E. T. Carlson, J. L. Wollock, and P. S. Noel, eds., *Benjamin Rush's [*unpublished*] Lectures* (1981), p. 404: "the science to which I have given that simple name . . . "

50. J. C. Spurzheim, *Observations sur la Phraenologie* (1818).

51. G. Combe, *Essays on Phrenology* (1819), p. xxiv: "The real subject of the system is the Human Mind. I have, therefore adopted the term *Phrenology* . . . as the most appropriate, and that which Dr. SPURZHEIM has for some years employed."

52. S. R., "Observations" (1817), p. 367.

53. J. C. Spurzheim, *Essai Philosophique* (1820). "Phraenologie" seems only to have been used in the "Préface," p. v.

54. J. C. Spurzheim, *Phrenology* (1825), p. 1. Only the 3d ed. was available, but there is no evidence that earlier ones existed. This is only one of many problems in the bibliography of phrenology. Also in idem, *Outlines* (1827), p. 1.

55. A distinguished historian of psychology, for example, did not differentiate adequately between Gall's and Spurzheim's systems. See E. G. Boring, *A History* (1957), p. 53.

56. An excellent account of Gall's anatomico-physiological relationships is in E. Lesky, "Structure and function" (1970). We have found it most useful and are grateful for Professor Lesky's characteristic scholarship.

57. F. J. Gall and J. C. Spurzheim, *Anatomie et Physiologie* (1810–1819), 1 (1810):XV.

58. F. J. Gall and J. C. Spurzheim, *Recherches* (1809), p. 246.

59. F. J. Gall, *Revue Critique* (1825), p. 118.

60. For F. Vicq d'Azyr's anatomical work, see Clarke and O'Malley (1968), pp. 268–270, 590–594, and elsewhere.

61. F. J. Gall and J. C. Spurzheim, *Anatomie et Physiologie* (1810–1819), 2 (1812):254. For Gall's work on the convolutions, see Clarke and O'Malley (1968), pp. 392–395. For an excellent discussion of the convolutions in the nineteenth century, see F. Schiller, "The rise" (1965).

62. O. Temkin, "Gall" (1947), p. 314.

63. F. J. Gall, *Philosophisch-medizinsche Untersuchungen* (1791).

64. F. J. Gall and J. C. Spurzheim, *Anatomie et Physiologie* (1810–1819), 2 (1812):5.

65. F. J. Gall and J. C. Spurzheim, *Recherches* (1809), p. 273. It should be noted, however, that Cabanis (and others later, see chap. 7) held that the passions were seated in the viscera.

66. Ibid., pp. 228–230. Swazey's similar quotation is corrupt in several places (J. P. Swazey, "Action propre" [1970], p. 215).

67. E. Lesky, "Structure and function" (1970). M. Bentley also discussed Gall's predecessors in "The psychological antecedents" (1916).

68. F. J. Gall and J. C. Spurzheim, *Recherches* (1809), p. 248.

69. C. Bonnet, *La Palingénésie* (1770), 1, pt. 9:234. See J. Hunt, "On the localisation" (1868–1869), 7 (1869):113–115.

70. C. Bonnet, *La Palingénésie* (1770), 1:27.

71. F. J. Gall and J. C. Spurzheim, *Recherches* (1809), pp. 248–249.

72. É. J. Georget, *De la Physiologie* (1821), 1:78–79, 104–112, 124–136, 141–144.

73. F. J. Gall, *Organologie* (1825), 5:519–525. This included Gall's response to other criticisms of Georget.

74. See E. Clarke, "The doctrine" (1968); and E. Clarke and J. G. Bearn, "The spiral bands" (1972). See also chap. 3 n. 10.

75. F. J. Gall, *Philosophisch-medizinische Untersuchungen* (1791), pp. 197–198. We wish to thank Professor Lesky for drawing our attention to this passage. The Wellcome Institute Library is fortunate in possessing a copy of this very rare book.

76. Both the original edition (1784–1791) and a modern reprint of it (1965) were used.

77. See E. Lesky, "Gall und Herder" (1967).

78. E. Lesky, "Structure and function" (1970), p. 304.

79. F. J. Gall and J. C. Spurzheim, *Anatomie et Physiologie* (1810–1819), 1 (1810):218.

80. J. G. Herder, *Ideen* (1965), vol. 1, bk. 4, pt. 1, "Der Mensch ist zur Verunftfährigkeit organisieret," p. 91. See also idem, *Ideen* (1784–1791), vol. 1, bk. 3, pt. 2, "Vergleichung der mancherlei organischen Kräfte, die im Tier wirken," pp. 111–180.

81. Ibid. (1784–1791), vol. 1, bk. 4, pt. 1, "Der Mensch ist zur Verunftfährigkeit organisieret," p. 201.

82. Ibid., p. 203.

83. Ibid., p. 204.

84. Ibid., p. 205.

85. L. F. Lélut, *Qu'est-ce que la Phrénologie?* (1836), sect. 3, "Comparaison du système de Gall et de la phrénologie avec les systèmes antérieurs, et appréciation de ce système," pp. 359–405. See also tables 1–3 listing the active and fundamental faculties of Hutcheson, Gall, Reid, and Spurzheim.

86. [F. Hutcheson], *An Essay* (1728), Treatise I, "Sect III. Particular divisions of the affections and passions," pp. 58–87.

87. See H. D. Spoerl, "Faculties" (1935–1936), p. 222.

88. Ibid.

89. Ibid.

90. L. F. Lélut, *Qu'est-ce que la Phrénologie?* (1836), p. 361.

91. A. Garnier, *La Psychologie* (1839), chap. 2. "Parallèle des théories psychologiques de Gall, de Spurzheim et des philosophes écossais," pp. 16–48.

92. For the history of physiognomy, see J. Graham,"Lavater's physiognomy" (1961); and idem, *Lavater's Essays* (1979).

93. G. B. della Porta, *De Humana Physiognomonia* (1586).

94. J. C. Lavater, *Von der Physiognomik* (1772). There have been many translations into English as, for example, *Essays on Physiognomy* (1797).

95. In 1817 Dr. J. Cross, in *An Attempt* (1817), defined the objects of physiognomy as follows: "To divide and arrange the body into organs, and to ascribe to each its functions, its physiology. To view all these organs in connexion, and to compute the influence of each, and the concentrated influence of the whole, in determining the great movements of the individual among other individuals, all acting their respective parts in the great struggle and bustle of life, is physiognomy. Physiognomy is just a system of corollaries arising out of physiology" (pp. 6–7). This broader view of physiognomy would have pleased Gall, but Cross was not in any way concerned with organology or phrenology. See R. P., "Quotations" (1929).

96. A. Froriep (1849–1917), *Die Lehren Franz Joseph Galls* (1911), p. 38. We are indebted to Professor O. Temkin for this reference (O. Temkin, "Gall" [1947], p. 277).

97. F. J. Gall, "Lettre" (1835). Cited by J. Létang, *Gall* (1906), p. 99. A full translation of this letter is in N. Capen, *Reminiscences* (1881), pp. 70–86; our quotation is from p. 85.

98. O. Temkin, "Gall" (1947), p. 277.

99. See E. Lesky, "Der angeklagte Gall" (1981), pp. 307–331.

100. For an account of the play, see C. G. Cumston, "An analysis" (1900).

101. C. W. Hufeland, "Remarks" (1807), pp. 137–138. The same comments have apparently been attributed to C. H. E. Bischoff in *Exposition* (1809), but this was not seen. G. Combe in *On the Functions* (1838), pp. 179–180, cited yet another version.

102. G. Cuvier et al., "Rapport" (1808). For trans. of this report, see Anonymous, "Report on a memoir" (1809).

103. F. J. Gall and J. C. Spurzheim, *Recherches* (1809).

104. F. J. Gall and J. C. Spurzheim, *Anatomie et Physiologie* (1810–1819).

105. F. J. Gall, *Sur les Fonctions du Cerveau* (1825). Each of the five volumes has its own subtitle. The volumes first appeared in 1822–1825, but were reprinted in 1825, and we have used this latter version throughout.

106. See n. 5 above.

107. For a recent account of phrenology, see F. Hedderly. *Phrenology* (1970), a practicing phrenologist.

108. J. D. Davies, *Phrenology* (1955), p. 172.

109. F. Hedderly, *Phrenology* (1970).

110. T. I. M. Forster, *Sketch* [1815], "Section VI. Of the application of the new zoonomy to education, founded on the supremacy of the will," pp. 84–98; and "Section VII. Of punishment," p. 99; and elsewhere. Note that he did not use "phrenology" in the title of this book, although it appeared in his text (see n. 47 above).

111. F. J. Gall, "Petition" (1838), pp. 325–326. This was first published in 1804 (see p. 309n).

112. M.J.A.N. de C. Condorcet, *L'Atlantide* (1968); and P. J. G. Cabanis, "Rapports" (1956), pt. 1, pp. 353–358 and 618–631. V. L. Hilts, "Obeying the laws" (1982), p. 62, drew our attention to these sources.

113. V. L. Hilts, "Obeying the laws" (1982).

114. The only bibliography of this vast literature is described by A. A. Walsh, "Contributions" (1971). But see "References" in R. J. Cooter, "Phrenology: The provocation of progress" (1976), pp. 228–234; and in his book *The Cultural Meaning* (1985).

115. R. J. Cooter, "Phrenology. The provocation of progress" (1976), pp. 213–214. In this article and in his book *The Cultural Meaning* (1985), all the literature on this wider view of phrenology is cited. Of this see, in particular, D. de Guistino, *Conquest of Mind* (1975); T. M. Parssinen, "Popular science" (1974) for an analysis of phrenology as a popular social movement in early Victorian Britain; A. McLaren, "Phrenology" (1974) deals with the audience phrenology found among British artisans; G. N. Cantor, "The Edinburgh phrenology debate" (1975), and S. Shapin, "Phrenological knowledge" (1975) together with Cantor's response, "A critique" (1975), show the value of phrenology in the illumination of wider aspects of nineteenth-century intellectual thought and social action. In par-

ticular, Shapin has revealed it to be a mediator of social values. R. J. Cooter's excellent study *The Cultural Meaning* (1985) is a scholarly discussion of phrenology's impact on Victorian society, its central concern being with "the social and ideological functions of science during the consolidation of urban industrial society" (dust jacket). It is claimed to be "the first extended treatment of the place and role of science among working-class radicals" (ibid.). For Gall as a Romantic, see J. Y. Hall, "Gall's phrenology" (1977).

116. C. W. Hufeland, "Remarks" (1807), p. 162.

117. F. J. Gall, *Organologie* (1825), vol. 5, "XVI [*sic;* should be XIV] Sens des mots, sens des noms, mémoire des mots, mémoire verbale. (*Wort-Gedaechtniss*)," pp. 12–29, see p. 18.

118. Ibid., "XV Sens du language de parole; talent de la philologie, etc. (*Sprach-Forschungs-sinn*)," pp. 30–75, see p. 30.

119. Ibid., pp. 30–31.

120. J. B. Bouillaud, "Recherches cliniques propres" (1825), p. 30. For a history of the early study of speech function (1825–1865), see H. Hécaen and J. Dubois, *La Naissance* (1969).

121. S. A. E. Aubertin, "Discussion" (1861); and idem, "Reprise" (1861). See Clarke and O'Malley (1968), pp. 492–494.

122. P. Broca, "Remarques" (1861). See Clarke and O'Malley (1968), pp. 494–497; and F. Schiller, *Paul Broca* (1979), pp. 165–211.

123. G. T. Fritsch and E. Hitzig, "Über die elektrische Erregbarkeit" (1870). See n. 5 above.

124. G. Cuvier, *Leçons* (1800–1805), 1 (1800):22.

125. C. Bell, *Idea* (1811), p. 17.

126. Ibid. The three extracts are on pp. 27, 36, and 23, respectively. See also J. M. D. Olmsted, "The aftermath" (1943).

127. H. M. Ducrotay de Blainville, "Considérations générales" (1821), p. 40.

128. For excellent studies of this episode, see J. M. D. Olmsted, "Historical note" (1944); and M. Neuburger (1981), pp. 201–208. See also C. Richet, *Dictionnaire* (1895–1928), 2 (1897):299–300.

129. J.B.P.A. de M. de Lamarck, *Histoire Naturelle des Végétaux* (1802), p. 225.

130. P. Flourens, *Recherches* (1824), p. 241. In 1825 he confirmed the existence of a respiratory center in the fish ("Nouvelles expériences" [1825], p. 423), and in 1828 repeated the statement quoted here ("Nouvelles expériences" [1828], p. [22]). See also, *Recherches* (1842): "the medulla oblongata, therefore, constitutes the real central point, the common bond, the *noeud* that unites all parts of the nervous system to each other" (p. 195).

131. Galen, *De Anatomicis Administrationibus,* bk. 8, chap. 9. In C. G. Kühn, ed., *[Galen] Medicorum Graecorum Opera* (1821–1833), 2 (1821):696–697. See also C. Singer, *Galen* (1956), p. 221. For a history of

the medulla oblongata up to the eighteenth century, see M. Neuburger (1981), pp. 93–100.

132. A. C. Lorry, "Sur les movemens" (1760), p. 367.

133. J. J. C. Legallois, *Expériences* (1812), pp. 37–39, see p. 37. See M. Neuburger (1981), pp. 204–206 for this research, and that of those who checked it.

134. J. J. C. Legallois, *Expériences* (1812), pp. 148–149.

135. P. Flourens, "Note" (1851).

136. Ibid., p. 437.

137. P. Flourens, "Nouvelles expériences" (1825). This was his first paper dealing with the respiratory center. See n. 130 above.

138. They are detailed in J. M. D. Olmsted, "Historical note" (1944), pp. 347–350. See also M. Neuburger (1981), p. 208.

139. C. Bell, "Of the nerves which associate" (1822).

140. H. Mayo, "On the cerebral nerves" (1823), pp. 4–6; and "Remarks" (1823), p. 136. Also cited n. 4.33

141. E. R. A. Serres, *Anatomie Comparée* (1824–1826), 2 (1826):717.

142. A. L. Dugès, *Traité* (1838–1839), 1 (1838):360.

143. K. F. Burdach, *Von Baue und Leben* (1819–1826), vol. 3 (1826).

144. Ibid., respectively § 938 (pp. 448–449); ibid., § 972 (p. 462); ibid., § 959 (pp. 457–458).

145. Ibid., §§ 944–953 (pp. 452–455). For a history of coenesthesia, see F. Schiller, "Coenesthesia" (1984).

146. Ibid., § 1011 (p. 484).

147. Ibid., § 887 (p. 413).

148. G. R. Treviranus, *Biologie* (1802–1822), 6 (1822):141–145.

149. G. R. Treviranus and L. C. Treviranus, *Vermischte Schriften* (1816–1821), 3 (1820):87.

150. G. R. Treviranus, *Biologie* (1802–1822), 6 (1822):145–146.

151. C. G. Carus, *Versuch einer Darstellung* (1814), p. 290. See also K. Feremutsch, "Die Grundzuege" (1951).

152. J. L. Schönlein, *Von der Hirnmetamorphose* (1816), p. 57.

153. A. K. A. Eschenmayer, *Psychologie* (1817), §§ 241–247 (pp. 210–216).

154. F. A. M. Mignet, "Réponse de M. Mignet" (1840), p. 25: "As they [Bell and Magendie] have done for the functions of nerves you have attempted for the functions of the nervous centers, and you have discovered the peculiar character and precise limits of their general activities."

155. For accounts of Flourens and of his work on the brain, see: M. Neuburger (1981), pp. 259–282, who gave an excellent account of his background; J. Soury, "Cerveau [cerebrum]" (1897), pp. 616–619, but unfortunately, he gave no general appraisal of Flourens's work nor assessed its significance, and the many quotations he provided are mostly faulty in

location or in content, or in both; J. M. D. Olmsted, "Pierre Flourens" (1953); E. G. Boring, *A History* (1957), pp. 62–67; R. M. Young, *Mind, Brain and Adaptation* (1970), pp. 57–74; Clarke and O'Malley (1968), pp. 656–662, 483–488. A paper by J. P. Swazey, "Action propre" (1970), should be used critically (see n. 4 above).

156. G. Legée, "M.J.P. Flourens" (1974). The announcement of the course was as follows: "The theory of sensations, or of the sensitive and intellectual faculties, is the real bond . . . between philosophy and physiology. . . . Thus, between physiologies and philosophies properly called, there arises a new science, indicated in turn by Locke, Condillac, Cabanis, Bichat, M. M. Gall, de Tracy, etc., and this science is the object of this course" (p. 95).

157. P. Flourens, *Recherches* (1824), p. XXV.

158. His memoir was read on 4, 11, 25, and 31 March and 29 April 1822, and reported briefly in P. Flourens, ["Des observations"] (1822). Its title was "Détermination des propriétés du système nerveux, ou recherches physiques sur l'irritabilité et la sensibilité."

159. G. Cuvier, "Rapport" (1822). Review in Anonymous, "Recent discoveries" (1824).

160. P. Flourens, "Recherches physiques" (1823). Review in Anonymous, "Recent discoveries" (1824).

161. P. Flourens, *Recherches* (1824). Translations of parts are in G. von Bonin, *Some Papers* (1960), pp. 3–21; J. F. Fulton, *Selected Readings* (1966), pp. 286–288; Clarke and O'Malley (1968), pp. 483–488. A second edition with additional experimental findings appeared as P. Flourens, *Recherches* (1842).

162. P. Flourens, ["Review of F.J. Gall"] (1819–1820). A two- part review of Gall's classic *Anatomie et Physiologie* (1810–1819).

163. He described his methods in *Recherches* (1842), pp. 502–511. See R. M. Young, *Mind, Brain and Adaptation* (1970), pp. 58–63; and M. Neuburger (1981), pp. 276–279; and Clarke and O'Malley (1968), pp. 483–488. See also 1.2.2.

164. P. Flourens, *Recherches* (1824), p. x.

165. Ibid., p. 236.

166. Ibid.

167. Ibid., p. 122.

168. P. Flourens, "Recherches physiques" (1823), p. 368.

169. P. Flourens, *Recherches* (1824), p. 122. See the section on "De l'unité du système nerveux," pp. 236–241. As E. G. Boring (*A History* [1957], pp. 65–66) has pointed out, Flourens's concept anticipated by a century Lashley's theory of equipotentiality and mass action and the views of Gestalt psychologists.

170. P. Flourens, "Recherches physiques" (1823), p. 352.

171. P. Flourens, *Recherches* (1824), p. 122.

172. Ibid., p. 99, para 4.

173. P. Flourens, *Recherches* (1842), pp. 99–100. The same statement was made in 1824 (*Recherches* [1824], p. 100), and we shall quote it below (n. 316), the only difference being that in 1842 "sensations" and "feeling" were replaced by "perceptions" and "perceiving" respectively. He explained that these substitutions were necessary because of difficulties aroused by earlier statements: "The animal that has lost its cerebral hemispheres has not lost its *sensibility;* it is fully preserved; it has lost only *perception* of its *sensations,* it has lost *intelligence* only." (Ibid., [1842], p. 79n.) In modern terms, removal of the cerebral hemispheres abolishes perception, but sensory discrimination remains. Perception has the same superordinate relation to sensation or mere sensitivity that volition occupies to the immediate cause of movement.

174. Ibid., (1824), pp. 34–35, paragraphs 6–7.

175. In the proceedings of the Académie des Sciences for 1822, the report that follows that of Flourens (["Des observations"] 1822) described Magendie's experiments on the spinal roots (pp. 358–359). It had been presented to the Académie in June of the same year: F. Magendie, [no title] (1822). For the Magendie-Flourens relationship, see n. 201 below.

176. P. Flourens, *Recherches* (1824), p. 234.

177. For a discussion of compensation of nervous function, see W. Riese, "The principle of compensation" (1944). He did not refer to Flourens.

178. P. Flourens, *Recherches* (1824), pp. 18–23.

179. Ibid. In the Preface he stated that he was planning to publish in another work his observations on galvanizing the brain (p. v), but this does not seem to have appeared. He deliberately avoided chemical irritation (pp. iv–v). In an account of his experimental methods in *Recherches* (1842, pp. 502–511), he made no reference to stimulation techniques. See 1.2.2.

180. P. Flourens, *Recherches* (1824), p. 20.

181. Ibid., § 4, pp. 101–102. This had been reported first in a communication to the Académie Royale des Sciences de l'Institut on 15 September 1823.

182. Ibid., p. 101.

183. David Ferrier reported in 1876 (*The Functions* [1876]) that electrical stimulation of the pigeon's brain was mainly negative (pp. 159–160).

184. G. von Bonin, *Some Papers* (1960), p. ix. For a modern discussion of this problem, see R. Pearson, *The Avian Brain* (1972), pp. 482–491.

185. F. Vicq d'Azyr, "Mémoire sur la structure du cerveau des animaux, comparée avec celle du cerveau de l'homme," in idem, *Oeuvres* (1805), *Sciences Physiologiques Médicales,* 6:211–220, see p. 215. Date of publication unknown, but probably the 1780s.

186. F. Magendie, *Leçons* (1841), 2:12.

187. M. Schiff, *Lehrbuch* (1858–1859), p. 336. However, although decorticating a pigeon might just be possible, Flourens could not have carried this out successfully in an animal with a convoluted cerebrum.

188. P. Flourens, *Recherches* (1824), p. 35.

189. F. A. Lange, *The History of Materialism* (1925), 3d sect., p. 137.

190. He reported the ten-month survival of one of his animals, a chicken after bilateral cerebral hemispherectomy, P. Flourens, *Recherches* (1824), pp. 87–93.

191. G. Cuvier, "Rapport" (1822), p. 378.

192. P. Flourens, *Recherches* (1842), "Chapitre XXXII. Méthode expérimentale employée dans mes recherches sur l'encéphale," pp. 502–511.

193. Ibid., p. 502. Also in chap. 1 n. 73.

194. M. Neuburger (1981), p. 276.

195. P. Flourens, ["Des observations"] (1822), pp. 357–358. Precisely how Rolando had heard of Flourens's studies is not clear, but presumably news of what he claimed to be plagiarism may have come from Flourens's lectures before submitting this communication to the Académie.

196. P. Flourens, "Recherches physiques" (1823).

197. J. Coster, "Expériences" (1823). For review, see Anonymous, "Recent discoveries" (1824).

198. L. Rolando, "Expériences" (1823).

199. In his *Recherches* (1824), pp. 273–302, Flourens reproduced L. Rolando, "Expériences" (1823) from Magendie's journal, except for the last section, "Expériences tentées également sur les animaux invertébrés," pp. 111–113. This is referred to as L. Rolando, "Expériences" (1824).

200. Flourens presented his defense in footnotes to the French translation of Rolando's experimental protocols in his *Recherches* (1824), pp. 273–302.

201. F. Magendie, in L. Rolando, "Expériences" (1823), pp. 95, n. (1), and 113–114 n. (1). His purpose for publishing this translation was so that "The public will judge," but he seemed to have no doubt of Flourens's innocence. For the relations between the rivals Magendie and Flourens, see J. M. D. Olmsted, *François Magendie* (1944), pp. 123–125, 165, 218–219.

202. P. Flourens, *Recherches* (1824), p. 274 n. 1.

203. L. Rolando, *Saggio* (1809); for example, "Sperienze sul cervello dei mammiferi," pp. 481–483; and idem, "Expériences" (1824), pp. 273–282.

204. P. Flourens, ["Des observations"] (1822), pp. 357–358.

205. F. Magendie, "Note sur le siège" (1823), p. 155.

206. P. Flourens, *Recherches* (1824), p. 274 n. 1.

207. M. Foderà, "Recherches" (1823). His results were reported to the Académie des Sciences on 31 December 1822. The merit of his work is shown by his award, shared with Flourens, of "the de Montyon prize for the encouragement of experimental physiology" for 1822, given by the Académie des Sciences. See N. Egli, *Der "Prix Montyon"* (1970); and M. Crosland, "From prizes to grants" (1979).

208. F. Magendie, *Leçons* (1841). Sensation and movement not localized in cerebral hemispheres, 1:172–211, 279–281, and elsewhere. Vision is discussed in 2:324–336.

209. Ibid., 2:336.

210. Ibid., 1:175–185.

211. F. Magendie, "Note sur les fonctions" (1823), p. 379.

212. F. A. Longet, *Anatomie et Physiologie* (1842), 1:643. This is the title of a section, pp. 643–644.

213. Ibid., p. 661. It is interesting to note that in 1842 sympathy was still being recruited to explain clinicopathological enigmas. For discussions of sympathy, see chaps. 4.2 and 7.3.

214. J. L. Budge, *Untersuchungen* (1841–1842), 2 (1842):84. See Anonymous ["Volkmann"] (1844).

215. C. Matteucci, *Traité* (1844), pt. 2, chap. 5, "Action du courant électrique sur les parties centrales du système nerveux," pp. 242–244.

216. E. F. W. Weber, "Muskelbewegung" (1846), p. 16.

217. D. Ferrier, *The Functions* (1876), p. 160.

218. J. M. Schiff, *Lehrbuch* (1858–1859), "3) Gibt es motorische Hirntheile?," p. 362.

219. I. van Deen, "Ueber die Unempfindlichkeit" (1860).

220. R. D. Grainger, *Observations* (1837), p. 68.

221. For example, W. B. Carpenter, *Principles of Human Physiology* (1846), § 459 (pp. 344–345): "The investigations of Flourens are the most clear and decisive in their results; and of these we shall accordingly take a general survey" (p. 344). Carpenter's original acceptance of Flourens's views on the cerebrum was in part due to his belief, along with Hall, that it was not involved in the reflex. However, under the influence of Laycock's studies on the cerebral reflexes (see 4.5.2), he later recanted (W. B. Carpenter, *Principles of Human Physiology* [1853], p. 672).

222. L. L. Rostan, *Recherches* (1823), p. 247. For a contemporary account of his work, see F. J. V. Broussais, *Examen* (1829–1834), 4 (1834):646–662.

223. J. B. Bouillaud, *Traité* (1825), p. 279.

224. G. Andral, *Clinique Médicale* (1829–1833), *Maladies de l'Encéphale,* 5 (1833):569. For a contemporary account of his work, see F. J. V. Broussais, *Examen* (1829–1834), 4 (1834):523–600.

225. For an account of Jackson's contribution to cortical localization, see Clarke and O'Malley (1968), pp. 499–505.

226. A. L. Foville and F. Pinel-Grandchamp, *Recherches* (1823), referred to by J. B. Bouillaud, *Traité* (1825), pp. 275–277.

227. E. R. A. Serres, *Anatomie Comparée* (1824–1826), "Action et maladies des hémisphères cérébraux," 2 (1826):653–719, see p. 689.

228. Ibid., pp. 689–694.

229. J. B. Lacrampe-Loustau, *Recherches* (1824). Cited by E. R. A. Serres, *Anatomie Comparée* (1824–1826), 2 (1826):690.

230. P. Flourens, *Recherches* (1824), p. 275 n. 1.

231. E. R. A. Serres, *Anatomie Comparée* (1824–1826), 2 (1826):715.

232. Ibid., pp. 716–718.

233. Ibid., p. 718.

234. Ibid., p. 717.

235. C. F. Lallemand, *Recherches* (1830–1834), "Huitième lettre," vol. 3 (1834), no. 51, § 6, p. 319.

236. Ibid., pp. 319–320.

237. Ibid., p. 320.

238. L. A. Desmoulins, *Anatomie* (1825), 2:606.

239. Ibid., p. 611.

240. J. B. M. Parchappe, *Deuxième Mémoire* (1838). See pp. 141–176 in particular. There is an excellent historical introduction on the morbid anatomy of mental disease, pp. 13–67.

241. J. B. M. Parchappe, *Du Siège Commun* (1856), p. 121.

242. J. B. M. Parchappe, *Deuxième Mémoire* (1838), p. 219.

243. J. B. Bouillaud, "Exposition" (1839–1840), p. 283.

244. Ibid., p. 334.

245. J. P. Damiron, *Essai* (1834), 1:11. For more recent accounts, see G. Boas, *French Philosophies* (1925); E. Haigh, "Medicine and ideology" (1984).

246. L. G. A. de Bonald, *Recherches Philosophiques* (1838), 1:295–296.

247. Ibid. See also M. S. Staum, "Medical components" (1978); idem, *Cabanis* (1980); G. Boas, *French Philosophies* (1925), pp. 25–26, 31; J. Kitchin, *Un Journal* (1965), p. 117.

248. G. Boas, *French Philosophies* (1925), p. 26.

249. N. Massias, *Rapport* (1821–1822), pp. 77–78.

250. Ibid., p. 118.

251. G. Boas, *French Philosophies* (1925), p. 203.

252. V. Cousin, *Cours* (1836), pp. xiii–iv.

253. V. Cousin, *Fragments* (1845), p. vi.

254. See F. J. Gall, *Sur L'Origine* (1825), pp. 62–63, 66–67. See also O. Temkin, "Gall" (1947), pp. 282–283; and R. M. Young, *Mind, Brain and Adaptation* (1970), pp. 15–16.

255. J. P. Damiron, *Essai* (1834), 1:185.

256. E. F. Dubois d'Amiens, *Philosophie Médicale* (1845), pp. 2–3.

257. L. F. Lélut, *Rejet de L'Organologie* (1843), pp. 361–363.

258. P. Flourens, *Examen* (1845), p. 14. See C. Blondel, *La Psycho-Physiologie* (1914), pp. 55–56; R. M. Young, *Mind, Brain and Adaptation* (1970), p. 19.

259. See C. Blondel, *La Psycho-Physiologie* (1914), pp. 50–51; R. M. Young, *Mind, Brain and Adaptation* (1970), pp. 34–35; O. Temkin, "Gall" (1947), pp. 283–284.

260. F. J. Gall, *Sur L'Origine* (1825), pp. 13–14, 21–22, 48–49, 56.

261. H. Gouhier, *La Jeunesse d'Auguste Comte* (1933–1941), 2:198.

262. A. Comte, *Cours* (1830–1842), 3:765, 774, 776–777.

263. L. G. A. de Bonald, *Du Divorce* (1818), p. 22.

264. F. J. Bérard, *Doctrine des Rapports* (1823), pp. 494–497.

265. L. F. Lélut, *Rejet de L'Organologie* (1843), pp. 367–368.

266. J. L. Moreau de la Sarthe, ["Review of *Traité* . . . of Pinel"] (An. IX [1800–1801]), pp. 458–459. See also P. Delaunay, "La médicine" (1929).

267. J. Burdin, *Cours* (1803), 1:xxxix–xl, xlv–xlvi; 3:109–110.

268. M. H. de Saint-Simon, *Oeuvres Choisis* (1859), 2:20–23, 50–52.

269. Ibid., p. 6.

270. F. J. Gall and J. C. Spurzheim, *Anatomie et Physiologie* (1810–1819), 1 (1810):iv–v.

271. F. J. Gall, *Sur L'Origine* (1825), pp. 15, 18–20.

272. P.-D. M., ["Review of . . . Gall"] (1819), p. 426.

273. L. G. A. de Bonald, *Recherches Philosophiques* (1838), 2:4–5.

274. M.F.P.G. Maine de Biran, "Observations" (c. 1808), p. 70. For his psychology, see T. C. T. Moore, *The Psychology* (1970).

275. M.F.P.G. Maine de Biran, "Observations" (c. 1808), pp. 71–74.

276. [L. J.] Bégin, "Discours" (1841), p. 384.

277. E. F. Dubois d'Amiens, "Broussais" (1864), p. 91n. See also M. Lévy, "Éloge de Broussais" (1839), p. 387.

278. P. Flourens, *Examen* (1845), p. lii.

279. F. J. V. Broussais, *De L'Irritation* (1828), pp. xiii, xvii–xix, xxiv–xxv. For biography of Broussais, see J.L.H.P., *Sketches* (1831), pp. 22–70; and *DSB*.

280. T. S. Jouffroy, "Du spiritualisme" (1825), pp. 121–161.

281. L. F. Lélut, *Rejet de L'Organologie* (1843), pp. viii–xi.

282. A. H. Kératry, *Inductions* (1817), p. 121.

283. Ibid., p. 132.

284. M.F.P.G. Maine de Biran, "Observations" (c. 1808), pp. 74–75.

285. Ibid., pp. 80–82.

286. J. P. Damiron, *Essai* (1834), 1:86 and also 186; and 2:19, 33.

287. Ibid., 2:274–275. Similarly, the influential theologian, M. D. Frayssinous (1765–1841), had declared that death was merely "a derangement of material parts: but the soul has neither parts, nor form, nor [a] situation of parts in relation to each other; and if the body can perish [,if] this arrangement of distinct parts [can] disintegrate and die, the soul, which has nothing comparable in its mode of existence, naturally cannot experience a comparable destruction" (*Défense du Christianisme* [1825], 1:382–383).

288. E. J. Georget, *De la Physiologie* (1821), 1:135–136.

289. F. J. Bérard, *Doctrine des Rapports* (1823), pp. 253, 499.

290. Ibid., pp. 632–633, 409–410.

291. G. Cuvier et al., *Rapport* (1808), pp. 49–50.

292. M.F.P.G. Maine de Biran, "Observations" (c. 1808), p. 81.

293. Maine de Biran's address of c. 1808 remained unpublished until 1887. However, it seems to have circulated in Parisian medical society. For a further example of unacknowledged quotation from this address, see [F.J.J.E.] Delpit, "Organoscopie" (1819), p. 255.

294. E. F. Dubois d'Amiens, *Philosophie Médicale* (1845), p. 343.

295. F. J. V. Broussais, *Cours* (1836), pp. 72, 118.
296. F. J. V. Broussais, *De L'Irritation* (1839), p. 523.
297. F. J. Gall and J. C. Spurzheim, *Anatomie et Physiologie* (1810–1819), 1 (1810):16.
298. F. J. Gall, *Sur L'Organe* (1825), pp. 405–406.
299. P. Flourens, ["Review of F.J. Gall"] (1819–1820), pt. 2 (1820), p. 455.
300. See G. Legée, "M.J.P. Flourens" (1974), p. 95.
301. P. Flourens, ["Review of F.J. Gall"] (1819–1820), pt. 1 (1819), p. 439.
302. Ibid., p. 443.
303. Ibid., pp. 443, 445, 451.
304. Ibid., pp. 443, 449; pt. 2 (1820), pp. 454–457.
305. Ibid., p. 466.
306. T. A. Appel, *The Cuvier-Geoffroy Debate* (1975), p. 195.
307. P. Flourens, "Essai sur l'espirit" (1820).
308. R. M. Young, *Mind, Brain and Adaptation* (1970), p. 56.
309. P. Flourens, *Cuvier* (1845), pp. 272–273, 275–276.
310. G. Cuvier et al., *Rapport* (1808), p. 50.
311. T. A. Appel, *The Cuvier-Geoffroy Debate* (1975), p. 91.
312. P. Flourens, ["Review of F.J. Gall"] (1819–1820), pt. 1 (1819), p. 452.
313. F. J. Gall, *Revue Critique* (1825), pp. 262–265.
314. R. M. Young, "The functions of the brain" (1968), p. 263.
315. R. M. Young, *Mind, Brain and Adaptation* (1970), pp. 72–73.
316. P. Flourens, *Recherches* (1824), p. 100. See n. 173 above.
317. E. F. Dubois d'Amiens, *Philosophie Médicale* (1845), p. 3.
318. J. P. Damiron, *Essai* (1834), 2:11–13.
319. F. J. Bérard and H. de Montègre, "Cranioscopie" (1813), pp. 314–315.
320. Ibid., pp. 316–317.
321. F. J. Bérard, *Doctrine des Rapports* (1823), p. 511.
322. E. F. Dubois d'Amiens, *Philosophie Médicale* (1845), pp. 241–243, 361–363.
323. P. Flourens, "Histoire des études" (1862), pp. 226–227.
324. P. Flourens, *Examen* (1845), pp. 8–9.
325. Ibid., p. 14.
326. Ibid., pp. 27–28.
327. Ibid., pp. 36–38.
328. Ibid., pp. 49, 56.
329. Ibid., pp. 52–53.
330. R. M. Young, "The functions of the brain" (1968), p. 263.
331. F. A. Longet, *Anatomie et Physiologie* (1842), 1:769.

332. L. Luciana, *Fisiologia* (1901–1911), 2, pt. 1 (1905):442. Also in idem, *Human Physiology* (1911–1921), *Muscular and Nervous Systems* 3(1915):430.

333. F. M. R. Walshe, "On disorders" (1921), p. 539.

334. The best accounts are in M. Neuburger (1981). Chap. 2 ("Experiments on the cerebellum," pp. 214–245) deals with the opinions of Thomas Willis; and chap. 18 ("Experiments on the cerebellum and the cerebrum," pp. 259–282), with the early nineteenth century; and passim. There is no comprehensive history of cerebellar anatomy and physiology, but see also F. A. Longet, *Anatomie et Physiologie* (1842), 1:703–769; A. Thomas, *Le Cervelet* (1897), pp. 1–40; C. S. Sherrington, "The cerebellum" (1900), pp. 893–910; L. Luciani, *Human Physiology* (1911–1921), 3 (1915):418–485; R. S. Dow and G. Moruzzi, *The Physiology* (1958), pp. 3–7; Clarke and O'Malley (1968), pp. 643–697.

335. Aristotle, *Historia Animalium* (1910), bk. 1, chap. 16 (494. b. 31–32): "Behind this [the cerebrum], right at the back, comes what is termed the 'cerebellum,' differing in form from the brain [cerebrum] as we may both feel and see."

336. He also thought the vermis of the cerebellum controlled the flow of animal spirits between the third and fourth ventricles. See Clarke and O'Malley (1968), pp. 629–631.

337. C. Varolio, *Anatomiae* (1591), p. 37.

338. T. Willis, *Cerebri Anatome* (1664), chap. 15, "De cerebelli . . . ," pp. 99–100. For an excellent analysis of his work, see M. Neuburger (1981), pp. 21–45. The reception of his notions is also discussed.

339. T. Willis, *Cerebri Anatome* (1664), chap. 17, p. 113.

340. For Haller's opinions, together with those of his followers Johann Georg Zimmermann (1728–1795) and J. G. Zinn, see M. Neuburger (1981), pp. 41–44.

341. A. C. Lorry, "Sur les mouvemens" (1760), p. 363.

342. M. Neuburger (1981), p. 40.

343. J. Mehée de la Touche, *Traité* (1773), pt. 1, Expts. XIII–XIV (pp. 84–89); pt. 2, "Suite des expériences: 1° Sur le cervelet," pp. 139–147. See M. Neuburger (1981), pp. 177–180. The head positioning is part of the palaeocerebellar syndrome mentioned below (6.6.4 and nn. 438–441).

344. M. V. G. Malacarne, *Nuova Esposizione* (1776). See Clarke and O'Malley (1968), pp. 643–646.

345. Anonymous, ["Researches of Malacarne"] (1824), see p. 121, and pp. 120–125.

346. M. V. G. Malacarne, *Encefalotomia* (1780), pt. 2, "Lettere del Signor Carlo Bonnet . . . all'autore relative all'encefalatomia." See letter dated 12 May 1779, pp. 11–12. See also L. Belloni, "Charles Bonnet" (1977).

347. Erasistratus's opinion was cited by Galen, *De Usu Partium*, bk. 8,

chap. 13, in C. G. Kühn, ed., *[Galen] Medicorum Graecorum Opera* (1821–1833), 3 (1822):673. See M. T. May, *Galen* (1968), 1:418; and Clarke and O'Malley (1968), pp. 385, 630–631.

348. Reil's six relevant papers were: "Fragmente" (1807–1808); "Erste Fortsetzung" (1807–1808); "Untersuchungen . . . Zweyte Fortsetzung" (1807–1808); "Nachtrag" (1809); "Das verlängerte Rückenmark. Fünfte Fortsetzung" (1809); "Nachträge . . . Achte Fortsetzung" (1812). English versions, not accurate translations, are in H. Mayo, *Anatomical* (1822–1823).

349. J. C. Reil, "Untersuchungen . . . Vierte Fortsetzung" (1809), pp. 136–143. See H. Mayo, *Anatomical* (1822–1823), Number I, pp. 48–51. Clarke and O'Malley (1968), pp. 830–842. Earlier methods, including that of Gall, had been much less successful. See 1.2.1.

350. J. C. Reil, "Untersuchungen . . . Vierte Fortsetzung" (1809), p. 137.

351. B. Stilling, *Neue Untersuchungen* (1878), p. 352. For Stilling's research on cerebellar anatomy, see this, and his *Untersuchungen* (1864–1878).

352. Anonymous, ["Mr Solly"] (1837), p. 487. It is ironical that 100 years later this comment could have been leveled at anatomy as it was being taught in Britain, under the influence of the Edinburgh school of anatomy! The critic also condemned Reil's nomenclature, some of which, like Malacarne's, is still in use today.

353. J. Gordon, *Observations* (1817), pp. 48–61.

354. H. Mayo, *Anatomical* (1822–1823). These are not accurate translations and must not be relied upon.

355. J. C. Reil, "Das verlängerte Rückenmark" (1809).

356. See M. Neuburger (1981), p. 312.

357. Ibid., pp. 626–627.

358. G. R. Treviranus, *Biologie* (1802–1822), vol. 6 (1822), pt. 1, chap. 3, pp. 141–145.

359. C. G. Carus, *Versuch* (1814), p. 207.

360. J. L. Schönlein, *Von der Hirnmetamorphose* (1816) [pt.] 25, pp. 124–125.

361. K. F. Burdach, *Vom Baue und Leben* (1819–1826), vol. 3 (1826) §§ 928–930 (pp. 442–444). In §§ 892–933 (pp. 417–446), he gave an excellent survey of theories of cerebellar function already proposed and also discussed comparative, developmental, and pathological anatomy.

362. Ibid., § 925 (pp. 440–441).

363. One of the Hippocratic Writers described this as follows: "This [spermatic] fluid is diffused from the brain into the loins and the whole body, but in particular into the spinal marrow [cord]." (Hippocrates, "The seed . . . " [1978], p. 317). From the spinal cord it passed through the veins of the kidney and in the case of the male, via the testicles into the penis (ibid., pp. 317–318). Aristotle reported that Diogenes of Apollonia in the fifth

century B.C. also held this opinion (Aristotle, *Historia Animalium* [1910], bk. 3, chap. 2, 512.b.1–2).

364. E. Swedenborg, *The Generative Organs* (1852), chap. 2, para. 32, p. 31: "*all the fibre [used as a collective noun] that flows into the testicles, descends from the medulla of the cerebellum, but not from that of the cerebrum: hence that the innermost and vital essence of the seed* owes its origin, not to the cerebrum, but to the *cerebellum.*" The ancient anatomists, he claimed, were aware of this.

365. (1) F. J. Gall and J. C. Spurzheim, *Anatomie et Physiologie* (1810–1819), "Section III, I. De l'instinct de la propagation," 3 (1818):61–99.
(2) F. J. Gall, *Influence du Cerveau* (1825), pp. 224–377.
(3) Both (1) and (2) above were translated into English: F. J. Gall et al., *On the Functions* (1838). Combe added his own supporting clinical material.
(4) R. B. Todd, ed., *The Cyclopaedia* (1835–1859), 3 (1839–1847):722S–722X. An excellent critical review of Gall's concept, which he rejected.
(5) Another critical review is in F. A. Longet, *Anatomie et Physiologie* (1824), 1:757–769.

366. The well-recognized association between cerebellar and testicular atrophy has not, however, been elucidated yet. See G. M. Holmes, "A form" (1907).

367. E. R. A. Serres, "Recherches" (1822); "Suite des recherches" (1822), pp. 249–257; and "Suite des recherches" (1823), pp. 114–123.

368. E. R. A. Serres, *Anatomie Comparée* (1824–1826), 2 (1826):595–613, see p. 597.

369. Ibid., p. 607.

370. Ibid., p. 612.

371. P. S. Ségalas d'Etchepare, "Note" (1824), pp. 292–294. The capybara, the largest living rodent, is allied to the guinea pig and is a native of South America.

372. É. J. Georget, *De la Physiologie* (1821), 2:164. There was sufficient to warrant a whole book on it, the only work devoted to one of Gall's "organs": F. J. Gall et al., *On the Functions* (1838). A booklet by H. Davies, *The Cerebellum* (1898), was a product of late nineteenth-century phrenology and cannot be considered a serious contribution to our subject. B. Hollander's *Scientific Phrenology* (1902) was part of the process of revitalization of phrenology after 1870, and he discussed the cerebellum in chap. 11; "The cerebellum and libido sexualis," pp. 180–189.

373. F. Hedderly, *Phrenology* (1970), pp. 59–60.

374. In 1826 K. F. Burdach gave a thorough review of the topic (*Vom Baue und Leben* [1819–1826], vol. 3 [1826], §§ 902–903 [pp. 423–426]). Of 178 cases of cerebellar disease or injury, only 10 had abnormal sexual function. In 1839, F. Leuret (F. Leuret and L. P. Gratiolet, *Anatomie Comparée* [1839–1857], 1 [1839]:425–430 [by Leuret], using quantitative

techniques, showed that castration of horses had no effect on the cerebellum.

375. [?] Combette. Cited by G. Andral, "Lectures" (1835–1836), pp. 842–843. Quote on p. 843. The original article was in "*Revue médicale,* April 1831," but this was not available. See also D. Ferrier, *The Functions* (1886), p. 180.

376. P. Flourens, *Recherches* (1842), pp. 163–164 n (1).

377. W. B. Carpenter, *Principles of Human Physiology* (1846), p. 351, para. 470.

378. W. A. Hammond, "The physiology" (1869). He also rejected Flourens's idea of the cerebellum as a coordinator of voluntary movements and favored Rolando's conclusions.

379. A. Flint, *The Physiology* (1872), p. 392. This appears in a section on "Connection of the cerebellum with the generative function," pp. 388–392.

380. D. Ferrier, *The Functions* (1886), p. 174 n. 1. This comment was not in the 1876 edition, perhaps because by 1886 there had been a resurgence of phrenology following Fritsch's and Hitzig's discovery of the dog's motor cortex in 1870. We should mention here the contribution of phrenology to sexual ethics and education during the nineteenth century: e.g., L. N. Fowler, *The Principles* (1842); and L. N. Fowler and O. S. Fowler, *Amativeness* (1889). These are reprinted in Anonymous, *Sex and Science* (1974). See also M. B. Stern, *Heads & Headlines* (1971).

381. For a discussion of the problems faced by the early experimenters on the cerebellum, see M. Neuburger (1981), pp. 18–19.

382. P. Flourens, *Recherches* (1824), p. 326.

383. P. Flourens, "[Des observations]" (1822). See nn. 158–161 above.

384. G. Cuvier, "Rapport" (1822), pp. 382–383. As we have noted, Cuvier's glowing report was largely responsible for Flourens's early reputation as a scientist. See J. M. D. Olmsted, "Pierre Flourens" (1953), p. 294.

385. P. Flourens, "Recherches physiques" (1823), pp. 355–359, 366–367.

386. P. Flourens, *Recherches* (1824), "Expériences relatives à la détermination du rôle et des fonctions du cervelet," pp. 36–42; and "Expériences sur le cervelet," pp. 137–149. And in idem, *Recherches* (1842), pp. 37–43; and "Chapitre VI. Fonctions du cervelet," pp. 133–141; and pp. 146–149, 400–404, 405–411. For English trans. see G. von Bonin, *Some Papers* (1960), pp. 12–21; J. F. Fulton, *Selected Readings* (1966), pp. 286–288; and Clarke and O'Malley (1968), pp. 656–661.

387. J. C. Dalton, "On the cerebellum" (1861), p. 83.

388. P. Flourens, ["Des observations"] (1822), p. 357.

389. P. Flourens, *Recherches* (1824), p. 37.

390. Ibid., "Préface," p. x.

391. Ibid., p. 297 n. 1.

392. Ibid., p. 148.

393. C. S. Sherrington, "The cerebellum" (1900), p. 909.

394. L. Luciani, *Il Cervelletto* (1891), p. 256.

395. Ibid.

396. L. Rolando, *Saggio* (1809): structure of cerebellum, pp. 24–28; experiments on cerebellum, pp. 44–51; functions of cerebellum, pp. 52–66. The book was reviewed in Anonymous, ["Recent discoveries"] (1824) and a French translation of the experiments was published by Magendie: L. Rolando, "Expériences" (1823), with section on cerebellum, pp. 107–111. Also in Flourens's *Recherches* (1824), pp. 273–302, with Flourens's comments in footnotes; section on cerebellum, pp. 293–302. See also E. Fadiga, "The first Italian" (1963), pp. 204–214; also Clarke and O'Malley (1968), pp. 653–656.

397. L. Rolando, *Saggio* (1809), pp. 59–64. See 5.3.2.

398. L. Rolando, *Saggio* (1809), p. 47.

399. Ibid., p. 44.

400. Ibid., p. 59.

401. Ibid.

402. R. S. Dow and G. Moruzzi, *The Physiology* (1958), p. 4.

403. P. Flourens, *Recherches* (1842), pp. 507–508.

404. L. Rolando, *Saggio* (1828).

405. L. Rolando, "Della struttura" (1831). See fig. 1, p. 132. It was named after him by Leuret in 1839; see F. Leuret and L. P. Gratiolet, *Anatomie Comparée* (1839–1857), 1 (1839):398 (by Leuret): "I have called this fissure the fissure of Rolando, because this anatomist described it in man, in whom it is even more developed than in the monkey." See Clarke and O'Malley (1968), p. 400.

406. F. J. Gall, *Influence du Cerveau* (1825), p. 414.

407. Ibid., p. 415.

408. Anonymous, ["Recent discoveries"] (1824), p. 153.

409. Ibid., p. 154.

410. F. J. V. Broussais, *Cours* (1836), p. 166. For English version of this lecture, see idem, "Lectures" (1836).

411. F. J. V. Broussais, *Cours* (1836), p. 169.

412. F. A. Longet, *Anatomie et Physiologie* (1842), 1:769.

413. A. L. Foville and F. Pinel-Grandchamp, *Recherches* (1823).

414. J. Soury, *Le Système Nerveux* (1899), 1:529.

415. F. Pourfour du Petit, *Lettres* (1710), "Lettre II, Observations," pp. 18–20. See S. Duckett "Étude" (1964). Also supported by J. Sabouraut, "Mémoire [1768]" (1778), pp. 501–502. See M. Neuburger (1981), pp. 271–272.

416. F. Pourfour du Petit, *Lettres* (1710), p. 18.

417. Ibid., p. 20.

418. C. Bell in J. and C. Bell, *The Anatomy* (1829), 2:388. See J. M. D. Olmsted, "The aftermath" (1943).

419. A. L. Foville, "Encéphale" (1831), pp. 202–205.

420. Ibid., p. 205.

421. Ibid.

422. R. B. Todd, *The Cyclopaedia* (1835–1859), 3 (1839–1847):722R. For a history of muscle sense, see E. G. Jones, "The development" (1972).

423. R. B. Todd, ed., *The Cyclopaedia* (1835–1859), 3 (1839–1847):722R–722S.

424. See J. F. Fulton, *Physiology* (1949), pp. 533–534; V. B. Mountcastle, ed., *Medical Physiology* (1980), pp. 837–858.

425. J. C. Prichard, *A Treatise on Insanity* (1835), p. 481.

426. Ibid., p. 482.

427. A. Dugès, *Traité* (1838–1839), 1 (1838):355–356.

428. J. B. Bouillaud, *Traité Clinique* (1825), p. 293.

429. P. Flourens, *Recherches* (1842), p. 18.

430. F. A. Longet, *Anatomie et Physiologie* (1842), 2:733–734. Subsequently Vulpian and Luciani did likewise, and D. Ferrier (*The Functions* [1886], p. 206) stated that he had never observed cutaneous anesthesia in monkeys or humans with extensive damage or disease of the cerebellum.

431. F. Magendie, *Leçons* (1841), 1:179–181, 215–217.

432. C. Bell, "On the functions" (1834), p. 482.

433. Ibid.

434. C. W. H. Nothnagel, *Topische Diagnostik* (1879), p. 15.

435. G. Andral, *Clinique Médicale* (1829–1833), "Livre troisième. Maladies du cervelet," 5 (1833):658–735.

436. A. Flint, *The Physiology* (1872), pp. 372–388. In fact, they favored Flourens's doctrine rather than opposing it.

437. M. Foderà, "Recherches expérimentales" (1823). The promised continuation did not appear in this journal. Review in Anonymous, ["Recent discoveries"] (1824).

438. R. S. Dow and G. Moruzzi, *The Physiology* (1958), p. 5.

439. M. Foderà, "Recherches expérimentales" (1823), p. 193. See also graphic account of pigeon after cerebellum completely removed, ibid., pp. 211–212.

440. J. Mehée de la Touche, *Traité* (1773). See n. 343 above. Neuburger referred to this curious phenomenon (M. Neuburger [1981], pp. 178–179), but believed it was produced by concomitant damage to the medulla oblongata, the palaeocerebellar syndrome being then unknown. This is a good example of the hazard of attempting to explain the findings of earlier authors on the basis of incorrect modern knowledge.

441. L. S. Saucerotte, "Mémoire [1768]" (1778), "XVIIIe observation," p. 405. See M. Neuburger (1981), p. 174. Others in the eighteenth century such as J. G. Zimmermann and J. G. Zinn had also observed this phenomenon. See M. Neuburger (1981), pp. 135 and 137.

442. For localization of functions in the cerebellum, see Clarke and O'Malley (1968), pp. 689–700.

443. M. Foderà, "Lettre" (1826), "Cervelet," p. 107.

444. F. Magendie, "Mémoire" (1824). See Clarke and O'Malley (1968), pp. 682–683; see pp. 683–689 for subsequent studies.

445. F. Magendie, "Mémoire" (1824), p. 402.

446. Ibid., p. 405.

447. H. Hertwig, *Experimenta* (1826).

448. J. Bouillaud, "Recherches expérimentelles" (1827).

449. Ibid., p. 89.

450. J. Bouillaud, "Recherches cliniques" (1827).

451. J. J. C. Legallois, *Oeuvres* (1830), "Avant-propos," 1:17. It has been suggested that Bell also approved of a coordinating force for the components of the respiratory mechanism, but it seems that he was seeking a process that would integrate rather than coordinate, in the true sense of the word.

452. J. Bostock, *An Elementary System* (1828–1830), 3 (1830):374–375.

453. Ibid., p. 374.

454. J. C. Dalton, "On the cerebellum" (1861), p. 83.

455. L. Luciani, *Il Cervelletto* (1891).

456. R. S. Dow and G. Moruzzi (in *The Physiology* [1958], pp. 6–7) divide modern research on cerebellar physiology into three lines of investigation: (1) of its equilibratory function; (2) of its functional localization; (3) of its electrophysiology. See Clarke and O'Malley (1968), pp. 681–707.

457. J. B. Bouillaud, "Recherches cliniques" (1825).

458. J. B. Bouillaud, *Traité Clinique* (1825).

459. J. B. Bouillaud, "Recherches cliniques" (1825), p. 26. See Clarke and O'Malley (1968), pp. 489–491.

460. T. Hood, "Notice of a case" (1824). It was continued in idem, "Continuation" (1826).

461. J. B. Bouillaud, "Recherches cliniques" (1825), p. 30.

462. J. B. Bouillaud, *Traité Clinique* (1825), "Préface," p. xxi. The motto on the title page of this book is "Pathology is the physiology of the diseased man," and is attributed to F. Magendie (*Précis* [1825], vol. 1, "Préface," pp. xi–xii). The original, however, reads: ". . . Medicine, which is only the PHYSIOLOGY OF THE DISEASED MAN . . . "

463. M. Neuburger (1981), pp. 2, 6, 68, 89, 151, 170–171. See also 1.2.5. above.

464. J. B. Bouillaud, *Traité Clinique* (1825), p. 291.

465. Ibid., p. 279.

466. L. A. Desmoulins, *Anatomie* (1825), 2:611.

467. J. B. M. Parchappe de Vinay, *Deuxième Mémoire* (1838), p. 160.

468. F. A. Longet, *Anatomie et Physiologie* (1842), 1:661. The quotation in n. 213 above should also be cited here.

469. J. Cruveilhier, "La faculté" (1839–1840).

470. C. F. Lallemand, *Recherches* (1830–1834). See for example: vol. 1 (1830), "Lettre première," case 8 (pp. 25–28), case 11 (pp. 34–38), and

"Lettre troisième," case 21 (pp. 406–411); vol. 2 (1830), "Cinquième lettre," case 3 (pp. 257–262), "Sixième lettre," case 7 (pp. 434–442).

471. G. Andral, *Clinique Médical* (1829–1833), 5 (1833):382.

472. J. B. Bouillaud, "Recherches cliniques" (1847–1848), p. 813 (7 March 1848). As we have noted, he had continued to amass data supporting his original opinion: idem, "Exposition de nouveaux faits" (1839–1840).

473. For this debate, see B. Stookey, "A note" (1954); and idem, "Jean-Baptiste Bouillaud" (1963); Clarke and O'Malley (1968), pp. 492–497; R. M. Young, *Mind, Brain and Adaptation* (1970), pp. 134–149; F. Schiller, *Paul Broca* (1979), pp. 165–211.

474. For these revolutionary events, see Clarke and O'Malley (1968), pp. 497–518; and R. M. Young, *Mind, Brain and Adaptation* (1970), pp. 150–248. For an excellent account of the present day position concerning cortical localization, see C. G. Phillips et al., "Localization" (1984).

7. THE VEGETATIVE NERVOUS SYSTEM

1. There is only one reliable general history of the autonomic nervous system: D. Sheehan, "Discovery" (1936). It is supplemented by his "The autonomic nervous system" (1941). E. H. Ackerknecht's brief survey, "The history" (1974) can also be recommended. Most later authors have followed Sheehan: J. C. White and R. H. Smithwick, *The Autonomic Nervous System* (1941), pp. 7–12; J. Pick, *The Autonomic Nervous System* (1970), pp. 3–21. G. A. G. Mitchell in *Anatomy* (1953), pp. 1–10 did likewise, but added material of his own, which is not always trustworthy. We, too, are grateful to Sheehan for his pioneer study. For the period before 1800, see J. N. Langley, "Sketch of the progress" (1916); R. French, "The origins" (1971); Neuburger (1981) deals with a number of autonomic functions, but not with the system as a whole. There is a thorough survey of developments before 1830 in F. Arnold, *Der Kopftheil* (1831), pp. 15–71, 127–146. Another excellent survey of the earlier literature on the autonomic ganglia is in K. W. Wutzer, *De Corporis Humani* (1817), pp. 1–46; each contribution is considered in detail and extensive quotations from original sources given.

2. For biography of Gaskell, see *DSB;* and G. L. Geison, *Michael Foster* (1978).

3. For biography of Langley, see G. L. Geison, ibid.; and *DSB*.

4. K. Koizumi and M. Brooks, *The Autonomic System* (1980), p. 893.

5. Galen, *De Usu Partium*, bk. 16, chap. 5. In C. G. Kühn, ed., *[Galen] Medicorum Graecorum Opera* (1821–1833), 2 (1822):289–291; see M. T. May, *Galen* (1968), 2:694–696. See also E. S. Smith, "Galen's account" (1971), pp. 178–181, 183–188. This is the best assessment so far of Galen's enumeration of the cranial nerves, and it differs somewhat from previous accounts.

6. See the following: C. Daremberg, *Exposition* (1841), "Anatomie des nerfs," pp. 43–61; T. Beck, "Die Galenischen Hirnnerven" (1909); E. S. Smith, "Galen's account" (1971), especially "Sixth pair [our glossopharyngeal, vagus, and accessory nerves]," pp. 183–188, and pp. 178–181.

7. Galen, *De Usu Partium,* bk. 16, chap. 5, in C. G. Kühn, ed., *[Galen] Medicorum Graecorum Opera* (1821–1833), 4 (1822):289–290. Also in M. T. May, *Galen* (1968), 2:695. He described the thoraco-lumbar rami communicantes as follows: "for some nerves from the thoracic spinal medulla [cord] itself and from two or three vertebrae below the thorax are added to the nerves passing to the roots of the ribs [i.e., the sympathetic trunk]."

8. C. Stephanus, *De Dissectione* (1545), bk. 2, chap. 49, "Nerui sensorii, tum motores, à cerebro," pp. 248–249. As with Galen and Vesalius, his sixth cranial nerve was composed of our glossopharyngeal, vagus, and accessory nerves, and included the sympathetic trunk. He did, however, differentiate between the components, and, for example, described the sympathetic separately.

9. B. Eustachius, *Tabulae Anatomicae* (1714), table 18, pp. 45–47. The illustrations had been completed in 1552, and this one shows the sympathetic trunk arising from the sixth cranial nerve, thus indicating its intracranial origin.

10. T. Willis, *Cerebri Anatome* (1664). A description of the great intercostal nerve is in chaps. 25–27. It arose from the fifth (trigeminal) and sixth (abducens) cranial nerves of his enumeration: "Concerning this intercostal nerve, which is formed from the lower branches of the fifth and sixth pair" (p. 153). See also ibid., chap. 22, pp. 152–156. For "intercostal nerve," see nn. 18, 21 below.

11. This exceptional discovery will be discussed later. See n. 52.

12. There is no comprehensive, scholarly history of sympathy, although R. Y. Meier's "Sympathy" (1979) deals with some of it. A good nineteenth-century account is in J. B. Monfalcon (1792–1874), "Sympathie" (1821). For the earlier period see T. Weidlich, *Die Sympathie* (1894); for a brief but valuable history up to the mid-seventeenth century, see R. Y. Meier, "'Sympathy'" (1982), which is part of his "Sympathy" (1979). For eighteenth-century ideas, see S. H. Jackson, *A Treatise* (1787).

13. For an account of Galen's concept of sympathy, see R. E. Siegel, *Galen's System* (1968), "V. Sympathy as a diagnostic concept," pp. 360–382. Siegel also traced sympathy to the nineteenth century. See also idem, *Galen on Sense Perception* (1970). Galen's ideas on sympathetic transmission are in Galen, *De Locis Affectis,* bk. 5, chap. 6, in C. G. Kühn, ed. *[Galen] Medicorum Graecorum Opera* (1821–1833), 8 (1824):341–342; English trans. in R. E. Siegel, *Galen on the Affected Parts* (1976), p. 153. Willis's account of sympathy is in his *Cerebri Anatome* (1664); for details, see R. Y. Meier, "'Sympathy'" (1982).

14. J. B. Monfalcon, "Sympathie" (1821), p. 620.

15. C. E. Brown-Séquard, *Course of Lectures* (1860), pp. 168 ff.

16. J. B. Monfalcon, "Sympathie" (1821), p. 617. For a thoughtful correlation of "Sympathy" with Scottish society of the eighteenth century, see C. Lawrence, "The nervous system" (1979).

17. The best account of the early etymology of "Sympathicus" is in J. Hyrtl, *Onomatologia* (1880), pp. 514–517. For a brief general survey, see M. P. M. Laignel-Lavastine, "Note sur l'histoire" (1923).

18. T. Willis, *Cerebri Anatome* (1664), p. 180.

19. [H. Crooke], *Somatographia Anthropine* [Greek] (1616), "Tabula XXVI, Fig. 1, iii," on leaf [61[R]]: "An inner branch [of the vagus] hanging unto the rackebones, and strengthening the intercostall Nerves, and is therefore called *Intercostalis.*"

20. H. Crooke, *Mikrokosmographia* [Greek] (1615), p. 893: "And because it runneth almost through all the bowels of the body it is therefore called *Coniugatio vaga,* the gadding or wandering coniugation."

21. T. Willis, *Cerebri Anatome* (1664), p. 180.

22. Ibid., chap. 25, "Nervi intercostalis descriptio," p. 182: "like *the sun* in the midst of *the planets* and from which numerous branches and fibers radiate into all parts of the mesentery."

23. J. B. Winslow, *Exposition Anatomique* (1732), "Traité des nerfs," p. 462, para. 361: "These nerves are usually called Intercostals. This name by no means corresponds with their situation or with the extent of their distribution, as will presently be seen. I believe that the great Sympathetic Nerves suits them better, because of their very frequent communications with most of the other main Nerves of the whole human body." See D. M. Blair, "Winslow" (1932); and J. Adler, "Winslow" (1971). For biography of Winslow, see E. Snorrason, *L'Anatomiste J.-B. Winslow* (1969).

24. J. Johnstone, "Essay" (1764) and J. Johnston [sic] "History" (1768) were incorporated into *An Essay* (1771), with a German translation, *Versuch* (1787). He also published *Medical Essays* (1795), which contained a revised version of *An Essay* (1771). For biography of Johnstone, see Anonymous, "Memoirs of the life of James Johnstone" (1817); and M. Neuburger (1981), p. 332.

25. F. Chaussier, *Exposition Sommaire* (1807), pp. 12–13, 152, 195.

26. K. F. Burdach, *Vom Baue und Leben* (1819–1826), 1 (1819):70. He was an ardent inventor of anatomical terms, but this one is rarely encountered.

27. S. Solly, *The Human Brain* (1836). He suggested this term for the human autonomic nervous system, because he thought the latter corresponded anatomically to "the nervous system of the cyclo-gangliated or molluscous division of the animal kingdom" (p. 28).

28. Anonymous, "Dr. de Chaumont on the sympathetic" (1854).

29. H. F. Campbell, *Essays* (1857). He thought the autonomic system was

concerned with secretion and nutrition and intimately connected with sensory nerves.

30. L. R. Müller, *Die Lebensnerven* (1924) and *Lebensnerven und Lebenstriebe* (1931). These books illustrate the excesses indulged in by modern clinicians when dealing with the role of the autonomic nervous system in disease, both functional and organic. They represent twentieth-century equivalents of the treatises on sympathy by earlier writers.

31. A. C. Guillaume, *Vagotonies* (1925), "Système des nerfs organo-végétatifs," p. 20.

32. M. P. M. Laignel-Lavastine, "Thérapeutique chimique" (1923–1924), p. 3. Here the author's terminology is said to have increased confusion, and it was denounced as being based on "The claims of the French language and French priority (Winslow)." (W. Sachs, *The Vegetative Nervous System* [1936], p. 8.)

33. E. Schilf, *Das autonome Nervensystem* (1926), p. 6.

34. J. C. Reil, "Ueber die Eigenschaften" (1807), p. 229.

35. For example, Association of Research in Nervous and Mental Diseases (vol. 9), *The Vegetative Nervous System* (1930); W. Sachs, *The Vegetative Nervous System* (1936); E. H. Ackerknecht, "The history" (1974). The periodical, *Acta Neurovegetativa,* begun in Vienna in 1950, carried articles on "neurovegetative anatomy, physiology, pharmacology and pathology." It changed its name to *Journal of Neuro-visceral Relations* in 1970, with the subtitle "journal for the study of the autonomic nervous system and of neuroendocrinology."

36. A. C. Eycleschymer, *Anatomical Names* (1917), pp. 93–94: "Systema nervorum sympathicum."

37. A. Dastre and J. P. Morat, "Sur l'expérience" (1880). See also their *Recherches Expérimentales* (1884), pp. 330–338. See W. Timme, "The vegetative nervous system" (1930), p. 4.

38. J. Johnstone, "Cui bono?" (1795). "Visceral" was also used in embryology after 1838. See R. A. Dart, "The misuse" (1922).

39. J. N. Langley, "On the union" (1898–1899), p. 241. See also, idem, "The nomenclature" (1913). It had been recommended by a colleague at the University of Cambridge, Sir Richard C. Jebb (1841–1905), Regius Professor of Greek.

40. In fifteen recent textbooks of anatomy or physiology published in Britain and the United States, "autonomic" is used in all of them. "Visceral" is often applied to autonomic nerve fibers.

41. H. Gray, *Gray's Anatomy* (1980), p. 1121.

42. W. H. Gaskell, *The Involuntary Nervous System* (1916), p. 1.

43. J. A. H. Murray et al., *A New English Dictionary* (1888–1928). See also *Supplement* (1972).

44. J. N. Langley, *The Autonomic Nervous System* (1921), p. 6.

45. J. N. Langley, in an address to students of medicine and natural philosophy in Amsterdam, 1905. Also in "On the reaction of cells" (1905), p. 403 n. 1.

46. See, for example, S. W. Ranson, "On the use" (1917); and E. Sharpey-Schafer, "The nomenclature" (1931).

47. E. Schilf, *Das autonome Nervensystem* (1926), p. 5.

48. H. Gray, *Gray's Anatomy* (1980), p. 1121.

49. J. E. Neubauer, *Descriptio Anatomica* (1772).

50. A. Scarpa, *Tabulae Nevrologicae* (1794).

51. S.A.A.D. Tissot, *Traité des Nerfs* (1800), vol. 1, chap. 5, § 95 (pp. 154–155). He called the rami "filets collatéraux" and discussed the ganglia (pp. 155–174). First edition was 1778.

52. F. Pourfour du Petit, "Sur ce que le nerf intercostal" (1729). This is a brief account of his researches. Its expanded form is "Mémoire" (1729). His experiments had been carried out at Namur in 1712 and repeated at Paris in 1725. See A. E. Best, "Pourfour du Petit's experiments" (1969).

53. Galen, *De Usu Partium,* bk. 16, chap. 5, in C. G. Kühn ed., *[Galen] Medicorum Graecorum Opera* (1821–1833), 4 (1822):289–291. And in M. T. May, *Galen* (1968), 2:694–696 n. 5.

54. For an excellent discussion of them, see M. Neuburger (1981), pp. 163–168.

55. T. Willis, *Cerebri Anatome* (1664), chap. 26, "Nervorum paris intercostales . . . ," pp. 184–185. His lengthy description of the intercostal nerve is in chaps. 25–27 (pp. 179–206).

56. Ibid., p. 184.

57. J. F. Meckel, the Elder, "Observation anatomique" (1749). See also J. F. Meckel, the Younger, *De Ganglio* (1795).

58. J. F. Meckel, the Younger, *Handbuch* (1815–1820), vol. 1, *Allgemeine Anatomie* (1815), § 182.4 (p. 313).

59. J. G. Zinn, "De l'enveloppe" (1753), pp. 137–138; A. von Haller, *Elementa* (1757–1766), vol. 4 (1762), bk. 10, sect. 6, § 12 "Ganglia," p. 203; J. G. Haase, "De gangliis" (1772), § 21. "Quae de gangliis dicta sunt sympathia nervorum illustratur" (pp. 85–86); A. Scarpa, *Anatomicarum Annotationum* (1779), chap. 2, "De usu gangliorum"; J. Pfeffinger, "De structura nervorum" (1791), "Ganglia nervorum," pp. 18–30, see pp. 20–21, 23; A. Monro, *secundus, Observations* (1783), chap. 19, "Of the ganglia of the nerves," pp. 50–58; J. F. Blumenbach, *Institutiones Physiologicae* (1787), sect. 15, "De sensoris et nervis," § 207 (pp. 170–171); E. H. Weber, *Anatomia Comparata* (1817), pt. 2, "Physiologica," sect. 2, "De gangliis," 4 (p. 150).

60. J. B. Winslow, *Exposition Anatomique* (1732), "Traité des nerfs," p. 462: "364. These ganglioform tumours, or ganglions, differ more or less in volume, color, and consistency; & one may regard them as so many

dispersed origins or sources of this great Pair of Sympathetic Nerves, and consequently as so many little brains."

61. J. Johnstone, *An Essay* (1771).

62. M. F. X. Bichat, *Recherches Physiologiques* (An VIII [1800]). There were further editions in 1802, 1805, 1822, and 1844. English trans., *Physiological Researches,* London (1815); and Boston (1827). The book comprises two parts: the first is theoretical, and here Bichat distinguished between animal and organic life; the second is experimental and he endeavored to determine the relative roles of the brain, heart, and lungs in producing death. It is a remarkable collection of physiological observations, experimental methods, and theories. Although several of these have since been disproved, Bichat's treatise remains an outstanding classic of medical science.

63. M. F. X. Bichat, *Anatomie Générale* (1801). Further Paris editions in 1812, 1821, and an English trans. of the latter: *General Anatomy* (1824).

64. M. F. X. Bichat, *Traité d'Anatomie* (1801–1803). Further Paris editions in 1819, 1823, and 1829.

65. E. H. Ackerknecht in "The history" (1974) claims that it "is still rather influential even today, although it has been officially to a large extent abandoned" (p. 3), but gives no evidence for this.

66. Bichat first discussed his physiological system in *Recherches Physiologiques* (An VIII [1800]). He elaborated it further in *Anatomie Générale* (1801), vol. 1, "Considérations générales," see § 8. "Remarques sur la classification des functions," pp. cii–civ. See also "Système nerveux de la vie animale," 1:115–212; and ibid., "Système nerveux de la vie organique," pp. 213–244. There is a good account of Bichat's system in W. R. Albury, "Experiment and explanation" (1977). For Bichat's vitalism, see P. L. Entralgo, "Sensualism" (1948); E. Haigh, "The roots" (1975); see also, idem, *Xavier Bichat* (1984). One of the most recent accounts of Bichat's physiology is in J. E. Lesch, *Science and Medicine in France* (1984), pp. 50–79, and it is probably the best. The genesis, influence, and background of his studies are also discussed.

67. However, the word "animal" used in the English trans. of Galen's Greek means "soul," being derived from its Latin form *animus*. Thus, "animal spirits" were spirits of the psyche or soul.

68. T. de Bordeu, *Recherches Anatomiques* (1751), § 110, p. 381.

69. Ibid., p. 382.

70. J.C.M.G. de Grimaud, *Mémoire sur la Nutrition* (1787), pp. 2–3.

71. For biography see [?] Hoefer, ed., *Nouvelle Biographie* (1858–1866), vol. 6 (1862); and *DSB*.

72. M. F. X. Bichat, *Anatomie Générale* (1801), 1:civ, 115–212, 213–244. See also, idem, *Traité d'Anatomie* (1801–1803), 3 (1802):143–318, 319–368.

73. See nn. 58, 59.

74. M. F. X. Bichat, *Anatomie Générale* (1801), 1:223–224.

75. H. Power and L. W. Sedgwick, *The New Sydenham Society's Lexicon* (1879–1899), "C. abdominale . . . The solar plexus"; and T. L. Stedman, *Illustrated Stedman's* (1982). It was first used by Heinrich August Wrisberg (1739–1808) in "Observationes anatomicae" (1780), p. 69.

76. M. F. X. Bichat, *Recherches Physiologiques* (An VIII [1800]), "Article onzième, De l'influence que la mort du cerveau exerce sur celle de touts les organes," § 1, 8°, pp. 415–416.

77. J. Johnstone, *An Essay* (1771), pp. 70–71: "The great sympathetic nerves being truly derived from the spinal marrow, have in their numerous ganglions proper to them, so many receptacles of nervous energy, so many subordinate Brains, which continue to dispense the nervous energy to the vital organs, long after they cease to have communication with the Brain."

78. M. F. X. Bichat, *Anatomie Générale* (1801), 1:115.

79. S. T. Soemmerring, *De Corporis Humani* (1794–1801), vol. 4, *De Cerebro et de Nervis* (1798). See "Nervorum ganglia," "Usu gangliorum," § 161, p. 151. Also in German, *Hirnlehre* (1791), § 161, p. 131.

80. J. F. Meckel, the Elder, "Observation anatomique" (1749).

81. J. B. Winslow, *Exposition Anatomique* (1732), "Traité des nerfs," para. 363 (p. 462), see also "Nota," p. 468.

82. F. J. Gall and J. C. Spurzheim, *Recherches* (1809), pp. 129–133; idem, *Anatomie et Physiologie* (1810–1819), 1 (1810):192–194 and pl. 5. See H. M. Thomas, "Decussation" (1910); Clarke and O'Malley (1968), pp. 280–284; and M. Neuburger (1981), pp. 53–63.

83. We can assume that J. Johnstone in *An Essay* (1771, p. 28) implied this when referring to the spinal cord: "from which the intercostal, or great sympathetic nerves which supply the Heart and the Intestines truly arise."

84. F. Pourfour du Petit, "Sur ce que le nerf intercostal" (1729), and idem, "Mémoire" (1729); see n. 52 above.

85. This and other evidence is listed in M. F. X. Bichat, *Anatomie Générale* (1801), 1:214–215.

86. E. H. Weber, *Anatomia Comparata* (1817), pt. 2, "Physiologica," sect. 1, 1), 5 (pp. 122–123).

87. A. Portal, "Description" (1801), p. 188.

88. J.G.C.F.M. Lobstein, *De Nervi Sympathetici* (1823), sect. I, chap. 2, pp. 32–47. (The English trans., *A Treatise* [1831], was not seen.) This man is usually referred to as Jean Frédéric Lobstein, the Younger, to differentiate him from Jean Frédéric Lobstein, the Elder (1736–1784), both of Strasbourg, but not related. There was also Jean Frédéric Daniel Lobstein (1777–c. 1840). To avoid confusion, the Lobstein to whom we shall be making frequent reference below will invariably be given his full initials, J.G.C.F.M. See n. 119 below, and chap. 1 n. 42.

89. G. Cuvier, *Leçons* (1800–1805), vol. 2 (1800), "Dixième leçon," "Article XVI, Du nerf grand sympathique, appelé encore grand intercostal

ou tri-spanchnique." "C. Dans les oisseaux," p. 294. This series of lectures had begun in 1795 at the Musée d'Histoire Naturelle and may well have been attended by Bichat. For accounts of them, see W. Coleman, *Georges Cuvier* (1964), pp. 44–73; R. Dujarric de la Rivière, *Cuvier* (1969); and *DSB*.

90. For example, by J. F. Meckel, the Younger, *Handbuch* (1815–1820), vol. 1, *Allgemeine Anatomie* (1815), § 182, 4, p. 313; F. Tiedemann, *Zoologie* (1808–1810), vol. 2, *Anatomie und Naturgeschichte der Vögel* (1810), § 39, p. 45; and Augustus Gottfried Ferdinand Emmert (1777–1819), "Beobachtungen" (1811).

91. G. Cuvier, *Leçons* (1800–1805), vol. 2 (1800), "Dixième leçon," art. 16, p. 285. See n. 89 above.

92. M. F. X. Bichat, *Anatomie Générale* (1801), 1:215–216.

93. Ibid., p. 242.

94. C. Bell, in J. Bell and C. Bell, *The Anatomy* (1829), 2:571.

95. J. B. Winslow, *Exposition Anatomique* (1732), para. 364, p. 462. See n. 60 above for quote.

96. See M. Neuburger (1981), pp. 166–168, for the work of other eighteenth-century investigators of this topic.

97. J. Johnstone, *An Essay* (1771), p. 80: "GANGLIONS seem analogous to the brain in their office: subordinate springs, and reservoirs of nervous power, they seem capable of dispensing it long after all communication with the brain is cut off. And tho' they ultimately depend upon the brain for its emanations, it appears from facts, that, *that* dependence is far from being immediate and instantaneous."

98. J. Johnstone, "History" (1768), p. 131: "As different sources of nervous power, *ganglions* are analagous to the brain in their office, though they derive their nervous filaments (to be new arranged in them), and consequently their power ultimately from it."

99. J. F. Meckel, the Elder, "Observation anatomique" (1749), p. 95. He did not accept that a ganglion was a source of nervous matter or energy (p. 91), and both Haller and Zinn agreed with him.

100. A. Monro, *secundus, Observations* (1783), p. 56.

101. Ibid., p. 57.

102. C. Bell, in J. Bell and C. Bell, *The Anatomy* (1823), 2:364: "I conceive that these bodies consist of the same matter with the brain."

103. See quote in n. 98 above. See also ibid., pp. 70–71.

104. J. Johnstone, *An Essay* (1771), p. 19: "MAY we not reasonably conclude that Ganglions are the Instruments, by which the motions of the Heart and Intestines are from the *earliest* to the *latest periods* of animal life, *rendered uniformly involuntary;* and that this *is their use?*"

105. Ibid., p. 81. There is also on p. 66: "Ganglions are organic parts of great importance in the nervous system, and animal machine . . . they limit the powers of volition, will."

106. J. Johnstone, *Medical Essays* (1795), p. 108 (first numbering).

107. Ibid., p. 100.

108. A. B. Richerand, *Nouveaux Élémens* (1801). This is the first edition, but it was not seen. For biography of Richerand, see J.L.H.P., *Sketches* (1831), pp. 101–119.

109. There were thirteen French and seventeen Belgian editions, as well as seven English, together with trans. into Chinese, Dutch, German, Italian (two editions), Russian, and Spanish. For an English edition, see A. B. Richerand, *Elements* (1829).

110. A. B. Richerand, *Nouveaux Élémens* (An XII–1804), vol. 1, "Prolégomenes," § 10, "Du systême des grands nerfs sympathiques," pp. 97–108.

111. A. B. Richerand, "Essai" (An VII [1799]).

112. A. B. Richerand, *Nouveaux Élémens* (An XII–1804), 1:102.

113. C. Bernard, *La Science Expérimentale* (1878), p. 155.

114. W. M. Bayliss, *Principles* (1931), p. 484; J. Learmonth, ["Recent advances"] (1938), p. 154; and idem, "The surgery" (1950), p. 505.

115. J. F. Meckel, the Elder, "Observation anatomique" (1749); and J. G. Haase, "De gangliis nervorum" (1772), § 13, pp. 76–77.

116. J. Johnstone, *An Essay* (1771), p. 79. Morgagni was the first to describe them thus: *Adversaria Anatomica Omnia* (1719), wherein see *Adversaria Anatomica Altera* (1717), "Animadversio XXXIV," pp. 70–71. See also idem, *De Sedibus* (1761), bk. 1, letter 12, article 14, p. 95.

117. J. Johnstone, *An Essay* (1771), p. 80. See quotations in nn. 97 and 98 above. See also ibid., p. 73 where he stated that ganglia were "subordinate origins of nerves sent to the intestines, yet, ultimately derived from the Brain."

118. S.A.A.D. Tissot, *Traité des Nerfs* (1800), vol. 2, article 11, "Des ganglions," § 248, pp. 205–212.

119. F. Vicq d'Azyr, "Lobstein" (1805). See J. F. Lobstein, the Elder, "De nervo spinali" (1760). This J. F. Lobstein must not be confused with J.G.C.F.M. Lobstein (1777–1835), also known as J. F. Lobstein, the Younger. See n. 88 above.

120. G. Cuvier, *Leçons* (1800–1805). See n. 89 above.

121. Ibid., "Première leçon," 1 (1800):26. His accounts of the sympathetic trunk in humans, mammals, reptiles, and fish are in ibid., vol. 2 (1800). "Dixième leçon," "Du nerf sympathique appelé encore grand intercostal ou trisplanchnique," pp. 285–297. His reference in this title to alternative nomenclature is worthy of note.

122. J. Fletcher, *Rudiments* (1835–1837), *Part IIa. On life, as Manifested in Irritation* (1836), chap. 4, sect. 2. "On the ganglionic nervous system in particular, regarded as the immediate seat of irritability," p. 66 n. This must be one of the few books in which the title page presents the author's thesis in symbolic form: the vital activity of the animal body.

123. J. Wilkes, *Essays, I* (1833). According to him, A. P. Wilson Philip "grants that Bichat derived his theory from Johnstone" (p. 33), but this could not be verified in Wilson Philip's writings.

124. M. F. X. Bichat, *Anatomie Générale* (1801), 1:242.

125. J. C. Reil, "Ueber die Eigenschaften" (1807).

126. Ibid., p. 192. We should note that like Johnstone, Jiří Procháska had already made a similar suggestion with regard to the ganglia (*Adnotationum* [1784], pp. 126–129). Impulses from the brain met resistance in the ganglia, which acted like semiconductors, either allowing messages to pass through or preventing them from doing so. This mechanism thus provided the ganglionic system with a degree of autonomy. Whether or not Procháska's and Reil's ideas were formulated independently and whether Procháska was copying Johnstone has not been discovered, but this clearly deserves further investigation.

127. D. Sheehan, "Discovery" (1936), p. 1097.

128. J. C. Reil, "Ueber die Eigenschaften" (1807), p. 225.

129. Ibid. He discussed this mechanism on pp. 200–205, 225–230, 242–243, and elsewhere.

130. Ibid., p. 242.

131. Ibid., p. 227.

132. J. Johnstone, *An Essay* (1771), p. 27.

133. J. C. Reil, "Ueber die Eigenschaften" (1807), pp. 210–225.

134. Ibid., p. 229.

135. Ibid., p. 210.

136. Ibid., p. 235.

137. Ibid., pp. 200–205, 225–237.

138. Ibid., pp. 237–254.

139. K. W. Wutzer, *De Corporis Humani* (1817), pp. 35–36, 119, 126.

140. Ibid., pp. 121–129.

141. F. J. Gall and J. C. Spurzheim, *Recherches* (1809), sect. 7, p. 153.

142. F. J. Gall and J. C. Spurzheim, *Anatomie et Physiologie* (1810–1819), vol. 1 (1810), sect. I, "Du nerf intercostal, ou du grand nerf sympathique," pp. 21–33.

143. Ibid., p. 21.

144. Ibid., pp. 31–32.

145. F. Chaussier, *Exposition Sommaire* (1807), p. 13 n. For biography of Chaussier, see J.L.H.P., *Sketches* (1831), pp. 71–76.

146. J. J. C. Legallois, *Expériences* (1812), pp. 150–151. See G. Legée, "M.J.P. Flourens" (1975).

147. J. J. C. Legallois, *Expériences* (1812), p. 151. Part of this quotation has been cited in chap. 1 n. 65.

148. A. P. Wilson Philip, *An Experimental Inquiry* (1817), chap. 9, pp. 203–204. This book was based on two papers presented to the Royal Society: "Experiments" (1815); and "Some additional experiments" (1815).

149. A. Scarpa, *Anatomicarum Annotationum* (1779), chap. 2, § 10, pp. 49–50.

150. J.G.C.F.M. Lobstein, *De Nervi Sympathetici* (1823), pp. 70–71.

151. A. P. Wilson Philip, "Some additional experiments" (1815), p. 438.

152. J. M. Good, *The Study of Medicine* (1822), 3:10.

153. J. M. Good, *The Study of Medicine* (1840), 3:8–9.

154. P. J. Barthez, *Nouveaux Élémens* (1806), vol. 2, chap. 10, "Des sympathies . . . ," 184, pp. 61–63.

155. Ibid., "Notes," p. 30.

156. P. A. Béclard, *Élémens* (1823), § 813, p. 690. For biography of Béclard, see R. Knox's trans. of the above: *Elements* (1830), pp. vii–xxiv. He stated that "Bichat . . . wrote the romance of the science [of anatomy]; Béclard labored to trace its code" (p. xix). The work of J. L. Brachet should be mentioned, because Béclard was probably referring to it here. It concerned the influence of the ganglionic system on the sympathies, but was of much less importance than that of Béclard. See J. L. Brachet, *Recherches Expérimentales* (1830), chap. 8, pp. 285–367. See also chap. 4 for additional nineteenth-century consideration of the Willisian theory.

157. P. A. Béclard, *Élémens* (1823), § 816, p. 696.

158. Ibid., p. 697.

159. J. N. Langley, "On the union" (1898–1899), p. 241.

160. J.G.C.F.M. Lobstein, *De Nervi Sympathici* (1823), pp. 32–47, 78–84, see also, idem, "Trisplanchnique (nerf)" (1821). Lobstein's ganglion is the accessory ganglion of the great splanchnic nerve above the diaphragm; see idem, *De Nervi Sympathici* (1823), § 29, pp. 20–21.

161. J.G.C.F.M. Lobstein, "Trisplanchnique (nerf)" (1821), p. 36.

162. Ibid.

163. Ibid., pp. 42–43.

164. F. J. V. Broussais, "Réflexions" (1818), pp. 31–43.

165. Ibid., pp. 137–148.

166. Ibid., pp. 166–167.

167. F. Fletcher, *Rudiments* (1836–1837), *Part IIa* (1836), chap. 4, sect. 2, pp. 61–94. See n. 122 above.

168. M. F. X. Bichat, *Anatomie Générale* (1801), 1:230–232.

169. J. F. Ackermann, "De nervei systematis" (1813), §§ 3–4 (pp. 77–87).

170. The most notable of these was J. F. Meckel, the Younger, in *Handbuch* (1815–1820), vol. 1, *Allgemeine Anatomie* (1815), pt. 2, sect. 3, § 198, see pp. 339–342.

171. J.G.C.F.M. Lobstein, *De Nervi Sympathetici* (1823), chap. 3, "De nervi sympathetici in foetu evolutione," pp. 47–56.

172. F. J. V. Broussais, "Réflexions" (1818), pp. 130–159.

173. For example, J. Clarke, "Description" (1793). In the case he reported there was no trace of a nervous system, but instead of a monster, the lesion could have been a hydatiform mole.

174. J.G.C.F.M. Lobstein, *De Nervi Sympathetici* (1823), §§ 65–69, pp. 52–55.

175. G. Breschet, "Recherches anatomiques" (1836), pp. 366–367.

176. M. Hall, *The Gulstonian Lectures* (1842), p. 33. He used the term "cerebrum," but presumably meant brain.

177. S. L. Parker, "Lectures" (1831), pp. 65–68, 70.

178. J.G.C.F.M. Lobstein, *De Nervi Sympathetici* (1823), p. 88.

179. [?] Cayre, "Note" (1819).

180. A. B. Richerand, "Essai" (An VII–[1799]), p. 309.

181. M. F. X. Bichat, *Anatomie Générale* (1801), 1:225. See also references to Cabanis on this topic in chap. 6.5.

182. Ibid. The possibility that the vegetative nervous system was involved in mesmerism was also proposed and this led to wild speculations that we have not, however, explored.

183. P. Pinel, *Traité* [1801], sect. I, 13, p. 38.

184. J.G.C.F.M. Lobstein, *De Nervi Sympathetici* (1823), pp. 125–129.

185. J. Waugh, *The Science* (1838), p. xx. This work is distinguished not only by its fanciful speculations but also by its outrageous terminology, which is never fully elucidated. See *BFMR* (1839), 7:228–229.

186. J.G.C.F.M. Lobstein, *De Nervi Sympathetici* (1823), sect. 3. "Pathologica," pp. 125–167.

187. A. Eulenberg and P. Guttmann, *Die Pathologie* (1873).

188. E. L. Fox, *The Influence* (1885).

189. E. H. Ackerknecht, "The history" (1974), p. 7.

190. M. F. X. Bichat, *Anatomie Générale* (1801), 1:220.

191. Ibid., p. 227.

192. J. C. Reil, "Ueber die Eigenschaften" (1807), p. 230.

193. F. J. Gall and J. C. Spurzheim, *Anatomie et Physiologie* (1810–1819), 1 (1810):30.

194. J. M. Dupuy, "Observations" (1816).

195. K. W. Wutzer, *De Corporis Humani* (1817), §§ 107–108, pp. 125–128.

196. J.G.C.F.M. Lobstein, *De Nervi Sympathetici* (1823), sect. 2. "Physiologica," p. 94.

197. Ibid., p. 95.

198. J. L. Brachet, *Recherches Expérimentales* (1830). See, for example, "Exp. CXXX," p. 305.

199. Ibid.

200. Ibid., pp. 307–308.

201. J. Müller, *Handbuch* (1835–1840), vol. 1 (1835, 2d ed.), bk. 3, pt. 2, chap. 3, 1, "Der Sympathicus hat Empfindung," p. 646.

202. E. H. Weber, *Das Gefäss-und Nervensystem* (1831), p. 335.

203. P. Flourens, *Recherches* (1824), pp. 204–206. See G. Legée, "M.J.P. Flourens" (1975).

204. P. Flourens, *Recherches* (1824), p. 214.

205. F. A. Longet, *Traité de Physiologie* (1850–1861), "I. Sensibilité du grand sympathique," 2 (1850):373–375. This section was almost unchanged in the 3d ed. (1868–1869), 3 (1869):593–594.

206. F. A. Longet, *Traité de Physiologie* (1850–1861), 2 (1850):374.

207. F. Arnold, *Der Kopftheil* (1831), pp. 149–150.

208. C. G. Ehrenberg, "Nothwendigkeit" (1833), "Ganglien," p. 458. Summary of a paper presented to the academy of science in Berlin, 29 April 1833. See Clarke and O'Malley (1968), pp. 39–43. See also chap. 3.1 above.

209. C. G. Ehrenberg, "Nothwendigkeit" (1833), p. 459. He discussed the cerebral cortex in greater detail on p. 451.

210. G. B. Morgagni, *Adversaria Anatomica Altera* (1717). See n. 116 above.

211. J. Johnstone, *Medical Essays* (1795), p. 85 (first numbering).

212. G. G. Valentin, "Über den Verlauf" (1836). See Clarke and O'Malley (1968), pp. 43–46.

213. G. G. Valentin, "Über den Verlauf" (1836), pp. 157–158.

214. Ibid., p. 138.

215. R. Remak, *Observationes Anatomicae* (1838), chap. 2, "De fibris organicis nervi sympathici et nervorum cerebrospinalium," § 6, p. 5. For review of this book, see ["Remak on the structure"] (1839). For his work on the vegetative ervous system, see 3.5.2 above; B. Kisch, "Forgotten leaders" (1954), pp. 250–254; and Clarke and O'Malley (1968), pp. 48–52.

216. R. Remak, *Observationes Anatomicae* (1838), p. 5.

217. Ibid. This is the title of chap. 1 of sect. 2, on p. 8.

218. Ibid., sect. 2, chap. 1, § 13, p. 9.

219. Ibid., § 15, p. 10.

220. Ibid., § 15, p. 11.

221. A. W. Volkmann, "Ueber die Faserung" (1838). For review see *BFMR* (1839), 7:541–544.

222. K. W. Wutzer, *De Corporis Humani* (1817), § 80, pp. 95–97. See also idem, "Ueber den Zusammenhang" (1834).

223. J. Müller, "Ueber das Ganglion" (1832), p. 85.

224. A. Scarpa, "De gangliis nervorum" (1831).

225. A. A. Retzius, "Ueber den Zusammenhang" (1832). A letter to J. Müller (3 August 1832) concerning the latter's article, n. 223 above.

226. A.F.J.C. Mayer, "Ueber das Gehirn" (1832).

227. These statements are not in the 2d edition of Müller's *Handbuch* (vol. 1, 1835), and where they first appeared has not been determined. They are in the 4th edition (vol. 1, 1840–1844), the only other edition of vol. 1 available to us: idem, *Handbuch* (1840–1844–?), vol. 1 (1840–1844), bk. 3, sect. 1, chap. 1, "b. Von dem feinern Bau der Nerven," "Weisse und graue Bündel in den Nerven," p. 520.

228. R. Remak, *Observationes Anatomicae* (1838), p. 11.

229. The 1st edition of vol. 1 of J. Müller's *Handbuch*, published 1833–

1834, was not available to us, but see vol. 1 of 2d edition (1835): bk. 3, pt. 2, chap. 3, "Von den Eigenschaften der Nervus sympathicus," pp. 646–652; and bk. 3, pt. 4, chap. 2, "Von den Eigentümlichkeiten anderer Nerven," "Nervus sympathicus," pp. 778–782. These sections also give details of Müller's opinions on the histology of the vegetative nervous system up to 1835.

230. This is from J. Müller, *Elements* (1838–1843), 1 (1838):670. The passage could not be located in the limited number of German editions available to us, but presumably it appeared in vol. 1 of the 1st edition (1833–1834).

231. F. G. J. Henle, *Allgemeine Anatomie* (1841), "Vom Nervengewebe," "Organischen Nerven," pp. 632–666.

232. F. G. J. Henle, *Pathologische Untersuchungen* (1840), p. 106.

233. R. Remak, "Ueber die physiologische Bedeutung" (1840).

234. Ibid., pp. 257–263.

235. Ibid., pp. 263–265.

236. B. Kisch, "Forgotten leaders" (1954), p. 251.

237. As in nn. 229 and 230, vol. 1 of Müller's *Handbuch,* 1st edition (1833–1834), in which this statement presumably appeared, was not available. It is in idem, *Elements* (1838–1843), 1 (1838):608.

238. J. Johnstone, *An Essay* (1771), p. 76. He expanded this in his *Medical Essays* (1795), p. 77 (first numbering).

239. J. Johnstone, *An Essay* (1771), p. 39.

240. R. Remak, "Ueber die physiologische Bedeutung" (1840), pp. 251–252.

241. A. W. Volkmann, "Nervenphysiologie" (1844), "C. Motorisches Vermögen des sympathischen Nervensysteme," pp. 604–612, see p. 605.

242. Ibid., pp. 604 et seq.

243. G. G. Valentin, *De Functionibus* (1839).

244. G. G. Valentin, "Über den Verlauf" (1836).

245. G. G. Valentin, *De Functionibus* (1839), bk. 2, "De nervo sympathico," pp. 61–73. He gave an excellent account of the literature, §§ 158–163, pp. 66–69.

246. Ibid., bk. 4, "De nervorum periphericorum in singulus functiones imperio," pp. 104–161.

247. Anonymous, "Valentin" (1841), p. 305.

248. G. G. Valentin, *De Functionibus* (1839), bk. 2, chap. 1, "De vera n. sympathici natura," §§ 144–145, p. 61. See also idem, "Ueber die Scheiden" (1839).

249. G. G. Valentin, *De Functionibus* (1839), bk. 2, chap. 1, §§ 144–145, p. 61. See also idem, "Ueber die Scheiden" (1839).

250. G. G. Valentin, *A Textbook* (1853), chap. 8, "Innervation," para. 1772, p. 525.

251. F. G. J. Henle, "Ueber Nervensympathien" (1840), p. 106.

252. G. G. Valentin, *De Functionibus* (1839), bk. 3, chap. 4, "De ortu fibrarum nervosarum n. sympathici," pp. 72–73.

253. Ibid., bk. 4, chap. 3, "De formatione gangliosa," §§ 222–228, pp. 92–95.

254. G. G. Valentin, "Nervensystem der Wirbelthiere" (1842), pp. 119–123, 128, 135.

255. Anonymous, ["Volkmann, Bidder"] (1844), p. 380.

256. F. H. Bidder and A. W. Volkmann, *Die Selbständigkeit* (1842).

257. Anonymous, ["Volkmann, Bidder"] (1844), p. 386.

258. As noted above (n. 221), Volkmann had already published some of his findings on sympathetic nerve fibers in the frog: "Ueber die Faserung" (1838).

259. Ibid.

260. W. H. Gaskell, "On the structure" (1885–1886).

261. F. H. Bidder and A. W. Volkmann, *Die Selbständigkeit* (1842), § 47, V, p. 66.

262. Ibid., p. 67.

263. J. F. Meckel, the Elder, "Observation anatomique" (1749). It is now well established that one preganglionic fiber may relate to up to fifteen or twenty postganglionic neurons so that a wide diffusion of autonomic effects is possible. See G. A. Wolff, "The ratio" (1941).

264. F. J. Bidder and A. W. Volkmann, *Die Selbständigkeit* (1842).

265. R. A. von Koelliker, *Die Selbständigkeit* (1844).

266. Ibid., pp. 5–31.

267. For a discussion of Remak's fibers some ten years later, see R. A. von Koelliker, *Manual* (1853–1854), 1 (1853):485–487.

268. R. A. von Koelliker, *Die Selbständigkeit* (1844), pp. 10 et seq.

269. Ibid., p. 10.

270. Part 2 of his *Die Selbständigkeit* (1844), pp. 31–40, is a discussion of ideas of function, arising from his microscopical findings.

271. Ibid., p. 31.

272. M. J. S. Schultze, "Allgemeines" (1871). In S. Stricker, ed. *Handbuch* (1871–1872).

273. T. S. Beck, "On the nerves of the uterus" (1846), pp. 215–216n, 223–224.

274. Ibid., pp. 215–216n.

275. T. S. Beck, "On the structure and function" (1847).

276. Ibid., p. 617.

277. R. Remak, "Über multipolare Ganglienzellen" (1854). An unreliable English version is in idem, "Professor Remak" (1854).

278. A. Monro, *secundus, Observations* (1783), p. 56. See n. 100 above referring to quote in text.

279. R. B. Todd, *The Cyclopaedia,* ed. R. B. Todd (1835–1859), 3 (1839–1847):723F.

280. Ibid. For a midcentury survey of the vegetative nervous system, see J. Drummond, "Sympathetic nerve" (1859).

281. Johann Gottlieb Walter (1734–1818) is said to have described this ganglion ("ganglion impar" or "the unpaired coccygeal ganglion of Walter"). His *Tabulae Nervorum* (1783) did not describe it, but it is noted in the modified English version, idem, *John Gottlieb Walter's Plates* (1804), p. 46.

282. Said to have been described by A. A. Retzius c. 1840, but this could not be verified. See n. 285 below.

283. J. F. Meckel, the Elder, *Tractatus* (1748); and idem, "Observations anatomique" (1749).

284. F. Arnold, *Ueber den Ohrenknoten* (1828); and "Mémoire" (1829).

285. F. Arnold discussed all these ganglia in *Observationes* (1826); and in "Beschreibung des Kopftheils" (1826), §§ 3–16, pp. 130–147; §§ 27–29, pp. 161–164; §§ 31–32, pp. 166–167.

286. For the early history of *piqûre diabètique,* see M. Laffont, "Recherches expérimentales" (1880), pp. 347–363; and M. D. Grmek, "Examen critique" (1966). For detailed accounts of it by Bernard, see his *Leçons de Physiologie* (1855–1856), 1 (1855):288–373; his *Leçons sur la Physiologie* (1858), "Piqûre du plancher du quatrième ventricule," 1:397–462; and his *Leçons sur le Diabète* (1877), pp. 369–400. For Magendie's reaction to this discovery, see his "Annonce d'une découverte" (1849).

287. J. L. Budge and A. V. Waller, "Recherches" (1851); and J. L. Budge, "Observations" (1851).

288. J. Müller, *Handbuch* (1835–1840), 1 (1835, 2d ed.):690, 717–720. See n. 145, chap. 4 above.

289. R. D. Grainger, "*Observations*" (1837), p. 57. See n. 213 chap. 4 above.

290. C. Bernard studied reflex action in the ganglionic system, and one of his early papers was "Sur les phénomènes reflexes" (1853). See chap. 4.3.

291. See, for example, L. T. Bochefontaine, "Étude expérimentale" (1876), "Points dont la faradisation agit sur la circulation sanguine," pp. 142–159. For a survey of this early research, see E. A. Schäfer, "The cerebral cortex" (1900), pp. 713–718.

292. The most important at that time was by Francis Maitland Balfour (1851–1882): "The development" (1876–1878), see 1877, 11:406–490. "Development of the spinal nerves and of the sympathetic nervous system" is on pp. 438–439.

293. For Gaskell's work, see his most important paper: "On the structure" (1885–1886). His studies were summarized in *The Involuntary Nervous System* (1916). For a summary of Langley's work, see "The sympathetic" (1900); and his *The Autonomic Nervous System* (1921). See also D. Sheehan, "Discovery" (1936).

294. J. Johnstone, *Medical Essays* (1795), p. 103 (first numbering).

295. Chap. 1 n. 12, above.

Bibliographical Notes

Interest in the history of the neurosciences both basic and clinical, as well as in related disciplines such as psychiatry and psychology, has always been active and today it continues to grow. It follows that the literature thereby generated is extensive, and we wish to mention and assess the publications that we have found of special value in our research. We hope our comments will be of assistance to others in coping with a rich store of source material.

I. GENERAL BACKGROUND

1. Unfortunately there is no entirely satisfactory history of nineteenth-century medicine available. There is, however, W. Coleman's *Biology in the Nineteenth Century* (1971) that can be strongly recommended. It is one of a series of books the aims of which are "to synthesize the discoveries and conclusions of recent scholarship in the history of science and present the general reader with an accurate, short narrative and analysis of the scientific activity of major periods in western history" (p. v). With the topics selected, none of which concerns the nervous system directly, he has been highly successful in his review of them. The "Bibliography" (pp. 167–182) is of particular interest.

2. K. E. Rothschuh's *History of Physiology* (1973) is a good survey of the problems of physiology and the various schools of the discipline that have evolved. Out of 368 pages, 218 deal with the nineteenth and twentieth centuries. Rothschuh's many writings on neurophysiology are referred to in the notes. See also G. J. Goodfield, *The Growth of Scientific Physiology* (1960); and E. Mendelsohn, "Physical models" (1965).

3. T. S. Hall's *Ideas of Life and Matter* (1969) is a scholarly and reliable survey of general physiology, 600 B.C. to A.D. 1900. It contains several topics that are relevant to the history of the neurosciences.

4. Gerald L. Geison in *Michael Foster and the Cambridge School of Physiology* (1978) examined a special topic: the stagnation of British physiology between 1840 and 1870, a curious situation to which we make reference below. Before 1840 the position was no better, although this period needs further study.

5. J. E. Lesch's *Science and Medicine in France* (1984) deals effectively with the development of French experimental physiology (1790–1855) and can be highly recommended.

6. J. T. Merz's *A History of European Thought in the Nineteenth Century* (1907–1914) is still of value as an introduction to our subject.

7. Another elderly classic is also worth consulting: F. A. Lange, *The History of Materialism* (1925), 2d book, pp. 153–362.

8. Concerning the philosophical backgrounds of German and British biology in the nineteenth century, two recent books are required reading, respectively, T. Lenoir, *The Strategy of Life* (1982) and P. F. Rehbock, *The Philosophical Naturalists* (1983).

II. HISTORY OF THE NEUROSCIENCES

Bibliographical sources are both primary and secondary.

1. Primary Sources

Many textbooks on the anatomy and physiology of the nervous system published in the first half of the nineteenth century contain historical material, varying considerably in quantity and quality. Those that are mentioned below are only a few of the ones available, and we have included later publications also. On the whole they are competent reviews of the literature but few include historical insights of note. Nevertheless they can be valuable sources, especially when compiled in critical vein by an eminent expert in the subject being discussed.

(a) K. F. Burdach in his *Vom Baue und Leben* (1819–1826) provides a remarkable reference work for the late eighteenth and early nineteenth centuries, as well as for earlier periods, quite apart from the book's importance as a presentation of current ideas, many of them his own. Alfred Meyer, the most outstanding modern historian of neuroanatomy who in particular has helped us to appreciate the important studies of German neuroanatomists, has described Burdach's book as "an unrivalled source of historical information on macroscopical neuroanatomy" (A. Meyer, "Karl Friedrich Burdach" [1970], p. 553). The only setback is that Burdach's German is difficult to comprehend, in part due to new terms he introduced.

(b) Possibly the best review of physiological literature during the first four decades of the nineteenth century is contained in Johannes Müller's *Handbuch*. He was particularly interested in the nervous system. We shall explore its bibliographical details shortly. Unfortunately, the English translator did not reproduce all the citations and also made other omissions so that his work is a version of the original and not a true translation.

(c) For English readers, R. B. Todd's edited *The Cyclopaedia* (1835–1859) is a splendid overview of midcentury opinion. The sections on neurophysiology and neuroanatomy provide excellent surveys. See, in particular, R. B. Todd, "Nervous system" (1847), published separately as *Physiology of the Nervous System* (1847).

(d) The outstanding French physiologist F. A. Longet, in *Recherches Expérimentales* (1841), presents us with a detailed and critical account of the experimental investigation of the form and function of the spinal cord and its roots, arranged chronologically from Lamarck (1809) to Valentin (1839) on pp. 4–86. He gives details of experiments and liberal quotations.

(e) F. A. Longet's *Anatomie et Physiologie* (1842) is primarily a textbook on the nervous system, but he presents a detailed survey of the literature and his references are mostly correct. He does, however, favor French authors.

(f) The Dutch anatomist and physiologist, J. L. C. Schroeder van der Kolk, in his *Professor J.L.C. Schroeder* (1859), begins his book with a good historical account of the spinal cord (pp. 1–28). His further descriptions of cord and medulla oblongata give us an excellent summary of midcentury opinion.

(g) E. A. Schäfer's edited *Text-book of Physiology* (1898–1900) is a majestic end-of-century survey of physiological knowledge, with full reference to Continental, British, and American literature by its distinguished contributors. Although some of the earlier research is discussed, the book is naturally concerned chiefly with the last two or three decades of the nineteenth century.

(h) Austin Flint (*The Physiology of the Nervous System* [1872]) also included historical material, but he favored unfairly the French school of physiology and neglected the German. His references are not always accurate.

(i) Luigi Luciani in *Human Physiology* (1911–1921) likewise included informative discussions of historical developments, often, however, revealing nationalistic bias. His references are few, rudimentary in content, and often inaccurate. Volume 3 deals with *Muscular and Nervous Systems* (1915).

(j) John F. Fulton's concern with the history of the neurosciences is evident in his textbook, *Physiology of the Nervous System* (1949), as well as in the many papers he contributed to the subject. Following in the Osler-Cushing tradition, he inspired many to study the history of medicine in general and the history of the neurosciences in particular.

The above are but a few of the primary sources that can be used as a guide to the appropriate "internal" literature when the historian needs it. But the historical assessments made by these authors are not always reliable, and all the literature they cite must be examined in the original in order to form an objective assessment.

2. Secondary Sources

(a) Of the older secondary literature, Max Neuburger's *Die historische Entwicklung* (1897) is by far the most important. He dealt only with experimental physiology of the brain and spinal cord up to the early 1820s, but his scholarly and penetrating analysis has not been surpassed. There is now an English translation, to which we make frequent reference, identifying it as "M. Neuburger (1981)."

(b) Jules Soury's *Le Système Nerveux Centrale* (1899) is also noteworthy, and its two large volumes are concerned with many aspects of the history of nervous system anatomy and physiology from Greek antiquity to the end of the nineteenth century. However, whereas Neuburger was concerned with identifying dominant neuroscientific concepts refined from a mass of primary material by means of analysis and synthesis in the best historical style, Soury preferred to present a chronological survey of individuals' achievements. He made less attempt to highlight the ideas they were creating and nurturing, so that his book is more like a vast review of the literature than a true historical exercise. By far the larger part ("Époque contemporaire," pp. 633–1782) is, in fact, a detailed survey of end-of-century opinions on the structure and function of the nervous system, with little or no historical perspective possible or attempted. Moreover, Soury's references are frequently faulty and there is no index. The historical part (pp. 1–631) is based on his essay of 1897 on "Cerveau [cerebrum]," at which the same criticisms can be leveled. However, each of these works can be consulted with profit, if their limitations are kept in mind.

(c) During the present century a large volume of secondary literature has appeared. It is uneven in quality, but the more important contributions to the themes we have selected are referred to in the foregoing chapters. However, we should point out that in the last few decades certain authors, mostly involved with the basic or clinical neurosciences and related disciplines, have published noteworthy books and articles on the history of the nervous system. These, too, have been cited, but we should list here the names of the more outstanding contributors and their special fields of research. We can state that all of their writings without exception are of estimable value and can be strongly recommended: Mary A. B. Brazier, neurophysiology; Paul F. Cranefield, neurophysiology; Hebbel E. Hoff, neurophysiology; Alfred Meyer, neuroanatomy, Thomas Willis; the late Walter Riese, neurology, neurophysiology; the late K. E. Rothschuh, neurophysiology (for bibliography, see idem, *Bibliographie* [1973] and *Bibliographie* [1983]); Francis Schiller, neuroanatomy, neurology, Paul Broca, etc.; and Owsei Temkin, many aspects of the basic and clinical neurosciences, as well as classic books and paper on other aspects of the history of medicine and biology, and their associations with philosophy (today's most eminent and distinguished historian of medicine).

Of these experts, Dr. Brazier's "The historical development" (1959) is the best short history of the neurosciences in English and the first volume of her work, *A History of Neurophysiology* (1984), which reaches to 1800 is an excellent introduction to our book, especially our chapter on nerve function. Her forthcoming second volume will presumably cover the nineteenth century. See also Dr. Brazier's "Rise of neurophysiology" (1957); "The growth of concepts" (1965); "La neurobiologie" (1977); and "Challenges from the philosophers" (1979). A. T. Rasmussen's *Some Trends in Neuroanatomy* (1947) is a useful survey mainly of neurohistology, but there are no references. The late John F. Fulton also merits individual mention because of his many historical publications and the interest he evoked. Unfortunately, we were not aware of the excellent book by Marc Jeannerod on the evolution of ideas concerning movement and the brain (*Le Cerveau Machine* [1983]) until the recent translation of it appeared (*The Brain Machine* [1986]). We have, therefore, been unable to incorporate his interesting arguments and conclusions.

(d) We should also call attention to the noteworthy historical studies of those in areas bordering upon the neurosciences: E. G. Boring, psychology; his *A History* (1957); and *A Source-book* (1965), with R. J. Herrnstein; K. E. Dewhurst, psychiatry, neuropsychiatry, Thomas Willis, John Hughlings Jackson; R. A. Hunter and I. MacAlpine, psychiatry; L. C. McHenry, *Garrison's History of Neurology* (1969), with good bibliographies; and R. M. Young, psychology, phrenology.

(e) Attention should also be drawn to certain collections of essays on neuroscientific topics that could easily be overlooked: F. N. L. Poynter, ed., *The History and Philosophy* (1958); L. Belloni, ed., *Essays on the History* (1963); K. E. Rothschuh, ed., *Von Boerhaave bis Berger* (1964).

(f) Finally, there is the extensive anthology of writings on neuroanatomy and neurophysiology from antiquity to the twentieth century compiled by one of us (E. C.) and the late Professor C. D. O'Malley, *The Human Brain and Spinal Cord* (1968). It is referred to frequently in the chapters above, as "Clarke and O'Malley (1968)," and we hope that its excerpts will complement the material we have amassed in our attempts to trace the few selected neuroscientific concepts discussed above.

III. BIOGRAPHY

1. General

There are several noteworthy and trustworthy general sources for biographical information on individuals, or that provide references to book and periodical literature on them:

(a) The various national biographies, some of which (the Italian, for example) are not yet completed.

(b) A. J. L. Jourdan, ed., *Dictionaire des Sciences Médicales* (1820–1825).

(c) J. B. Dezeimeris et al., eds., *Dictionaire Historique* (1828–1839).

(d) I. Fischer, ed., *Biographisches Lexikon* (1932–1933).
(e) A. Hirsch et al., eds., *Biographisches Lexikon* (1962). The best source available.
(f) *Dictionary of Scientific Biography* (1970–1980).
(g) M. Whitrow, ed., *Isis Cumulative Bibliogoraphy* (1971–1984), vols. 1–2 (1971) *Personalities.*
(h) J. Neu, ed., *Isis Cumulative Bibliography* 2 vols. (1980–1985), vol. 1 *Personalities* (1980).
(i) Wellcome Institute, *Subject Catalogue* (1980), *Biographical Section.*

2. Books On Neuroscientists

In addition to the above, there are a few special biographical source books.

(a) B. Kisch, "Forgotten leaders" (1954).
(b) K. Kolle, ed., *Grosse Nervenärzte* (1956–1963).
(c) W. Haymaker and F. Schiller, eds., *The Founders of Neurology* (1970). The best source available.
(d) L. Zusne, *Names in the History of Psychology* (1975).

IV. MÜLLER'S "HANDBUCH DER PHYSIOLOGIE"

During our studies the only bibliographical problem of any magnitude that we encountered concerns Johannes Müller's treatise on physiology. This classic appeared in various editions and translations during the 1830s and 1840s, and it is considered to be the first modern, systematic textbook on the subject. It represents an authoritative and discerning survey of each aspect of physiology, with plentiful references to the preceding literature, in particular to that from the first three or four decades of the nineteenth century. Peter Schmidt has analyzed carefully the origins of Müller's material, using the quantitative and graphic methods that the late Professor K. E. Rothschuh introduced into medical history (P. Schmidt, *Zu den geistigen Wurzeln* [1973]). This is a most informative study that tells us a great deal about early nineteenth-century physiology and its practitioners as well as revealing the formative influences that affected Müller.

Despite the popularity of Müller's textbook among students, teachers, and researchers, and the fact that many copies must have been disseminated throughout the Western world, it is difficult to establish the precise dates of the several editions that were published. There seem to be three reasons for this confusion. First, the original German editions were issued in parts, so that in the case, for example, of volume 1 of the 1st edition, the first of these appeared in the spring of 1833 and the last in the following year. This has allowed writers to cite it as 1833 or 1834. Similarly, the parts of volume 2 appeared between 1837 and 1840, thus again providing two alternative dates. We have given both dates where this is necessary to avoid confusion. Unfortunately, in the case of the *Handbuch*'s first edition, we could not locate a copy of the first volume and the copy we cite throughout our book is as follows: volume 1, 2d ed., 1835; volume 2, 1st ed., 1837–1840. The other edition we used was the fourth, also imperfect: volume 1 only, 1841–1844.

The following is an incomplete list of editions: 1st edition, vol. 1 (1833–1834); vol. 2 (1837–1840); 2d edition, vol. 1 (1835); vol. 2 (?1840); 3d edition, vol. 1 (1837–1838); vol. 2 (?); and 4th edition, vol. 1 1841–1844); vol. 2 (?1844). It seems that the only edition of the second volume was the first, 1837–1840 (E. du Bois-Reymond and P. Diepgen, eds., *Two Great Scientists* [1982], p. 134 n. 77).

The second reason for the confusion is the practice of issuing reprints of volumes having identical contents, but bearing dates that differ from the original. This is mainly true of the English, so-called translations which were also issued in parts. It is always difficult to discover the German editions from which they were prepared. Moreover, they are not faithful translations and must not be relied upon. Unfortunately, the translator took it upon himself to act also as an editor, and thus portions have been omitted (see chap. 4 n. 106) as have many of the references, which as indicated above are one of the main attractions of the work, for they reveal Müller's familiarity with, and evaluation of contemporary literature on physiology and allied sciences. The English version by William Baly appeared as follows: 1st edition, London, 1838–1842; and 1839–1843, presumably reprints; 2d edition, London, 1840–1843. There is also an American edition by John Bell (Philadelphia, 1843) from the 2d London edition. A French translation is *Manuel de Physiologie*, Paris (1845 and 1851) by A. J. L. Jourdan from the 4th (1844) German edition.

The third factor responsible for the difficulty with Müller's treatise is the paucity of copies available for inspection. It is possible that many were thumbed out of existence, but it is curious, as well as frustrating, to discover that few examples of Müller's classic treatise are to be found in libraries that were collecting actively in the first half of the nineteenth century. In the case of Britain, the stagnation of physiological research known to be present during this period no doubt had its effect (G. L. Geison, *Michael Foster* [1978]) as well as linguistic deficiencies. A wider study of the impact of Müller's treatise is clearly needed as well as further bibliographical elucidation of it.

Abbreviations

In the nineteenth century, Continental periodicals were often known by the name of their editor, and these have been included below in parentheses where appropriate.

AAP	*Archiv für Anatomie und Physiologie* ([J. F.] Meckel [the Younger]'s *Archiv*), Halle & Berlin, 1826–1832. Continued as *AAPM*
AAPM	*Archiv für Anatomie, Physiologie und wissenschaftliche Medizin* (Müller's *Archiv*), Berlin & Leipzig, 1834–1876.
ACP	*Annales de Chimie et de Physique,* Paris, 1816–1897. Continuation of *Annales de Chimie,* 1789–1815.
AGM	*Archives Générales de Medécine . . . ,* Paris, 1823–1879.
AP	*Archiv für die Physiologie* (Reil's *Archiv*), Halle, 1795–1815. Continued as *DAP.*
APC	*Annalen der Physik und Chemie* (Poggendorff's *Annalen*), Leipzig, 1824–1900.
BFMR	*British and Foreign Medical Review,* London, 1836–1847. Continued as *BFMCR.*
BFMCR	*British and Foreign Medico-Chirurgical Review,* London, 1848–1877.
BHM	*Bulletin of the History of Medicine,* Baltimore Md., 1933– .
CRAS	*Comptes Rendus Hebdomadaires des Séances de l'Académie des Sciences,* Paris.
DAP	*Deutsches Archiv für die Physiologie* ([J. F.] Meckel [the Younger]'s *Archiv*), Halle & Berlin, 1815–1825. Continued as *AAP.*

DNB	*Dictionary of national biography,* 22 vols., London: Smith Elder, 1908–1909.
DSB	*Dictionary of scientific biography,* 16 vols., New York: C. Scribner's, 1970–1980.
EMSJ	*Edinburgh Medical and Surgical Journal,* 1805–1855.
JHB	*Journal of the History of Biology,* Boston, Mass., 1968– .
JHM	*Journal of the History of Medicine and Allied Sciences,* New Haven, Conn., 1946– .
JP	*Journal of Physiology,* Cambridge & London, 1883–1884– .
JPEP	*Journal de Physiologie Expérimentale et Pathologique* (Magendie's *Journal*), Paris, 1821–1831.
MH	*Medical History,* London, 1957– .
PM	*The Philosophical Magazine,* 1798–1813; *The Philosophical Magazine and Journal,* 1814–1826, and a variety of similar titles thereafter. London & Edinburgh.
PRS	*Abstracts of Papers Printed in the Philosophical Transactions,* 1800–1854; and then *Proceedings of the Royal Society,* 1856–1904.
PT	*Philosophical Transactions of the Royal Society of London,* 1665– .
SAGM	*Sudhoff's Archiv für Geschichte der Medizin,* Leipzig, 1908– .

Bibliography

Abernethy, John.

1822 *Physiological lectures, exhibiting a general view of Mr Hunter's physiology, and of his researches in comparative anatomy. . . .* 2d ed. London: Longman et al.

Abrams, M. H.

1953 *The mirror and the lamp. Romantic theory and the literary tradition.* New York: Oxford University Press.

Achard, Thomas.

1969 *Die Physiologe F. Bidder 1810–1894.* Zürich: Juris.

Ackerknecht, Erwin H.

1959 *A short history of psychiatry.* New York & London: Hafner.

1964 "Johann Lucas Schoenlein," *JHM,* 19:13–38.

1967 *Medicine at the Paris Hospital 1794–1848.* Baltimore: Johns Hopkins Press.

1974 "The history of the discovery of the vegetative (autonomic) nervous system," *MH,* 18:1–18.

Ackerknecht, Erwin H., and Henri V. Vallois.

1956 *Franz Joseph Gall, inventor of phrenology and his collection.* Madison: University of Wisconsin Medical School.

Ackermann, Jacob Fidelis.

1813 *De nervei systematis primordiis commentatio.* Mannheim & Heidelberg: Schwann & Goetz.

Adanson, Michel.

1759 *A voyage to Senegal, the Isle of Goree and the River Gambia.* London: J. Nourse & W. Johnston.

Addison, Thomas.

1837 "On the influence of electricity as a remedy in certain convulsive and spasmodic diseases," *Guy's Hospital Reports,* 2:493–507.

Adelon, [Nicolas Philibert] et al., eds.
1812– 1822 *Dictionaire des sciences médicales, par une société de médecins et de chirurgiens.* 60 vols. Paris: C. L. F. Panckoucke.

Adler, J.
1971 "Winslow und das vegetative Nervensystem." Inaugural-Dissertation, University of Zürich.

Aesch, Alexander Gode-von (*see* Gode-von Aesch, Alexander).

Agassi, Joseph.
1969 "Sir John Herschel's philosophy of success," *Historical Studies in the Physical Sciences.* 1:1–36.

Akert, Konrad, and Michael P. Hammond.
1962 "Emanuel Swedenborg (1688–1772) and his contributions to neurology," *MH,* 6:255–266.

Albury, William Randall.
1974 "Physiological explanation in Magendie's manifesto of 1809," *BHM,* 48:90–99.
1977 "Experiment and explanation in the physiology of Bichat and Magendie." *Studies in History of Biology.* 1:47–131.

Aldini, Giovanni.
1794 *De animali electricitate dissertationes duae.* Bologna: ex Typographia Instituti Scientiarum.
1803 *An account of the late improvements in galvanism . . .* London: Cuthell & Martin.
1804 *Essai théoretique et expérimental sur la galvanisme . . .* Paris: Fournier.

Alison, William Pulteney.
1826 "Observations on the physiological principle of sympathy. Chiefly in reference to the peculiar doctrines of Mr Charles Bell." *Transactions of the Medico-Chirurgical Society of Edinburgh.* 2:165–228.
1831 *Outline of physiology.* Edinburgh: Blackwood.

[Alison, W. P.]
1837 "Travers, Mayo, Ley, Hall, &c. on the physiology and pathology of their nervous system." *BFMR,* 3:1–39.

Amacher, M. Peter.
1964 "Thomas Laycock, I. M. Sechenov, and the reflex arc concept." *BHM,* 38:168–183.

Amici, Giovanni Battista.
1818 *De' microscopii catadiottrici memoria.* Modena: Società Tipografica.

Ampère, André Marie.
1820 "Mémoire . . . sur les effets des courans électriques," *ACP,* 2d series, 15:59–76. Continued as "Du mémoire sur l'action mutuelle entre deux courans électriques, entre un courant

électrique et un aimant ou le globe terrestre, et entre deux aimans [*sic*]," pp. 170–218.

Ampère, A. M., and J. Babinet.

1822 *Exposé des nouvelles découvertes sur l'électricité et le magnetisme* . . . , Paris: Méquignon-Marcis.

Anderson, John.

1837 *Sketch of the comparative anatomy of the nervous system; with remarks on the development of the human embryo.* London: Sherwood, Gilbert, and Piper.

Andral, Gabriel.

1829–1833 *Clinique médicale, ou choix d'observations recueillies à l'Hôpital de la Charité. . . .* 2d ed. 5 vols. Paris: Gabon; Cavellin.

1835–1836 "Lectures on diseases of the brain and nervous system . . . Lecture XIII. Atrophy of the brain and spinal marrow." *Lancet* (27 February), 1:841–846.

Andral, Gabriel et al., eds.

1829–1836 *Dictionnaire de médecine et de chirurgie pratiques.* 15 vols. Paris: Méquignon & J. B. Baillière.

Andreoli, Armando.

1961 *Zur geschichtlichen Entwicklung der Neuronentheorie.* Basel: B. Schwabe.

Anonymous.

1803 [an XII] *Exposition de la doctrine physionomique du Docteur Gall, ou nouvelle théorie du cerveau, considérée comme le siége des facultés intellectuelles et morales.* Paris: Henrichs.

1806 "Prof. Bischoff's account of Dr. Gall's cranioscopy," *EMSJ*, 2:345–366.

1807*a* *Craniologie, ou découvertes nouvelles du Docteur F.J. Gall, concernant le cerveau, le crâne, et les organes. Ouvrage traduit de l'Allemand.* Paris: H. Nicolle.

1807*b* *Some account of Dr. Gall's new theory of physiognomy, founded upon the anatomy and physiology of the brain, and the form of the skull.* London: Longman et al.

1807*c* ["Review of *Darstellungen des Gegensatzes* (1805) by J. W. Ritter"], *EMSJ*, 3:228–241.

1809 "Report on a memoir of Drs Gall and Spurzheim, relative to the anatomy of the brain [15 April 1808]. By M. M. Tenon, Portal, Sabatier, Pinel, and Cuvier . . . ," *EMSJ*, 5:36–66.

1817 "Memoirs of the life of James Johnstone M.D. . . . " *Transactions of the Medical Society of London,* 1 (part 2):301–309.

1823 "Dr Gall's second dissection of the brain," *Weekly Medico-chirurgical and Philosophical Magazine,* 1:317–318.

1824*a* ["Researches of Malacarne and Reil. Present state of cerebral anatomy"], *EMSJ,* 21:98–141.

1824*b* ["Recent discoveries on the physiology of the nervous system"], *EMSJ,* 21:141–159.

1836*a* ["Review of *Illustrations of the comparative anatomy of the nervous system* by Joseph Swan"]. *BFMR,* 2:192–196.

1836*b* ["Review of *Report on animal physiology; comprising a review of the progress and state of theory, and of our information respecting the blood and the powers which circulate it,* by William Clark"]. *BFMR,* 1:379–396.

1837*a* ["Review of *The human brain* (1836) by Samuel Solly"]. *EMSJ,* 47:477–485.

1837*b* ["Mr. Solly on the human brain"]. *BFMR,* 4:485–488. A review of S. Solly, *The human brain* (1836).

1839*a* ["Review of *Histoire générale et particulière des anomalies de l'organisation* by Isidore Geoffroy St. Hilaire"]. *BFMR,* 8:1–36.

1839*b* ["Review of *On the physiological inferences to be deduced from the structure of the nervous system in the invertebrated classes of animals* by William B. Carpenter"]. *BFMR,* 8:506–511.

1840 ["Review of *Illustrations of the comparative anatomy of the nervous system* by Joseph Swan"]. *EMSJ,* 53:228–235.

1841*a* "Rapport des Commissaires chargés par le Roi de l'examen du magnétisme animal." In C. Burdin jeune and F. Dubois (d'Amiens), *Histoire académique* (1841). Pp. 26–91.

1841*b* "Valentin on the functions of the nerves." *BFMR,* 11:277–305.

1842 "Versuch einer kritischen Beleuchtung der Lex Belliana." *Archiv für physiologische Heilkunde* (W. Roser et al.: Stuttgart), 1:295–310.

1844 ["Volkmann, Bidder, Stilling, van Deen, Budge: anatomy and physiology of the nervous system"]. *BFMR,* 17:379–403.

1854 "Dr. de Chaumont on the sympathetic nervous system." *Monthly Journal of Medical Science* (Edinburgh), 19:179–183.

1962 *Jan Evangelista Purkyně.* Prague: State Medical Publishing House.

1974 *Sex and science. Phrenological reflections on sex and marriage in nineteenth century America.* New York: Arno Press.

Appel, Toby Anita.

1975 "The Cuvier-Geoffroy debate on unity of composition." Ph.D. Dissertation, Princeton University.

Appleyard, R.
1930 *Pioneers of electrical communication.* London: Macmillan.

Aristotle.
1910 *Historia animalium by D'Arcy Wentworth Thompson.* In J. A. Smith and W. D. Ross, eds. *The works of Aristotle* (1908–1931). Vol. 4.
1921 *De motu animalium . . . by A.S.L. Farquharson.* In J. A. Smith and W. D. Ross, eds., *The works of Aristotle* (1908–1931). Vol. 5.

Arnett, L. D.
1904 "The soul—a study of past and present beliefs." *The American Journal of Psychology,* 15:121–200, 347–382.

Arnold, Friedrich.
1826*a* "*Observationes nonnullis neurologicas de parte cephalica nervi sympathici in homine.*" Inaugural-Dissertation, Heidelberg University.
1826*b* "Beschreibung des Kopftheils der sympathischen Nerven beim Kalb, nebst einigen Beobachtungen über diesen Theil beim Menschen." *Zeitschrift für Physiologie* (F. Tiedemann & G. R. Treviranus: Heidelberg), 2:125–172.
1828 *Ueber den Ohrenknoten. Eine anatomisch-physiologische Abhandlung.* Heidelberg: C. F. Winter.
1829 "Mémoire sur le ganglion otique." *Repertoire générale d'Anatomie et de Physiologie pathologique et de Clinique chirurgicale.* (G. Breschet: Paris), 8:1–31.
1831 *Der Kopftheil des vegetativen Nervensystems beim Menschen, in anatomischer und physiologischer Hinsicht bearbeitet.* Heidelberg & Leipzig: K. Groos.
1851 *Handbuch der Anatomie des Menschen mit besonderer Rücksicht auf Physiologie und praktische Medicin.* 3 vols. Freiburg: Herder'sche Verlagshandlung.

Arnold, Johann Wilhelm.
1842 *Die Lehre von der Reflex-Function für Physiologen und Aerzte.* Heidelberg: K. Groos.

Asratyan, Ezras Asratovich.
1953 *I. P. Pavlov. His life and work.* Moscow: Foreign Languages Publishing House.

Association for Research in Nervous and Mental Diseases.
1930 *The vegetative nervous system. An investigation of the more recent advances.* Vol. 9. Baltimore: Williams & Wilkins.

Aubertin, Simon Alexandre Ernest.
1861*a* "Discussion." *Bulletin de la Société d'Anthropologie de Paris,* 2:66–67.

1861*b* "Reprise de la discussion sur la forme et le volume du cerveau." *Bulletin de la Société d'Anthropologie de Paris,* 2:209–220.

Aumueller, G.
1984 "Benedict Stillings (1810–1879) Untersuchungen über das Rückenmark—ein Wendepunkt in der neuroanatomischen Forschung." *Medizinhistorisches Journal,* 19:53–59.

Autenrieth, Johann Friedrich Ferdinand von.
1807 "Bemerkungen über die Verschiedenheit beyder Geschlechter und ihrer Zeugungsorgane, als Beitrag zu einer Theorie der Anatomie," *AP,* 7:1–139.

Baader, Joseph.
1762 *Observationes medicae, incisionibus cadaverum anatomicis illustratae.* In E. Sandifort, *Thesaurus dissertationum* (1768–1778). 3 (1778):1–62.

Bacq, Z. M.
1975 *Chemical transmission of nerve impulses. A historical sketch.* Oxford: Pergamon Press.

Baillarger, Jules Gabriel François.
1840 "Recherches sur la structure de la couche corticale des circonvolutions du cerveau." *Mémoires de l'Académie Royale de Médecine* (Paris), 8:149–183.

Baker, John Randall.
1945 *The discovery of the uses of colouring agents in biological micro-technique.* London: Williams & Norgate.
1948–1955 "The cell-theory: a restatement, history and critique." *Quarterly Journal of Microscopical Science,* 1948, 89:103–125; 1949, 90:87–108; 1952, 93:157–190; 1953, 94:407–444; 1955, 96:449–481.

Balfour, Francis Maitland.
1876–1878 "The development of the elasmobranch fishes." *Journal of Anatomy and Physiology,* 1876, 10:377–411, 517–570, 672–688; 1877, 11:128–172, 406–490, 674–706; 1878, 12:177–216.

Barker, Lewellys F.
1898 "On the validity of the neurone doctrine." *American Journal of Insanity,* 55:31–49.
1899 *The nervous system and its constituent neurones. Designed for the use of practitioners of medicine and of students of medicine and psychology.* New York: D. Appleton.

Barnes, Barry, and Steven Shapin, eds.
1979 *Natural order. Historical studies of scientific culture.* Beverly Hills & London: Sage.

Barthez, Paul Joseph.
1806 *Nouveaux élémens de la science de l'homme*. 2d ed. 2 vols. Paris: Goujon & Brunot.
Baxter, Alice, and John Farley.
1979 "Mendel and meiosis." *JHB*, 12:137–173.
Bayliss, Sir William Maddock.
1931 *Principles of general physiology*. 4th ed. London: Longman, Green.
Bayne, David.
1739 *A new essay on the nerves, and the doctrine of the animal spirits rationally considered* . . . 2d ed. London: W. Innys & J. Manby.
Beccario, Giambattista.
1753 *Dell'elettricismo artificiale e naturale libri due*. Turin: F. A. Campana.
1776 *A treatise upon artificial electricity*. London: J. Nourse.
Beck, Theodor.
1909 "Die Galenischen Hirnnerven in moderner Beleuchtung," *SAGM*, 3:110–114.
Beck, Thomas Snow.
1846 "On the nerves of the uterus." *PT*, 136:213–222, 233–235.
1847 "On the structure and function of the sympathetic nervous system, as distinct from, and independent of, the cerebro-spinal system," *Lancet*, i:615–617.
Béclard, Pierre Augustin.
1821 "Additions au système de la vie organique." In M. F. X. Bichat, *Anatomie générale* (1821). 1:398–409.
1823 *Eléméns d'anatomie général, ou description de tous les genres d'organes qui composent le corps humain*. Paris: Béchet Jeune.
1830 *Elements of anatomy*. Trans. Robert Knox. Edinburgh: Maclachland & Stewart.
Becquerel, Antoine César.
1834–1840 *Traité expérimental de l'électricité et du magnétisme et de leurs rapports avec les phénomènes naturels*. 6 vols. Paris: F. Didot.
1849 "Note relative au developpement de l'electricité dans l'acte de la contraction musculaire." *CRAS*, 28:663–664.
Bégin, [Louis Jacques].
1841 "Discours prononcé par M. Bégin." *Recueil de Mémoires de Médecine, de Chirurgie et de Pharmacie Militaires*, 51:361–385.

Bell, Sir Charles.
[1811] *Idea of a new anatomy of the brain; submitted for the observations of his friends.* [London: Strahan & Preston].
1821 "On the nerves; giving an account of some experiments on their structure and functions, which lead to a new arrangement of the system." *PT.* Part I. Pp. 398–424.
1822 "Of the nerves which associate the muscles of the chest, in the actions of breathing, speaking, and expression. Being a continuation of the paper on the structure and functions of the nerves," *PT.* Part II. Pp. 284–312.
1826 "On the nervous circle which connects the voluntary muscles with the brain." *PT.* Part II. Pp. 163–173.
1830 *The nervous system of the human body. . . .* London: Longman.
1834 "On the functions of some parts of the brain, and on the relations between the brain and nerves of motion and sensation." *PT.* Part I. Pp. 471–483.

Bell, John, and Sir Charles Bell.
1823 *The anatomy and physiology of the human body . . .* 5th ed. 3 vols., London: Longman et al. (Charles Bell wrote the section on the nervous system.)
1829 *The anatomy and physiology of the human body.* 7th ed. 3 vols. London: Longman et al. (This was the last edition.)

Belloni, Luigi.
1968 "Die Neuroanatomie von Marcello Malpighi." *Analecta Medico-Historica,* 3:193–206.
1977 "Charles Bonnet et Vincenzo Malacarne sur le cervelet siège de l'âme et sur l'impression du crâne dans le crétinisme." *Gesnerus,* 34:69–81.

Belloni, Luigi, ed.
1963 *Essays on the history of Italian neurology. Proceedings of the International Symposium on the History of Neurology. Varenna. 30. VII./ 1. IX. 1961,* Milan: Studi e Testi 6, Università degli Studi.

Benassi, Enrico.
1963 "Ipotesi elettropathogenetiche e proposte elettroterapiche nell'opera di Luigi Galvani." In L. Belloni, ed. *Essays* (1963). Pp. 131–138.

Bennett, John Hughes.
1837 *Inaugural dissertation on the physiology and pathology of the brain: Being an attempt to ascertain what portions of that organ are more immediately connected with motion, sensa-*

tion, and intelligence . . . Edinburgh: J. Carfrae & Son.
1860 [Letter from J. H. Bennett to Mrs. Marshall Hall, 18 March 1860], Edinburgh University Library manuscripts, 2007/1–4(2).

Bentley, Madison.
1916 "The psychological antecedents of phrenology," *Psychological Monographs* (Princeton & Lancaster, Pa.) 21:102–115.

Bérard, Frédéric Joseph.
1823 *Doctrine des rapports du physique et du moral, pour servir de fondement à la physiologie dite intellectuelle et à la métaphysique.* Paris: Gabon.

Bérard, Frédéric Joseph, and Horace de Montègre.
1813 "Cranioscopie." In F. P. Chauventon and F. V. Mérat de Vaumartoise, eds. *Dictionnaire* (1812–1822). 7:300–318.

Berg, Alexander.
1942 "Die Lehre von der Faser als Form-und Funktionselement des Organismus. Die Geschichte des biologisch-medizinischen Grundproblems vom kleinsten Bauelement des Körpers bis zur Begründung der Zellenlehre." *Archiv für pathologische Anatomie und Physiologie* (R. Virchow: Berlin), 309:333–460.

Bernard, Claude.
1853 "Sur les phénomènes réflexes." *Comptes-Rendus des Seances de la Société de Biologie* (Paris), 4 (Comptes rendus):149–151.
1855–1856 *Leçons de physiologie expérimentale appliquée à la médecine, faites au Collège de France.* 2 vols. Paris: J. B. Baillière.
1858 *Leçons sur la physiologie el la pathologie du système nerveux.* 2 vols. Paris: J. B. Baillière.
1865 *Introduction à l'étude de la médecine expérimentale.* Paris: J. B. Baillière. English trans. *An introduction* (1927).
1877 *Leçons sur le diabète et la glycogenèse animale.* Paris: J. B. Baillière.
1878 *La science expérimentale.* Paris: J. B. Baillière.
1927 *An introduction to the study of experimental medicine, translated by Henry Copley Greene* . . . New York: Macmillan.

Berzelius, Jöns Jacob.
1817–1830 *Läerbobk i Kemien* . . . *Andra upplagan* . . . 6 vols., Stockholm. (Not seen.)
1818 *A view of the progress and present state of animal chemistry.* Trans. from Swedish, Gustavus Brunnmark. London: J. Callow.

Best, A. E.
1969 "Pourfour du Petit's experiments on the origin of the sympathetic nerve." *MH,* 13:154–174.

Bianchi, Nicomede.
1874 *Carlo Matteucci e l'Italia del suo tempo. Narrazione di . . . Corredata di documenti inediti.* Rome, Turin, and Florence: Bocca.

Bichat, Marie François Xavier.
An VIII [1800*a*] *Recherches physiologiques sur la vie et la mort.* Paris: Brosson, Gabon.
1800*b* *Traité des membranes en géneral et de divers membranes en particulier.* Paris: Richard, Caille et Ravier.
1801 *Anatomie générale, appliquée à la physiologie et la médecine.* 4 vols. Paris: Brosson, Gabon. English trans. *General anatomy* (1824).
1801–1803 *Traité d'anatomie descriptive.* 5 vols. Paris: Gabon, Brosson. (Bichat wrote the first three volumes, but the fourth was prepared by Mathieu-François Buisson, and the fifth by Philibert-Joseph Roux, both posthumously.)
1815 *Physiological researches on life and death by Xavier Bichat.* Trans. F. Gold. London: Longman et al.
1821 *Anatomie générale, appliquée à la physiologie et à la médecine. [notes and additions by P. A. Béclard].* 4 vols. Paris: J. A. Brosson & J. S. Chaudé.
1824 *General anatomy, applied to physiology and the practice of medicine.* Trans. C. Coffyn, rev. G. Calvert. 2 vols. London: S. Highley.
1827 *Physiological researches upon life and death.* Trans. F. Gold, with notes by F. Magendie. Boston: Richardson & Card.

Bidder, Friedrich Heinrich.
1847 *Zur Lehre von dem Verhältniss der Ganglienkörper zu den Nervenfasern.* Leipzig: Breitfopf & Haertel.

Bidder, Friedrich Heinrich, and A. W. Vollkmann.
1842 *Die Selbständigkeit des sympathischen Nervensystems durch anatomische Untersuchungen nachgewiesen.* Leipzig: Breitkopf & Härtel.

Bischoff, Christian Heinrich Ernst.
1809 *Exposition of Gall's system.* Berlin: 1809. (Not seen.)

Bischoff, Christian Heinrich Ernst, and C. W. Hufeland.
1805 *Darstellung der Gallschen Gehirn-und Schädel-Lehre . . . nebst Bemerkungen über diese Lehre, von C.W. Hufeland.* . . . Berlin: L. W. Wittich.

Blainville, Henri Marie de Ducrotay.
1821 "Considérations générales sur le système nerveux." *Nouveau Bulletin des Sciences de la Société Philomatique de Paris.* Pp. 39–58.
1829 *Cours de physiologie générale et comparée.* 3 vols. Paris: Rouen Frères.
1845 *Histoire des sciences de l'organisation et de leurs progrés, comme base de la philosophie.* 3 vols. Paris & Lyon: Perisse Frères.
Blair, D. M.
1932 "Winslow and the sympathetic system." *British Medical Journal.* ii:1200.
Blane, Sir Gilbert.
[1788] *A lecture on muscular motion, read at the Royal Society, the 13th and 20th of November, 1788.* London: J. Murray.
1822 *Select dissertations on several subjects of medical science.* London: T. & G. Underwood.
Blondel, Charles.
1914 *La psycho-physiologie de Gall: Ses idées directrices.* Paris: F. Alcan.
Blumenbach, Johann Friedrich.
1787 *Institutiones physiologicae.* Göttingen: J. C. Dieterich.
1805 *Handbuch der vergleichenden Anatomie.* Göttingen: Dietrich.
1815 *The elements of physiology.* Trans. with notes by John Elliotson. 4th ed. London: Longman.
Boakes, Robert.
1984 *From Darwin to behaviourism: Psychology and the minds of animals.* Cambridge: Cambridge University Press.
Boas, George.
1925 *French philosophies of the Romantic period.* Baltimore: Johns Hopkins Press.
Bochefontaine, L. T.
1876 "Étude expérimentale de l'influence exercée par la faradisation de l'écorce grise du cerveau sur quelques fonctions de la vie organique." *Archives de Physiologie normale et pathologique* (Paris), 2d series, 3:140–172.
Boerhaave, Herman.
1742–1746 *Academical lectures on the theory of physic.* 4 vols. London: W. Innys.
Bonald, Louis Gabriel Ambroise de.
1818 *Du divorce consideré au XIXe siècle, relativement à l'état domestique et à l'état public de société.* 3d ed. Paris: Le Clerc.

1838 *Recherches philosophiques sur les premiers objets de connoisances morales.* 3d ed. 2 vols. Paris: Le Clerc.

Bonin, Gerhardt von, trans.

1960 *Some papers on the cerebral cortex.* Springfield, Ill.: C. C Thomas.

Bonnet, Charles.

1770 *La palingénésie philosophique ou ideés sur l'état passé et sur l'état futur des êtres vivans. . . .* 2 vols. Geneva: J. M. Bruyset, C. Philibert & B. Chirol.

Bordeu, Théophile de.

1751 *Recherches anatomiques sur la position des glandes et sur leur action.* Paris: G. F. Quillan.

Boring, Edwin G.

1957 *A history of experimental psychology.* 2d ed. New York: Appleton-Century-Crofts.

1961 "The beginning and growth of measurement in psychology." *Isis,* 52:238–257.

Boruttau, Heinrich.

1922 *Emil du Bois-Reymond.* Vienna: Rikola.

Bostock, John.

1818 *An account of the history and present state of galvanism.* London: Baldwin, Cradock, & Joy.

1828–1830 *An elementary system of physiology.* 2d ed. 3 vols. London: Baldwin & Cradock.

Bouillaud, Jean Baptiste.

1825*a* "Recherches cliniques propres à démontrer que la perte de la parole correspond à la lésion des lobules antérieurs du cerveau, et à confirmer l'opinion de M. GALL, sur le siège de l'organe du langage articulé." *AGM,* 1st series, 8:25–45.

1825*b* *Traité clinique et physiologique de l'encéphalite, ou inflammation du cerveau, et de ses suites. . . .* Paris: J. B. Baillière.

1827*a* "Recherches expérimentelles tendant à prouver que le cervelet préside aux actes de la station et de la progression, et non à l'instinct de la propagation," *AGM,* 1st series, 15:64–91.

1827*b* "Recherches cliniques tendant à réfuter l'opinion de M. Gall sur les fonctions du cervelet, et à prouver que cet organe préside aux actes de l'équilibration, de la station et de la progression." *AGM,* 1st series, 15:225–247.

1839–1840 "Exposition de nouveaux faits à l'appui de l'opinion qui localise dans les lobules antérieures du cerveau le principe législateur de la parole; examen préliminaire des objections dont cette opinion a été le sujet," *Bulletin de l'Académie*

Royale de Médecine (Paris), 4:282–328, 333–349, 353–369.

1847–1848 "Recherches cliniques propres à démontrer que le sens du langage articulé est le principe coordinateur des mouvements de la parole resident dans les lobules antérieures du cerveau," ibid., 13:699–719 (22 February 1848); and ibid., pp. 778–808 and discussion, pp. 808–816 (7 March 1848).

Bowman, I. A.

1975 "William Cullen (1710–1790) and the primacy of the nervous system." Ph.D. Dissertation, Indiana University.

Bracegirdle, Brian.

1978 *A history of microtechnique. The evolution of the microtome and the development of tissue preparation.* London: Heinemann.

Brachet, Jean Louis.

1830 *Recherches expérimentales sur les fonctions du système nerveux ganglionaire, et sur leur application à la pathologie.* Paris: Gabon.

Bradbury, Savile.

1967 *The evolution of the microscope.* Oxford: Pergamon.

Brazier, Mary A. B.

1957 "Rise of neurophysiology in the 19th century." *Journal of Neurophysiology,* 20:212–226.

1958 "The evolution of concepts relating to the electrical activity of the nervous system. 1600–1800." In F. N. L. Poynter, ed. *The history and philosophy* (1958). Pp. 191–222.

1959 "The historical development of neurophysiology." In J. Field, ed. *Handbook of physiology* (1959–1977), Section I. Neurophysiology. Vol. 1. Pp. 1–58.

1963 "Felice Fontana." In L. Belloni, ed. *Essays* (1963). Pp. 107–116.

1965 "The growth of concepts relating to brain mechanisms," *Journal of the History of the Behavioral Sciences,* 1:218–234.

1977 "La neurobiologie, du vitalisme au matérialisme." *La Recherche,* 8:965–971.

1979 "Challenges from the philosophers to the neuroscientists." *Brain and mind, Ciba Foundation Symposium.* No. 69. Pp. 5–43.

1982 "The problem of neuromuscular action: two 17th century Dutchmen." In F. C. Rose and W. F. Bynum, eds. *Historical aspects* (1982). Pp.13–22.

1984 *A history of neurophysiology in the 17th and 18th centuries. From concept to experiment.* New York: Raven Press.

Breschet, Gilbert.

1836 "Recherches anatomiques et physiologiques sur l'organe de l'ouïe et sur l'audition dans l'homme et les animaux vertébrés." *Mémoires de l'Académie Royale de Médecine* (Paris), 5:229–523.

Brigham, Amariah.

1840 *An inquiry concerning the diseases and functions of the brain, the spinal cord and the nerves.* New York: G. Adlard.

Brissenden, R. F., and J. C. Eade, eds.

1976 *Studies in the eighteenth century III.* Canberra: Australian National University Press.

Broca, Pierre Paul.

1861 "Remarques sur le siège de la faculté du langage articulé; suivies d'une observation d'aphémie (perte de la parole)." *Bulletin de la Société de l'Anatomie de Paris,* 36:330–357. Trans. in G. von Bonin, *Some papers* (1960). Pp. 49–72.

Brooks, Chandler M., and Paul F. Cranefield.

1959 *The historical development of physiological thought.* New York: Hafner.

Broussais, François Joseph Victor.

1818 "Réflexions sur les fonctions du systême nerveux en général, sur celles du grand sympathique en particulier, et sur quelques autres points de physiologie." *Journal Universel des Sciences Médicales* (Paris), 12:5–43, 129–167.

1828 *De l'irritation et de la folie, ouvrage dans lequel les rapports du physique et du moral sont établis sur les bases de la médecine physiologique . . .* Brussels: Laurent.

1829–1834 *Examen des doctrines médicales et des systèmes de nosologie, précédé de propositions renfermant la substance de la médecine physiologique.* 3d ed. 4 vols. Paris: Mlle. Delaunay.

1836*a* *Cours de phrénologie.* Paris: J. B. Baillière.

1836*b* "Lectures on phrenology delivered in 1836 in the University of Paris. Lecture VI. The functions of the cerebellum," *Lancet,* ii:577–583.

1839 *De l'irritation et de la folie . . .* 2d ed. 2 vols. Paris: J. B. Baillière.

Brown, J. M.

1969 "The electric current in early nineteenth-century French physics." *Historical Studies in the Physical Sciences,* 1:61–103.

Brown-Séquard, Charles Édouard.

1860 *Course of lectures on the physiology and pathology of the central nervous system. Delivered at the Royal College of Surgeons of England in May, 1858.* Philadelphia: Collins.

Bruford, W. H.

1962 *Culture and society in classical Weimar.* Cambridge: Cambridge University Press.

Brunschwig, Alexander.

1933 "Jean Fréderic [*sic*] Lobstein. The first professor of pathology." *Annals of Medical History,* 2d series, 5:82–84.

Büchner, Georg.

1836 "Probevorlesung ueber Schädelnerven gehalten in Zürich 1836." In W. R. Lehmann, ed. *Georg Büchner* (1967–) Vol. 2 (1971). Pp. 291–301.

Budge, Julius Ludwig.

1841–1842 *Untersuchungen über das Nervensystem.* 2 vols. Frankfurt am Main: Jäger.

1851 "Observations sur la partie intercranienne du nerf sympathique, et sur l'influence qu'exercent les troisième, quatrième, cinquième et sixième paires sur les mouvements de l'iris," *CRAS,* 33:418–423.

Budge, Julius Ludwig, and Augustus Volney Waller.

1851 "Recherches sur le système nerveux . . . Première partie. Action de la partie cervicale du nerf grand sympathique et d'une portion de la moelle épinière sur la dilatation de la pupille," *CRAS,* 33:370–374.

Buess, Heinrich.

1964 "Vom Beitrag der Schweizer Ärzte zur Geschichte der Neuronentheorie." In K. E. Rothschuh, ed. *Von Boerhaave bis Berger* (1964). Pp. 186–210.

Burdach, Karl Friedrich.

1819–1826 *Vom Baue und Leben des Gehirns.* 3 vols. Leipzig: Dyk.

Burdach, Karl Friedrich et al.

1826–1840 *Die Physiologie als Erfahrungswissenschaft . . .* 6 vols. Leipzig: L. Voss.

Burdin, C. jeune and E. F. Dubois (d'Amiens).

1841 *Histoire académique du magnétisme animal . . .* Paris: J. B. Baillière.

Burdin, Jean.

1803 *Cours d'études médicales, ou exposition de la structure de l'homme comparée à celle des animaux; de l'histoire de ses maladies; des connaissances acquises sur l'action régulière de ses organes, etc., etc.* 3 vols. in 5. Paris: L. Duprat, Letellier.

Burr, H. S., and F. S. C. Northrop.

1935 "The electrodynamic theory of life." *Quarterly Review of Biology,* 10:322–333.

Bynum, William F.

1973 "The anatomical method, natural theology, and the functions of the brain." *Isis,* 64:445–468.

Cabanis, Pierre Jean George.

1805 *Rapports du physique et du moral de l'homme.* 2d ed. 2 vols.

Paris: Crapart, Caille & Ravier. 1st ed., 1802. 3d ed., 1815 with same imprint. 4th ed. revised and extended by Étienne Pariset. 2 vols. Paris: Bechet Jeune, 1824.

1956*a* *Rapports du physique et du moral de l'homme.* In *Oeuvres* (1956). Part 1. Pp. 105–631.

1956*b* *Oeuvres philosophiques de Cabanis.* Paris: Presses Universitaires de France.

Cailliet, Emile.

1943 *La tradition littéraire des idéologues.* Philadelphia: The American Philosophical Society. Vol. 19.

Caldani, Leopoldo Marco Antonio.

1762*a* "Lettre . . . à Mr. Albert de Haller. Sur l'insensibilité & l'irritabilité de quelques parties des animaux." In A. von Haller, *Mémoires* (1762), 3:1–56. Also in G. B. Fabri, *Sulla insensitività* (1757–1759), 1 (1757):269–336.

1762*b* "Sur l'insensibilité et l'irritabilité de Mr. Haller. Seconde lettre." In A. von Haller, *Mémoires* (1762), 3:343–485.

Calmeil, Louis Florentin.

1828 "Sur la structure, les fonctions et le ramollissement de la moelle épinière." *Journal des Progrès des Sciences et Institutions Médicales . . .* (Paris), 11:77–124.

Cameron, G. R.

1955 "Rudolf Albert Kölliker (1817–1905)." *Annals of Science,* 11:167–172.

Campbell, Henry Fraser.

1857 *Essays on the secretory and the excito-secretory system of nerves.* Philadelphia: J. B. Lippincott. (This was not seen.)

Camper, Pieter.

1778 "Deux discours sur l'analogie qu'il y a entre la structure du corps humain et celle des quadrupèdes, des oisseaux et des poissons." In *Oeuvres* (1803), 3:327–370.

1803 *Oeuvres de Pierre Camper, qui ont pour objet l'histoire naturelles, la physiologie et l'anatomie comparée . . .* 3 vols. Ed. and trans. H. J. Jansen. Paris: H. J. Jansen.

Canguilhem, Georges.

1955 *La formation du concept de rèflexe aux XVIIe et XVIIIe siècles.* Paris: Presses Universitaires. 2d ed. Paris: J. Vrin, 1977.

1964 "Le concept de réflexe au XIXe siècle." In K. E. Rothschuh, ed. *Von Boerhaave bis Berger* (1964). Pp. 157–167.

Cantor, G. N.

1975*a* "The Edinburgh phrenology debate: 1803–1828." *Annals of Science,* 32:195–218.

1975*b* "A critique of Shapin's social interpretation of the Edinburgh phrenology debate." *Annals of Science,* 32:245–256.

Capen, Nahum.
1881 *Reminiscences of Dr. Spurzheim and George Combe: and a review of the science of phrenology . . .* New York: Fowler & Wells.

Carlson, Eric T., Jeffrey L. Wollock, and Patricia S. Noel, eds.
1981 *Benjamin Rush's* [unpublished] *lectures on the mind.* Philadelphia: American Philosophical Society.

Carmichael, Andrew.
1833 *A memoir of the life and philosophy of Spurzheim.* Dublin: W. F. Wakeman.

Carmichael, Leonard.
1927 "Robert Whytt: A contribution to the history of physiological psychology." *Psychological Review,* 34:287–304.

Carpenter, William Benjamin.
1837 "On the voluntary and instinctive actions of living beings." *EMSJ,* 48:22–44.
1839*a* *Principles of general and comparative physiology, intended as an introduction to the study of human physiology, and as a guide to the philosophical pursuit of natural history.* London: J. Churchill.
1839*b* *Prize Thesis. Inaugural dissertation on the physiological inferences to be deduced from the structure of the nervous system in the invertebrated classes of animals.* Edinburgh: J. Carfrae.
1841 *Principles of general and comparative physiology, intended as an introduction to the study of human physiology, and as a guide to the philosophical pursuit of natural history.* 2d ed. London: J. Churchill.
1846*a* *Principles of human physiology, with their chief applications to pathology, hygiene and forensic medicine.* 3d ed. London: J. Churchill.
1846*b* *A manual of physiology, including physiological anatomy for the use of the medical student.* London: J. Churchill.
1853 *Principles of human physiology, with their chief applications to psychology, pathology, therapeutics, hygiene, and forensic medicine.* 4th ed. London: J. Churchill.
1855 *Principles of human physiology: with their chief applications to psychology, pathology, therapeutics, hygiene, and forensic medicine.* 5th ed. London: J. Churchill.

[Carpenter, William B.]
1846 ["Review of *The brain and its physiology* by Daniel Noble"], *BFMR,* 22:488–544.

Carus, Carl Gustav.
1814 *Versuch einer Darstellung des Nervensystems und insbesondere des Gehirns, nach ihrer Bedeutung, Entwickelung und*

Vollendung im thierischen Organismus. Leipzig: Breitkopf & Härtel.

1827 *An introduction to the comparative anatomy of animals; compiled with reference to physiology* . . . Trans. R. T. Gore. 2 vols. London: Longman et al. This is a trans. of 1st ed. of *Lehrbuch* (Dresden, 1818). (Not seen.)

1834 *Lehrbuch der vergleichenden Zootomie. Mit stäter Hinsicht auf Physiologie ausgearbeitet* . . . 2d ed. 2 vols. Leipzig: E. Fleischer; Vienna: C. Gerold. The 1st ed. (Dresden, 1818) was not seen.

1835 *Traité élémentaire d'anatomie comparée, suivi de recherches d'anatomie philosophique ou transcendante sur les parties primaires du système nerveux et du squelette intérieur et extérieur*. Trans. A. J. L. Jourdan from the 2d ed. 2 vols. Paris: J. B. Baillière.

Cavendish, Henry.

1776 "An account of some attempts to imitate the effects of the Torpedo by electricity." *PT*. Part I. Pp. 196–225.

Cayre, [?].

1819 "Note sur le plus grand développement du nerf appelé grand sympathique, rencontré sur des cadavres de personnes mortes dans un état d'idiotisme." *Nouveau Journal de Médecine, Chirurgerie et Pharmacie* (Béclard et al: Paris), 6:40–45.

Charbonnel-Duteil, Edmond.

1943 *Les débuts de l'électrothérapie en France*. Thèse, University of Paris. Paris: Jouve.

Chaumont, Dr. de. See Anonymous, "Dr. de Chaumont" (1854).

Chaussier, François.

1807 *Exposition sommaire de la structure et des différentes parties de l'encéphale ou cerveau* . . . Paris: T. Barrois.

Chauventon, F. P., and F. V. Mérat de Vaumartoise, eds.

1812–1822 *Dictionnaire des sciences médicales*. 60 vols. Paris: Panckoucke.

Chevalier, Vincent, and Charles Louis Chevalier.

1827 *Microscopes catadioptriques et achromatiques de M. le Professeur J.-B. Amice, construits, pour la première fois, en France, en 1827* [Paris: H. Balzac].

Churchill, Frederick B.

1976 "Rudolf Virchow and the pathologist's criteria for the inheritance of acquired characteristics." *JHM*, 31:117–148.

Clarke, Edwin.

1968 "The doctrine of the hollow nerve in the seventeenth and eighteenth centuries." In L. G. Stevenson and R. P. Multhauf, eds. *Medicine science and culture* (1968). Pp. 123–141.

1978 "The neural circulation; the use of analogy in medicine." *MH,* 22:291–307.

Clarke, Edwin, and J. G. Bearn.

1968 "The brain 'glands' of Malpighi elucidated by practical history." *JHM,* 23:309–330.

1972 "The spiral nerve bands of Fontana." *Brain,* 95:1–20.

Clarke, Edwin, and K. E. Dewhurst.

1972 *An Illustrated history of brain function.* Oxford: Sandford Publications.

Clarke, Edwin, and John L. Laidlaw.

1958 "Silent hydrocephalus," *Neurology* (Minneapolis), 8:382–386.

Clarke, Edwin, and C. D. O'Malley.

1968 *The human brain and spinal cord. A historical study illustrated by writings from Antiquity to the Twentieth century.* Berkeley and Los Angeles: University of California Press. (Referred to in notes as Clarke and O'Malley [1968].)

Clarke, John.

1793 "Description of an extraordinary production of human generation, with observations." *PT.* Part II, pp. 154–263.

Clarke, J. F.

1874 *Autobiographical recollections of the medical profession.* London: J. & A. Churchill.

Cohen, I. Bernard.

1952 "The two hundredth anniversary of Benjamin Franklin's two lightning experiments and the introduction of the lightning rod." *Proceedings of the American Philosophical Society,* 96:331–366.

1953 "Introduction" to L. Galvani. *Luigi Galvani* (1953). Pp. 9–41.

Coldstream, J.

[1837] "Electricity, animal." In R. B. Todd, ed. *The cyclopaedia* (1835–1859). 2 (1836–1839):81–98. (Completed in 1837.)

Coleman, William.

1964 *Georges Cuvier zoologist. A study in the history of evolution theory.* Cambridge, Mass.: Harvard University Press.

1971 *Biology in the nineteenth century: Problems of form, function, and transformation.* New York: John Wiley.

1976 "Morphology between type concept and descent theory." *JHM,* 31:149–175.

Combe, George.

1819 *Essays on phrenology, or an inquiry into the principles and utility of the system of Drs. Gall and Spurzheim, and into the objections made against it.* Edinburgh: Bell & Bradfute.

1826 *Letter from George Combe to Francis Jeffrey, Esq. in answer to his criticism on phrenology . . .* 2d ed. Edinburgh: J. Anderson.

1838 *On the functions of the cerebellum,* by Drs. Gall, Vimont, and Broussais . . . Edinburgh: Maclachlan & Stewart.

Combette, [?].

1831 *Revue médicale,* April. Cited by G. Andral, *Lectures* (1835–1836). Pp. 842–843.

Comparetti, Andrea.

1780. *Occursus medici de vaga aegrititudine infirmitatis nervorum.* Venice: Typis Francisci ex N. Pezzana.

Comte, Isidore Auguste Marie François Xavier.

1830–1842 *Cours de philosophie positive.* 6 vols. Paris: Bachelier.

Condorcet, Marie Jean Antoine Nicolas de Caritat, Marquis de.

1968*a* *Atlantide* in *Oeuvres* (1968). Part VI. Pp. 618–631.

1968*b* *Oeuvres,* reprint of 1847–1849 ed. Stuttgart: F. Frommann.

Conn, H. J.

1946 "Development of histological staining." *Ciba Symposium* (Summit, N.J.), 7:270–300.

Conn, H. J., ed.

1933 *The history of staining.* Geneva, N.Y.: Biological Stain Commission.

Cooter, Roger J.

1976*a* "Phrenology and British alienists c. 1825–1845. Part I: Converts to a doctrine." *MH,* 20:1–21. "Part II: Doctrine and practice." Pp. 135–151.

1976*b* "Phrenology: The provocation of progress." *History of Science,* 14:211–234.

1985 *The cultural meaning of popular science: Phrenology and the organization of consent in nineteenth-century Britain.* Cambridge: Cambridge University Press.

Copland, J.

1829 "Appendix." In A. B. Richerand, *Elements of physiology* (1829). Pp. 531–738.

Corti, Marquese Alfonso.

1851 "Recherches sur l'organe de l'ouïe des mammifères." *Zeitschrift für wissenschaftliche Zoologie,* 3:109–169.

Costa, A. Masucco.

1977 *Psychologie soviétique.* Paris: Payot.

Coster, Jacques.

1823 "Expèriences sur le système nerveux de l'homme et des animaux; publiées en Italie, en 1809, et repétées en France en 1822," *AGM,* 1st series, 1:359–418.

Cousin, Victor.

1836 *Cours de philosophie.* Paris: L. Hachette.

1845 *Fragments de philosophie cartésienne.* Paris: Charpentier.

Craig, William.

1859 *On the influence of variations of electric tension as the remote cause of epidemic and other diseases.* London: J. Churchill.

Cranefield, Paul F.

1957 "The organic physics of 1847 and the biophysics of today." *JHM,* 12:407–423.

1966 "The philosophical and cultural interests of the biophysics movement of 1847." *JHM,* 21:1–7.

1974 *The way in and the way out: François Magendie, Charles Bell and the roots of the spinal nerves.* Mount Kisco, N.Y.: Futura.

Creed, R. S., D. Denny-Brown, J. C. Eccles, E. G. T. Lidell, and C. S. Sherrington.

1932 *Reflex activity of the spinal cord.* London: Oxford University Press. There is a 1972 reprint with annotations by D. P. C. Lloyd.

Critchley, Macdonald, ed.

1978 *Butterworths medical dictionary.* 2d ed. London: Butterworth.

Crooke, Helkiah.

1615 *Mikrokosmographia* [Greek]. *A description of the body of man . . .* London: W. Jaggard.

[Crooke, Helkiah.]

1616 *Somatographia anthropine* [Greek]. *Or a description of the body of man . . .* London: W. Jaggard.

Crosland, Maurice.

1979 "From prizes to grants in support of scientific research in France in the nineteenth century: the Montyon legacy." *Minerva,* 17:355–380.

Cross, John.

1817 *An attempt to establish physiognomy upon scientific principles. Originally delivered in a series of lectures.* Glasgow: A. & J. M. Duncan et al.

Cruveilhier, Jean.

1829–1842 *Anatomie pathologique du corps humain, ou descriptions, avec figures lithographiées et calorées, des diverses altérations morbides dont le corps humain est susceptible.* 3 vols. Paris: J. B. Baillière.

1839–1840 "La faculté du langage a-t-elle un siège dans le cerveau, et ce siège est-il dans les lobes antérieurs de cet organe?" [5 December 1839], *Bulletin de l'Académie de Médecine* (Paris), 4:334–342.

Cullen, William.
1785 *Institutions of medicine. Part I. Physiology . . .* 3d ed., Edinburgh: C. Elliot. (All published.)
1789 *A treatise of the materia medica.* 2 vols. Edinburgh: C. Elliot.
1827 *The works of William Cullen, M.D. . . . containing his physiology, nosology, and first lines of the practice of physic . . .* Ed. John Thomson. 2 vols. Edinburgh: W. Blackwood.

Culotta, Charles A.
1974 "German biophysics, objective knowledge, and romanticism." *Historical Studies in the Physical Sciences,* 4:3–38.

Cumston, Charles Greene.
1900 "An analysis of Kotzebue's 'Die Organe des Gehirns.'" *The St. Paul Medical Journal,* November. (Reprint only seen.)

Cuvier, Georges, Baron.
1800–1805 *Leçons d'anatomie comparée de G. Cuvier.* 5 vols., Paris: Baudouin. Vols. 1–2 (1800) ed. by C. Duméril and vols. 3–5 (1805) by G. L. Duvernoy, but Cuvier took full responsibility for the contents.
1817 *Le régne animal distribué d'apres son organisation.* 4 vols. Paris: Deterville.
1822 "Rapport fait á l'Académie des Sciences sur des expériences relatives aux fonctions du systeme nerveux." *JPEP,* 2:372–384. Also in: *Mémoires du Muséum d'Histoire Naturelle* (Paris), 1822, 9:120–138; *Revue Encyclopédie* (47ième Cahier), November 1822, pp. 1–18 (see in reprint form only); *PM,* 1823, 61:114–125; *Journal Complémentaire du Dictionaire des Sciences Médicales* (Paris), 1823, 15:44–57; P. Flourens, *Recherches* (1824), pp. 59–84; *Recherches* (1842), pp. 60–84.

Cuvier, Georges, J. R. Tenon, R. B. Sabatier, A. Portal, and P. Pinel.
1808 "Rapport sur un mémoire de MM. Gall et Spurzheim sur l'anatomie du cerveau." In "Séance du lundi 25 avril 1808," *Procès-verbaux des Séances de l'Académie* (Paris) [1795–1835], 4:48–63.

Dale, Sir Henry Hallam.
1938 "Acetylcholine as a chemical transmitter of the effects of nerve impulses. History of ideas and evidence . . . " *Journal of the Mount Sinai Hospital,* 4:401–415.

Dalton, John Call.
1861 "On the cerebellum, as the centre of co-ordination of the voluntary movements." *American Journal of Medical Science,* 9th ser., 41:83–88.
1875 *Experimentation on animals, as a means of knowledge in physiology, pathology, and practical medicine.* New York:

F. W. Christern. Reprinted by Arno Press (New York), 1980.
1882 *The experimental method in medical science* . . . New York: G. P. Putnam. Reprinted New York: Arno Press, 1980.

Damiron, Jean Philibert.
1834 *Essai sur l'histoire de la philosophie en France, au XIXe siècle.* 2 vols. 3d ed. Paris: L. Hachette.

Daremberg, Charles.
1841 "Exposition des connaisances de Galien sur l'anatomie, la physiologie et la pathologie du système nerveux . . . " Paris: Rignoux. This was his M.D. thesis.

Daremberg, Charles, trans.
1854–1856 *Oeuvres anatomiques, physiologiques et médicales de Galien* . . . 2 vols. Paris: J. B. Baillière.

Darnton, R.
1968 *Mesmerism and the end of the Enlightenment in France.* Cambridge, Mass.: Harvard University Press.

Dart, Raymond A.
1922 "The misuse of the term visceral." *Journal of Anatomy* (London), 56:177–188.

Darwin, Erasmus.
1794–1796 *Zoonomia; or, the laws of organic life.* 2 vols. London: J. Johnson.

Dastre, A., and J. P. Morat.
1880 "Sur l'expérience du grand sympathique cervical." *CRAS,* 91:393–395.
1884 *Recherches expérimentales sur le système nerveux vasomoteur.* Paris, G. Masson.

David, Isidore Bernard.
1830 "Identité du fluide nerveux et du fluide électrique." Thèse de Paris, No. 196. (Not seen.)

Davies, H.
1898 *The cerebellum.* London: Nichols.

Davies, John D.
1955 *Phrenology, fad and science. A 19th-century American crusade.* New Haven: Yale University Press.

Davy, Sir Humphry.
1829 "An account of some experiments on the Torpedo," *PT.* Part I, pp. 15–18.

Davy, John.
1832 "An account of some experiments and observations on the Torpedo *(Raia Torpedo, Linn.).*" *PT.* Part II, pp. 259–278.
1834 "Observations on the Torpedo, with an account of some additional experiments on its electricity," *PT.* Part II, pp. 531–550.

Deen, Izaak van.
1841 *Traités et découvertes sur la physiologie de la moelle épinière.* Leyden: S. & J. Luchtmans.
1860 "Ueber die Unempfindlichkeit der Cerebrospinalcentra für elektrische Reize," *Untersuchungen zur Naturlehre des Menschen und der Thiere* (Moleschott: Frankfurt am Main), 7:380–392.

Deiters, Otto Friedrich Karl.
1865 *Untersuchungen über Gehirn und Rückenmark des Menschen und der Säugethiere.* Braunschweig: Vieweg.

Delaunay, Paul.
1920 "La médecine et les idéologues: L. J. Moreau de la Sarthe." *Bulletin de la Société Française d'Histoire de la Médecine,* 14:24–70.

Delpit, [Félix Jean Jacques Édouard].
1819 "Organoscopie." In F. P. Chaumenton and F. V. Mérat de Vaumartoise, eds. *Dictionnaire* (1812–1822). Vol. 38. Pp. 254–269.

Desmoulins, Louis Antoine.
1825 *Anatomie des systèmes nerveux des animaux à vertèbres, appliquée à la physiologie et à la zoologie. Ouvrage dont la partie physiologique est faite conjointement avec F. Magendie.* 2 vols. Paris: Méquignon-Marvis.

Dewhurst, K. E.
1980 *Thomas Willis's Oxford lectures.* Oxford: Sandford Publications.
1981 *Willis's Oxford casebook (1650–1652).* Oxford: Sandford Publications.
1982 *Hughlings Jackson on psychiatry.* Oxford: Sandford Publications.

Dezeimeris, J. B., C. P. Ollivier, and J. Raige-Delorme, eds.
1828–1839 *Dictionnaire historique de la médecine ancienne et moderne* . . . 4 vols. in 7. Paris: Béchet Jeune.

Dibner, Bern.
1952 *Galvani-Volta. A controversy that led to the discovery of useful electricity.* Norwalk, Conn.: Burndy Library.
1954 *Ten founding fathers of the electrical science.* Norwalk, Conn.: Burndy Engineering Co.
1961 *Oersted and the discovery of electromagnetism.* Norwalk, Conn.: Burndy Library. Also published in 1962 at New York: Blaisdell.
1964 *Alessandro Volta and the electric battery.* New York: F. Watts.
1969 *Heralds of science as represented by two hundred epochal*

books and pamphlets selected from the Burndy Library. Cambridge, Mass.: M.I.T. Press.

Dictionary of national biography. 22 vols. London: Smith, Elder.
1908–
1909

Dictionary of scientific biography. 16 vols. New York: C. Scribner's.
1970–
1980.

Dingwall, Eric J.
1967 "The French commissions of the 1780s," In E. J. Dingwall, ed. *Abnormal hypnotic phenomena* (1967–1968). Vol. 1. *France* (1967), pp. 6–21.

Dingwall, Eric J., ed.
1967–
1968 *Abnormal hypnotic phenomena. A survey of nineteenth-century cases*. 4 vols. London: J. & A. Churchill.

Dobell, Clifford.
1932 *Anton van Leeuwenhoek and his little animals*. London: Bale & Danielsson.

Döllinger, Ignaz.
1805 *Grundriss der Naturlehre des menschlichen Organismus*. Bamberg & Wirzburg [*sic*]: J. A. Goebhardt.
1824 *Von den Fortschritten, welche die Physiologie seit Haller gemacht hat*. Munich: M. Lindauer.

Donné, Alfred.
1834 "Recherches sur quelques unes des propriétés chimiques des sécrétions et sur les courants électriques qui existent dans les corps organisés." *ACP*, 57:398–416.

Dorsman, C., and C. A. Crommelin.
1957 "The invention of the Leyden jar." *Janus*, 46:275–280.

Dow, Robert Stone.
1940 "Thomas Willis (1621–1675) as a comparative neurologist." *Annals of Medical History*, 3d ser., 2:181–194.

Dow, Robert Stone, and Giuseppe Moruzzi.
1958 *The physiology and pathology of the cerebellum*. Minneapolis: University of Minnesota Press.

Drummond, J.
1859 "Sympathetic nerve." In R. B. Todd, ed. *The Cyclopaedia* (1835–1859). *Supplement* (1859): anatomy of nerve, pp. 423–455; physiology, pp. 455–473.

Dubois d'Amiens, E. Frédéric.
1845 *Philosophie médicale. Examen des doctrines de Cabanis et de Gall*. Paris: J. B. Baillière.
1864*a* "Broussais." In *Éloges lus* (1864). 2:53–110.

1864*b* *Éloges lus dans les séances publiques de l'Académie de Médecine (1845–1863).* 2 vols. Paris: Didier.

du Bois-Reymond, Emil.

1843 "Vorläufiger Abriss einer Untersuchung über den sogenannten Froschstrom und über die elektromotorischen Fische." *APC* (January), 58:1–30.

1848–1884 *Untersuchungen über thierische Elektricität.* 2 vols. Berlin: G. Reimer. Vol. 1 (1848); vol. 2, part 1 (1849); vol. 2, part 2, pp. 1–384 (1860); vol. 2, part 2, pp. 385–579 (1884).

1853 *On Signor Carlo Matteucci's letter to H. Bence Jones, M.D., F.R.S. &c. editor of an abstract of Dr. du Bois-Reymond's researches in animal electricity.* London: J. Churchill.

du Bois-Reymond, Estelle, and Paul Diepgen, eds.

1927 *Zwei grosse Naturforscher des 19. Jahrhunderts: Ein Briefwechsel zwischen Emil du Bois-Reymond und Karl Ludwig* [1847–94]. Leipzig: J. A. Barth.

1982 *Two great scientists of the nineteenth century. Correspondence of Emil du Bois-Reymond and Carl Ludwig* [1847–1894]. Trans. S. Lichtner-Ayèd. Ed. P. F. Cranefield. Baltimore: Johns Hopkins University Press.

Duckett, S.

1964 "Étude de la fonction cérébelleuse par François Pourfour du Petit (1710)." *Encéphale,* 53:291–297.

Dugès, Antoine.

1826 "Mémoire sur les fonctions du système nerveux." *Éphémérides médicales de Montpellier,* 1:42–63.

1832 *Mémoire sur la conformite organique dans l'échelle animale.* Montpellier: A. Ricard.

1838–1839 *Traité de physiologie comparée de l'homme et des animaux.* 3 vols. Montpellier: L. Castel.

Dujarric de la Rivière, R.

1969 *Cuvier, sa vie, son oeuvre; Pages choisies.* Paris: J. Peyronnet.

Dupré, A.

1843 "Expériences sur les fonctions de la moelle épinière et de ses racines." *CRAS,* 17:204–206.

Dupuy, J. M.

1816 "Observations et expériences sur l'enlèvement des ganglions gutturaux des nerfs trisplanchniques, sur des chevaux." *Journal de Médecine, Chirurgie, Pharmacie, etc., contenant les Travaux de la Société Médicale d'Émulation* (Leroux: Paris), December 1816, 37:340–350. Also published in *Bulletin de la Société Médicale d'Emulation* (G. Breschet: Paris), 1816, 1:581–591. Also reported in "Versuche" (1818).

1818 "Versuche über die Wegnahme des ersten Halsknotens des Gangliennerven bei Pferden." *DAP,* 4:105–108.

Dutrochet, René Joachim Henri.

1824 *Recherches anatomiques et physiologiques sur la structure intime des animaux et des végétaux.* Paris: J. B. Baillière.

Eccles, John C., and William C. Gibson.

1979 *Sherrington. His life and thought.* Heidelberg: Springer International.

Eckhard, Carl.

1881 "Beiträge zur Geschichte der Experimentalphysiologie des Nervensystems . . . Geschichte der Entwickelung der Lehre von den Reflexerscheinungen." *Beiträge zur Anatomie und Physiologie* (C. Eckhard: Giessen), 9:29–192.

Edwards, Henri Milne. See Milne-Edwards, Henri.

Egli, N.

1970 *Der "Prix Montyon des physiologie expérimentale" im 19 Jahrhundert.* Zürich: Juris. (*Zürcher Medizingeschichtliche Abhandlungen,* new series 72.)

Ehrenberg, Christian Gottfried.

1833 "Nothwendigkeit einer feineren mechanischen Zerlegung des Gehirns und der Nerven vor der chemischen, dargestellt aus Beobachtungen von C. G. Ehrenberg." *APC,* 28:449–465, 471–473.

1836 *Beobachtung einer auffallenden bisher unerkannten Struktur des Seelenorgans bei Menschen und Thieren.* Berlin: Königlichen Akademie der Wissenschaften. English trans. in *EMSJ* (1837), 48:258–304.

Ehrlich, Paul.

1886 "Über die Methylenblaureaction der lebenden Nervensubstanz." *Deutsche medizinische Wochenschrift,* 12:49–52.

Elliot, Sir John.

1786 *Elements of the branches of natural philosophy connected with medicine . . .* 2d ed. London: J. Johnson.

Elliotson, John, trans.

1815 J. F. Blumenbach's *The elements of physiology.*

Emmert, Augustus Gottfried Ferdinand.

1811 "Beobachtungen über einige anatomische Eigenheiten der Vögel." *AP,* 10:377–392.

Engelhardt, Dietrich von.

1972*a* "Gründzüge der wissenschaftlichen Naturforschung um 1800 und Hegels spekulative Naturwissenschaft." *Philosophia naturalis,* 13:290–315.

1972*b* "Einheitliche und umfassende Naturdarstellungen in der Naturwissenschaft um 1800 und Hegels Philosophie der Natur." *Rete,* 1:167–192.

1975 "Naturphilosophie im Urteil der 'Heidelberger Jahrbücher der Literatur' 1808–1832." *Heidelberger Jahrbücher,* 19: 53–81.

Engelhardt, H. T.
1975 "John Hughlings Jackson and the mind-body relationship." *BHM,* 49:137–151.

Entralgo, Pedro Lain.
1948 "Sensualism and vitalism in Bichat's 'Anatomie générale.'" *JHM,* 3:47–64.

Ernst, Benjamin Gottlob.
1847 *Neues Planetenbuch oder Mikro- und Makrokosmos. Hypothese von Ernst.* Breslau: J. U. Kern.
1850 *Planetogenesis; neues Planetenbuch, oder Mikro- und Makrokosmos, eine These von Ernst. 2. verm. Aufl . . . Nebst einem Anhange: Papierstreifen aus dem Portefeuille eines verstorbenen Naturforschers* [J. E. Purkyně]. Breslau: J. U. Kern.

Eschenmayer, Adam Karl August.
1817 *Psychologie in drei Theilen als empirische, reine und angewandte.* Stuttgart & Tübingen: J. G. Cotta.

Esposito, Joseph L.
1977 *Schelling's idealism and philosophy of nature.* Lewisburg, Pa.: Buchnell University Press.

Estienne, Charles. See Stephanus, Carolus.

Eulenberg, Albert, and Paul Guttmann.
1873 *Die Pathologie des Sympathicus auf physiologischer Grundlage.* Berlin: A. Hirschwald.

Eustachius, Bartholomaeus.
1714 *Tabulae anatomicae . . . B. E. . . . praefatione, notisque illustravit . . . J. M. Lancisi.* Rome: R. Gonzaga.

Eycleschymer, A. C.
1917 *Anatomical names; especially the Basle Nomina Anatomica ("BNA").* New York: W. Wood.

Fabbroni [erroneously Fabroni], Giovani Valentino Mattia.
1799 "Sur l'action chimique des différens métaux." *Journal de Physique, de Chimie, et d'Histoire Naturelle* (Paris), 49:348–357.

Fabri, Giacinto Bartolomeo.
1757–1759 *Sulla insensitività ed irritabilità Halleriana. Opuscoli di varii autori raccolti da G.B.F.* 2 vols. & suppl. Bologna: G. Corciolani.

Fadiga, Ettore.
1963 "The first Italian contributions to the study of cerebellar functions and the work of Luigi Luciani. I- Researches accomplished before Luciani." In L. Belloni, ed. *Essays* (1963). Pp. 203–223.

Fahie, John Joseph.
1884 *A history of electric telegraphy to the year 1837* . . . London: E. & F. N. Spon.

Faraday, Michael.
1839 "Experimental researches in electricity.—Fifteenth series." "§ 23. Notice of the character and direction of the electric force of the Gymnotus" [15 November, 1838]. *PT,* Part I, pp. 1–12.

Farrar, Clarence B.
1905 "The growth of [neuro-] histological techniques during the nineteenth century." *Review of Neurology and Psychiatry,* 3:501–515, 573–594.

Fearing, Franklin.
1929 "René Descartes. A study in the history of reflex action." *Psychological Review,* 36:375–388.
1930 *Reflex action. A study in the history of physiological psychology.* London: Baillière, Tindall & Cox.

Feremutsch, K.
1951 "Die Grundzuege der Hirnanatomie bei Carl Gustav Carus (1789–1869). Ein Beitrag zur Geschichte der Medizin und der Naturwissenschaft des beginnenden 19. Jahrhunderts," *Centaurus,* 2:52–85.

Ferrier, Sir David.
1876 *The functions of the brain.* London: Smith, Elder.
1883 "An address on the progress of knowledge in the physiology and pathology of the nervous system." *British Medical Journal,* ii:805–808.
1886 *The functions of the brain.* 2d ed. London: Smith, Elder.

Fichtel, K.
1965 "Wilhelm Griesinger—ein Vorläufer der materialistischen Reflextheorie." *Zeitschrift für ärztliche Fortbildung,* 59: 1032–1037.

Field, John, ed.
1959–1977 *Handbook of physiology: a critical, comprehensive presentation of physiological knowledge and concepts.* 25 vols., Washington, D.C.: American Physiological Society.

Figlio, Karl M.
1975 "Theories of perception and the physiology of mind in the late eighteenth century." *History of Science,* 12:177–212.

Finger, Otto, and Friedrich Herneck, eds.
1963 *Von Liebig zu Laue: Ethos und Weltbild grosser deutscher Naturforscher und Ärtze.* Berlin: Veb deutscher Verlag der Wissenschaften.

Finn, Bernard S.
1971 "Output of eighteenth century electrostatic machines." *British Journal of the History of Science,* 5:289–291.

Fischer, I., ed.
1932–1933 *Biographisches Lexikon der hervorragenden Ärzte der letzten fünfzig Jahre.* 2 vols. Berlin & Vienna: Urban & Schwarzenberg.

Fisher, J.
1956 "The history of electricity in Germany during the first half of the eighteenth century." *Bulletin of the British Society of the History of Science,* 2:49–51.

Flemyng, Malcolm.
1751 *The nature of the nervous fluid, or animal spirits, demonstrated: with an introductory preface.* London: A. Millar.

Fletcher, John.
1835–1837 *Rudiments of physiology, in the three parts . . .* Edinburgh: J. Carfrae. Part III (1837) was edited by Robert Lewins after the author's death.

Flint, Austin, Jr.
1868–1875 *The physiology of man . . .* 5 vols. New York: D. Appleton.
1872 *The physiology of the nervous system.* In *The physiology of man* (1868–1875). Vol. 4.

Flourens, Pierre.
1819–1820 ["Review of F. J. Gall, *Anatomie et physiologie du système nerveux*"]. *Révue Encyclopédique,* 3:437–452; 5:454–466.
1820 "Essai sur l'espirit et sur l'influence de la *Philosophie anatomique,*" *Révue Encyclopédique,* 5:217–232.
1822 ["Des observations pleines d'intérêt sur les fonctions des parties centrales du système nerveux"]. *Histoire de l'Académie Royale des Sciences,* 5:355–359.
1823 "Recherches physiques sur les propriétés et les fonctions du système nerveux dans les animaux vertébrés." *AGM,* 1st series, 2:321–370.
1824 *Recherches expérimentales sur les propriétés et les fonctions du système nerveux, dans les animaux vertébrés.* Paris: Crevot.
1825 "Nouvelles expériences sur le système nerveux." *AGM,* 1st series, 8:422–426.
1828 "Nouvelles expériences sur le système nerveux." *Annales des Sciences naturelles* (Paris), January, 13:86–108. (Seen only in reprint of 22 pp.)
1842 *Recherches expérimentales sur les propriétés et les fonctions*

du système nerveux dans les animaux vertébrés. 2d ed. Paris: J. B. Baillière.

1845*a* *Examen de la phrénologie.* Paris: Paulin.

1845*b* *Cuvier. Histoire de ses travaux.* Paris: Paulin.

1847*a* "Note touchant les effets de l'inhalation étherée sur la moelle épinière." *CRAS,* 24:161–162, 253–259.

1847*b* "Note touchant les effets de l'éther sur les centres nerveux." *CRAS,* 24:340–344.

1851 "Note sur le point vital de la medulla allongée." *CRAS,* 33:437–439.

1860 "Éloge historique de Henri-Marie Ducrotay de Blainville." *Mémoires de l'Academie des Sciences,* 27:I–LX.

1862*a* "Histoire des études sur le cerveau humain." *Journal des Savants,* pp. 221–234, 406–417, 453–463.

1862*b* *Recueil des éloges historiques lus dans les séances publiques de l'Académie des Sciences.* Paris: Garnier Frères.

Foderà, Michele.

1823 "Recherches expérimentales sur le système nerveux." *JPEP,* 3:191–217. (Presented to the Académie des Sciences, 31 December 1822.)

1826 "Lettre de M. Foderà au Rédacteur général (premier extrait)." *Journal Complémentaire du Dictionaire des Sciences Médicales* (Paris), 26:101–110.

Fodor, J.

1974 *The language of thought.* Cambridge, Mass.: Harvard University Press.

Fontana, Felice Gaspar Ferdinand.

1762 "Dissertation epistolaire." In A. von Haller, *Mémoires* (1762). Vol. 3. Pp. 157–243.

1781 *Traité sur le vénin de la vipère.* 2 vols. Florence: n.p.

Forel, August Henri.

1887 "Einige hirnanatomische Betrachtungen und Ergebnisse." *Archiv für Psychiatrie und Nervenkrankheiten,* 18:162–198.

Forster, Thomas Ignatius Maria.

1815*a* "Sketch of the new anatomy and physiology of the brain and nervous system of Drs. Gall and Spurzheim, considered as comprehending a complete system of phrenology." *The Pamphleteer Respectfully Dedicated to both Houses of Parliament,* 5:219–243.

[1815*b*] *Sketch of the new anatomy and physiology of the brain and nervous system of Drs. Gall and Spurzheim, considered as a comprehending system of zoonomy. With observations on its tendency to the improvement of education, of punishment,*

and of the treatment of insanity. London: Law & Whittaker et al.; Edinburgh: Macredie.

Fossati, Jean Antoine Laurent.

1858 "GALL (François-Joseph)." [?] Hoefer, *Nouvelle biographie générale* (1858–1866). Vol. 19. Columns 271–284.

Foville, Achille Louis.

1829 "Researches on the anatomy of the brain." *PM*, New series, 5:278–286, 331–339 (April and May).

1831 "Encéphale." In G. Andral et al., eds. *Dictionnaire* (1829–1836), 7:191–250.

1844 *Traité complet d'anatomie, de la physiologie et de la pathologie du système nerveux cérébro-spinale, Part 1, Anatomie*. Paris: Fortin, Masson.

Foville, Achille Louis, and Félix Pinel-Grandchamp.

1823 *Recherches sur le siège spécial de différentes fonctions du système nerveux*. Paris: A. Borée. Cited by J. B. Bouillaud, *Traité* (1825). Pp. 275–277.

Fowler, Lorenzo Niles.

1842 *The principles of phrenology and physiology applied to man's social relations; together with an analysis of domestic feelings*. New York: L. N. Fowler & O. S. Fowler. Reprinted in Anonymous, *Sex and science* (1974).

Fowler, Lorenzo Niles, and Orson Squire Fowler.

1889 *Amativeness; embracing the evils and remedies of excessive and perverted sexuality, including warning and advice to the married and single*. Revised ed. New York: Fowler & Wells. Reprinted in: Anonymous, *Sex and society* (1974).

Fox, Edward Long.

1885 *The influence of the sympathetic on disease*. London: Smith, Elder.

Frank, Johann Peter.

1791 "Untersuchungen über die Krankheiten des Rückgrats, und des in ihm befindlichen Rückenmarkes." In *Kleine Schriften* (1797), pp. 277–324.

1797 *Kleine Schriften praktischen Inhalts*. Vienna: T. Edler.

Frankenberger, Zderăk.

1959 "J. E. Purkyně und die Zellenlehre." *Nova Acta Leopoldina*, 24:47–55.

Franklin, B., et al.

1785 *Report of Dr. Benjamin Franklin, and other commissioners, charged by the King of France, with the examination of the animal magnetism, as now practised at Paris*. Trans. from the French. London: J. Johnson.

Frayssinous, M. D.

[1825] *Défense du Christianisme ou conférences sur la réligion.* 2d ed. 3 vols. Paris: Le Clerc.

French, Roger K.

1969 *Robert Whytt, the soul and medicine.* London: Wellcome Institute of the History of Medicine.

1971 "The origins of the sympathetic nervous system from Vesalius to Riolan." *MH,* 15:45–54.

Fried, Ruth Leys.

1976 "Alison versus Hall: Aspects of the formation and reception of the reflex concept in Britain," Ph.D. Dissertation, Harvard University.

Fried, R. Leys [Ruth Leys].

1980 "Background to the reflex controversy: William Alison and the doctrine of sympathy before Hall." *Studies in History of Biology,* 4:1–66.

Fritsch, Gustav Theodor, and Eduard Hitzig.

1870 "Über die elektrische Erregbarkeit des Grosshirns." *AAPM,* pp. 300–332. English translation in G. von Bonin, *Some papers* (1960), pp. 73–96; in H. Wilkins "Neurosurgical classics XII" (1963); and H. Wilkins, *Neurosurgical classics* (1965). Pp. 15–27.

Froriep, August.

1911 *Die Lehren Franz Joseph Galls beurteilt nach dem Stand der heutigen Kenntnisse.* Leipzig: Barth. (Not seen.)

Fulton, John F.

1926*a* "The history of the physiology of muscle." In idem, *Muscular contraction* (1926). P. 1–55.

1926*b* *Muscular contraction and the reflex control of movement.* Baltimore: Williams & Wilkins.

1949 *Physiology of the nervous system.* 3d ed. New York: Oxford University Press.

1966 *Selected readings in the history of physiology,* with Leonard G. Wilson. 2d ed. Springfield, Ill.: C. C Thomas.

Fulton, John F., and Harvey Cushing.

1936 "A bibliographical study of the Galvani and the Aldini writings on animal electricity." *Annals of Science,* 1:239–268.

Galaty, David H.

1974 "The philosophical basis of mid-nineteenth century German reductionism." *JHM,* 29:295–316.

Galen.

See Kuhn, C. G. *[Galen] medicorum graecorum opera* (1821–1823).

1916 *Galen on the natural faculties with an English translation by Arthur John Brock M.D. Edinburgh.* London: W. Heinemann (Loeb Library).

Gall, Franz Joseph.

1791 *Philosophisch-medizinische Untersuchungen über Natur und Kunst im Kranken und gesunden Zustande des Menschen.* Vol. 1 (all published). Vienna: R. Gräffer.

1825*a* *Sur les fonctions du cerveau et celles de chacune de ses parties, avec des observations sur la possibilité de reconnaitre les instincts, les pechans, les talens, ou les dispositions morales et intellectuelles des hommes et des animaux, par la configuration de leur cerveau et du leur tête.* 6 vols. Paris: J. B. Baillière. Each volume has its own subtitle. English trans. in F. J. Gall, *On the functions* (1835).

1825*b* *Sur l'origine des qualités morales et des facultés intellectuelles de l'homme, et sur les conditions de leur manifestation.* Vol. 1 of F. J. Gall, *Sur les fonctions* (1825).

1825*c* *Sur l'organe des qualités morales et des facultés intellectuelles, et sur la pluralité des organes cérébraux.* Vol. 2 of F. J. Gall, *Sur les fonctions* (1825).

1825*d* *Influence du cerveau sur la forme du crâne, difficultés et moyens de déterminer les qualités et les facultés fondamentales, et de découvrir le siége de leurs organes. Exposition des qualités et des facultés fondamentales et de leur siége, ou organologie.* Vol. 3 of F. J. Gall, *Sur les fonctions* (1825).

1825*e* *Organologie ou exposition des instincts, des penchans, des sentimens et des talens, ou des qualités morales et des facultés intellectuelles fondamentales de l'homme et des animaux, et du siége de leurs organes.* Vols. 4 and 5 of F. J. Gall, *Sur les fonctions* (1825).

1825*f* *Revue critique de quelques ouvrages anatomico-physiologiques, et exposition d'une nouvelle philosophie des qualités morales et des facultés intellectuelles.* Vol. 6 of F. J. Gall, *Sur les fonctions* (1825).

1835*a* *On the functions of the brain of each of its parts: with observations on the possibility of determining the instincts, propensities, and talents . . . of men and animals, by the configuration of the brain and head.* Trans. Winslow Lewis, Jr. 6 vols. Boston: Marsh, Capen, & Lyon.

1835*b* "Lettre au Baron Joseph Fr. de Retzer." *Journal de la Société Phrénologique de Paris.* P. 134. (Not seen.) Cited by J. Létang, *Gall* (1906). P. 99. Full trans. in N. Capen, *Reminiscences* (1881). Pp. 70–86.

1838 "Petition and remonstrance by Dr. Gall against an order by Francis the First, Emperor of Germany . . . Translated from the German." In F. J. Gall, et al., *On the functions of the cerebellum* (1838). Pp. 309–339. Details of German original of 1804 given on p. 309n.

Gall, F. J., et al.

1838 *On the functions of the cerebellum by Drs Gall, Vimont, and Broussais, transl. G. Combe. . . .* Edinburgh: Maclachlan & Stewart, pp. 1–94.

Gall, F. J., and J. C. Spurzheim.

1809 *Recherches sur le système nerveux en général, et sur celui du cerveau en particulier; Mémoire présenté à l'Institut de France, le 14 mars, 1808; suivi d'observations sur le Rapport qui en à été fait à cette compagnie par ses Commissaires.* Paris: F. Schoell & H. Nicolle. Reprinted in 1967 by Bonset of Amsterdam.

1810–1819 *Anatomie et physiologie du systême nerveux en général, et du cerveau en particulier, avec des observations sur la possibilité de reconnoitre plusieurs dispositions intellectuelles et morales de l'homme et des animaux, par la configuration de leur têtes.* 4 vols. and atlas. Vols. 1–2 and atlas, Paris: F. Schoell, 1810–1812; vol. 3, Paris: Libraire Grecque-Latine-Allemande, 1818; vol. 4, Paris: N. Maze, 1819. The first volume was by both authors. In vol. 2 a note on p. 147 states that Spurzheim had left Paris. The rest of this volume and vols. 2 and 4 are, therefore, by Gall alone, and in them he used the first person singular throughout.

Galvani, Luigi.

1791*a* "De viribus electricitatis in motu musculari. Commentarius." *De Bononiensi Scientiarum et Artium Instituo atque Academia, Commentarii,* 7:363–418. (Not seen.)

1791*b* *De viribus electricitatis in motu musculari. Commentarius.* Bologna: ex Typographia Instituti Scientiarum.

1953*a* *Luigi Galvani. Commentary on muscular motion, translated by M. G. Foley, notes and critical introduction by I.B. Cohen and a bibliography of the editions and translations by J.F. Fulton and M.E. Stanton.* Norwalk, Conn.: Burndy Library.

1953*b* *A translation of Luigi Galvani's "De viribus electricitatis in motu musculari commentarius . . .* By R. M. Green. Cambridge, Mass.: E. Licht.

[Galvani, Luigi].

1794 *Dell'uso e dell'attività dell'arco conduttore nelle contrazioni dei muscoli.* Bologna: T. d'Aquino. (Not seen.)

Garnier, A.
1839 *La psychologie et la phrénologie comparées.* Paris: L. Hachette.

Garrison, Fielding H.
1931 "The Romantic period in the history of German medicine." *Bulletin of the New York Academy of Medicine,* 7:841–864.

Gartrell, Ellen G.
1975 *Electricity, magnetism and animal magnetism. A checklist of printed sources 1600–1850.* Wilmington, Del.: Scholarly Resources.

Gaskell, Walter Holbrook.
1885–1886 "On the structure, distribution and function of the nerves which innervate the visceral and vascular systems." *JP,* 7:1–80.
1916 *The involuntary nervous system.* London: Longman, Green.

Gault, Robert H.
1904 "A sketch of the history of reflex action in the latter half of the nineteenth century." *American Journal of Psychology,* 15:526–568.

Geddes, L. A.
1984 *A short history of the electrical stimulation of excitable tissue including electrotherapeutic applications.* Supplement 1 of *Physiologist,* 27:S.1–S.47.

Geddes, L. A., and H. E. Hoff.
1961 "The capillary electrometer. The first graphic recorder of bioelectric signals." *Archives Internationales d'Histoire des Sciences* (Paris), 14:275–290.

Geison, Gerald L.
1972 "Social and institutional factors in the stagnancy of English physiology, 1840–1870." *BHM,* 46:30–58.
1978 *Michael Foster and the Cambridge School of Physiology. The scientific enterprise in late Victorian society.* Princeton: Princeton University Press.

George, John Durrance.
1837–1838 "Contribution to the history of the nervous system." [1838], *London Medical Gazette,* new series, ii:40–47, 93–96.

Georget, Étienne Jean.
1821 *De la physiologie du système nerveux, et spécialemente du cerveau. Recherches sur les maladies nerveuses en général . . .* 2 vols. Paris: J. B. Baillière.

Gerlach, Joseph von.
1865 *Mikroscopische Studien aus dem Gebiete der menschlichen Morphologie.* Erlangen: F. Enke.

1872 "Über die Structur der grauen Substanz des menschlichen Grosshirns. Vorläufige Mittheilung." *Centralblatt für die medizinischen Wissenschaften,* 10:273–275.

Gerland, Ernst, and F. Traumüller.

1899 *Geschichte der physikalischen Experimentierkunst.* Leipzig: W. Engelmann.

Gieve, Ronald N., and Richard S. Westfall, eds.

1973 *Foundations of scientific method: The nineteenth century.* Bloomington: Indiana University Press.

Gill, Sydney.

1976 "A Voltaic enigma and a possible solution to it." *Annals of Science,* 33:351–370.

Gliozzi, M.

1935 "Giambattista Beccaria nella storia dell'elettricità." *Archeion,* 17:15–47.

Gode-von Aesch, Alexander.

1966 *Natural science in German Romanticism.* New York: AMS Press.

Golgi, Camillo.

1875 "Sulla fina struttura dei bulbi olfattoria." *Rivista Sperimentale di Freniatria e di Medicia Legale,* 1:66–78. Also in *Opera Omnia* (1903–1929). Vol. 1 (1903), "Istologie normale 1870–1883." Pp. 113–132.

1883–1884 "Recherches sur l'histologie des centres nerveux." *Archives italienne de Biologie,* 3:285–317; 4:92–123.

1886 "Professor Golgi's method of black coloring of the central nervous organs." *Alienist and Neurologist* (St. Louis), 7:127–131.

1903–1929 *Opera omnia.* 4 vols. Milan: Hoepli.

Good, J. M.

1822 *The study of medicine.* 4 vols. 1st ed. London: Baldwin, Cradock, & Joy.

1840 *The study of medicine.* 4 vols. 4th ed. London: Longman.

Goodfield, G. J.

1960 *The growth of scientific physiology . . .* London: Hutchinson.

Goodsir, John.

1856 "On the morphological relations of the nervous system in the annulose and vertebrate types of organisation." In *The anatomical memoirs* (1868). Vol. 2. Pp. 78–87.

1868 *The anatomical memoirs.* Ed. William Turner. 2 vols. Edinburgh: A. & C. Black.

Gordon, John.
1817 *Observations on the structure of the brain, comprising an estimate of the claims of Drs. Gall and Spurzheim to discovery in the anatomy of that organ.* Edinburgh: W. Blackwood.

Gordon-Taylor, Sir Gordon, and E. W. Walls.
1958 *Sir Charles Bell: His life and times.* London & Edinburgh: E. S. Livingstone.

Gouhier, Henri.
1933–1941 *La jeunesse d'Auguste Comte et la formation du positivisme.* 3 vols. Paris: J. Vrin.

Gould, Stephen Jay.
1977 *Ontogeny and phylogeny.* Cambridge, Mass.: Belknap Press.

Gower, Barry.
1973 "Speculation in physics: The history and practice of *Naturphilosophie.*" *Studies in the History and Philosophy of Science,* 3:301–356.

Gräfe, Carl Ferdinand von, C. W. Hufeland et al., eds.
1828–1849 *Encyclopädisches Wörterbuch der medicinischen Wissenschaften.* 37 vols. Berlin: J. W. Boike & Veit. (Early volumes had different editors and publishers.)

Graham, John.
1961 "Lavater's physiognomy in England," *Journal of the History of Ideas,* 22:561–572.
1979 *Lavater's essays on physiognomy. A study in the history of ideas.* Frankfurt-am-Main & Las Vegas. (Not seen.)

Grainger, Richard Dugard.
1829 *Elements of general anatomy, containing an outline of the organization of the human body.* London: S. Highley.
1837 *Observations on the structure and functions of the spinal cord.* London: S. Highley.
1842–1843 "Illustrations of the medical uses of comparative anatomy." *Lancet,* i:93.

Granit, Ragnar.
1966 *Charles Scott Sherrington. An appraisal.* London: Nelson.
1982 "Interactions between Pavlov and Sherrington." *Trends in Neuroscience,* 5:184–186.

Gratiolet, Louis Pierre.
1852 "Structure de la moelle épinière." *L'Institut,* 20:272–273.
1857 *Anatomie comparée du système nerveux considéré dans ses rapports avec l'intelligence.* Paris: J. B. Baillière. This is vol. 2 of F. Leuret and P. Gratiolet, *Anatomie comparée* (1839–1857).

Gray, Henry.
1980 *Gray's anatomy*. 36th ed. Peter L. Williams and Roger Warwick, eds. Edinburgh: Churchill Livingstone.

Gregory, Frederick.
1977 *Scientific materialism in nineteenth century Germany*. Dordrecht & Boston: D. Reidel.

Gregory, John.
c. 1770 "Lectures on the practice of medicine." Edinburgh. Wellcome Institute for the History of Medicine, manuscript 2616.

Griesinger, Wilhelm.
1843 "Ueber psychische Reflexactionen. Mit einem Blick auf das Wesen der psychischen Krankheiten." *Archiv für physiologische Heilkunde,* 2:76–113.
1844 "Neue Beiträge zur Physiologie und Pathologie des Gehirns," *Archiv für physiologische Heilkunde,* 3:69–98.
1845 *Die Pathologie und Therapie der psychischen Krankheiten, für Aerzte und Studierende.* Stuttgart: A. Krabbe.
1867 *Mental pathology and therapeutics.* Trans. by C. L. Robertson & J. Rutherford. London: The New Sydenham Society. Facsimile reprint, New York: Hafner, 1965; see *BHM* (1968), 42:286–287.

Grimaud, Jean Charles Marguerite Guillaume de.
1787 *Mémoire sur la nutrition.* Montpellier: J. Martel, Snr.

Grisolía, S., et al., eds.
1983 *Ramón y Cajal's contribution to the neurosciences.* Amsterdam: Elsevier.

Grmek, M. D.
1966 "Examen critique de la genèse d'une grande découverte: 'la piqûre diabétique' de Claude Bernard," *Clio Medica,* 1:341–350.
1970 "La notion de fibre chez les médecins de l'école iatrophysique." *Clio Medica,* 5:297–318.

Grohmann, Johann C. A.
1820 "Physiologie des menschlichen Geistes nach allgemeinen Naturgesetzten." *Zeitschrift für psychischen Aerzte,* 3 (1):284–332; 449–504.

Gross, Michael.
1979 "The lessened locus of feelings: A transformation in French physiology in the early nineteenth century." *JHB,* 12:231–271.

Gruithuisen, Franz von Paula.
1810 *Anthropologie: Oder von der Natur des menschlichen Lebens*

und Denkens; für angehende Philosophen und Aertze. Munich: I. J. Lentner.

1811 *Organozoonomie, oder: Ueber das niedrige Lebensverhältniss, als Propädeutik zur Anthropologie . . .* Munich: I. J. Lentner.

Guericke, Otto von.

1672 *Experimenta nova (ut vocantur) Magdeburgica de vacuo spatio, primum à R.P. Gaspare Schotto . . .* Amsterdam: J. Jansson-Waesberg.

Guillaume, A. C.

1925 *Vagotonies sympathicotonies neurotonies. Les états de déséquilibre du système nerveux organo-végétatif.* Paris: Masson.

Guistino, D. de.

1975 *Conquest of mind: Phrenology and Victorian social thought.* London: Croom Helm.

Guyton, Arthur C.

1976 *Textbook of medical physiology.* 5th ed. Philadelphia: W. B. Saunders.

Haase, Johann Gottlob.

1772 "De gangliis nervorum. Lipsiae 1772." In C. F. Ludwig, *Scriptores nevrologicae minores* (1791–1795). Vol. 1 (1791). Pp. 61–88.

Haberling, Wilhelm.

1924 *Johannes Müller: Das Leben des rheinischen Naturforschers auf Grund neuer Quellen und seiner Briefe.* Leipzig: Akademische Verlagsgesellschaft M.B.H.

1926 "du Bois-Reymond in Paris 1850." *Deutsche medizinische Wochenschrift* (5 February), 52:251–252.

Hackmann, W. D.

1972 "The researches of Dr. Martinus van Marum (1750–1837) on the influence of electricity on animals and plants." *MH,* 16:11–26.

1973 *John and Jonathan Cuthbertson. The invention and development of the eighteenth century plate electrical machine.* Leyden: Rijksmuseum voor de Geschiedenis der Natuurwetenschappen.

1978 *Electricity from glass. The history of the frictional electrical machine 1600–1850.* Alphen aan den Rijn: Sijthoff & Noordhoff.

Haigh, Elizabeth.

1975 "The roots of the vitalism of Xavier Bichat." *BHM,* 49: 72–86.

1984*a* "Medicine and ideology: The methodology and epistemology of the sensationalists," in E. Haigh, *Xavier Bichat* (1984), pp. 66–86.

1984*b* *Xavier Bichat and the medical theory of the eighteenth century*. London: Wellcome Institute for the History of Medicine. Suppl. 4 of *MH.*

Hales, Stephen.

1733 *Statical essays: containing haemostaticks . . .* Vol. 2. [*Vegetable staticks* being vol. 1, 1727], London: W. Innys et al.

[Hall, Charlotte].

1861 *Memoirs of Marshall Hall, M.D., F.R.S. . . . by his widow.* London: R. Bentley.

Hall, Jason Y.

1977 "Gall's phrenology: A Romantic psychology." *Studies in Romanticism,* 16:305–317.

Hall, Marshall.

1832*a* "Theory of the inverse ratio which subsists between the respiration and irritability, in the animal kingdom." *PT.* Part II, pp. 321–334.

1832*b* " . . . a brief account of a particular function of the nervous system." *Proceedings of the Committee of Science and Correspondence of the Zoological Society of London,* Part 2, pp. 190–192. Reprinted in idem, *Memoirs* (1837), pp. v–ix.

1833*a* "On the reflex function of the medulla oblongata and spinalis, or the principle of tone in the muscular system." *Abstracts of the papers printed in the Philosophical Transactions . . . 1880 to 1884,* 3 [1830–1837]:210.

1833*b* "On the reflex function of the medulla oblongata and medulla spinalis." *PT.* Part II, pp. 635–665.

1836 *Lectures on the nervous system and its diseases.* London: Sherwood, Gilbert, & Piper [April].

1837*a* *Memoirs on the nervous system.* London: Sherwood, Gilbert, & Piper.

1837*b* *Principles of the theory and practice of medicine . . .* London: Sherwood, Gilbert, & Piper.

1837*c* "On the function of the medulla oblongata and medulla spinalis, and on the excito-motory system of nerves." [*PRS*], *Abstracts of the Papers printed in the Philosophical Transactions . . . 1880 to 1884,* 3 [1830–1837]:463–464. The full paper was published in *Annales des Sciences Naturelles . . .* (Zoologie) series 1, 7:321–370, 1837; and noted in *Notizen aus dem Gebiete der Natur-und Heilkunde* (L. F. von Froriep: Erfurt, Weimar) (1837), 1: columns 211–213.

1837*d* "On the reflex function of the spinal marrow; by Prof. Müller." *PM,* 10(i):51–57, 124–129, 187–193.

1840*a* "Memoirs on some principles of pathology in the nervous system. Memoir III. On the distinct influence of volition, of emotion, and of the vis nervosa." *Medico-Chirurgical Transactions* (London), 22:168–191.

1840*b* "Briefe über das Nervensystem am Prfessor [*sic*] J. Müller. Erster Briefe. Ueber die Vis nervosa Haller's." *AAPM* pp. 451–466.

1841 *On the diseases and derangements of the nervous system . . .* London: H. Baillière.

1842 *The Gulstonian Lectures for MDCCCXLII. On the mutual relations between anatomy, physiology, pathology, and therapeutics, and the practice of medicine.* London: H. Baillière.

1843 *New memoir on the nervous system.* London: H. Baillière.

1846 "On the anatomy of the excito-motory system." *Lancet,* ii:147.

1848 *A letter addressed to the Earl of Rosse, President-elect of the Royal Society.* 2d ed. London: [presumably published privately], November.

1850 *Synopsis of the diastaltic nervous system.* London: J. Mallett.

1856 "The true spinal marrow the true sympathetic. Observations and suggestions." *Lancet,* ii:38–39, see p. 38.

Hall, Thomas S.

1969 *Ideas of life and matter. Studies in the history of general physiology 600* B.C.*–1900* A.D. 2 vols. Chicago & London: University of Chicago Press.

Haller, Albrecht von.

1747 *Primae lineae physiologiae in usum praelectionum academicarum.* Göttingen: A. Vandenhoeck.

1751 *Primae lineae physiologiae in usum praelectionum academicarum.* 2d ed. Göttingen: A. Vandenhoeck.

1753 "De partibus corporis humani sensibilibus et irritabilibus." *Commentarii Societatis Regiae Scientiarum Gottingensis* [22 April, 6 May 1752], 2:114–158.

1754 *Dr Albert Haller's physiology; being a course of lectures upon the visceral anatomy and vital oeconomy of human bodies . . .* 2 vols. London: W. Innys & J. Richardson.

1755 *A dissertation on the sensible and irritable parts of animals* [trans. from S.A.A.D. Tissot's French version, and not from the original Latin], London: J. Nourse. See "A dissertation" (1936).

1757–1766 *Elementa physiologiae corporis humani.* 8 vols., Lausanne: M. M. Bousquet; S. d'Arnay; F. Grasset. Leyden: C. Haak.

1762 *Mémoires sur la nature sensible et irritable, des parties du corps animal.* 4 vols. Lausanne: F. Grasset. All editions have identical pagination.

1767 *Primae lineae physiologiae in usum praelectionum academicarum.* 3d ed., Edinburgh: G. Drummond, & Kincaid & Bell.

1936 "A dissertation on the sensible and irritable parts of animals . . . [London, J. Nourse, 1755]. Introduction by Owsei Temkin," *BHM,* 4:651–699.

Hammond, William A.

1869 "The physiology and pathology of the cerebellum." *Quarterly Journal of Psychological Medicine and Medical Jurisprudence* (New York), April, 3:5–20. (Seen in reprint form only.)

Hannover, Adolph.

1840 "Die Chromsäure, ein vorzügliches Mittel bei mikroscopischen Untersuchungen." *AAPM,* pp. 549–558.

Harless, Emil.

1846 "Briefliche Mittheilung über die Ganglienkugeln der Lobe electrici von Torpedo Galvani." *AAPM,* pp. 283–291.

Harvey, E. Ruth.

1975 *The inward wits. Psychological theory in the Middle Ages and the Renaissance.* London: Warburg Institute.

Harvey, William.

1651 *Exercitationes de generatione animalium.* London: O. Pulleyn.

Hassall, Arthur Hill.

1849 *The microscopic anatomy of the human body, in health and disease.* 2 vols. London: S. Highley.

Hastings, Hester.

1936 *Man and beast in French thought of the eighteenth century.* Baltimore: Johns Hopkins Press.

Hausen, Christian August.

1743 *Novi profectus in historia electricitatis, post obitum auctoris . . .* Leipzig: T. Schwan.

Hawkins, Francis Bisset.

1829 *Elements of medical statistics; containing the substance of the Gulstonian Lectures . . .* London: Longman et al.

Haymaker, Webb, and Francis Schiller, eds.

1970 *The founders of neurology. One hundred and forty-six biographical sketches by eighty-nine authors.* 2d ed. Springfield, Ill.: C. C Thomas.

Head, Sir Henry.

1926 *Aphasia and kindred disorders of speech.* 2 vols. Cambridge: Cambridge University Press.

Hécaen, Henri, and J. Dubois.

1969 *La naissance de la neuropsychologie du langage (1825–1865).* Paris: Flammarion.

Hedderly, Frances.
1970 *Phrenology. A study of mind.* London: L. N. Fowler.

Heilbron, J. L.
1966*a* "À propos de l'invention de la bouteille de Leyde." *Revue de l'Histoire des Sciences* (Paris), 19:133–142.
1966*b* "G. M. Bose. The prime mover in the invention of the Leyden jar?" *Isis,* 57:264–267.
1979 *Electricity in the 17th and 18th centuries. A study of early modern physics.* Berkeley, Los Angeles, London: University of California Press.

Helmholtz, Hermann Ludwig Ferdinand von.
1842 "De fabrica systematis nervosi evertebratorum." Berlin: typis Nietackianis. Inaugural-Dissertation. (Not seen.)
1850 "Vorläufiger Bericht über die Fortpflanzungsgeschwindigkeit der Nervenreizung," *AAPM,* pp. 71–73.

Henle, Friedrich Gustav Jakob.
1840*a* "Ueber Nervensympathie," in F. G. H. Henle, *Pathologische Untersuchungen* (1840), pp. 83–165.
1840*b* "Krankhafte Sympathien," in ibid., pp. 121–165.
1840*c* *Pathologische Untersuchungen.* Berlin: A. Hirschwald. Reviewed in *BFMR,* 1840, 9:404–410.
1841 *Allgemeine Anatomie. Lehre von den Mischungs-und Formbestandtheilen des menschlichen Körpers.* Leipzig: L. Voss.
1846–1853 *Handbuch der rationellen Pathologie.* 2 vols. Braunschweig: F. Vieweg.

Herder, Johann Gottfried.
1784–1791 *Ideen zur Philosophie der Geschichte der Menschheit.* 4 vols. Riga & Leipzig: J. F. Hartknoch.
1965 *Ideen zur Philosophie der Geschichte der Menschheit.* Heinz Stolpe ed. 2 vols. Berlin & Weimar: Aufbau Verlag.

Hermann, Ludimar.
1863 *Grundriss der Physiologie des Menschen.* Berlin: A. Hirschwald.
1892 *Lehrbuch der Physiologie.* 10th ed. Berlin: A. Hirschwald.

Herrnstein, Richard J., and Edwin G. Boring, eds.
1965 *A source book in the history of psychology.* Cambridge, Mass.: Harvard University Press.

Herschel, Frederick William.
1831 *A preliminary discourse on the study of natural philosophy.* London: Longman et al.

Hertwig, Heinrich.
1826 *Experimenta quaedam de effectibus laesionum in partibus encephali singularibus et de verosimili eorum partium func-*

tione [Inaugural Dissertation]. Berlin: Feister & Eisersdorff.

Hildebrandt, Georg Friedrich.

1830–1832 *Handbuch der Anatomie des Menschen.* 4 vols. E. H. Weber, ed. Brunswick: Schulbuchhandlung.

Hilts, Victor L.

1982 "Obeying the laws of hereditary descent: phrenological views on inheritance and eugenics." *Journal of the History of the Behavioral Sciences,* 18:62–77.

Hintzsche, Erich.

1943 "Die Entwicklung der histologischen Farbetechnik." *Ciba Zeitschrift,* 8:3074–3109.

Hintzsche, Erich, ed.

1963 *Zellen und Gewebe in G. Valentin's 'Histogenia comparata' von 1835 und 1838.* Bern: P. Haupt.

Hintzsche, Erich, and W. Rytz.

1953 *Gustav Gabriel Valentin (1810–1883): Versuch einer Bio- und Bibliographie.* Bern: P. Haupt.

Hippocrates (Hippocratic Writers).

1978*a* "The seed . . . " Trans. I. M. Lonie. In Hippocrates, *Hippocratic writings* (1978). Pp. 317–323.

1978*b* *Hippocratic writings. Edited with an introduction by G.E.R. Lloyd.* Harmondsworth: Penguin.

Hirsch, August et al., eds.

1962 *Biographisches Lexikon der hervorragenden Ärzte aller Zeiten und Völker,* 3d ed. 5 vols. and Suppl. Munich & Berlin: Urban & Schwarzenberg.

His, Wilhelm.

1887 "Zur Geschichte des menschlichen Rückenmarkes und der Nervenwurzeln," *Abhandlungen der Königlich Sächsischen Gesellschaft der Wissenschaft. Mathematisch-Physicalische Klasse,* 13:477–514.

Hodge, C. F.

1890 "A sketch of the history of reflex action." *American Journal of Psychology,* 3:149–167, 343–363.

Hodgkin, Alan L. et al.

1977 *The pursuit of nature. Informal essays on the history of physiology.* Cambridge: Cambridge University Press.

Hodgkin, Thomas, and J. J. Lister.

1827 "Notice of some microscopical observations of the blood and animal tissues." *PM,* 2:130–138.

Hoefer, [?], ed.

1855– *Nouvelle biographie générale . . .* 46 vols. Paris: Firmin

1866 Didot.

Hoff, H. E.

1936 "Galvani and the pre-Galvanian electrophysiologists." *Annals of Science,* 2:157–172.

Hoff, H. E., and L. A. Geddes.

1957 "The rheotome and its prehistory: a study in the historical interrelation of electrophysiology and electromechanics." *BHM,* 31:212–234, 327–347.

1960 "Ballistics and the instrumentation of physiology: The velocity of the projectile and of the nerve impulse." *JHM,* 15:133–146.

Hoff, H. E., and Peter Kellaway.

1952 "The early history of the reflex." *JHM,* 7:211–249.

Hollander, Bernard.

1902 *Scientific phrenology. Being a practical mental science and guide to human character . . .* London: G. Richards.

1909 *The unknown life & works of Dr. Francis Joseph Gall the discoverer of the anatomy and physiology of the brain.* London: Gall Society.

Holmes, Sir Gordon M.

1907 "A form of familial degeneration of the cerebellum." *Brain,* 30:466–489.

Home, Sir Everard.

1799 "The Croonian Lecture. Experiments and observations upon the structure of nerves" [1798]. *PT.* 98:1–12.

1814–1828 *Lectures on comparative anatomy in which are explained the preparations in the Hunterian Collection.* 6 vols. London: G. & W. Nichol.

Home, Roderick W.

1970 "Electricity and the nervous fluid." *JHB,* 3:235–251.

Hood, Alexander.

1824 "Notice of a case in which the patient suddenly forgot the use of spoken and written language." *Transactions of the Phrenological Society* (Edinburgh), 1:235–246.

1826 "Continuation of the singular and important case of R.W." *Phrenological Journal and Miscellany* (Edinburgh), 3:26–36.

Hoppe, Brigitte.

1968 "Discussions histologiques et physico-chimiques au commencement de la cytologie au XIXe siècle." In *XIIe Congrès International d'Histoire des Sciences,* 8:73–83.

1971 "Le concepte de biologie chez G.R. Treviranus." *Collogue International "Lamarck."* Paris: A. Blanchard.

Horsley, Victor, and Edward Albert Schäfer.
1888 "A record of experiments upon the functions of the cerebral cortex" [17 February 1887]. *PT*, 179B:1–45.

Hufeland, Christoph Wilhelm.
1807 "Remarks on Dr. Gall's theory concerning the organs of the brain." In Anonymous, *Some account* (1807). Pp. 137–162.

Hüffmeier, Dorothee.
1961 "Johann Wilhelm Ritter, Naturforscher oder Naturphilosoph?" *SAGM*, 45:225–234.

Hüffmeier-von Hagen, Dorothee.
1964 "J.W. Ritter und die Anfänge der Elektrophysiologie." In K. E. Rothschuh, ed. *Von Boerhaave bis Berger* (1964). Pp. 48–61.

Hughes, Arthur.
1959 *A history of cytology*. New York: Abelard-Schuman.

Humboldt, Friedrich Heinrich Alexander, Baron von.
1797 *Versuche über die gereizte Muskel-und Nervenfaser nebst Vermuthungen über den chemischen Process des Lebens in der Thier-und Pflanzenwelt.* 2 vols. Posen: Decker. Berlin: H. A. Rottmann.
1806 *Versuche über die electrischen Fische . . . Aus einem Briefe an den Präsidenten Freyherrn von Dachroeden. Rom im August 1805.* Erfurt: Beyer & Maring.
1849 *Aspects of nature in different lands and . . . climates.* Trans. Mrs. Sabine. 2 vols. London: Longman & J. Murray.

Humphreys, A. W.
1937 "The development of the conception of measurement of electric current," *Annals of Science,* 2:164–178.

Hunt, James.
1868–1869 "On the localisation of the functions of the brain, with special reference to the faculty of language," *Anthropological Review,* 6:329–345; 7:100–116, 201–214.

Hunter, John.
1774 "Anatomical observations on the Torpedo." *PT,* 63:Part II, 481–489.
1775 "An account of the Gymnotus electricus." *PT,* 65:Part II, 395–407.

Huschke, Emil.
1854 *Schaedel, Hirn und Seele des Menschen und der Thiere nach Alter, Geschlecht und Raçe. Dargestellt nach neuen Methoden und Untersuchungen.* Jena: F. Mauke.

[Hutcheson, F.].
1728 *An essay on the nature and conduct of the passions and*

affections. With illustrations on the moral sense. London: T. Smith & W. Bruce.

Huxley, Thomas Henry.

1854–1858 "On the present state of knowledge as to the structure and function of nerves." *Notice of the Proceedings at the Meetings of the Members of the Royal Institution of Great Britain,* 2:432–437.

Hydén, H., ed.

1967 *The neuron.* Amsterdam: Elsevier.

Hyrtl, Jószef.

1880 *Onomatologia anatomica. Geschichte und Kritik der anatomische Sprache der Gegenwart . . .* Vienna: W. Braumüller.

Ischlondsky, N.

1958 "The life and activity of I.M. Sechenov." *Journal of Nervous and Mental Diseases,* 126:367–391.

Jackson, John Hughlings.

1876 "On the scientific and empirical investigation of epilepsies." In J. H. Jackson, *Selected writings* (1931), 1:162–273.

1931–1932 *Selected writings of John Hughlings Jackson,* James Taylor, ed. 2 vols. London: Hodder & Stoughton.

Jackson, Seguin Henry.

1787 *A treatise on medical sympathy, and on the balance and connection of the extreme vessels of the human body . . .* 2d ed. London: J. Robson & W. Clarke.

Jackson, Stanley W.

1970 "Force and kindred notions in eighteenth-century neurophysiology and medical psychology." *BHM,* 44:397–410, 539–554.

Jacyna, L. S.

1983 "John Goodsir and the making of cellular reality." *JHB,* 16:75–99.

1984 "Principles of general physiology: The comparative dimension to British neuroscience in the 1830s and 1840s," *Studies in History of Biology,* 7:47–92.

Jahn, Ilse.

1971 "Ehrenberg, Christian Gottfried," *DSB,* 4:288–292.

Jeannerod, Marc.

1983 *Le cerveau-machine: Physiologie de la volonté.* Paris: Librairie Arthème Fayard. Translation:

1985 *The brain machine: The development of neurophysiological thought.* Cambridge, Mass.: Harvard University Press.

Jefferson, Sir Geoffrey.

1953 "Marshall Hall, the grasp reflex and the diastaltic spinal cord." In E. A. Underwood, ed. *Medicine, science, and history* (1953), 2:303–320.

Jeffress, L. A., ed.
1951 *Cerebral mechanisms in behavior*. The Hixon Symposium. New York: John Wiley.

[Jeffrey, Francis, Lord].
1826 [Review of *A system of phrenology* by George Combe], *Edinburgh Review,* 44:1253–1318.

John, Henry J.
1959 *Jan Evangelista Purkyně: Czech scientist and patriot (1787–1869)*. Philadelphia: American Philosophical Society.

Johnstone, James.
1764 "Essay on the use of the ganglions of the nerves" [24 November 1763]. *PT,* 54:177–184.
1768 "History of a foetus born with a very imperfect brain; to which is subjoined a supplement of the essay on the use of ganglions, published in Philos. Trans. for 1764" [20 December 1766]. *PT,* [Part I for 1767], 57:118–131. His name is here spelled Johnston.
1771 *An essay on the use of the ganglions of the nerves*. Shrewsbury: Printed by J. Eddowes and sold by T. Becket et al.
1787 *Versuch über den Nutzen der Nervenknoten. Aus dem Englischen übersetzt,* [trans. A. Kolpin]. Stettin: J. S. Kaffka.
1795*a* "Cui bono? or, physiological and pathological observations on the functions of the visceral nerves . . . " In J. Johnstone, *Medical essays* (1795). Pp. 97–189.
1795*b* *Medical essays and observations, with disquisitions relating to the nervous system. And an essay on mineral poisons.* Evesham: J. Agg.

Jones, E. G.
1972 "The development of the 'muscular sense' concept during the nineteenth century and the work of H. Charlton Bastian." *JHM,* 27:298–311.

Jones, Henry Bence, ed.
1852 *On animal electricity; being an abstract of the discoveries of Emil du Bois-Reymond . . .* London: J. Churchill.

Jouffroy, Theodore Simon.
1825 "Du spiritualisme et du matérialisme." In *Mélanges philosophiques* (1866). Pp. 121–161.
1866 *Mélanges philosophiques*. 4th ed. Paris: L. Hachette.

Jourdan, Antoine Jacques Louis, ed.
1820– *Dictionaire des sciences médicales. Biographie médicale.*

1825 7 vols. Paris: C. L. F. Panckoucke.

Kellaway, Peter.

1946 "The part played by electric fish in the early history of bioelectricity and electrotherapy." *BHM,* 20:112–137.

Kellner, C.

1963 *Alexander von Humboldt.* London: Oxford University Press.

Kératry, A. H.

1817 *Inductions morales et physiologiques.* Paris: Marachan.

Keuffel, G. G. T.

1811 "Ueber das Rückenmark," *AP,* 10: 123–202.

Keynes, Richard D.

1956 "The generation of electricity by fishes." *Endeavour,* 15:215–222.

1979 "Ion channels in the nerve-cell membrane." *Scientific American,* March, 240:98–107.

Keynes, R. D., and D. J. Aidley.

1981 *Nerve and muscle.* Cambridge: Cambridge University Press.

Kinneir, Doctor. See Bayne, David.

Kirschner, G., trans.

1840 *M. Hall. Abhandlungen über das Nervensystem. Aus dem Englischen mit Erläuterungen und Zusätzen.* Marburg. (Not seen.)

Kisch, Bruno.

1954 "Forgotten leaders in modern medicine. Valentin, Gruby, Remak, Auerbach." *Transactions of the American Philosophical Society,* new ser., 44:139–317, see pp. 227–296.

Kitchin, Joanna.

1965 *Un journal philosophique: La Décade (1794–1807).* Paris: M. J. Minard.

Knight, David M.

1970 "The physical sciences and the Romantic movement." *History of Science,* 9:54–75.

Knoefel, P. K.

1980 *Felice Fontana, 1730–1805: An annotated bibliography.* Trento: Società di Studi Trentini di Scienze Storiche.

Kock, Andreas.

1715 *De generatione febrium . . . Praeside Friderico Hoffmanno . . .* Halle: C. A. Zeitler.

Koelliker, Rudolph Albert von.

1844 *Die Selbständigkeit und Abhängigkeit des sympathischen Nervensystems, durch anatomische Beobachtungen bewiesen.* Zürich: Meyer & Zeller.

1848 "Neurologische Bemerkungen." *Zeitschrift für wissenschaftliche Zoologie,* 1:135–163.

1850–1854 *Mikroskopische Anatomie oder Gewebelehre des Menschen.* Leipzig: W. Engelmann. Vol. 2, part 1, 1850; vol. 2, part 2, sect. 1, 1852; vol. 2, part 2, sect. 2, 1854. Vol. 1 never published.

1853–1854 *Manual of human histology.* Trans. G. Buck and T. Huxley. 2 vols. London: Sydenham Society. Trans. of *Handbuch der Gewebelehre des Menschen* (1852). 2 vols. Leipzig: W. Engelmann.

1892 "Nervenzellen und Nervenfasern." *Biologisches Centralblatt,* 12:33–51.

1896 *Handbuch der Gewebelehre des Menschen.* 6th ed. 2 vols. Leipzig: W. Engelmann.

1899 *Erinnerungen aus meinem Leben.* Leipzig: W. Engelmann.

Koizumi, Kiyomi, and Chandler M. Brooks.

1980 "The autonomic nervous system and its role in controlling body functions." In V. B. Mountcastle, ed. *Medical physiology* (1980), 1:893–922.

Kolle, Kurt, ed.

1956–1963 *Grosse Nervenärzte; Lebensbilder.* 3 vols. Stuttgart: G. Thieme.

Koller, Gottfried.

1958 *Das Leben des Biologen Johannes Müller, 1801–1858.* Stuttgart: Wissenschaftliche Verlagsgesellschaft.

Krishaber, Maurice.

1864 *Considérations sur l'historique et le développement de l'encéphale.* Paris: A. Parent.

Kronenberg, [?].

1839 "Versuche über motorische und sensible Nervenwurzeln." *AAPM,* pp. 360–362.

Kruger, L.

1963 "François Pourfour du Petit 1664–1741," *Experimental Neurology,* 7:iii–v.

Kruta, Vladislav.

1962*a* "J.E. Purkyně—a creative scientist." In Anonymous, *Jan Evangelista Purkyně* (1962). Pp. 13–116.

1962*b* "The physiologist George Procháska (1749–1820) and the reflex theory." *Epilepsia,* 3:446–456.

1964 "G. Prochaska's and J.E. Purkyně's contributions to neurophysiology." In K. E. Rothschuh, ed. *Von Boerhaave bis Berger* (1964). Pp. 134–156.

1966 "Les relations entre G.-G. Valentin et J.-E. Purkinje." In *Proceedings XIXth International Congress of the History of Medicine*. Basel: S. Karger. Pp. 436–440.

1968 *The poet and the scientist: Johann Wolfgang Goethe, Jan Evangelista Purkyně*. Prague: Academia.

1971*a* "J.E. Purkyně's contribution to the cell theory." *Clio Medica*, 6:109–120.

1971*b* "J.E. Purkyně's conception of physiology." In V. Kruta, ed. *Jan Evangelista Purkyně* (1971). Pp. 27–33.

1971*c* "A note on the history of Purkyně cells. In V. Kruta, ed. *Jan Evangelista Purkyně* (1971). Pp. 125–136.

1971–1972 "K.E. von Baer and J.E. Purkyně: An analysis of their relations as reflected in their unpublished letters." *Lychnos*. Pp. 93–120.

Kruta, Vladislav, ed.

1971 *Jan Evangelista Purkyně 1787–1869*. Brno: Universita Jan Evangalisty Purkyně.

Kühn, Carl Gottlob, trans. and ed.

1821–1833 *[Galen] Medicorum graecorum opera quae exstant . . . Claudii Galeni*. 20 vols. in 22. Leipzig: C. Cnobloch.

Lacrampe-Loustau, J. B.

1824 *Recherches pathologiques et expérimentales sur différentes fonctions du système nerveux et en particulier sur la siège des causes de la paralysie des membres*. Paris: Gueffler. (Not seen.)

Laffont, M.

1880 "Recherches expérimentales sur la glycosurie considerée dans ses rapports avec le système nerveux." *Journal de l'Anatomie et de la Physiologie Normales et Pathologiques de l'Homme et des Animaux* (Paris), 16:347–433.

Laignel-Lavastine, Maxime Paul Marie.

1923 "Note sur l'histoire du sympathique." *Bulletin de la Société Française d'Histoire de la Médecine* (Paris), 17:401–406.

1923–1924 "Therapeutique chimique du sympathique." *La Médecine* (Paris), 5 (Suppl. for Oct. 1923):1–32.

Lallemand, Claude François.

1818 *Observations pathologiques propres à éclairer plusieurs points de physiologie*. Paris: Didot.

1820–1821 *Recherches anatomico-pathologiques sur l'encéphale et ses dépendances*. [Vol. 1]. Paris. Baudouin Bros. [Gabon Snr.; Bechet Jnr.]

1830– *Recherches anatomico-pathologiques sur l'encéphale et ses*

1834 *dépendances*. 3 vols. Paris: Béchet Jeune.

Lamarck, Jean Baptiste Pierre Antoine Monet de.

1802 *Histoire naturelle des végétaux*. Paris. (Not seen.) Cited by J. M. D. Olmsted, "Historical note" (1944). P. 343.

Lange, Frederick Albert.

1925 *The history of materialism and criticism of its present importance*. Trans. E. C. Thomas. London: Kegan Paul et al.

Langley, John Newport.

1898–1899 "On the union of cranial autonomic (visceral) fibres with the nerve cells of the superior cervical ganglion." *JP*, 23:240–270.

1900 "The sympathetic and other related systems of nerves." In E. A. Schäfer, ed. *Text-book* (1898–1900). 2:616–696.

1905 "On the reaction of cells and of nerve-endings of certain poisons, chiefly as regards the reaction of striated muscle to nicotine and to curari." *JP*, 33:374–413.

1913 "The nomenclature of the sympathetic and of the related systems of nerves." *Zeitschrift für Physiologie*, 27:149–152.

1916 "Sketch of the progress of discovery in the eighteenth century as regards the autonomic nervous system." *JP*, 50:225–258.

1921 *The autonomic nervous system, Part I*. Cambridge: W. Heffer.

Lanteri-Laura, Georges.

1970 *Histoire de la phrénologie: L'homme et son cerveau selon F.J. Gall*. Paris: Presses Universitaires de France.

Larrey, Baron Dominique Jean.

1829–1836 *Clinique chirurgicale, exercée particulièrement dans les camps et les hôpitaux militaires, depuis 1792 jusq'en 1829 [1832, 1836]*. 5 vols. Paris: Gabon (and J. B. Baillière).

Larrey, H.

1871 [Obituary of F. A. Longet]. *Bulletin de l'Académie de Médecine*, 36:1063–1077.

Lashley, Karl Spencer.

1933 "Integrative functions of the cerebral cortex." *Physiological Review*, 13:1–42.

1937 "Functional determinants of cerebral localization." *Archives of Neurology and Psychiatry*, 38:371–387.

Laurentius, Paul.

1936 *Geschichte der Krankenbehandlung mittels Elecktrizität*. Inaugural-Dissertation, University of Düsseldorf. Krefeld: W. Greven.

Lavater, Johann Caspar.

1772 *Von der Physiognomik*. 2 parts in 1 vol. Leipzig: Weidmanns Erben.

1797 *Essays on physiognomy; calculated to extend the knowledge and the love of mankind . . .* Trans. C. Moore, 3 vols. London: H. D. Symonds.

Lawrence, Christopher.

1979 "The nervous system and society in the Scottish enlightenment." In B. Barnes and S. Shapin, eds. *Natural order* (1979). Pp. 19–40.

Lawrence, Sir William.

1819 *Lectures on physiology, zoology, and the natural history of man. Delivered at the Royal College of Surgeons [1818].* London: J. Callow.

1822 *Lectures on physiology, zoology, and the natural history of man.* London: Benbow.

Laycock, Thomas.

1833–1857 "A journal, 1833–1857." Edinburgh University Library, Manuscripts, Gen. 1813.

1839 "Analytical essay on irregular and aggravated forms of hysteria." *EMSJ,* 52:43–86.

1840 *A treatise on the nervous diseases of women: comprising an inquiry into the nature, causes, and treatment of spinal and hysterical disorders.* London: Longmans.

1845*a* "Letter to George Combe, 27 February 1845." *Combe Manuscripts,* National Library of Scotland, 7276, ff. 3–4.

1845*b* "Letter to George Combe, 3 June 1845." *Combe Manuscripts,* National Library of Scotland, 7276, ff. 10–13.

1845*c* "On the reflex function of the brain." *BFMR,* 19:298–311.

1855 "Further researches into the functions of the brain," *BFMCR,* 16:155–187.

1859 "Phrenology." In *Encyclopaedia Britannica,* 8th ed. 17:556–558.

1860 *Mind and brain: or, the correlations of consciousness and organisation.* 2 vols. Edinburgh: Sutherland and Knox.

1876 "Reflex, automatic, and unconscious cerebration," *Journal of Mental Science,* 21:477–498.

Learmonth, Sir James.

1938 ["Recent advances in surgery of the sympathetic nervous system."] *Transactions of the Medical Society of London,* 61: [in a symposium] 154–162.

1950 "The surgery of the sympathetic nervous system." *Lancet,* ii:505–508.

Lee, Edwin.

1849 "The brain the sole centre of the human nervous system," *EMSJ,* 71:60–70. Paper read to Royal Society, May 1848.

Leeuwenhoek, Antoni van.

1685 "An abstract of a letter from Mr Anthony Leeuwenhoeck, Fellow of the Royal Society; concerning the parts of the brain of severall animals . . . " *PT*, 15:883–895.

1722 "De structura cerebri diversorum animalium . . . " In A. van Leeuwenhoek, *Opera omnia* (1722–1730. [Vol. 1]. Pp. 29–41.

1722–1730 *Opera omnia seu arcana naturae* . . . [Vol. 1] ed. novissima. Leyden: J. A. Langerak.

Legallois, Eugéne.

1830 "Notice sur l'auteur." In J. J. C. Legallois, *Oeuvres* (1830). 1:1–11.

Legallois, Julien Jean César.

1812*a* "Rapport fait à la Classe des Sciences Pysiques [*sic*] et Mathématiques de l'Institut impérial de France . . . [1811]" In J. J. C. Legallois, *Expériences* (1812). Pp. 252–326.

1812*b* *Expériences sur le principe de la vie, notamment sur celui des mouvemens du coeur, et sur le siége de ce principe* . . . Paris: D'Hautel.

1830 *Oeuvres de C*[ar] *Legallois* . . . 2 vols. Paris: Le Rouge.

Legée, Georgette.

1974 "M.J.P. Flourens (1794–1867) et Destutt de Tracy (1754–1836)." *Histoire et Nature* (Paris), 4:95–98.

1975 "M.J.P. Flourens (1794–1867), C. Legallois (1770–1814) et les fonctions du système nerveux vegetatif." *Histoire et Nature* (Paris), No. 7:59–73.

Lehmann, Werner R., ed.

1967– *Georg Büchner sämtliche Werke und Briefe*. 4 vols. Hamburg: Christian Wegner. (In progress. Vols. 3–4 still unpublished.)

Leibowitz, Joshua O.

1957 "Electroshock therapy in Ibn-Sina's Canon." *JHM*, 12:71–72.

Lélut, Louis Francisque.

1836 *Qu'est-ce que la phrénologie? Ou essai sur la significance et la valeur des systèmes de psychologie en général, et de celui de Gall en particulier*. Paris: Trinquart.

1843 *Rejet de l'organologie phrénologique de Gall, et de ses successeurs*. Paris: Fortin, Masson.

Lenoir, Timothy.

1978 "Generational factors in the origin of *Romantische Naturphilosophie*." *JHB*, 11:57–100.

1981 "Teleology without regrets. The transformation of physiology in Germany: 1790–1847." *Studies in the History and Philosophy of Science,* 12:293–354.

1982 *The strategy of life: Teleology and mechanics in nineteenth century German biology.* Dordrecht: D. Reidel.

Lesch, John E.

1984 *Science and medicine in France. The emergence of experimental physiology, 1790–1855.* Cambridge, Mass.: Harvard University Press.

Lesky, Erna.

1967 "Gall und Herder." *Clio Medica,* 2:85–96.

1970 "Structure and function in Gall." *BHM,* 44:297–314.

1981 "Der angeklagte Gall." *Gesnerus,* 38:301–311.

Lesky, Erna, ed.

1979 *Franz Joseph Gall 1758–1828: Naturforscher und Anthropologe.* Bern: H. Huber.

Létang, Jean.

1906 *Gall et son oeuvre.* Thèse de Lyon. Paris & Lyon: A. Maloine.

Leuckhart, Karl George Friedrich Rudolf. See Wagner, Richard (1850).

Leuret, François.

1839 *Anatomie comparée du système nerveux considéré dans ses rapports avec l'intelligence . . .* Paris: Baillière. This is vol. 1 of F. Leuret and P. Gratiolet, *Anatomie comparée* (1839–1857), 2 vols.

Leuret, François, and Louis Pierre Gratiolet.

1839–1857 *Anatomie comparée du système nerveaux considéré dans ses rapports avec l'intelligence . . .* 2 vols. Paris: J. B. Baillière.

Lévy, Michel.

1839 "Éloge de Broussais," *Recueil de Mémoires de Médecine, de Chirurgie et de Pharmacie Militaires,* 46:363–392.

Lewes, George Henry.

1877 *The physical basis of mind. With illustrations. Being the second series of problems of life and mind.* London: Trübner.

Lewis, Sir Aubrey.

1958 "J.C. Reil's concept of brain function." In F. N. L. Poynter, ed. *The history and philosophy* (1958). Pp. 154–166.

1965 "J.C. Reil: innovator and battler." *Journal of the History of the Behavioral Sciences,* 1:178–190.

Ley, Hugh.

1836 *An essay on laryngismus stridulus . . . and of the functions and diseases of the par vagum* [vagus]. London: J. Churchill.

Leys, Ruth. See Fried, Ruth Leys.

Liddell, E. G. T.
1960 *The discovery of reflexes.* Oxford: Clarendon Press.
Lindeboom, Gerrit A.
1982 "Jan Swammerdam (1637–1680) and his Biblia naturae." *Clio Medica,* 17:113–131.
Lister, Joseph Jackson.
1830 "On some properties in achromatic object-glasses applicable to the improvement of the microscope" [21 January, 1830]. *PT.* Part I, pp. 187–200.
Lister, Joseph, Lord.
1870 "Of the late Joseph Jackson Lister, F.R.S., F.Z.S., with special reference to his labours in the improvement of the achromatic microscope." *The Monthly Microscopical Journal (Transactions of the Microscopical Society of London),* 3:134–143.
Lobstein, Johann Friedrich, the Elder.
1760 "De nervo spinali ad par vagum accessorio. Argentorati 1760." In C. F. Ludwig, ed. *Scriptores nevrologici minores* (1791–1795). 2 (1792): 219–241.
Lobstein, Johann Georg Christian Friedrich Martin
(also known as Johann Friedrich Lobstein, the Younger).
1821*a* *Discours sur la prééminence du système nerveux dans l'économie animale, et l'importance d'une étude approfondie de ce système . . .* Strasbourg: F. G. Levrault.
1821*b* "Trisplanchnique (nerf)." In Adelon [N.P.] et al., eds. *Dictionaire des sciences médicales* (1812–1822), 56 (1821):9–43.
1823 *De nervi sympathetici humani fabrica usu et morbis. Commentatio anatomico-physiologico-pathologica . . .* Paris: F. G. Levrault.
1831 *A treatise on the structure, functions and diseases of the human sympathetic nerve.* Trans. J. Pancoast. Philadelphia: J. G. Auner. (Not seen.)
1835 *Essai d'une nouvelle théorie des maladies, fondée sur les anomalies de l'innervation.* Paris & Strasbourg. (Not seen. Cited by G. Rath, "Neural pathology" [1959].)
Long, Esmond R.
1965 *A history of pathology.* New York: Dover.
Longet, François Achille.
1841 *Recherches expérimentales et pathologiques sur les propriétés et les fonctions des faisceaux de la moelle épinière et des racines des nerfs rachidiens précédées d'un examen historique et critique des expériences faites sur ces organes depuis Sir Ch. Bell, et suivies d'autres recherches sur diverses parties du système nerveux.* Paris: Bechet Jeune & Labé.
1842 *Anatomie et physiologie du système nerveux de l'homme et*

des animaux vertébrés. 2 vols. Paris: Fortin, Masson.

1850–1861 *Traité de physiologie*. 2 vols. in 3. Paris: V. Masson (vol. 1, 1861; vol. 1, pt. 2, 1852; vol. 2, 1850). At least four editions.

1868–1869 *Traité de physiologie*. 3d ed. 3 vols. Paris: Germer Baillière.

Lorry, Anne Charles de.

1760 "Sur les mouvemens du cerveau. Second mémoire. Sur les mouvemens contre nature de ce viscère, & sur les organes qui sont le principe de son action," *Mémoires de Mathématique et de Physique, presentés à l'Académie Royale des Sciences . . .* (Paris), 3:344–377.

Lovejoy, Arthur.

1961 *The reason, the understanding, and time*. Baltimore: Johns Hopkins Press.

Luciani, Luigi.

1891 *Il cervelletto. Nuovi studi di fisiologia normale e patologica*. Florence: successori le Monnier.

1901–1911 *Fisiologia dell'uomo*. 2 vols. in 3. Milan: Società Editrice Libraria.

1911–1921 *Human physiology*. Trans. F. A. Welby. 5 vols. London: Macmillan.

Ludwig, Carl.

1852–1856 *Lehrbuch der Physiologie des Menschen*. 2 vols. Heidelberg: C. F. Winter.

Ludwig, Christian Friedrich, ed.

1791–1795 *Scriptores nevrologici minores selecti sive opera minora ad anatomiam physiologiam et pathologiam nervorum spectantia*. 4 vols. Leipzig: J. F. Junius; J. G. Feind.

M., P.-D.

1819 ["Review of *Anatomie et physiologie du système nerveux*, by F.J. Gall"]. *Revue Encyclopédique*, 1:417–426.

McCulloch, Warren S.

1951 "Why the mind is in the head." In L. A. Jeffress, ed. *Cerebral mechanisms* (1951). Pp. 42–111.

McFarland, David, ed.

1981 *The Oxford companion to animal behaviour*. Oxford: Oxford University Press.

McHenry, Lawrence C.

1969 *Garrison's History of Neurology revised and enlarged with a bibliography of classical, original and standard works in neurology*. Springfield, Ill.: C. C Thomas.

McIlwain, Henry.

1958 "Chemical contributions, especially from the nineteenth century, to knowledge of the brain and its functioning." In

F. N. L. Poynter, ed. *The history and philosophy* (1958). Pp. 167–186.

McLaren, Angus.

1974 "Phrenology: Medium and message," *Journal of Modern History,* 46:86–97.

Macleod, Kenneth.

1908 *Laycock*. Glasgow: A. Macdougall.

McMenemey, William H.

1958 "Alexander Philips Wilson Philip (1770–1847 [*sic*]), physiologist and physician." *JHM,* 13:289–328.

Magendie, François.

1809 "Quelques idées générales sur les phénomènes particuliers aux corps vivans." *Bulletin des Sciences Médicales de la Société Médicale d'Émulation de Paris,* 4:145–170.

1816–1817 *Précis élémentaire de physiologie.* 2 vols. Paris: Méquignon-Marvis.

1822*a* [No title], *Histoire de l'Académie Royale des Sciences* (Paris), 5:358–359.

1822*b* "Expériences sur les fonctions des racines des nerfs rachidiens," *JPEP,* 2:276–279.

1823*a* "Note sur le siège du mouvement et du sentiment dans la moelle épinière," *JPEP,* 3:153–161.

1823*b* "Note sur les fonctions des corps striés et des tubercules quadrijumeaux," *JPEP,* 3:376–381.

1823*c* *Mémoire sur quelques découvertes récentes relatives aux fonctions de système nerveux*. Paris: Méquignon-Marvis. (Read to Académie Royale des Sciences, 2 June 1823.)

1824 "Mémoire sur les fonctions de quelques parties du système nerveux." *JPEP,* 4:399–407.

1825 *Précis élémentaire de physiologie,* 2d ed. 2 vols. Paris: Méquignon-Marvis.

1841 *Leçons sur les fonctions et les maladies du système nerveux, professées au Collège de France.* C. James, ed. 2 vols. Paris: Lecaplain.

1849 "Annonce d'une découverte physiologique récente de Claude Bernard consistant en ce fait, que la blessure d'un certain point de l'encéphale donne lieu à la formation du sucre dans le sang et dans les urines." *CRAS,* 28:393–394.

Maine de Biran, Marie François Pierre Gauthier.

c. 1808 "Observations sur les divisions du cerveau, considerés comme sièges des différentes facultés intellectuelles et morales, des rapports qu'on peut établir entre l'analyse des facultés de l'entendement et cette sorte de division: Examen du système du Docteur Gall à ce sujet." In *Oeuvres* (1920–1949), 5 (1925):69–129.

1920–1949 *Oeuvres de Maine de Biran*. P. Tisserand, ed. 14 vols. Paris: Alcan.

Malacarne, Michele Vincenzo Giacinto.

1776 *Nuova esposizione della vera struttura del cervelletto umano*. Turin: G. Briolo. Reprinted in M. V. G. Malacarne, *Encefalotomia* (1780), Part 3, pp. 17–129 under the title: "Notizie generali intorno a tutte le parti che entrano nella composizione del cervelletto umano."

1780 *Encefalotomia nuova universale*. 3 parts. Turin: G. Briolo.

Malpighi, Marcello.

1666 *De viscerum structura exercitatio anatomica*. Bologna: J. Monti.

Manni, E.

1973 "Luigi Rolando, 1773–1831." *Experimental Neurology*, 38:1–5.

Manuel, Diana E.

1980 "Marshall Hall, F. R. S. (1790–1857). A conspectus of his life and work." *Notes and Records of the Royal Society of London*, 35:135–166.

Marjoribanks, Edward.

1929 *The life of Sir Edward Marshall Hall (1858–1927)* . . . London: Gollancz.

Marx, Otto M.

1970 "Nineteenth-century medical psychology: Theoretical problems in the work of Griesinger, Meynert, and Wernicke." *Isis*, 61:355–370.

Massias, Nicolas.

1821–1822 *Rapport de la nature à l'homme, et de l'homme à la nature*. 3 vols. Paris: Firman Didot.

Matoušek, Otakar.

1970 "Purkinje's contributions and views before and after the foundation of the cellular theory," *Svenska Medicinhistoriska Sällskapets Årsskrift*, 7:31–52.

Matteucci, Carlo.

1836 "Expériences sur la Torpille." *CRAS*, 3:430–431.

1837*a* "Recherches physiques, chimiques, et physiologiques sur la Torpille." *ACP*, 66:396–437. Also in *PM* (1838), 12:196—201, 256–258.

1837*b* "Nouvelle expériences sur la Torpille." *CRAS*, 5:501–504.

1838 "Sur le courant électrique ou propre de la grenouille; second mémoire sur l'électricité animale, faisant suite à celui sur la torpille." *ACP,* 2d ser., 68:93–106.

1839 "Ueber die electrischen Erscheinungen beim Zitterrochen." *Neue Notizen aus dem Gebiete der Natur- und Heilkunde* (L. F. von and R. Froriep: Weimar), February, columns 129–133.

1840 *Essai sur les phénomènes électriques des animaux.* Paris: Carillian-Goeury & Dalmont.

1842*a* "Deuxième mémoire sur le courant électrique propre de la grenouille et sur celui des animaux à sang chaud [1841]." *ACP,* 3d ser. 6:301–339.

1842*b* [Report on muscle contraction current read by J. M. Dumas on 24 October 1842]. *CRAS,* 15:797–798.

1842*c* "Sur un phénomène physiologique produit par les muscles en contraction" [1841]. *ACP,* 3d ser., 6:339–342. (The sealed-packet paper.)

1844 *Traité des phénomènes électro-physiologiques des animaux.* Paris: Fortin, Masson.

1845*a* "Expériences sur les phénomènes de la contraction induite (Lettre à M. Dumas)." *ACP,* 15:64–70.

1845*b* "Electro-physiological researches.—First memoir. The muscular current." *PT,* Part II, pp. 283–295.

1845*c* "Electro-physiological researches.—Second memoir. On the proper current of the frog." *PT,* Part II, pp. 297–301.

1845*d* "Electro-physiological researches.—Third memoir. On induced contractions." *PT,* Part II, pp. 303–317.

1847 *Lectures on the physical phenomena of living beings.* Trans. J. Pereira. London: Longman et al.

1850*a* "Electro-physiological researches. Eighth series [1849]." *PT,* Part I, pp. 287–296.

1850*b* "Electro-physiological researches. On induced contraction. Ninth series." *PT,* Part II, pp. 645–649.

1861 *Corso di elettrofisiologia in sei lezioni.* Turin: Castellano & Vercellino. (Not seen.) English trans. in C. Matteucci, "Electro-physiology" (1866).

1866 "Electro-physiology: A course of lectures by Prof. Carlo Matteucci, Senator, &c. Turin, 1861." Trans. C. A. Alexander, *Annual Report of the Smithsonian Institution for 1865* (Washington, D.C.). Pp. 291–345.

Matteucci, C., and F. H. A. von Humboldt.

1843 "Sur le courant électrique des muscles des animaux vivants ou récemment tués." *CRAS,* 16:197–200.

Matteucci, C., and F. A. Longet.

1844 "Note sur l'hypothèse des courants électriques dans les nerves." *ACP,* 3d ser., 12:579–580.

Mauro, Alexander.

1969 "The role of the Voltaic pile in the Galvani-Volta controversy concerning animal *vs.* metallic electricity." *JHM,* 24:140–150.

May, Margaret Tallmadge, trans.

1968 *Galen on the usefulness of the parts of the body . . . "De usu partium." Translated from the Greek with an introduction and commentary by Margaret Tallmadge May.* 2 vols. Ithaca: Cornell University Press.

Mayer, August Franz Joseph Carl.

1832 "Ueber das Gehirn, das Rückenmark und die Nerven." [1833], *Nova Acta Physico-medica Academiae Caesareae Leopoldino-Carolinae Naturae Curiosorum* (Vratislava & Bonn), 16:679–770.

Mayo, Herbert.

1822–1823 *Anatomical and physiological commentaries.* London: T. & G. Underwood. Number I, August 1822; Number II, July 1823. Reprinted Metuchen, N.J.: Scarecrow Press, 1975, with introduction by Paul F. Cranefield.

1823*a* "On the cerebral nerves, with reference to sensation and voluntary motion." In H. Mayo, *Anatomical* (1822–1823), Number II (1823), pp. 1–21.

1823*b* "Remarks upon the spinal chord and the nervous system generally." In H. Mayo, *Anatomical* (1822–1823), Number II (1823), pp. 132–141.

1823*c* "Sur les nerf cérébraux, considérés dans leur rapport avec le sentiment et le mouvement voluntaire." JPEP, 3:345–361.

1827 *Outlines of human physiology.* London: Burgess & Hill.

1829 *Outlines of human physiology.* 2d ed. London: Burgess & Hill.

1842 *The nervous system and its functions.* London: J. W. Parker.

Mead, Richard.

1704 *De imperio solis ac lunae in corpora humana, et morbis inde oriundus.* London: R. Smith. English trans. in R. Mead, *Of the power* (1712).

1712 *Of the power and influence of the sun and moon on humane bodies; and of the diseases that arise from thence.* London: R. Wellington.

Meckel, Johann Friedrich, the Elder.

1748 *Tractatus anatomico-physiologicus de quinto pare nervorum cerebri*. Göttingen: A. Vandenhoek.

1749 "Observation anatomique sur un noeud [Meckel's ganglion] . . . avec l'examen physiologique du véritable usage des noeuds, ou ganglions des nerfs," *Histoire de l'Académie Royale des Sciences et Belle-Lettres de Berlin,* 5:84–102.

Meckel, Johann Friedrich, the Younger.

1795 "De ganglio secundi rami quinto paris nervorum cerebri nuper detecto, de que vera gangliorum nervosorum utilitate. Berolini, 1749." In C. F. Ludwig, ed. *Scriptores nevrologicae minores* (1791–1795), 4 (1795):7–9.

1808–1811 *Beyträge zur vergleichenden Anatomie*. 2 vols. Leipzig: C. H. Reclam.

1815–1820 *Handbuch der menschlichen Anatomie*. 4 vols. Halle & Berlin: Buchhandlung des Hallischen Maisenhauses.

Mehée de la Touche, Jean.

1773 *Traité des lesions de la tête, par contre-coup, avec des expériences propres à en éclairer la doctrine*. Meaux: L. A. Courtois.

Meier, Richard Y.

1979 "Sympathy as a concept in early neurophysiology," Ph.D. Dissertation, University of Chicago.

1982 "'Sympathy' in the neurophysiology of Thomas Willis." *Clio Medica,* 17:95–111.

Meissner, Paul Traugott.

1832 *System der Heilkunde aus den allgemeinsten Naturgesetzen*. Vienna: C. Gerold.

Mendelsohn, Everett.

1965 "Physical models and physiological concepts: Explanation in nineteenth-century biology." *British Journal of the History of Science,* 2:201–219.

Merton, Robert K.

1961 "Singletons and multiples in scientific discovery: a chapter in the sociology of science." *Proceedings of the American Philosophical Society,* 105:470–486.

Merz, John Theodore.

1907–1914 *A history of European thought in the nineteenth century*. 4 vols. 3d unaltered ed. Edinburgh & London: W. Blackwood.

Mesmer, Franz Anton.

1766 *Dissertatio physico-medica de planetarum influxu*. Vienna: Ghelenianis.

1779 *Mémoire sur la découverte du magnétisme animal*. Geneva & Paris: P. F. Didot jeune.

1948 *Mesmerism . . . Being the first translation of Mesmer's historic Mémoire sur la decouverte du magnétisme animal to appear in English* [by V. R. Myers]. London: Macdonald.

Mette, Alexander.
1963 "Wilhelm Griesinger." In O. Finger and F. Herneck, eds. *Von Liebig zu Laue* (1963). Pp. 52–85.

Meyer, Alfred.
1966 "Karl Friedrich Burdach on Thomas Willis." *Journal of the Neurological Sciences,* 3:109–116.
1970 "Karl Friedrich Burdach and his place in the history of neuroanatomy." *Journal of Neurology, Neurosurgery and Psychiatry,* 33:553–561.
1971 *Historical aspects of cerebral anatomy.* London: Oxford University Press.

Meyer, A., and R. Hierons.
1964 "A note on Thomas Willis' views on the corpus striatum and the internal capsule." *Journal of the Neurological Sciences,* 1:547–554.
1965 "On Thomas Willis's concepts of neurophysiology: Part II." *MH,* 9:142–155.

Meynell, G.
1983 "Francis Bauer, Joseph Banks, Everard Home and others." *Archives of Natural History,* 11:209–221.

Michelitz, Anton.
1782 "Scrutinium hypotheseos spirituum animalium. Pragae 1782." In C. F. Ludwig, ed. *Scriptores nevrologicae minores* (1791–1795). 3 (1793):209–239.

Mignet, François Auguste Marie.
1840 "Réponse de M. Mignet . . . au discours de M. Flourens." *Receuil des Discours de l'Académie Française,* 1:21–36.

Milne-Edwards, Henri.
1823 *Mémoire sur la structure élémentaire des principaux tissus organiques des animaux.* Paris: Didot. (His M.D. Thèse.) Also in *AGM* (1823), 3 1st series:165–184.
1826 "Recherches microscopiques sur la structure intime des tissus organiques des animaux." *Annales des Science Naturelles* (Paris), 9 1st series:362–394.

Mitchell, E.
1829 *Engravings of the cardiac nerves . . . copied from the "Tabulae neurologicae" of Antonio Scarpa.* 2d ed. Edinburgh: Maclachlan & Stewart.

Mitchell, G. A. G.
1953 *Anatomy of the autonomic nervous system.* Edinburgh & London: E. & S. Livingstone.

Monfalcon, Jean Baptiste.
1821 "Sympathie." In [N. P.] Adelon et al., eds. *Dictionaire des sciences médicales* (1812–1822). 53:537–621.

Monro, Alexander, *secundus*.
1783 *Observations on the structure and functions of the nervous system . . .* Edinburgh: W. Creech & J. Johnson.
1820 *The anatomy of the human bones and nerves . . .* 3d ed. Edinburgh: Bell & Bradfute, and A. Black.

Moore, T. C. T.
1970 *The psychology of Maine de Biran*. Oxford: Clarendon Press.

Moreau de la Sarthe, Jacques Louis.
An. IX [1800–1801] ["Review of *Traité medico-philosophique sur l'aliénation mentale* by Phillipe Pinel"]. *La Décade Philosophique, Littéraire et Politique*, 29:458–467.

Morgagni, Giovanni Baptista.
1717 *Adversaria anatomica altera . . .* Padua: J. Cominus.
1719 *Adversaria anatomica omnia . . .* Padua: J. Cominus.
1761 *De sedibus, et causis morborum . . .* Venice: Remondini.

Moruzzi, Giuseppe.
1963 "The electrophysiological work of Carl Matteucci." In L. Belloni, ed. *Essays* (1963). Pp. 139–147.
1964 "L'opera elettrofisiologica di Carlo Matteucci." *Physis*, 6:101–140.
1973 *L'opera elettrofisiologica di Carlo Matteucci*, and *Il contributo di Carlo Matteucci alla creazione del modello fisico del nervo*. Ferrara: Università degli Studi (*Quaderni di Storia della Scienza e della Medicina*, XII).

Mottelay, Paul Fleury.
1922 *Bibliographical history of electricity & magnetism chronologically arranged . . .* London: C. Griffin.

Mountcastle, Vernon B., ed.
1980 *Medical physiology*. 14th ed. 2 vols. St. Louis: C. V. Mosby.

Müller, Johannes (of Berlin).
1826 *Zur vergleichenden Physiologie des Gesichtssinnes der Menschen und der Thiere*. Leipzig: Cnobloch.
1828 "Ueber die Metamorphosen des Nervensystems in der Thierwelt." *AAP*, pp. 1–22.
1831 "Bestätigung des Bell'schen Lehrsatzes, dass die doppelten Wurzeln der Rückenmarksnerven verschiedene Functionen haben, durch neue und entscheidende Experimente." *Notizen aus dem Gebiete der Natur-und Heilkunde* (L. F. von Froriep: Erfurt, Weimar), 30:columns 113–117.

1832 "Ueber das Ganglion oticum Arnoldi." *AAP*, pp. 67–86.

1835 *Vergleichende Anatomie der Myxinoiden, der Cyclostomen mit durchbotem Gaumen.* Berlin: Druckerei der Königlichen Akademie.

1835 to 1837–1840 *Handbuch der Physiologie des Menschen für Vorlesungen.* 2 vols. Coblenz: J. Hölscher. This copy comprised vol. 1 of 2d ed. (1835) and vol. 2 of 1st ed. (1837–1840). See Bibliographical Notes.

1841–1844 to ? *Handbuch der Physiologie der Menschen für Vorlesungen.* 4th ed. 2 vols. Coblenz: J. Hölscher. Only vol. 1 of this ed. (1841–1844) was available. See Bibliographical Notes.

1838–1843 *Elements of physiology.* Trans. W. Baly. 2 vols. London: Taylor & Walton. The second vol. (1843) is a reprint of the 1842 printing. See Bibliographical Notes.

1845 *Manuel de physiologie.* Trans. A. J. L. Jourdan. 2 vols. Paris: J. B. Baillière. (2d ed., 1851.)

Müller, Johannes (of Freiburg-im-Breisgau).

1849 *Bericht über die neuesten Fortschritte der Physik,* Braunschweig. (Not seen.)

Müller, L. R.

1924 *Die Lebensnerven.* Berlin: J. Springer. (Not seen.)

1931 *Lebensnerven und Lebenstriebe.* Berlin: J. Springer. (Not seen.)

Murray, Sir James August Henry et al., eds.

1888–1928 *A new English dictionary on historical principles.* 10 vols. in 20, Oxford: Clarendon Press.

Musgrave, Samuel.

1776 *Speculations and conjectures on the qualities of the nerves.* London: P. Elmsly et al.

Nachmansohn, David.

1940 "Electricity elicited by an organic chemical process." *Science,* 91:405–406.

Neu, John, ed.

1980–1985 *Isis cumulative bibliography 1966–1975 . . .* 2 vols. London: Mansell.

Neubauer, Johann Ernest.

1772 *Descriptio anatomica nervorum cardiacorum. Sectio prima de nervo intercostalis cervicali, dextri imprimis lateralis.* Frankfurt & Leipzig: in off. Fleischariana.

Neuburger, Max.

1897 *Die historische Entwicklung der experimentellen Gehirn-und Rückenmarksphysiologie vor Flourens.* Stuttgart: F. Enke.

1909 "Streiflichter auf die neurologische Forschung in Wien während des 18. Jahrhunderts." *Wiener medicinische Wochenschrift,* 59:2132–2139.

1913 *Johann Christian Reil.* Stuttgart: F. Enke.

1981 *The historical development of experimental brain and spinal cord physiology before Flourens.* Trans. and ed., Edwin Clarke. Baltimore & London: Johns Hopkins University Press. Trans. of M. Neuburger, *Die historische Entwicklung* (1897). Referred to in notes as M. Neuburger (1981).

Newport, George.

1843 "On the structure, relations, and development of the nervous and circulatory systems, and on the existence of a complete circulation of the blood in vessels, in Myriapoda, and Macrourous Arachnida. First series." *PT,* Part II, pp. 243–302.

Nisbet, H. B.

1970 *Herder and the philosophy and history of science.* Cambridge: Modern Humanities Association.

1972 *Goethe and the scientific tradition.* London: Institute of Germanic Studies.

Nobili, Leopoldo.

1825 "Descrizione di un nuovo galvanometro." *Giornale di Fisica, Chimica, e Storia Naturale* (L. Brugnatelli: Pavia), 8:278–282. Also in *Quarterly Journal of Literature, Science and Arts* (London), 1826, 20:170–172.

1828 "Comparaison entre les deux galvanomètres les plus sensibles, la grenouille et le multiplicateur à deux aiguilles, suivie de quelques résultats nouveaux." *ACP,* 38:225–245.

1830 "Analyse expérimentale et théorique des effets électro-physiologiques de la grenouille, suivie d'un appendice sur la nature du tétanos et de la paralysie, et sur la manière de guérir ces deux maladies au moyen de l'électricité" [1829]. *ACP,* 44:60–94.

Noel, Patricia S., and Eric T. Carlson.

1970 "Origins of the word 'phrenology.'" *American Journal of Psychiatry,* 127:694–697.

Nothanagel, Carl Wilhelm Hermann.

1879 *Topische Diagnostik der Gehirnkrankheiten. Eine klinische Studie.* Berlin: A. Hirschwald.

Ochs, Sidney.

1975 "Waller's concept of the trophic dependence of the nerve fiber on the cell body in the light of early neuron theory." *Clio Medica,* 19:253–265.

Oersted, Hans Christian.

1820*a* *Experimenta circa effectum conflictus electrici in acum magneticam.* Copenhagen: Published privately, 21 July.

1820*b* "Experiments on the effect of a current of electricity on the magnetic needle." *Annals of Philosophy* (T. Thomson: London), 16:273–276.

Ollivier d'Angers, Charles Prosper.

1827 *Traité de la moelle épinière et de ses maladies. . . .* 2 vols., 2d ed., Paris: Crevot.

Olmsted, J. M. D.

1939 *Claude Bernard, physiologist.* London: Cassell.

1943 "The aftermath of Charles Bell's 'Idea.'" *BHM,* 14:341–351.

1944*a* "Historical note on the *noeud vital* or respiratory center." *BHM,* 16:343–350.

1944*b* *François Magendie. Pioneer in experimental physiology and scientific medicine in XIX century France.* New York: Schuman.

1953 "Pierre Flourens." In E. A. Underwood, ed. *Science medicine and history* (1953), 2:290–302.

Olmsted, J. M. D., and E. Harris Olmsted.

1952 *Claude Bernard & the experimental method in medicine.* London: Cassell.

Orbach, Jack, ed.

1982 *Neuropsychology after Lashley. Fifty years since the publication of "Brain mechanisms and intelligence."* Hillsdale, N.J.: L. Erlbaum.

Otto, Adolph Wilhelm.

1830 *Lehrbuch der pathologischen Anatomie des Menschen und der Thiere.* Vol. 1 only. Berlin: A. Rücker.

1831 *A compendium of human and comparative pathological anatomy, translated . . . by John F. South.* London: B. Fellowes.

Owen, Sir Richard.

1843 *Lectures on the comparative anatomy and physiology of the invertebrate animals.* London: Longman.

P., J. L. H.

1831 *Sketches of the character and writings of eminent living surgeons and physicians of Paris.* Trans. Elisha Bartlett. Boston: Carter, Hendee & Babcock. (Selections from French ed., *Les médicins français contemporains* [1827–1828].)

P., R.

1929 "Quotations. Dr. John Cross on physiognomy and constitution." *Human Biology. A Record of Research,* 1:426–430.

Paget, James.

1846 "Report on the progress of human anatomy and physiology in the years 1844–5." *BFMR,* 22:261–292.

Paine, Martyn.

1847 *The institutes of medicine.* New York: Harper.

1858 *The institutes of medicine.* 4th ed. New York: Harper.

Parchappe de Vinay, Jean Baptiste Maximilian.

1836–1838 *Recherches sur l'encéphale, sa structure, ses fonctions et ses maladies* [2 *mémoires* in one vol.], Paris: De Just Rouvier & E. le Bouvier.

1838 *Deuxième mémoire. Des altérations de l'encéphale dans l'aliénation mentale.* In *Recherches* (1836–1838).

1856 *Du siège commun de l'intelligence, de la volonté et de la sensibilité chez l'homme.* Paris: V. Masson.

Parker, G. H.

1900 "The neurone theory in the light of recent discoveries." *The American Naturalist,* 34:457–470.

Parker, S. Langston.

1831 "Lectures on comparative anatomy, as illustrative of general and human physiology . . . " *London Medical Gazette* [1830–1831], 7:65–70.

Parssinen, T. M.

1974 "Popular science and society: the phrenology movement in early-Victorian Britain." *Journal of Social History,* 7:1–20.

Pattie, Frank A.

1956 "Mesmer's medical dissertation and its debt to Mead's *De imperio solis ac lunae.*" *JHM,* 11:275–287.

Pavlov, Ivan Petrovich.

1928–1941 *Lectures on conditioned reflexes.* Trans. W. H. Gantt. London: Lawrence.

Pearson, Ronald.

1972 *The avian brain.* London: Academic Press.

Person, Charles Cléophas.

1830 "Sur l'hypothèse des courans électriques dans les nerfs." *JPEP,* 10:216–225. (Read to Académie des Sciences 25 October 1830.)

Petetin, Jacques Henri Desiré.

1808 *Électricité animale, prouvée par la découverte des phénomènes physiques et moraux de la catalepsie hystérique . . .* Paris: Brunot-Labbe and Gautier & Bretin.

Pfaff, Christoph Heinrich.

1795 *Über thierische Elektricität und Reizbarkeit. Ein Beytrag zu den neuesten Entdeckungen über diese Gegenstände.* Leipzig: S. L. Crusius.

Pfeffinger, Johann.

1791 "De structura nervorum. Sectio prima. Argentorati 1782." In C. F. Ludwig, *Scriptores nevrologicae minores* (1791–1795), 1 (1791):1–30.

Philip, Alexander Philips Wilson (known as Wilson Philip).

1815*a* "Experiments made with a view to ascertain the principle on which the action of the heart depends, and the relation which subsists between that organ and the nervous system." *PT,* Part I, pp. 65–90.

1815*b* "Some additional experiments and observations on the relation which subsists between the nervous and sanguiferous systems." *PT,* Part II, pp. 424–446.

1817*a* "On the effects of galvanism in restoring the due action of the lungs" [1816]. *PT,* Part I, pp. 22–31.

1817*b* *An experimental inquiry into the laws of the vital functions, with some observations on the nature and treatment of internal diseases.* London: T. & G. Underwood. In part republished from A. P. W. Philip, "Experiments made" (1815); "Some additional experiments" (1815); and "On the effects of galvanism" (1817).

1818 *An experimental inquiry into the laws of the vital functions . . .* 2d ed. London: T. & G. Underwood.

Philites, C. A.

1809 "Von dem Alter des Menschen überhaupt und dem Marasmus senilis inbesondere," *AP,* 9:1–128.

Phillips, C. G., S. Zeki, and H. B. Barlow.

1984 "Localization of function in the cerebral cortex. Past, present, and future." *Brain,* 107:327–361.

Picavet, François.

1891 *Les idéologues. Essai sur l'historie des idées et des théories scientifiques, philosophiques, religieuses, etc. en France depuis 1789.* Paris: F. Alcan.

Pick, J.

1970 *The autonomic nervous system.* Philadelphia: J. B. Lippincott.

Pickstone, John V.

1973 "Globules and coagula: concepts of tissue formation in the early nineteenth century." *JHM,* 28:336–356.

1981 "Bureaucracy, liberalism and the body in post-Revolutionary France: Bichat's physiology and the Paris medical school." *History of Science,* 19:115–142.

Pinel, Philippe.

[1801] *Traité médico-philosophique sur l'aliénation mentale ou la manie.* Paris: Richard, Caille & Ravier.

1822 "Recherches d'anatomie pathologique sur l'endurcissement du système nerveux," *JPEP,* 2:191–219.

Plarr, Victor G.

1930–1970 *Plarr's lives of the Fellows of the Royal College of Surgeons of England.* 4 vols. Bristol: J. Wright et al.

Plato.

1873 *Platonis opera omnia . . .* C. Tauchnit, ed. Leipzig: O. Holtze.

Poggendorff, Johann Christian.
1821 "Physikalisch-chemische Untersuchungen zur nähern Kenntniss des Magnetismus der voltaischen Säule." *Isis, oder Encyclopädische Zeitung* (L. Oken: Jena), columns 687–710.
1863–1926 *Biographisch-literarisches Handwörterbuch zur Geschichte der exacten Wissenschaften* . . . 5 vols. Leipzig: J. A. Barth.

Polaillon, J. F. B.
1865 *Étude sur les ganglions nerveux péripheriques.* Paris: A. Parent.

Porta, Giovanni Battista della.
1586 *De humana physiognomonia libri IIII.* Vico Aequense [Vico di Sorrento]: J. Cacchi.

Portal, Baron Antoine.
1801 "Description du nerf intercostal dans l'homme." *Mémoires de la Classe des Sciences mathématiques et physiques de l'Institut.* Pp. 151–208.

Pourfour du Petit, François.
1710 *Lettres d'un médecin des hôpitaux du Roi, à un autre médecin de ses amis.* Namur: C. G. Albert.
1729*a* "Sur ce que le nerf intercostal fournit des esprits aux yeux [1727]." *Histoire de l'Académie des Sciences.* Pp. 7–10. This is an abstract of "Mémoire" (1729).
1729*b* "Mémoire dans lequel il est démontré que les nerfs intercostaux fournissent des rameaux qui portent des esprits dans les yeux [1727]." *Memoires de Mathématique et de Physiologie,* in *Histoire de l'Académie des Sciences.* Pp. 1–19 (of the second numbering).

Power, Henry, and Leonard W. Sedgwick.
1879–1899 *The New Sydenham Society's lexicon of medicine.* 5 vols. London: New Sydenham Society.

Poynter, F. N. L., ed.
1958 *The history and philosophy of knowledge of the brain and its functions. An Anglo-American symposium, July 15th-17th, 1957.* Oxford: Blackwell.

Prévost, Jean Louis, and Jean Baptiste André Dumas.
1823 "Sur les phénomènes qui accompagnent la contraction de la fibre musculaire." *JPEP,* 3:301–338; with "Additions . . . ," pp. 339–344.

Prichard, James Cowles.
1829 *A review of the doctrine of a vital principle as maintained by some writers on physiology with observations on the causes of physical and animal life.* London: Sherwood et al., and J. & A. Arch.

1835 *A treatise on insanity and other disorders affecting the mind.* London: Sherwood et al.

Priestley, Joseph.

1767 *History and present state of electricity, with original experiments.* London: J. Dodsley. Further editions (2d–4th), in 1769, 1775, 1776. French trans. Paris, 1771.

Procháska, Jiří.

1779 *De structura nervorum. Tractatus anatomicus . . .* Vienna: R. Graeffer.

1784 *Adnotationum academicarum. Fasciculus tertius.* Prague: W. Gerle. English trans. in J. Procháska, *. . . and a dissertation* (1851).

1815 *Versuch einer empirischen Darstellung des polarischen Naturgesetzes und dessen Anwendung auf die Thätigkeiten der organischen und unorganischen Körper, mit einem Rückblick auf den thierischen Magnetismus.* Vienna: Camesina.

1820 *Physiologie oder Lehre von der Natur des Menschen.* Vienna: C. F. Beck.

1851 *. . . and a dissertation on the functions of the nervous system.* Trans. Thomas Laycock. London: Sydenham Society. Pp. 361–450. See J. A. Unzer, *The principles* (1851).

Pupilli, G. C. and Ettore Fadiga.

1963 "The origins of electrophysiology." *Journal of World History,* 7:547–589.

Purkyně, Jan Evangelista.

1828 ["Review of Carl Friedr. Burdach, *Vom Baue und Leben des Gehirns*"]. *Opera omnia.* 5:55–77.

1833 ["Review of K. F. Burdach, *Die Physiologie als Erfahrungswissenschaft*]." *Opera omnia.* 5:117–122.

1834*a* "Ei." *Opera omnia.* 4:152–193.

1834*b* "Einbildungskraft." *Opera omnia.* 4:193–203.

1837*a* "Neueste Beobachtungen über die Struktur des Gehirns." *Opera omnia.* 2:88.

1837*b* "Neueste Untersuchungen aus der Nerven-und Hirnanatomie." *Opera omnia.* 3:45–49.

1837*c* "Über den Bau der Magen-Drüsen und über die Natur des Verdauungsprocesses." *Opera omnia.* 3:43–45.

1839 "Ueber die Analogieen in den Struktur-Elementen des thierischen und pflanzlichen Organismus." *Opera omnia.* 2:90–91.

1842 "Ueber die Struktur des Herzens der Säugethiere nach dem Grundtypus der Formation der Muskelfasern desselben." *Opera omnia.* 2:95–96.

1843 "Ueber den Typus der Windungen des Grossen Hirns des Menschen und über dessen Ableitung aus der allgemeinen Faltentheorie." *Opera omnia.* 2:103–106.

1844 "Mikroskop." *Opera omnia.* 3:119–154.

1846 "Sinne im allgemeinen." *Opera omnia.* 3:155–163.

1850 "Papierstreifen aus dem Portefeuille eines verstorbenen Naturforschers." *Opera omnia.* 4:239–288. Originally in B. G. Ernst, *Planetogenesis* (1850).

1852 "Ueber den Begriff der Physiologie, ihre Beziehung zu den übrigen Naturwissenschaften, und zu andern wissenschaftlichen und Kunst-Gebieten, die Methoden ihrer Lehre und Praxis, über die Bildung zum Physiologen, über Errichtung Physiologischer Institute." *Opera omnia.* 3:64–79.

1918–1973 *Opera omnia.* 12 vols., Prague: Purkýnova Společnost.

Purkyně, J. E., and G. G. Valentin.

1835*a* *De motu vibratorio animalium vertebratorum. Observationes recentissimus.* In J. E. Purkyně. *Opera omnia.* 3:15–22.

1835*b* *De phaenomeno generali et fundamentali motus vibratorii continui in membranis cum externis tum internis animalium plurimorum et superiorum et inferiorum ordinum obvii.* In J. E. Purkyně. *Opera omnia.* 1:277–571.

Quain, Jones.

1837 *Elements of anatomy.* 4th ed. London: Taylor & Walton.

1848 *Elements of anatomy.* Ed. Richard Quain and William Sharpey. 5th ed. 2 vols. London: Taylor, Walton, & Maberly.

R., S.

1817 "Observations on the remarks of A. M. on the doctrines of Gall and Spurzheim." *Blackwood's Magazine,* 1:365–367.

Ramón y Cajal, Santiago.

1888 "Estruttura de los centros nerviosos de los aves." *Revista trimestral Histologia normal y patológica* (Barcelona), May, 1:305–315.

1933 "¿Neuronismo o reticularismo? Las pruebas objectivas de la unidad anátomica, de las celulas nerviosas." *Archivos Neurobiologia* (Madrid), 13:217–291, 579–646.

1954 *Neuron theory or reticular theory? Objective evidence of the anatomical unity of nerve cells.* Trans. M. U. Purkiss & C. A. Fox. Madrid: Instituto Ramón y Cajal.

Ramström, O. M.

1911 "Swedenborg on the cerebral cortex as the seat of psychical activity." In *Swedenborg Congress* (1911). Pp. 56–70.

Ranson, Stephen Walter.

1917 "On the use of the word 'sympathetic' in anatomical and

physiological nomenclature." *Anatomical Record,* 11:397–400.
1959 *The anatomy of the nervous system: Its development and function.* 10th ed. Philadelphia & London: W. B. Saunders.

Rapp, Dietmar.
1970 "Die Entwicklung der physiologischen Methodik von 1784 bis 1811. Eine quantitative Untersuchung," Münster (*Münstersche Beiträge zur Geschichte und Theorie der Medizin,* Nr. 2).

Rasmussen, A. T.
1947 *Some trends in neuroanatomy.* Dubuque, Iowa: W. C. Brown.

Rath, Gernot.
1958 "Albrecht Thaer als Neuralpathologe," *SAGM,* 42:65–70.
1959 "Neural pathology. A pathogenetric concept of the 18th and 19th centuries." *BHM,* 33:526–541.

Rather, Lelland J.
1958 *Disease, life, and man: Selected essays by Rudolf Virchow.* Stanford, Calif.: Stanford University Press.
1969 "Some relations between eighteenth-century fiber theory and nineteenth-century cell theory." *Clio Medica,* 4:191–202.
1978 *The genesis of cancer: A study in the history of ideas.* Baltimore: Johns Hopkins Press.

Rehbock, Philip F.
1983 *The philosophical naturalists: Themes in early nineteenth-century British biology.* Madison: University of Wisconsin Press.

Reichenbach, Baron Charles von.
1851 *Physico-physiological researches on the dynamics of magnetism, electricity, heat, light, crystallization, and chemism, in their relations to vital force.* London: H. Baillière.

Reil, Johann Christian.
1807 "Ueber die Eigenschaften des Ganglien-Systems und sein Verhältniss zum Cerebral-Systeme." *AP,* 7:189–254.
1807–1808*a* "Fragmente über die Bildung des kleinen Gehirns im Mensche." *AP,* 8:1–58. Trans. in H. Mayo, *Anatomical* (1822–1823), Number I (1822), pp. 19–55. See Clarke and O'Malley (1968). Pp. 647–651.
1807–1808*b* "Erste Fortsetzung der Untersuchungen über den Bau des kleinen Gehirns im Menschen." *AP,* 8:273–304. Trans. in H. Mayo. *Anatomical* (1822–1823), Number I (1822), pp. 56–73.
1807–1808*c* "Untersuchungen über den Bau des kleinen Gehirns im Menschen. Zweyte Fortsetzung. Ueber die Organisation der Lappen und Läppchen, oder der Stämme, Aeste, Zweige und

Blättchen des kleinen Gehirns, die auf dem Kern desselben aufsitzen." *AP,* 8:385–426. Trans. in H. Mayo. *Anatomical* (1822–1823), Number I (1822), pp. 74–101. See Clarke and O'Malley (1968). Pp. 651–652.

1809*a* "Nachtrag zur Anatomie des kleinen Gehirns. Dritte Fortsetzung." *AP,* 9:129–135. Trans. in H. Mayo, *Anatomical* (1822–1823), Number I (1822), pp. 102–106.

1809*b* "Untersuchungen über den Bau des grossen Gehirns im Menschen . . . Vierte Fortsetzung." *AP,* 9:136–208. Trans. in H. Mayo, *Anatomical* (1822–1823), Number II (1823), pp. 48–83.

1809*c* "Das verlängerte Rückenmark, die hinteren, seitlichen und vörderen Schenkel des kleinen Gehirns . . . Fünfte Fortsetzung." *AP,* 9:485–524. Trans. in H. Mayo, *Anatomical* (1822–1823), Number II (1823), pp. 84–112.

1812 "Nachträge zur Anatomie des grossen und kleinen Gehirns . . . Achte Fortsetzung." *AP,* 11:345–376. Trans. in H. Mayo, *Anatomical* (1822–1823), Number II (1823), pp. 119–131.

Remak, Robert.

1836 "Vorläufige Mittheilung mikroscopischer Beobachtungen über den innern Bau der Cerebrospinalnerven und über die Entwicklung ihrer Formelemente." *AAPM,* pp. 145–159.

1837 "Weitere mikroscopische Beobachtungen über die Primitivfasern des Nervensystems der Wirbelthiere." *Neue Notizen aus dem Gebiete der Natur-und Heilkunde* (L. F. & R. Froriep: Erfurt & Weimar), 3:columns 36–41.

1838*a* *Observationes anatomicae et microscopicae de systematis nervosi structura.* Berlin: G. Reimer.

1838*b* "Ueber die Verrichtungen des organischen Nervensystems." *Neue Notizen aus dem Gebiete der Natur-und Heilkunde* (L. F. & R. Froriep: Erfurt & Weimar), 7:columns 65–70.

1839 ["Remak on the structure of the nervous system"]. *BFMR,* 7:500–505.

1840 "Ueber die physiologische Bedeutung des organischen Nervensystems, besonders nach anatomischen Thatsachen." *Monatsschrift für Medicin, Augenheilkunde und Chirurgie* (F. A. von Ammon: Leipzig), 3:225–265.

1841*a* "Anatomische Beobachtungen über das Gehirn, das Rückenmark und die Nervenwurzeln." *AAPM,* pp. 506–522.

1841*b* "Nervensystem (histologisch)." In C. F. von Gräfe, C. W. Hufeland et al., eds. *Encyclopädisches Handwörterbuch* (1828–1849), 25:129–152.

1841*c* "Nervensystem (physiologisch)." Ibid., pp. 152–195.

1843 "Ueber den Inhalt der Nervenprimitivröhren." *AAPM*, pp. 197–201.

1854*a* "Ueber multipolare Ganglienzellen." *Bericht über die zur Bekanntmachung geeigneten Verhandlungen der Könige Preuss. Akademie der Wissenschaften zu Berlin*, 19:26–32. English version in R. Remak, "Professor Remak" (1854).

1854*b* "Professor Remak on multipolar ganglion-cells." *The Monthly Journal of Medical Sciences* (Edinburgh), 18:362–365.

Retzius, Anders Adolf.

1832 "Ueber den Zusammenhang der Pars thoracica nervi sympathici mit den Wurzeln der Spinalnerven." *AAPM*, pp. 260–262. (A letter to J. Müller dated 3 August 1832.)

Reuss, Franz Ambros.

1783 "Ergo spirituum animalium hypothesi carere possunt physiologi." M.D. Thesis, University of Prague.

Révész, Béla.

1917 *Geschichte des Seelenbegriffes und der Seelenlokalisation.* Stuttgart: F. Enke.

Rich, Arnold R.

1926 "The place of R. J. H. Dutrochet in the development of the cell theory." *Bulletin of the Johns Hopkins Hospital*, 39:330–365.

Richerand, Anthelme Balthasar.

An VII [1799] "Essai sur la connexion de la vie avec la circulation." *Mémoire de la Société Médicale d'Emulation, séante à l'École de Médecine de Paris*, 3:296–310.

1801 *Nouveaux élémens de physiologie*. Paris, 1801. (Not seen.)

An XII [1804] *Nouveaux élémens de physiologie*. 3d ed. 2 vols. Paris: Crapart, Caille & Ravier.

1829 *Elements of physiology*. 2d ed. Trans. G. J. M. De Lys, from the 5th French ed. London: Longman et al.

Richet, Charles.

1895–1928 *Dictionnaire de physiologie*. 10 vols. Paris: F. Alcan.

Riese, Walther.

1936*a* "F.-J. Gall et le problème des localisations cérébrales." *L'Hygiène Mentale*, 31:105–135.

1936*b* "Les discussions du problème des localisations cérébrales dans les sociétés savantes du XIXe siècle et leurs rapports avec des vues contemporaines." *L'Hygiène Mentale*, 31:137–158.

1944 "The principle of compensation of nervous function." *Journal of Nervous and Mental Disease,* 100:263–274.

Riese, Walther, and C. E. Arrington.

1963 "The history of Johannes Müller's doctrine of the specific energies of the senses: original and later versions." *BHM,* 39:179–183.

Ritter, Johann Wilhelm.

1798 *Beweis, dass ein beständiger Galvanismus den Lebensprozess im Thierreich begleitet.* Weimar. (Not seen.)

1800 "Beweis dass die Galvanische Action oder der Galvanismus auch in der anorganischen Natur möglich und wirklich sey." In J. W. Ritter, ed. *Beyträge* (1800–1805), vol. 1, part 2, §§ 87–88 (pp. 250–253).

1801 "Versuche und Bemerkungen über den Galvanismus der voltaischen Batterie." *Annalen der Physik* (L. W. Gilbert: Halle & Leipzig) 7:431–484; 8:385–473; 9:212–263, 265–352.

1802 "Von der Galvanischen Batterie nebst Versuchen und Bemerkungen den Galvanismus überhaupt betreffend." In J. W. Ritter, ed. *Beyträge* (1800–1805), vol. 2, part 4, pp. 195–290.

1805 "Darstellungen des Gegensatzes zwischen Flexoren und Extensoren und ihre Erregbarkeiten, wie ihn Galvanische Versuch gehen, und Reduction desselben auf einen andern neuen überall verbreiteten Gegensatz." In J. W. Ritter, ed. *Beyträge* (1800–1805), vol. 2, part 3.

1806 "New Galvanic discoveries. By M. Ritter. Extracted from a letter from M. Christ. Bernoulli." *PM,* 23:51–54.

Ritter, Johann Wilhelm, ed.

1800–1805 *Beyträge zur nähern Kenntniss des Galvanismus und der Resultate seiner Untersuchung.* 2 vols. Jena: F. Frommann.

Ritterbush, Phillip C.

1964*a* "Electricity: the soul of the universe." In P. C. Ritterbush, *Overtures to biology* (1964). Pp. 15–56.

1964*b* *Overtures to biology. The speculations of eighteenth-century naturalists.* New Haven & London: Yale University Press.

Rolando, Luigi.

1809 *Saggio sopra la vera struttura del cervello dell'uomo e degl'animali e sopra le funzioni del sistema nervoso.* Sassari: [no publisher]. Reprinted by A. Forni of Bologna (1974) with introduction by Ugo Stefanutti.

1823 "Expériences sur les fonctions du système nerveux." *JPEP,* 3:95–113.

1824 "Expériences sur les fonctions du système nerveux." In P. Flourens, *Recherches* (1824). Pp. 273–302.

1828 *Saggio sopra la vera struttura del cervello e sopra le funzioni del sistema nervoso*. Turin: P. Marietti.

1831 "Della struttura degli emisferi cerebrali." *Memorie della reale Accademia delle Scienze di Torino,* 35:103–146.

Rolleston, J. D.

1930–1931 "Jean-Baptiste Bouillaud (1796–1881). A pioneer in cardiology and neurology." *Proceedings of the Royal Society of Medicine,* 24:1255–1262.

Romagnosi, Gian Domenico.

1802 "Articulo sul Galvanismo." *Gazzetta di Trento,* 3 August. (Not seen.)

Romberg, Moritz Heinrich.

1840–1846 *Lehrbuch der Nervenkrankheiten des Menschen.* 2 vols. A. Duncker.

1853 *A manual of the nervous diseases of man.* Trans. and ed. E. H. Sieveking. 2 vols. London: Sydenham Society.

Romberg, Moritz Heinrich, trans.

1832 *Karl Bell's physiologische und pathologische Untersuchungen des Nervensystems.* Berlin: Stuhr.

Ronchi, V.

1969 "Giovanni Battista Amici's contribution to the advances of optical microscopy." *Physis,* 11:520–533.

Rose, F. Clifford, and W. F. Bynum, eds.

1982 *Historical aspects of the neurosciences. A Festschrift for Macdonald Critchley.* New York: Raven Press.

Rosen, George.

1946 "The philosophy of ideology and the emergence of modern medicine in France." *BHM,* 20:328–339.

1951 "Romantic medicine: A problem in historical periodization." *BHM,* 25:149–158.

Rosenmüller, T. C.

1806 "Account of Dr. Gall's discoveries regarding the structure of the brain." *EMSJ,* 2:320–324.

Rostan, Léon Louis.

1823 *Recherches sur le ramollissement du cerveau . . .* 2d ed. Paris: Béchet, Gabon & Crévot.

Rothschuh, K. E.

1958 "Vom spiritus animalis zum Nervenaktionsstrom." *Ciba Zeitschrift,* 8:2949–2978.

1959*a* "Aus der Frühzeit der Elecktrobiologie." *Elektromedizin und ihre Grenzgebiete* 4:201–217.

1959*b* "Friedrich Alexander von Humboldt: Versuche über die gereizte Muskel-und Nervenfaser . . . (1797)," *Neue Zeitschrift für ärztliche Fortbildung* (Berlin), 48:432–433.

1959*c* "Alexander von Humboldt und die Physiologie seiner Zeit." *SAGM,* 43:97–113. Other articles on Humboldt, *SAGM,* 43:114–171.

1960*a* "Alexander von Humboldt et l'histoire de la découverte de l'électricité animale." *Conférence faite au Palais de la Découverte le 5 mars 1960. Histoire des Sciences,* Alençon (Orne): Alençonnaise. P. 15.

1960*b* "Von der Idee bis zum Nachweis der tierischen Elektrizität." *SAGM,* 44:25–44.

1964 "Emil du Bois-Reymond (1818–1896) und die Electrophysiologie der Nerven." In K. F. Rothschuh, ed. *Von Boerhaave bis Berger* (1964). Pp. 85–105.

1966 "Zur Geschichte der physiologischen Reizmethodik im 17. und 18. Jahrhundert." *Gesnerus,* 23:147–160.

1971*a* "Von der Histomorphologie zur Histophysiologie." In V. Kruta, ed. *Jan Evangelista Purkyně.* Pp. 197–212.

1971*b* "Die Bedeutung apparativer Hilfsmittel für die Entwicklung der biologischen Wissenschaften im 19. Jahrhundert." In H. Schimank, ed. *Geschichte der Naturwissenschaften* (1971). Pp. 137–174.

1973*a* *History of physiology.* Trans. G. B. Risse, Huntington, N.Y.: R. E. Krieger.

1973*b* *Bibliographie 1935–1973.* Münster (*Münstersche Beiträge zur Geschichte und Theorie der Medicin.* Nr. 8).

1983 *Bibliographie 1974–1983,* 2d ed., Münster (*Münstersche Beiträge zur Geschichte und Theorie der Medicin.* Nr. 19).

Rothschuh, K. E., ed.

1964 *Von Boerhaave bis Berger. Die Entwicklung der kontinentalen Physiologie im 18. und 19. Jahrhundert mit besonderer Berücksichtigung der Neurophysiologie.* Stuttgart: G. Fischer.

Rothschuh, K. E., and Elisabeth Tutte.

1975 "Emil du Bois-Reymond (1818–1896). Bibliographie. Originalien und Sekundärliteratur." *Acta Historica Leopoldina.* Nr. 9. Pp. 113–136.

Rousseau, George S.

1976 "Nerves, spirits, and fibres: Towards defining the origins of sensibility." In R. F. Brissenden and J. C. Eade, eds. *Studies* (1976). Pp. 137–157.

Rowbottom, Margaret, and C. Susskind.

1984 *Electricity and medicine. History of their interaction.* London: Macmillan.

Rush, Benjamin.
1811*a* *On the utility of a knowledge of the faculties and operations of the human mind, to a physician, in sixteen introductory lectures*. Philadelphia: Bradford & Innskeep.
1811*b* *On the opinions and modes of practice of Hippocrates, in sixteen introductory lectures*. Philadelphia: Bradford & Innskeep.

Russell, E. S.
1916 *Form and function: A contribution to the history of animal morphology*. London: J. Murray.

Sabouraut, Jean.
1778 "Mémoire sur le même sujet [contre-coup head injuries] [1768]." *Mémoires sur les Sujets proposés pour le Prix de l'Académie Royale de Chirurgie* (Paris), 4 (Part I):439–518.

Sachs, W.
1936 *The vegetative nervous system: A clinical study*. London: Cassell.

Saint-Simon, Maximilien Henri de.
1859 *Oeuvres choisies*. 3 vols. Brussels: Fr. van Meenen.

Sanderson, Sir John Scott Burdon, ed.
1887 *Translations of foreign biological memoirs. I. Memoirs on the physiology of nerve, of muscle and of the electrical organ*. Oxford: Clarendon Press.

Sandifort, Eduard.
1768–1778 *Thesaurus dissertationum, programmatum, aliorumque opusculorum selectissimorum, ad omnem medicinae ambitum pertinentium*. 3 vols. Leyden: S. & J. Luchtmans; P.v.d. Eyk & D. Vygh.

Sarton, George.
1928 "The foundation of electromagnetism (1820)." *Isis*, 10:435–444.
1931*a* "The discovery of the electrical cell (1800)." *Isis*, 15:124–128.
1931*b* "The discovery of the mammalian egg and the foundation of modern embryology." *Isis*, 16:315–330.

Saucerotte, Louis Sebastian.
1778 "Mémoire sur les contre-coups dans les lésions de la tête" [1768]. *Mémoires sur les Sujets proposés pour le Prix de l'Académie Royal de Chirurgie* (Paris), 4 (Part I):368–438.

Scarpa, Antonio.
1779 *Anatomicarum annotationum liber primus. De nervorum gangliis, et plexibus*. Modena: heirs of B. Soliani.
1794 *Tabulae nevrologicae, ad illustrandum historiam anatomicam*

cardiacorum nervorum, noni nervorum cerebri, glossopharyngaei et pharyngaei ex octavo cerebri. Pavia: B. Comini. English version in E. Mitchell. *Engravings* (1829).

1831 "De gangliis nervorum deque origine et essentià nervi intercostalis." *Annali Universali di Medicina* (A. Omodei: Milan), 58:474–483. Also in *Transactions médicales. Journal de Médecine pratique* (Paris), 5:264–282.

Schäfer, Edward A. (See also Sharpey-Schafer, Sir Edward A.)

1893 "The nerve cell considered as the basis of neurology." *Brain,* 16:134–169.

1900 "The cerebral cortex." In E. A. Schäfer, ed. *Text-book* (1898–1900). 2:697–782.

Schäfer, Edward A., ed.

1898–1900 *Text-book of physiology.* 2 vols. Edinburgh & London: Y. J. Pentland.

Schelling, Friedrich Wilhelm Joseph.

1798 *Von der Weltseele: Eine Hypothese der höhern Physik zur Erklärung des allgemeinen Organismus.* Hamburg: F. Perthes.

1799 *Einleitung zu seinem Entwurf eines Systems der Naturphilosophie.* Jena & Leipzig: C. E. Gabler.

Schierbeek, A.

1967 *Jan Swammerdam (12 February 1637–17 February 1680). His life and works.* Amsterdam: Swets & Zeitlinger.

Schiff, Moritz.

1858–1859 *Lehrbuch der Physiologie des Menschen . . . I. Muskel- und Nervenphysiologie.* Lahr: M. Schauenburg.

Schilf, Erich.

1926 *Das autonome Nervensystem.* Leipzig: G. Thieme.

Schiller, Francis.

1965 "The rise of the 'enteroid process' in the 19th century: some landmarks in cerebral nomenclature." *BHM,* 39:326–338.

1969 "Stilling's nuclei—turning point in basic neurology." *BHM,* 53:67–84.

1974 "The intriguing nucleus of Deiters. Notes on an eponymn." *BHM,* 48:276–286.

1979 *Paul Broca. Founder of French anthropology, explorer of the brain.* Berkeley, Los Angeles, London: University of California Press.

1981 "Reverend Wesley, Doctor Marat and their electric fire." *Clio Medica,* 15:159–176.

1982 "Neurology: the electrical root." In F. C. Rose and W. F. Bynum, eds. *Historical aspects* (1982). Pp. 1–11.

1984 "Coenesthesia." *BHM,* 58:496–515.

Schiller, Joseph.
1967 "Claude Bernard and vivisection." *JHM,* 22:246–260.
1973 "The genesis and structure of Claude Bernard's experimental method." In R. N. Gieve and R. S. Westfall, eds. *Foundations* (1973). Pp. 133–160.
1980 *Physiology and classification: Historical relations.* Paris: Maloine.

Schimank, Hans.
1935 "Geschichte der Electrisiermaschine bis zum Beginn des 19. Jahrhunderts." *Zeitschrift für technische Physik,* 16:245–254.

Schimank, Hans, ed.
1971 *Geschichte der Naturwissenschaften und der Technik im 19. Jahrhundert . . .* N.p.: Verlag des Vereins deutscher Ingenieure.

Schmidt, Peter.
1973 "Zu den geistigen Wurzeln von Johannes Müller (1801–1858): Eine quantitative Analysis der im Handbuch der Physiologie von J. Müller (1840–1844) zitierten und verwerteten Autoren." Inaugural-Dissertation, Münster. (*Münstersche Beiträge zur Geschichte und Theorie der Medizin,* Nr. 9.)

Schönlein, Johann Lucas.
1816 *Von der Hirnmetamorphose. Inauguralabhandlung.* Würzburg: F. C. Nitribitt.

Schroeder van der Kolk, Jacob Ludwig Conrad.
1859*a* *Bau und Functionen der Medulla spinalis und oblongata und nächste Ursache und rationelle Behandlung der Epilepsie.* Trans. from Dutch by F. W. Theile. Braunschweig: F. Vieweg. English edition, *Professor Schroeder* (1859).
1859*b* *Professor Schroeder van der Kolk on the minute structure and functions of the spinal cord and medulla oblongata, and on the proximate cause and rational treatment of epilepsy.* Trans. W. D. Moore. London: New Sydenham Society.

Schultheisz, Emil.
1982 "The beginning of quantification in physiology." *Clio Medica,* 17:193–197.

Schultze, Maximilian Johann Sigismund.
1871 "Allgemeines über die Structurelemente des Nervensystems." In S. Stricker, ed. *Handbuch der Lehre von den Geweben* (1871–1872). Vol. 1 (1871), chap. 3, pp. 108–136.

Schulz, Benedict.
1842 *Die Physiologie des Rückenmarkes mit Berücksichtigung seiner pathologischen Zustände für praktische Aerzte.* Vienna: Pfautsch. Review in *BFMR,* 1844, 17:403.

Schwann, Theodor.
1839 *Mikroskopische Untersuchungen über die Übereinstimmung in der Struktur und dem Wachsthum der Thiere und Pflanzen.* Berlin: G. Reimer. English translation, T. Schwann, *Microscopical researches* (1847).
1847 *Microscopical researches into the accordance in the structure and growth of animals and plants.* Trans. Henry Smith. London: Sydenham Society.

Schweigger, Johann Salomo Christoph.
1821 "Electromagnetischer Multiplicator." *Journal für Chemie und Physik* (J. S. C. Schweigger: Nuremberg), 31:35–41.

Sechenov, Ivan Mikhailovich.
1863 *Physiologische Studien über die Hemmungsmechanismen für die Reflexthätigkeit des Rückenmarks im Gehirne des Frosches.* Berlin: A. Hirschwald. Reprinted in I. M. Sechenov, *I. Sechenov. Selected works* (1935). Pp. 153–176.
1935 *I. Sechenov. Selected works.* Ed. A. A. Subkov, Moscow & Leningrad: State Publishing House for Biological and Medical Literature. (Produced for the 15th Physiological Congress, Moscow, 1935.)
1962 *Selected physiological and psychological works.* London: Central Books.
1965 *Autobiographical notes.* Washington, D.C.: American Institute of Biological Sciences.

Ségalas d'Etchepare, Pierre Salomon.
1824 "Note sur quelques points de physiologie." *JPEP,* 4:284–293.

Serres, Étienne Reynaud Augustin.
1822*a* "Recherches sur les maladies organiques du cervelet." *JPEP,* 2:172–184.
1822*b* "Suite des recherches sur les maladies organiques du cervelet." *JPEP,* 2:249–269.
1823 "Suite des recherches sur les maladies organiques du cervelet." *JPEP,* 3:114–153.
1824–1826 *Anatomie comparée du cerveau, dans les quatres classes des animaux vertébrés, appliquée à la physiologie et la pathologie du système nerveux.* 2 vols. and atlas. Paris: Gabon.

Shapin, S.
1975 "Phrenological knowledge and the social structure of early nineteenth-century Edinburgh." *Annals of Science,* 32:219–243.

Sharpey-Schafer, Sir Edward A.
1931 "The nomenclature of the autonomic nervous system." *JP,* 71:362–363. (Known earlier as Edward A. Schäfer, *q.v.*)

Shaternikov, M. N.
1935 "The life of I.M. Sechenov." In I. M. Sechenov, *I.M. Sechenov. Selected works* (1935). Pp. IX–XXVI.

Sheehan, Donal.
1936 "Discovery of the autonomic nervous system." *Archives of Neurology and Psychiatry,* 35:1081–1115.
1941 "The autonomic nervous system prior to Gaskell." *New England Journal of Medicine,* 224:457–460.

Sherrington, Sir Charles S.
1900*a* "The spinal cord." In E. A. Schäfer, ed. *Text-book* (1898–1900). 2:783–883.
1900*b* "The cerebellum." In E. A. Schäfer, ed. *Text-book*(1898–1900). 2:893–910.
1942 *Goethe on nature & on science.* Cambridge: Cambridge University Press.

Sheynin, O. B.
1980 "On the history of the statistical method in biology." *Archives of the History of the Exact Sciences,* 22:323–371.

Siegel, Carl.
1913 *Geschichte der deutschen Naturphilosophie.* Leipzig: Akademische Verlagsgesellschaft.

Siegel, Rudolf E.
1968 *Galen's system of physiology and medicine: An analysis of his doctrines and observations on bloodflow, respiration, humors and internal diseases.* Basel: S. Karger.
1970 *Galen on sense perception.* Basel: S. Karger.
1973 *Galen on psychology, psychopathology, and function and diseases of the nervous system: An analysis of his doctrines, observations and experiments.* Basel: S. Karger.
1976 *Galen on the affected parts: Translation from the Greek text with explanatory notes.* Basel: S. Karger.

Siesser, William G.
1981 "Christian Gottfried Ehrenberg: Founder of micropalaeontology." *Centaurus,* 25:166–188.

Sigaud la Fond, Joseph Aignan.
1802 *De l'électricité médicale.* Paris: Delaplace & Goujon.

Singer, Bernard R.
1981 "History of the study of animal behaviour." In D. McFarland, ed. *The Oxford companion* (1981). Pp. 255–272.

Singer, Charles.
1956 *Galen on anatomical procedures . . . De anatomicis administrationibus. Translation by C. Singer.* London: Wellcome Historical Medical Museum.

Smee, Alfred.

1849 *Elements of electro-biology, of the voltaic mechanism of man; of electro-pathology, especially of the nervous system; and of electro-therapeutics.* London: Longman et al.

1850 *Instinct and reason: Deduced from electro-biology.* London: Reeve & Benham.

Smith, Emilie Savage.

1971 "Galen's account of the cranial nerves and the autonomic nervous system." *Clio Medica,* 6:77–98, 173–194.

Smith, J. A., and W. D. Ross, eds.

1908–1931 *The works of Aristotle translated into English . . .* 11 vols. Oxford: Clarendon Press. Vols. 6–11 were edited by W. D. Ross alone.

Snelders, H. A. M.

1971 "J.S.C. Schweigger: his Romanticism and his crystal electrical theory of matter." *Isis,* 62:328–338.

Snorrason, Egill.

1969 *L'anatomiste J.-B. Winslow (1669–1760).* Copenhagen: (n.p.).

1974 *C.G. Kratzenstein, professor physices experimentalis Petropol. et Havn. and his studies on electricity during the eighteenth century.* Odense: University Press.

Soemmerring, Samuel Thomas.

1791–1792 *Vom Baue des menschlichen Körpers.* 5 vols. Frankfurt am Main: Varrentrapp & Wenner.

1791 *Hirnlehre und Nervenlehre.* Frankfurt am Main: Varrentrapp & Wenner. Vol. 5, *Vom Baue* (1791–1792).

1794–1801 *De corporis humani fabrica. Latio donato abipso auctore aucta.* 6 vols. in 5. Frankfurt am Main: Varrentrapp & Wenner. Trans. of *Vom Baue* (1791–1792).

1811 *Über den Saft, welcher aus den Nerven wieder eingesaugt wird, im gesunden und kranken Zustande des menschlichen Körpers . . .* Landshut: P. Krüll.

1841 *Hirn und Nervenlehre.* Leipzig: L. Voss.

Solly, Samuel.

1836 *The human brain, its configuration, structure, development, and physiology; Illustrated by references to the nervous system in the lower order of animals.* London: Longman et al.

1847 *The human brain: its structure, physiology and diseases. With a description of the typical forms of brain in the animal kingdom.* 2d ed. London: Longman et al.

Solmsen, F.

1961 "Greek philosophy and the discovery of the nerves." *Museum Helvetica, Basel,* 18:150–167, 169–197.

Soury, Jules.

1897 "Cerveau [cerebrum]." In C. Richet, *Dictionnaire* (1895–1928). 2:547–670.

1899 *Le système nerveux centrale structure et fonctions. Histoire critique des théories et des doctrines.* 2 vols. Paris: G. Carré & C. Naud.

Spatz, H.

1952 "Neuronenlehre und Zellenlehre; zur 100. Wiederkehr des Geburtstages von S. Ramon y Cajal am 1. Mai 1952." *Münchener medizinische Wochenschrift,* 94: 1153–1164, 1209–1218, 1255–1262.

Spiess, Gustav Adolf.

1844 *Physiologie der Nervensystems, vom ärztlichen Standpunkte dargestellt.* Braunschweig: F. Vieweg.

Spillane, John D.

1981 *The doctrine of the nerves. Chapters in the history of neurology.* Oxford: Oxford University Press.

Spoerl, H. D.

1935–1936 "Faculties *versus* traits: Gall's solution." *Character and Personality* (Durham, N.C. & London), 4:216–231.

Spurzheim, Johann Caspar.

1815 *The physiognomical system of Drs Gall and Spurzheim founded on an anatomical examination of the nervous system in general, and of the brain in particular.* London: Baldwin, Cradock.

1818 *Observations sur la phraenologie, ou la connaissance de l'homme moral et intellectuel, fondée sur les fonctions du système nerveux.* Paris: Treuttel & Wurtz.

1820 *Essai philosophique sur la nature morale et intellectuelle de l'homme.* Paris: Treuttel & Würtz.

1825 *Phrenology, or, the doctrine of the mind; and of the relations between its manifestation and the body.* 3d ed. London: C. Knight.

1826 *The anatomy of the brain, with a general view of the nervous system.* Trans. R. Willis. London: S. Highley.

1827 *Outlines of phrenology; being also a manual of reference for the marked bust.* London: Treuttel, Wurtz, & Richter.

Stainbrook, Edward.

1948 "The use of electricity in psychiatric treatment during the nineteenth century." *BHM,* 22:156–177.

Stauffer, Robert C.

1953 "Persistent errors regarding Oersted's discovery of electromagnetism." *Isis,* 44:307–310.

1957 "Speculation and experiment in the background of Oersted's discovery of electromagnetism." *Isis,* 48:33–50.

Staum, Martin S.

1978 "Medical components in Cabanis's science of man." *Studies in History of Biology,* 2:1–31.

1980 *Cabanis: Enlightenment and medical philosophy in the French Revolution.* Princeton, N.J.: Princeton University Press.

Stedman, Thomas Lathrop.

1982 *Illustrated Stedman's medical dictionary.* 24th ed. Baltimore & London: Williams & Wilkins.

Steno, Nicolas.

1669 *Discours de Monsieur Stenon, sur l'anatomie du cerveau.* Paris: R. de Ninville. (A paper read in 1665.)

Stephanus, Carolus, or Charles Estienne.

1545 *De dissectione partium corporis humani libri tres.* Paris: S. Colinaeus.

Stern, Madeleine B.

1971 *Heads & headlines. The phrenological Fowlers.* Norman: University of Oklahoma Press.

Stevenson, Lloyd G.

1959 "Anatomical reasoning in physiological thought." In C. M. Brooks and P. F. Cranefield, eds. *The historical development* (1959). Pp. 27–38.

Stevenson, Lloyd G., and Robert P. Multhauf, eds.

1968 *Medicine science and culture. Historical essays in honor of Owsei Temkin.* Baltimore, Md.: Johns Hopkins Press.

Stieda, Christian Hermann Ludwig.

1899 "Geschichte der Entwickelung der Lehre von den Nervenzellen und Nervenfasern während des XIX. Jahrhunderts, I. Teil: von Sömmering bis Deiters." In *Festschrift zum 70. Geburtstag von Carl v. Kupffer.* Jena: G. Fischer. Pp. 79–196.

Stilling, Benedikt.

1842*a* "Fragmente zur Lehre von der Verrichtung des Nervensystems." *Archiv für physiologische Heilkunde* (W. Roser et al.: Stuttgart), 1:91–144.

1842*b* *Untersuchungen über die Functionen des Rückenmarks und der Nerven.* Leipzig: O. Wigand.

1843 *Ueber die Medulla oblongata.* Erlangen: F. Enke.

1846 *Über den Bau des Hirnknotens oder der Varolischen Brücke.* Jena: F. Mauke.

1856 *Anatomische und mikroskopische Untersuchungen über den feineren Bau der Nerven-Primitivfaser und der Nervenzelle.*

Frankfurt: Verlag von Literarischer Anstalt.

1856–1859 *Neue Untersuchungen über den Bau des Rückenmarks.* Kassel: Hotop.

1864–1878 *Untersuchungen über den Bau des kleinen Gehirns des Menschen.* 3 parts. Cassel: T. Kay.

1878 *Neue Untersuchungen über den Bau des kleinen Gehirns des Menschen, enthaltend Untersuchungen über den Bau . . .* Cassel: T. Fischer. This is to be considered the third part or volume of *Untersuchungen* (1864–1878).

Stilling, Benedikt, and Joseph Wallach.

1842 *Untersuchungen über den Bau des Nervensystems. Erstes Heft. Untersuchungen über die Textur des Rückenmarks.* Leipzig: O. Wigand.

Stirling, William.

1902 *Some apostles of physiology being an account of their lives and labours that have contributed to the advancemnt of the healing art as well as to the prevention of disease.* London: printed privately by Waterlow.

Stookey, Byron.

1954 "A note on the early history of cerebral localization." *Bulletin of the New York Academy of Medicine,* 30:559–578.

1963 "Jean-Baptiste Bouillaud and Ernest Aubertin. Early studies on cerebral localization and the speech center." *Journal of the American Medical Association,* 184:1024–1029.

Stricker, Salomon, ed.

1871–1872 *Handbuch der Lehre von den Geweben des Menschen und der Thiere.* 2 vols. Leipzig: W. Engelmann. English trans. in S. Stricker, *Manual* (1870–1873).

1870–1873 *Manual of human and comparative histology.* Trans. H. Power. 3 vols. London: New Sydenham Society.

Studnička, F. K.

1927 "Joh. Ev. Purkinje und seiner Schule Verdienste um die Entdeckung tierischer zellen und um die Aufstellung der 'Zellen'-Theorie." *Acta Societatis Scientiarum Naturalium Moravicae,* 4:1–168.

1931–1932 "Aus der Vorgeschichte der Zellentheorie, H. Milne Edwards, H. Dutrochet, F. Raspail, J.E. Purkinje." *Anatomischer Anzeiger* (Jena), 73:390–416.

1936*a* "J.E. Purkinje's 'physiology' and his services to science." *Osiris,* 2:472–483.

1936*b* "Joh. Ev. Purkinjes histologische Arbeiten." *Anatomischer Anzeiger* (Jena), 82:41–66.

Sudduth, William M.

1980 "The Voltaic pile and electro-chemical theory in 1800." *Ambix,* 27:26–35.

Sue, Pierre, aîné.

1802–1805 *Histoire du galvanisme; et analyse des différens ouvrages publiés sur cette découverte, depuis son origine jusqu'à ce jour.* 4 vols. Paris: Bernard.

Surr, Thomas Skinner.

1806 *A winter in London; or sketches of fashion: A novel . . .* 3 vols. London: R. Phillips.

Sutton, Geoffrey.

1981*a* "The politics of science in early Napoleonic France. The case of the Voltaic pile." *Studies in the History and Philosophy of Science,* 11:329–366.

1981*b* "Electric medicine and mesmerism." *Isis,* 72:375–392.

Swammerdam, Jan.

1737–1738 *Bybel der natuure . . . of historie der insecten . . .* Ed. H. Boerhaave. 2 vols. Leyden: I. Severinus, B. Vander Aa, & P. Vander.

1758 *The book of nature: or, the history of insects . . .* Trans. T. Floyd, revised J. Hill. London: C. G. Seyffert.

Swan, Joseph.

1835 *Illustrations of the comparative anatomy of the nervous system.* London: Longman.

Swazey, Judith P.

1969 *Reflexes and motor integration. Sherrington's concept of integrative action.* Cambridge, Mass.: Harvard University Press.

1970 "Action propre and action commune: the localization of cerebral function." *JHB,* 3:213–234.

Swedenborg, Emanuel.

1852 *The generative organs, considered physically and philosophically. A posthumous work.* Trans. J. J. G. Wilkinson. London: W. Newbery.

1882–1887 *The brain considered anatomically, physiologically and philosophically.* Ed., trans., annotator, R. L. Tafel. 2 vols. London: Swedenborg Society.

Swedenborg Congress.

1911 *Transactions of the International Swedenborg Congress . . . London, July 4 to 8, 1910.* 2d ed. London: The Swedenborg Society.

Taine, Hippolyte Adolphe [Henri].

1871 *On intelligence.* Trans. T. D. Haye. London: L. Reeve.

Teich, Mijulăs.

1962 "The world outlook of Jan Evangelista Purkyně." In Anon-

ymous, *Jan Evangelista Purkyně* (1962). Pp. 119–143.
1970 "Purkyně and Valentin on ciliary motion: An early investigation in morphological physiology." *British Journal for the History of Science,* 5:168–177.

Teichmann, Jürgen.
1974 "Beziehungen zwischen Johann Wilhelm Ritter und Alessandro Volta." *SAGM,* 58:46–59.

Temkin, Owsei.
1946*a* "The philosophical background of Magendie's physiology." *BHM,* 20:10–35.
1946*b* "Materialism in French and German physiology of the early nineteenth century." *BHM,* 20:321–327.
1947 "Gall and the phrenological movement." *BHM,* 21:275–321.
1950 "German concepts of ontogeny and history around 1800." *BHM,* 24:227–246.
1953 "Remarks on the neurology of Gall and Spurzheim." In E. A. Underwood, ed. *Science medicine and history* (1953), 2:282–289.

Thomas, André.
1897 *Le cervelet. Étude anatomique, clinique et physiologique.* Paris: G. Steinheil.

Thomas, Henry M.
1910 "Decussation of the pyramids—an historical enquiry." *Bulletin of the Johns Hopkins Hospital,* 21:304–311.

Tiedemann, Friedrich.
1808–1810 *Zoologie. Zu seinen Vorlesungen entworfen.* 2 vols. Landshut: Weber, 1808; Heidelberg: Mohr & Zimmer, 1810.
1816*a* *Anatomie und Bildungsgeschichte des Gehirns im Foetus des Menschen nebst einer vergleichenden Darstellung des Hirnbaues in den Thieren.* Nuremberg: Stein. English trans. F. Tiedemann, *The anatomy* (1826).
1816*b* *Anatomie der Röhren—Holothurie des Pomeranzfarbigen Seesterns und Stein-Seeigels.* Landshut: J. Thomannschen.
1824 "Beobachtung über Missbildung des Gehirns und seiner Nerven." *Untersuchungen über die Natur des Menschen, der Thiere, und der Pflanzen.* 1:56–110.
1825 "Über den Antheil des sympathischen Nervens an den Verrichtungen der Sinne." *Zeitschrift für Physiologie* (F. Tiedemann & C. R. & L. C. Treviranus: Heidelberg), 1:237–290.
1826 *The anatomy of the foetal brain.* Trans. William Bennett. Edinburgh: J. Carfrae.

Timme, Walter.
1930 "The vegetative nervous system. Historical retrospect." In *Association for Research* (1930). Vol. 9, pp. 1–10.

Tissot, Simon August André David.

1800 *Traité des nerfs et de leurs maladies*. 4 vols. Avignon: Chambeau.

Tizard, Barbara.

1959 "Theories of brain localization from Flourens to Lashley." *MH*, 3:132–145.

Todd, Robert Bentley.

1839–1847 "Physiology of the nervous system." In R. B. Todd, ed. *The cyclopaedia* (1835–1859), 3:720G–723G. (Article finished in 1847.)

1847 *Physiology of the nervous system*. London: Marchant Singer. Todd's article, "Physiology of the nervous system" (1839–1847), in his *The cyclopaedia* (1835–1859), published separately. Reviewed in *BFMCR* (1850), 5:1–18.

Todd, Robert Bentley, ed.

1835–1859 *The cyclopaedia of anatomy and physiology*. 5 vols. in 6. London: Longman et al.

Todd, Robert Bentley, and William Bowman.

1845–1856 *The physiological anatomy and physiology of man*. 2 vols. London: J. W. Parker.

Toellner, Richard.

1971 "Naturphilosophische Elemente im Denken Purkyně's." In V. Kruta, ed. *Jan Evangelista Purkyně* (1971). Pp. 35–41.

Torre, Giovanni Maria della.

1776 *Nuove osservazioni microscopiche*. Naples: n.p.

Towers, Donald B.

1958 "Origins and development of neurochemistry." *Neurology* (Minneapolis), vol. 8, suppl. 1.

Treviranus, Gottfried Reinhold.

1802–1822 *Biologie, oder Philosophie der lebenden Natur für Naturforscher und Aerzte*. 6 vols. Göttingen: J. F. Röwer.

1831 *Die Erscheinungen und Gesetzte des organischen Lebens*. Bremen: J. G. Heyse.

1835 *Neue Untersuchungen über die organischen Elemente der thierischen Körper und deren Zusammensetzungen*. Bremen: J. G. Heyse.

Treviranus, Gottfried Reinhold, and Ludolf Christian Treviranus

1816–1821 *Vermischte Schriften anatomischen und physiologischen Inhalts*. 4 vols. Vol. 1, Göttingen: J. F. Röwer; vols. 2–4, Bremen: J. G. Heyse.

Tsouyopoulos, Nelly.

1984 "German philosophy and the rise of modern clinical medicine." *Theoretical Medicine*, 5:345–357.

Underwood, Edgar Ashworth.

1953 *Science medicine and history. Essays on the evolution of scientific thought and medical practice written in honour of Charles Singer.* 2 vols. London: Oxford University Press.

Unzer, Johann August.

1771 *Erste Gründe einer Physiologie der eigentlichen thierischen Natur thierischer Körper.* Leipzig: Weidmanns, Erben & Reich. English trans. J. A. Unzer, *The principles of physiology* (1851).

1851 *The principles of physiology, by John Augustus Unzer; and a dissertation on the functions of the nervous system, by George Prochaska.* Trans. Thomas Laycock. London: Sydenham Society. Pp. 1–360.

Valentin, Gustav Gabriel.

1835 *Handbuch der Entwickelungsgeschichte des Menschen.* Berlin: A. Rücker.

1836*a* "Fortgesetzte Untersuchungen über die Flimmerbewegung." *Repertorium für Anatomie und Physiologie* (G. G. Valentin: Berlin, etc.) 1:148–159.

1836*b* "Feinere Anatomie der Sinnesorgane des Menschen und der Wirbelthiere," ibid., 1:300–316.

1836*c* "Über den Verlauf und die letzten Enden der Nerven." *Nova Acta Physico-medica Academiae Caesareae Leopoldino-Carolinae Naturae Curiosorum* (Vratislava & Bonn), 18 (Part I):51–240.

1837 "Die Entwickelung der Pflanzengewebe und Pflanzenorgane." In K. F. Burdach et al. *Die Physiologie* (1826–1840). 2:161–182.

1839*a* "Die Fortschritte der Physiologie im Jahre 1838." *Repertorium für Anatomie und Physiologie* (G. G. Valentin: Berlin, etc.), 4:1–358.

1839*b* "Ueber die Scheiden der Ganglienkugeln und deren Fortsetzungen." *AAPM,* pp. 139–164.

1839*c* *De functionibus nervorum cerebralium et nervi sympathici libri quattuor.* Berne & St. Gallen: Huber. Reviewed in Anonymous, "Valentin on the function of the nerves" (1841).

1842*a* "Nervensystem der Wirbelthiere." In "Die Fortschritte der Physiologie im Jahre 1841." *Repertorium für Anatomie und Physiologie* (G. G. Valentin: Berlin, etc.), 8:93–138.

1842*b* "Flimmerbewegung." In R. Wagner, ed. *Handwörterbuch* (1842–1853), 1:484–516.

1842*c* "Gewebe des menschlichen und thierischen Körpers." In R. Wagner, ed. *Handwörterbuch* (1842–1853). 1:617–797.

1842*d* "Über die Entwickelung der thierischen Gewebe." In R. Wagner, *Lehrbuch der Physiologie* (1842). Pp. 132–139.

1844 *Lehrbuch der Physiologie des Menschen. Für Aertze und Studirende.* 2 vols. Braunschweig: F. Vieweg.

[c. 1851] *Lehrbuch der Physiologie des Menschen für Aerzte und Studirende,* 3d ed. 2 vols. Braunschweig: F. Vieweg.

1853 *A textbook of physiology.* Trans. and ed. W. Brinton. London: H. Renshaw. This is an abridgement of his *Lehrbuch der Physiologie* [c. 1851].

Van der Loos, Hendrik.

1967 "The history of the neuron." In H. Hydén, ed. *The neuron* (1967). Pp. 1–48.

Varolio, Constanzo.

1591 *Anatomiae, sive de resolutione corporis humani . . .* Frankfurt: J. Wechel & P. Fischer.

Verworn, Max.

1899 *General physiology. An outline of the science of life.* London: Macmillan.

Vesalius, Andreas.

1543 *De humani corporis fabrica libri septem.* Basle: J. Oporini.

Vicq d'Azyr, Félix.

1784 "Recherches sur la structure du cerveau, du cervelet, de la moelle elongée, de la moelle épinière; et sur l'origine des nerfs de l'homme et des animaux [1781]." *Histoire de l'Académie Royale des Sciences* (Paris). Pp. 495–622.

1805*a* *Oeuvres de Vicq-d'Azyr,* 6 vols. Ed. J. L. Moreau. Paris: L. Duprat-Duverger. Vols. 1–3 contain *Éloges historiques par Vicq-d'Azyr.*

1805*b* "Lobstein" (1805). In F. Vicq-d'Azyr, *Oeuvres* (1805). *Éloges historiques par Vicq d'Azyr,* 3:34–45.

Viets, H. R., and F. H. Garrison.

1940 "Purkinje's original description of the pear-shaped cells in the cerebellum." *BHM,* 8:1397–1398.

Virchow, Rudolf.

1858*a* *Die Cellularpathologie in ihrer Begründung auf physiologische und pathologische Gewebelehre.* Berlin: A. Hirschwald.

1858*b* "Eulogy of Johannes Müller." *EMSJ,* 4:452–463, 527–544.

Virey, J. J.

1835 *Philosophie de l'histoire naturelle ou phénomènes de l'organisation des animaux et des végétaux.* Paris: J. B. Baillière.

Volkmann, Alfred Wilhelm.

1837 *Die Lehre von dem leiblichen Leben des Menschen. Ein*

anatomisch-physiologisches Handbuch zum Selbstunterricht für Gebildete. Leipzig: Breitkopf & Härtel.
1838*a* "On reflex motions." *BFMR,* 6:211–218.
1838*b* "Ueber Reflexbewegungen." *AAPM,* pp. 15–43. Summary in A. W. Volkmann, "On reflex motions" (1838).
1838*c* "Ueber die Faserung des Rückenmarkes und des sympathischen Nerven in Rana esculenta." *AAPM,* pp. 274–295.
1842 "Gehirn." In R. Wagner, ed. *Handwörterbuch* (1842–1853). 1:563–597.
1844 "Nervenphysiologie." In R. Wagner, ed. *Handwörterbuch* (1842–1853). 2:476–627.

Volta, Alessandro.
1792*a* "Memoria prima sull'elettricità animale." *Giornale Fisico-Medico* (L. Brugnatelli: Pavia), 2:146–192.
1792*b* "Memoria seconda sull'elettricità animale." *Giornale Fisico-Medico* (L. Brugnatelli: Pavia), 2:241–300.
1793 "Account of some discoveries made by Mr Galvani, of Bologna; with experiments and observations on them. In two letters from Mr. Alexander Volta, F.R.S. . . . to Mr Tiberius Cavallo, F.R.S.," *PT,* Part I, pp. 10–44. In French. Read 31 January 1793.
1800*a* "On the electricity excited by the mere contact of conducting substances of different kinds." *PT,* Part I, pp. 403–431. In French.
1800*b* "On the electricity excited by the mere contact of conducting substances of different kinds." *PM* (September), 7:289–311. Reprinted in *American Journal of Physics* (1945), 13:397–406.
1816 *Collezione dell'opere del Cavaliere Conte Alessandro Volta Patrizio Comasco*. 3 vols. in 5. Florence: G. Piatti.

Vulpian, Edme Félix Alfred.
1866 *Leçons sur la physiologie générale et comparée du système nerveux*. Paris: Germer Baillière.

Wagener, Samuel Christoph.
1828 *Das Leben des Erdballs und aller Welten. Neue Ansichten und Folgerungen aus Thatsachen*. Berlin: C. F. Amelang.

Wagner, Rudolph.
1846 "Sympathischen Nerv, Ganglienstructur und Nervenendigungen." In R. Wagner, ed., *Handwörterbuch* (1842–1853). Vol. 3, part I, pp. 360–406.
1847 *Neue Untersuchungen über den Bau und die Endigung der Nerven und die Struktur der Ganglien*. Leipzig: L. Voss.
1850 "Neurologische Untersuchungen." *Nachrichten von der*

Georg-Augustus Universität und der Königlich Gesellschaft der Wissenschaft zu Göttingen, pp. 41–56. Contains the findings of K.G.F.R. Leuckart.

1854*a* "Ueber den Bau des Rückenmarks und die daraus resultirende Grundlage zu einer Theorie der Reflexbewegungen, Mitbewegungen und Mitempfindungen." *Nachrichten von der Georg-Augustus Universität und der Königlich Gesellschaft der Wissenschaft zu Göttingen,* pp. 89–102.

1854*b* "Ueber die Elementar-Organisation des Gehirns." *Nachrichten von der Georg-Augustus Universität und der Königlich Gesellschaft der Wissenschaft zu Göttingen,* pp. 25–44.

Wagner, Rudolph, ed.

1842–1853 *Handwörterbuch der Physiologie mit Rücksicht auf physiologische Pathologie,* 4 vols. in 5. Braunschweig: F. Vieweg.

Wakley, Thomas Henry.

1846 [Review of M. Hall, *New memoir* (1843)]. *Lancet,* ii:154–157, 186–189, 244–247.

[Wakley, Thomas Henry].

1850 "Biographical sketch of Marshall Hall, M.D., F.R.S." *Lancet,* ii:120–128.

Waldeyer, Wilhelm.

1891 "Über einige neuere Forschungen im Gebiete der Anatomie des Centralnervensystems." *Deutsche medizinische Wochenschrift,* 17:1213–1218, 1244–1246, 1267–1269, 1287–1289, 1331–1332, 1352–1356.

Walker, A. Earl.

1957*a* "The development of the concept of cerebral localization in the nineteenth century." *BHM,* 31:99–121.

1957*b* "Stimulation and ablation. Their role in the history of cerebral physiology." *Journal of Neurosurgery,* 20:435–449.

Walker, W. Cameron.

1936 "The detection and estimation of electrical charges in the eighteenth century." *Annals of Science,* 1:66–100.

1937 "Animal electricity before Galvani." *Annals of Science,* 2:84–113.

Walsh, Anthony A.

1971 "Contributions to the history of psychology: XIII, Bibliographia phrenologica." *Psychology Reports,* 28:641–642.

Walsh, John.

1774 "Of the electric property of the torpedo. In a letter from John Walsh, Esq; F.R.S. to Benjamin Franklin, Esq; LL.D., F.R.S., Ac.R. Par. Soc. Ext., &c.," *PT.* 63 (Part II):461–480. Dated and read, 1 July 1773.

Walshe, Francis M. R.
1921 "On disorders of movement resulting from loss of postural tone, with special reference to cerebellar ataxy." *Brain,* 44:539–556.

Walter, Johann Gottlieb.
1783 *Tabulae nervorum thoracis et abdominis.* Berlin: G. J. Decker.
1804 *John Gottlieb Walter's plates of the thoracic and abdominal nerves . . . accompanied by coloured explanations and a description of the par vagum, great sympathetic and phrenic nerves.* London: J. Murray.

Watkins, R. L.
1906 "The brain: the dynamo-electric machine of the human body." *Medical Bulletin* (Philadelphia), 28:211.

Waugh, John.
1838 *The science of the cerebro-spinal phenomena attempted.* London: S. Highley.

Weaver, William D., ed.
1909 *Catalogue of the Wheeler Gift of books, pamphlets and periodicals in the Library of the American Institute of Electrical Engineers.* 2 vols. New York: American Institute of Electrical Engineers.

Weber, Eduard Friedrich Wilhelm.
1846 "Muskelbewegung." In R. Wagner, ed. *Handwörterbuch* (1842–1853). Vol. 3, part 2, pp. 1–122.

Weber, Ernst Heinrich.
1817 *Anatomia acomparata nervi sympathici.* Leipzig: C. H. Reclam.
1831 *Das Gefäss-und Nervensystem.* Vol. 3, of E. H. Weber, ed. *F. Hildebrandt, Handbuch* (1830–1832).

Weber, Ernst Heinrich, ed. See G. F. Hildebrandt.

Weidlich, T.
1894 *Die Sympathie in der antiken Literatur.* Stuttgart: C. Lieblich.

Weinhold, Karl August.
1817 *Versuche über das Leben und seine Grundkräfte, auf dem Wege der experimental-Physiologie.* Magdeburg: Creutz.

Weldon, W. F. R.
1898 "Albert von Kölliker." *Nature,* 58:1–4.

Wellcome Institute for the History of Medicine and Related Sciences.
1980 *Subject catalogue of the history of medicine and related sciences. Biographical section,* 5 vols. Munich: Kraus.

Wenzel, Joseph, and Carl Wenzel.
1812 *De penitiori structura cerebri hominis et brutorum.* Tübingen: Cotta.

W[erner], [Carl?] von.
1802 *Critische Darstellung der Gallschen anatomisch-physiologischen Untersuchungen des Gehirns und Schädelbaues.* Zurich: Ziegler.

Wharton, Thomas.
1656 *Adenographia: sive, glandularum totius corporis descriptio.* London: J. G. for the author.

White, James C., and R. H. Smithwick.
1941 *The autonomic nervous system: Anatomy, physiology, and surgical application.* 2d ed. New York: Macmillan.

Whitrow, Magda, ed.
1971–1984 *Isis cumulative bibliography . . . 1913–1965.* 6 vols. London: Mansell.

Whytt, Robert.
1751 *An essay on the vital and other involuntary motions of animals.* Edinburgh: Hamilton, J. Balfour & Neill.
1755 "Physiological essays. II. Observations on the sensibility and irritability of the parts of men and other animals. Occasioned by the late M. de Haller's late treatise on those subjects." In R. Whytt, *The works* (1768). Pp. 255–306.
1765 *Observations on the nature, causes, and cure of those disorders which have been commonly called nervous, hypochondriac, or hysteric, to which are prefixed some remarks on the sympathy of the nerves.* Edinburgh: T. Becket & P. A. De Hondt; & J. Balfour for London.
1768 *The works of Robert Whytt, M.D. . . . published by his son.* Edinburgh: T. Becket & P. A. De Hondt; & J. Balfour for London.

Wieberg, J.
1914 "The anatomy of the brain in the works of Galen and 'Ali 'Abbās, a comparative historical-anatomical study." *Janus,* 19:17–32.

Wilkes, James.
1833 *Essays, I.—on the anatomy, physiology, and pathology of the great sympathetic nerves . . .* Birmingham: J. C. Barlow.

Wilkins, George.
1822 *Body and soul.* London: Longman.

Wilkins, Robert H.
1963 "Neurosurgical classics XII." *Journal of Neurosurgery,* 29: 904–916.

Wilkins, Robert H., compiler.
1965 *Neurosurgical classics.* New York & London: Johnson Reprint.

Wilkinson, Charles Hunnings.
1804 *Elements of galvanism, in theory and practice; with a comprehensive view of its history, from the first experiments of Galvani to the present time . . .* 2 vols. London: J. Murray.

Will, J. G. Friedrich.
1844 "Vorläufige Mittheilung über die Structur der Ganglien und den Ursprung der Nerven bei wirbellosen Thieren." *AAPM*, pp. 76–93.

Williams, Billie Innes.
1975 "The conceptual and empirical basis of Luigi Galvani's work on muscular motion." Ph.D. Dissertation, University of London.

Williams, L. Pearce.
1965 *Michael Faraday. A biography.* London: Chapman and Hall.

Willis, Thomas.
1664 *Cerebri anatome: cui accessit nervorum descriptio et usus.* London: T. Roycroft, Impensis J. Martyn, & J. Allestry. The octavo edition, not the quarto, has been used throughout.
1672 *De anima brutorum quae "hominis" vitalis ac sensitiva est, exercitationes duae . . .* London: Typis E. F. Impensis Ric. Davis, Oxon., 1672.
1684 *Dr. Willis's practice of physick, being the whole works of that renowned and famous physician . . .* Trans. S. Pordage. London: T. Dring, C. Harper & J. Leigh.

Wilson, J. Walter.
1947*a* "Dutrochet and the cell theory." *Isis*, 37:14–21.
1947*b* "Virchow's contribution to the cell theory." *JHM*, 2:163–178.

Winslow, Jacques Benigne.
1732 *Exposition anatomique de la structure du corps humain.* Paris: G. Desprez & J. Desessartz.

Witte, Erich.
1942 "Beitrag zur Kenntnis der Bildung von Purkinjé." *SAGM*, 35:348–356.

Wolff, G. A., Jr.
1941 "The ratio of preganglionic neurons to postganglionic neurons in the visceral nervous system." *Journal of Comparative Neurology*, 75:235–243.

Wollaston, W. H.
1809 "On the agency of electricity on animal secretions." *PM*, 33:488–490.

Wrisberg, Heinrich August.
1780 "Observationes anatomicae de nervis viscerum abdomina-

lium. Particula prima de ganglio plexque semilunari. Gottingae 1780." In C. F. Ludwig, ed. *Scriptores nevrologici minores* (1791–1795), 4 (1795):50–69.

Wutzer, K. W.

1817 *De corporis humani gangliorum fabrica atque usu, monographia*. Berlin: F. Nicolai.

1834 "Ueber den Zusammenhang des sympathischen Nerven mit den Spinalnerven." *AAPM*, pp. 305–310.

Young, Robert M.

1968 "The functions of the brain: Gall to Ferrier (1808–1886)." *Isis*, 59:251–268.

1970 *Mind, brain and adaptation in the nineteenth century. Cerebral localisation and its biological context from Gall to Ferrier*. Oxford: Clarendon Press.

1972 "Franz Josef Gall." DSB, 5:250–256.

Zanobio, B.

1959 "Le osservazioni microscopiche di Felice Fontana sulla struttura dei nervi." *Physis*, 1:307–320.

Zehnder, E.

1968 *François Pourfour du Petit (1664–1741) und seine experimentelle Forschung über das Nervensystem*. Zurich: Juris.

Zinn, Johann Gottfried.

1749 "Experimenta quaedam circa corpus callosum, cerebellum, duram meningem, in vivis animalibus instituta. Gottingae 1749." In C. F. Ludwig, ed. *Scriptores nevrologici minores* (1791–1795), 4 (1795):106–132.

1753 "De l'enveloppe des nerfs." *Histoire de l'Académie Royale des Sciences et des Belles-Lettres de Berlin*. 9:130–144.

Zorab, George.

1967 "Electrical and galvanic theories." In E. J. Dingwall, ed. *Abnormal hypnotic phenomena* (1967–1968). *Belgium and the Netherlands, Germany and Scandinavia*, 2 (1967):21–35.

Zusne, Leonard.

1975 *Names in the history of psychology: A biographical sourcebook*. New York: J. Wiley.

Index

Designer: U.C. Press Staff
Compositor: Janet Sheila Brown
Text: 10/12 Sabon
Display: Sabon
Printer: The Murray Printing Company
Binder: The Murray Printing Company